ANNALS OF THE NEW YORK ACADEMY OF SCIENCES

Volume 1004

EDITORIAL STAFF

Director, Publishing and New Media
SARAH GREENE

Managing Editor
JUSTINE CULLINAN

Associate Editor
MARION L. GARRY

The New York Academy of Sciences
2 East 63rd Street
New York, New York 10021

THE NEW YORK ACADEMY OF SCIENCES
(Founded in 1817)

BOARD OF GOVERNORS, September 2003 – September 2004

TORSTEN N. WIESEL, *Chairman of the Board*
GERALD D. FISCHBACH, *Vice Chairman*
JOHN T. MORGAN, *Treasurer*
ELLIS RUBINSTEIN, *Chief Executive Officer* [ex officio]

Honorary Life Governors
WILLIAM T. GOLDEN   JOSHUA LEDERBERG

Governors

KAREN E. BURKE	PETER B. CORR	R. BRIAN FERGUSON
RONALD L. GRAHAM	MARNIE IMHOFF	WENDY EVANS JOSEPH
JACQUELINE LEO	RODERT W. LUCKY	PAUL MARKS
BRUCE McEWEN	RONAY MENSCHEL	JOHN F. NIBLACK
SANDRA PANEM	PETER RINGROSE	DAVID D. SABATINI
	LEE G. VANCE	DEBORAH WILEY

HELENE L. KAPLAN, *Counsel* [ex officio]   LARRY R. SMITH, *Secretary* [ex officio]

THE OCULOMOTOR AND VESTIBULAR SYSTEMS
THEIR FUNCTION AND DISORDERS

ANNALS OF THE NEW YORK ACADEMY OF SCIENCES
Volume 1004

THE OCULOMOTOR AND VESTIBULAR SYSTEMS
THEIR FUNCTION AND DISORDERS

Edited by Thomas Brandt, Bernard Cohen, and Christoph Siebold

The New York Academy of Sciences
New York, New York
2003

Copyright © 2003 by the New York Academy of Sciences. All rights reserved. Under the provisions of the United States Copyright Act of 1976, individual readers of the Annals are permitted to make fair use of the material in them for teaching or research. Permission is granted to quote from the Annals provided that the customary acknowledgment is made of the source. Material in the Annals may be republished only by permission of the Academy. Address inquiries to the Permissions Department (editorial@nyas.org) at the New York Academy of Sciences.

Copying fees: For each copy of an article made beyond the free copying permitted under Section 107 or 108 of the 1976 Copyright Act, a fee should be paid through the Copyright Clearance Center, Inc., 222 Rosewood Drive, Danvers, MA 01923 (www.copyright.com).

♾ The paper used in this publication meets the minimum requirements of the American National Standard for Information Sciences—Permanence of Paper for Printed Library Materials, ANSI Z39.48-1984.

Library of Congress Cataloging-in-Publication Data

International Ocular Motor Meeting (3rd : 2003 : Wildbad Kreuth, Germany)
 The oculomotor and vestibular systems : their function and disorders / edited by Thomas Brandt, Bernard Cohen, and Christoph Siebold.
   p. ; cm. — (Annals of the New York Academy of Sciences ; v. 1004)
 Includes bibliographical references and index.
   ISBN 1-57331-482-X (cloth : alk. paper) — ISBN 1-57331- 483-8 (paper : alk. paper)
   1. Eye—Movements—Congresses. 2. Vestibular apparatus—Congresses.
    [DNLM: 1. Ocular Physiology—Congresses. 2. Eye Diseases—therapy—Congresses. 3. Vestibular Diseases—therapy—Congresses. 4. Vestibule–physiology—Congresses WW 103 I56o 2003] I. Brandt, Thomas, 1943– II. Cohen, Bernard, 1929– III. Siebold, Christoph. IV. Title. V. Series.
   Q11.N5 vol. 1004
   500 s—dc22
   [617.7   2003022864

GYAT/PCP
Printed in the United States of America
ISBN 1-57331-482-X (cloth)
ISBN 1-57331-483-8 (paper)
ISSN 0077-8923

ANNALS OF THE NEW YORK ACADEMY OF SCIENCES

Volume 1004
October 2003

THE OCULOMOTOR AND VESTIBULAR SYSTEMS

THEIR FUNCTION AND DISORDERS

Editors
THOMAS BRANDT, BERNARD COHEN, AND CHRISTOPH SIEBOLD

Conference Organizers
CHRISTOPH SIEBOLD, ANDREAS STRAUBE, MICHAEL STRUPP,
UTE APPENDINO, AND THOMAS BRANDT

This volume is the result of a conference entitled **Physiology and Disorders of Oculomotor and Vestibular Control**, held April 3–5, 2003 at Wildbad Kreuth, Germany.

CONTENTS

Preface. A Tribute to Ulrich Büttner. *By* THOMAS BRANDT, BERNARD COHEN, AND CHRISTOPH SIEBOLD xiii

Historical Note on the Congress Venue: The Spa at Kreuth, or Why Did the Russian Czars Visit There? *By* WERNER GRAF xv

Part I. Basic Oculomotor Mechanisms

Physiology of the Eyelid Motor System. *By* JOSÉ M. DELGADO-GARCÍA, AGNÈS GRUART, AND JOSÉ A. TRIGO 1

Development of the Optokinetic Response in Macaques: A Comparison with Cat and Man. *By* C. DISTLER AND K.-P. HOFFMANN 10

GABAergic Neurons in the Rostral Mesencephalon of the Macaque Monkey That Control Vertical Eye Movements. *By* ANJA K.E. HORN, CHRISTOPH HELMCHEN, AND PETRA WAHLE 19

Shared Brainstem Pathways for Saccades and Smooth-Pursuit Eye Movements. By EDWARD L. KELLER AND MARCUS MISSAL 29

Motor and Sensory Innervation of Extraocular Eye Muscles. *By* J.A. BÜTTNER-ENNEVER, A. EBERHORN, AND A.K.E. HORN 40

Part II. Adaptation and Plasticity of the Vestibular and Oculomotor Systems

Activity-Related Postlesional Vestibular Reorganization.
  By NORBERT DIERINGER 50

Discharge Patterns of Cerebellar Output Neurons in the Caudal Fastigial Nucleus during Head-Free Gaze Shifts in Primates. *By* SANDRA C. BRETTLER, ALBERT F. FUCHS, AND LEO LING 61

Adaptation of Saccadic Eye Movements: Transfer and Specificity. *By* NADIA ALAHYANE AND DENIS PÉLISSON 69

Adaptive Changes in the Angular VOR: Duration of Gain Changes and Lack of Effect of Nodulo-Uvulectomy. *By* SERGEI B. YAKUSHIN, SVETLANA E. BUKHARINA, THEODORE RAPHAN, JEAN BÜTTNER-ENNEVER, AND BERNARD COHEN 78

Short-Term Adaptation of the VOR: Non-Retinal-Slip Error Signals and Saccade Substitution. *By* SCOTT D.Z. EGGERS, NICK DE PENNINGTON, MARK F. WALKER, MARK SHELHAMER, AND DAVID S. ZEE 94

Adaptations and Deficits in the Vestibulo-Ocular Reflex after Peripheral Ocular Motor Palsies. *By* JAMES A. SHARPE, DOUGLAS TWEED, AND AGNES M.F. WONG 111

Part III. Brainstem Control of Eye and Head Movements

Neural Control of Three-Dimensional Eye and Head Posture. *By* ELIANA M. KLIER AND J. DOUGLAS CRAWFORD 122

Dynamic Modulation of Ocular Orientation during Visually Guided Saccades and Smooth-Pursuit Eye Movements. *By* BERNHARD J.M. HESS AND DORA E. ANGELAKI 132

Mathematical Model Predicts Clinical Ocular Motor Syndromes.
  By MARIANNE DIETERICH, STEFAN GLASAUER, AND THOMAS BRANDT . 142

Examining the Paradoxical Relation between Number of Spikes and Gaze Amplitude in Abducens Neurons. *By* L. LING, J.O. PHILLIPS, AND C. SIEBOLD 158

Signal Processing of Semicircular Canal and Otolith Signals in the Vestibular Nuclei during Passive and Active Head Movements. *By* ROBERT A. MCCREA AND HONGGE LUAN 169

Morphological Properties of Vestibulospinal Neurons in Primates. *By* RICHARD BOYLE AND CURT JOHANSON 183

Role of the Dorsolateral Pontine Nucleus in Visual-Vestibular Behavior.
  By MICHAEL J. MUSTARI, SEIJI ONO, VALLABH E. DAS, AND RONALD J. TUSA 196

Part IV. Cerebellar Control of Vestibular Function and Eye Movements

Cerebellar Contribution to Saccades and Gaze Holding: A Modeling Approach. *By* STEFAN GLASAUER 206

Saccade Dysmetria during Functional Perturbation of the Caudal Fastigial Nucleus in the Monkey. *By* LAURENT GOFFART, LONGTANG L. CHEN, AND DAVID L. SPARKS 220

The Role of the Fastigial Nucleus in Saccadic Eye Oscillations. *By* CHRISTOPH HELMCHEN, HOLGER RAMBOLD, CHRISTIAN ERDMANN, CHRISTIAN MOHR, ANDREAS SPRENGER, AND FERDINAND BINKOFSKI 229

Multimodal Signal Integration in Vestibular Neurons of the Primate Fastigial Nucleus. *By* ULRICH BÜTTNER, S. GLASAUER, L. GLONTI, Y. GUAN, E. KIPIANI, J. KLEINE, C. SIEBOLD, T. TCHELIDZE, AND A. WILDEN 241

Discharge Properties of Saccade-Related Neurons in the Primate Fastigial Oculomotor Region. *By* J.F. KLEINE, Y. GUAN, AND U. BÜTTNER 252

Part V. Cortical Processing of Vestibular, Visual, and Oculomotor Function

Neurons in the Caudal Frontal Eye Fields of Monkeys Signal Three-Dimensional Tracking. *By* SERGEI KURKIN, NORIHITO TAKEICHI, TEPPEI AKAO, FUMIE SATO, JUNKO FUKUSHIMA, CHRIS R.S. KANEKO, AND KIKURO FUKUSHIMA 262

Vestibular Signals of Posterior Parietal Cortex Neurons during Active and Passive Head Movements in Macaque Monkeys. *By* FRANÇOIS KLAM AND WERNER GRAF 271

Inhibitory Interhemispheric Visuovisual Interaction in Motion Perception. *By* THOMAS BRANDT, ESTHER MARX, THOMAS STEPHAN, SANDRA BENSE, AND MARIANNE DIETERICH 283

Part VI. Spatial Orientation and Attention

Delayed Saccades, but Not Delayed Manual Aiming Movements Require Visual Attention Shifts. *By* HEINER DEUBEL AND WERNER X. SCHNEIDER 289

Prolonged Optokinetic Stimulation Generates Podokinetic after Rotation. *By* CARLOS R. GORDON, DROR TAL, NATAN GADOTH, AND AVI SHUPAK .. 297

A Modeling Approach to the Human Spatial Orientation System. *By* T. MERGNER AND W. BECKER 303

Spatial Memory Deficits in Patients with Chronic Bilateral Vestibular Failure. *By* FRANZ SCHAUTZER, DEREK HAMILTON, ROGER KALLA, MICHAEL STRUPP, AND THOMAS BRANDT 316

Part VII. Oculomotor and Vestibular Disorders

The Human Horizontal Vestibulo-Ocular Reflex in Response to Active and Passive Head Impulses after Unilateral Vestibular Deafferentation. *By* G.M. HALMAGYI, R.A. BLACK, M.J. THURTELL, AND I.S. CURTHOYS .. 325

Evaluating Small Eye Movements in Patients with Saccadic Palsies. *By* SIOBHAN GARBUTT, MARK R. HARWOOD, ARUN N. KUMAR, YANNING H. HAN, AND R. JOHN LEIGH 337

Incomitance of Ocular Rotation Axes in Trochlear Nerve Palsy. *By* KONRAD P. WEBER, ANTONELLA PALLA, KLARA LANDAU, THOMAS HASLWANTER, AND DOMINIK STRAUMANN 347

Eye Movements and Balance. *By* MICHAEL STRUPP, STEFAN GLASAUER, KLAUS JAHN, ERICH SCHNEIDER, SIEGBERT KRAFCZYK, AND THOMAS BRANDT 352

The Critical Role of Velocity Storage in Production of Motion Sickness. *By* BERNARD COHEN, MINGJIA DAI, AND THEODORE RAPHAN 359

Poster Papers

Visually Guided Saccade Adaptation: Transfer to Averaging Saccades Elicited by Double Visual Stimuli. *By* NADIA ALAHYANE AND DENIS PÉLISSON 377

Saccade Disconjugacy and Adaptation in Strabismic Monkeys. *By* VALLABH E. DAS, LAI NGOR FU, SEIJI ONO, RONALD J. TUSA, AND MICHAEL J. MUSTARI 381

Analysis of Saccades to Stationary and Moving Targets in the Monkey. *By* YANFANG GUAN, THOMAS EGGERT, OTMAR BAYER, AND ULRICH BÜTTNER 385

Accounting for Saccade Dysmetria after Cerebellar Lesion: A Modeling Approach. *By* ANSGAR KOENE AND LAURENT GOFFART 389

Characteristics of a Range Effect for Vergence Movements. *By* ARUN N. KUMAR, YANNING H. HAN, AND R. JOHN LEIGH 394

The Role of DLPN and NRTP in Visual-Vestibular Behavior. *By* SEIJI ONO, V.E. DAS, AND M.J. MUSTARI 399

Influence of Head Restraint on Visually Triggered Saccades in the Rhesus Monkey. *By* JULIE QUINET AND LAURENT GOFFART 404

Distribution of HSV-1 in Human Geniculate and Vestibular Ganglia: Implications for Vestibular Neuritis. *By* V. ARBUSOW, D. THEIL, P. SCHULZ, M. STRUPP, M. DIETERICH, E. RAUCH, AND T. BRANDT 409

Twitch and Non-Twitch Motoneurons of Extraocular Muscles Have Different Histochemical Properties. *By* ANDREAS C. EBERHORN, ANJA K.E. HORN, AHMED MESSOUDI, AND JEAN A. BÜTTNER-ENNEVER 414

Plasticity in Brainstem Motor Systems When Innervating a New Muscle in Adult Mammals. *By* AGNÈS GRUART, MICHAEL STREPPEL, ORLANDO GUNTINAS-LICHIUS, D.N. ANGELOV, WOLFRAM F. NEISS, AND JOSÉ M. DELGADO-GARCÍA 418

Vestibulo-Oculomotor Behavior in Rats after a Transient Unilateral Vestibular Loss Induced by Lidocaine. *By* ANNA K. MAGNUSSON AND RICHARD THAM 422

A Synaptic Mechanism on Prepositus Hypoglossi Neurons Underlying Eye Fixation. *By* JUAN D. NAVARRO-LOPEZ, JUAN CARLOS ALVARADO, MIGUEL ESCUDERO, JOSÉ M. DELGADO-GARCÍA, AND JAVIER YAJEYA. 424

Spatial Convergence Pattern of Canal and Macular Nerve Afferent Signals in Frog Second-Order Vestibular Neurons. *By* HANS STRAKA AND NORBERT DIERINGER 429

Acute Vestibular Nucleus Lesion Affects Cortical Activation Pattern during Caloric Irrigation in PET. *By* SANDRA BENSE, THOMAS STEPHAN, PETER BARTENSTEIN, MARKUS SCHWAIGER, THOMAS BRANDT, AND MARIANNE DIETERICH 434

Three Determinants of Vestibular Hemispheric Dominance during Caloric Stimulation: A Positron Emission Tomography Study. *By* SANDRA BENSE, PETER BARTENSTEIN, STEFFI LUTZ, THOMAS STEPHAN, MARKUS SCHWAIGER, THOMAS BRANDT, AND MARIANNE DIETERICH 440

Brain Activation Patterns during Fixation of a Central Target: A Functional Magnetic Resonance Imaging Study. *By* ANGELA DEUTSCHLÄNDER, THOMAS STEPHAN, ESTHER MARX, HARTMUT BRÜCKMANN, AND THOMAS BRANDT 446

Involvement of the Frontal Oculomotor Areas in Developmental Compensation for the Directional Asymmetry in Smooth-Pursuit Eye Movements in Young Primates. *By* JUNKO FUKUSHIMA, TEPPEI AKAO, NORIHITO TAKEICHI, CHRIS R.S. KANEKO, AND KIKURO FUKUSHIMA 451

Magnetoencephalography during Optokinetic and Vestibular Activation of the Posterior Insula. *By* S. HEGEMANN, M. PAWLOWSKI, R. HUONKER, J. HAUEISEN, C. FITZEK, AND M. FETTER 457

Impaired Representation of Saccadic Eye Displacement after Posterior Parietal Lesions: Is it a Craniotopic or a Directional Deficit? *By* WOLFGANG HEIDE, ANDREAS SPRENGER, BARBARA SACKERER, KLAUS G. ROTTACH, CHRISTIAN GAEBEL, AND DETLEF KÖMPF 465

Vestibular and Somatosensory Cortex Deactivation during Imagined Locomotion: A Functional Magnetic Resonance Imaging Study. *By* KLAUS JAHN, ANGELA DEUTSCHLÄNDER, THOMAS STEPHAN, HARTMUT BRÜCKMANN, MICHAEL STRUPP, AND THOMAS BRANDT 469

Head Impulses in Three Orthogonal Planes of Space: Influence of Age. *By* R. BRZEZNY, S. GLASAUER, O. BAYER, C. SIEBOLD, AND U. BÜTTNER . 473

Binocular Vertical-Torsional Spontaneous Nystagmus in a Midbrain Lesion Involving the Interstitial Nucleus of Cajal Indicates a Vestibular Imbalance of Vertical Semicircular Canals. *By* CHRISTOPH HELMCHEN, HOLGER RAMBOLD, AND ULRICH BÜTTNER 478

Vestibular Dysfunction in Acute Unilateral Hearing Loss. *By* J. BOENKI, H. RAMBOLD, G. STRITZKE, F. WISST, B. NEPPERT, AND C. HELMCHEN 482

Torsional Eye Movement Responses to Monaural and Binaural Galvanic Vestibular Stimulation: Side-to-Side Asymmetries. *By* KLAUS JAHN, ANDREA NAESSL, MICHAEL STRUPP, ERICH SCHNEIDER, THOMAS BRANDT, AND MARIANNE DIETERICH 485

Barbecue Whole-Body Position Modulates Cerebellar Downbeat Nystagmus. *By* SARAH MARTI, ANTONELLA PALLA, AND DOMINIK STRAUMANN ... 490

Two Opposite Effects of Nicotine on Downbeat Nystagmus: An Observation. *By* CRISTIANA BORGES PEREIRA, MICHAEL STRUPP, VERA CARINA ZINGLER, AND THOMAS BRANDT 492

Three-Dimensional Aspects of Spontaneous Nystagmus in Dorsolateral Medullary Infarction. *By* HOLGER RAMBOLD AND CHRISTOPH HELMCHEN . 497

Nonlinear Nystagmus Processing Causes Torsional VOR Nonlinearity. *By* E. SCHNEIDER, S. GLASAUER, T. BRANDT, AND M. DIETERICH 500

3,4-Diaminopyridine Improves Head-Shaking Nystagmus Caused by Neurovascular Cross-Compression. *By* M. STRUPP, V. QUERNER, T. EGGERT, A. STRAUBE, AND T. BRANDT 506

Solving the Redundancy Problem for Unrestricted Reaching Movements: A Comparison of Patients with Cerebral Infarcts and Healthy Controls. *By* THOMAS EGGERT, TEKLA TIHANYI, AND ANDREAS STRAUBE 511

Common Reference System for Estimation of the Postural and Subjective Visual Vertical. *By* K. JAGGI-SCHWARZ AND B.J.M. HESS 516

Lateropulsion in Wallenberg's Syndrome Decreases with Increasing Locomotion Speed. *By* KLAUS JAHN, MICHAEL STRUPP, AND THOMAS BRANDT 521

Eye–Head Coordination: Challenging the System by Increasing Head Inertia. *By* NADINE LEHNEN, STEFAN GLASAUER, AND ULRICH BÜTTNER 524

Perception and Pursuit: The Link between Object Motion Perception and the Motor Control of Ocular Pursuit. *By* G. SCHWEIGART, T. MERGNER, AND G.R. BARNES 527

Haptic Subjective Vertical Shows Context Dependence: Task and Vision Play a Role during Dynamic Tilt Stimulation. *By* WILLIAM GEOFFREY WRIGHT AND STEFAN GLASAUER 531

Index of Contributors 537

Financial assistance was received from:

- DEUTSCHE FORSCHUNGSGEMEINSCHAFT (SONDERFORSCHUNGSBEREICH 462)

> The New York Academy of Sciences believes it has a responsibility to provide an open forum for discussion of scientific questions. The positions taken by the participants in the reported conferences are their own and not necessarily those of the Academy. The Academy has no intent to influence legislation by providing such forums.

THE OCULOMOTOR AND VESTIBULAR SYSTEMS
THEIR FUNCTION AND DISORDERS

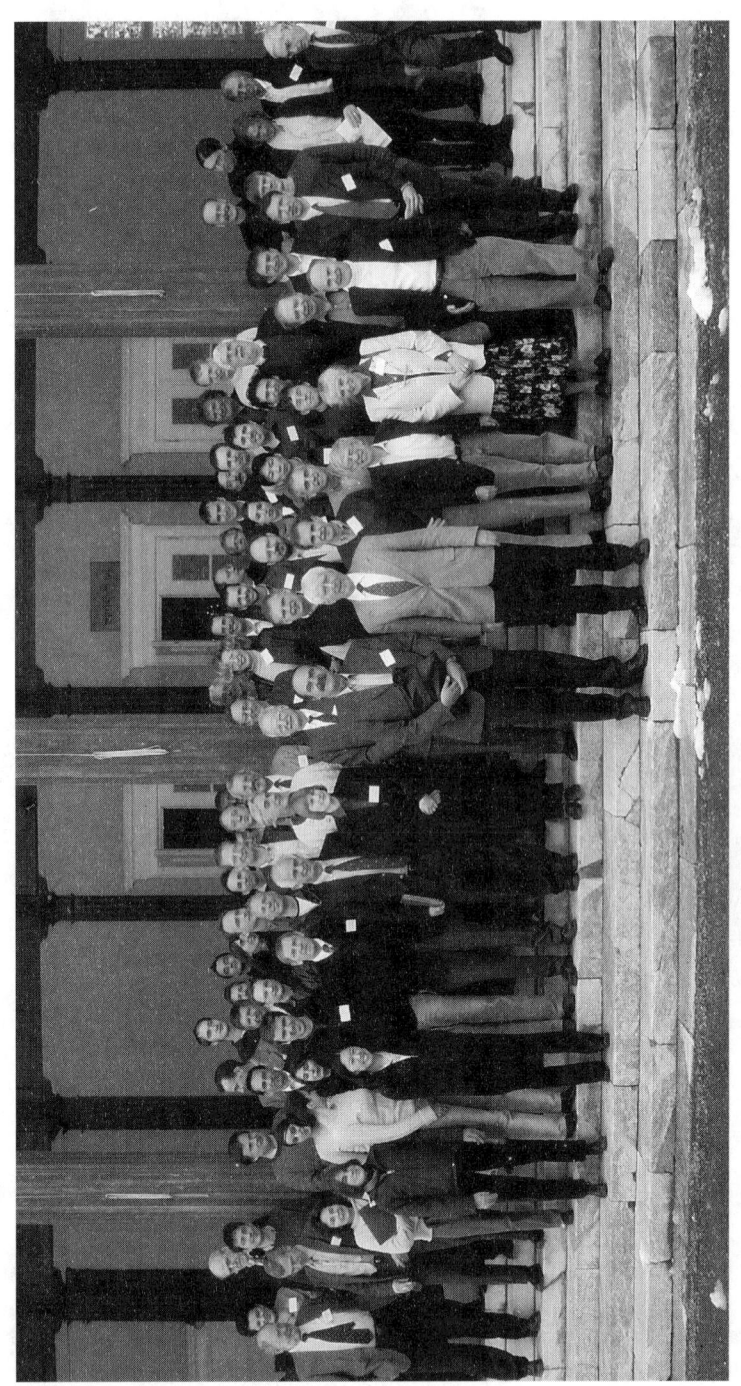

Contributors to the conference **Physiology and Disorders of Oculomotor and Vestibular Control**, held in Wildbad Kreuth, Germany, April 3–5, 2003, to honor Ulrich Büttner, M.D.

Preface

A Tribute to Ulrich Büttner

This volume contains proceedings from the Third International Ocular Motor Meeting, "Physiology and Disorders of Oculomotor and Vestibular Control," held in the Bavarian Alps from April 3–5, 2003. The meeting honored Ulrich Büttner, a leading scientist who has made many important contributions to our understanding of the control and disorders of eye movement. The first ocular motor meeting, "Contemporary Ocular Motor and Vestibular Research," was held in honor of David A. Robinson, and the second meeting, "The Vestibular and Ocular Motor Systems: Basic Mechanisms and Clinical Applications," was in honor of Bernard Cohen. All three scientists used a similar methodology, combining animal experiments with investigations of human neurophysiology to understand important problems of oculomotor control.

Ulrich Büttner was born in Berlin in 1943, but grew up in the city of Celle. It was Otto-Joachim Grüsser, a neurophysiologist in Berlin and a student of the famous neurologist Richard Jung, who made Ulrich aware of the importance of solving clinical problems using experimental neurophysiology. This was the starting point of his long, productive scientific career. Here we will cite just a few of the most important milestones.

Ulrich's background in the visual system and Albert Fuch's experience with the oculomotor system led them to collaborate in Seattle in 1971 to make single-cell recordings from the lateral geniculate body of alert monkeys. They found neurons that were modulated both by eye movements and visual stimuli. This combination of sensory and motor function in the same cell was most unusual at the time. For the first time, they had provided a physical basis for determining sensory-motor integration.

Later, in Volker Henn's laboratory in Zürich, Ulrich and Volker recorded from cells in the thalamus, which responded to natural vestibular stimulation and to large moving visual fields. Ulrich extended these studies to the parietal cortex (area 2v), where neurons in the behaving monkey also exhibited similar visual–vestibular interaction. While recording the activity of vestibular neurons in the thalamus, Ulrich and Volker encountered a number of neurons beneath the thalamus whose activity was correlated with vertical saccades. At that time, important strides had been made in understanding the neural organization for horizontal eye movements, but very little was known about how and where vertical eye movements were produced. At the same time, Jean Büttner-Ennever, also working in Zürich, was doing tracer studies to investigate projections from the paramedian pontine reticular formation (PPRF), a critical center for horizontal gaze. She found strong projections from the PPRF to a region of the midbrain she called the rostral interstitial nucleus of the median longitudinal fasciculus (riMLF). Recognizing the potential significance of the neural activity in this region, Ulrich, Volker, and Jean then localized and recorded from cells in this region, providing the first convincing evidence that the riMLF is a major center for vertical gaze in the monkey.

But did this region also play a similar role in the human? This question was answered when the group, working with Bernard Cohen, identified the same region in an American patient, who had come to the Zürich clinic with a vertical gaze palsy. The patient was transferred to the Mount Sinai Hospital, where he later died of unrelated causes. By studying the areas of the brain that were involved, they were able to combine neurophysiological and neuropathological findings to show that the riMLF had the same significance for vertical gaze in humans as in the monkey.

More recently, Professor Büttner turned his attention to understanding the role of the cerebellar nuclei in oculomotor control, a subject still under intense investigation. During a sabbatical in Seattle in 1989, he and Albert Fuchs succeeded in recording neural activity in the fastigial nucleus correlated with eye movements, especially smooth pursuit. Fastigial lesions were then shown to lead to saccadic dysmetria and smooth-pursuit deficits. Later, with Andreas Straube, Ulrich also described a corresponding clinical syndrome in neurological patients.

Professor Büttner's current work with Justus Kleine is still focused on defining neural activity in the fastigial nucleus. The aim is to understand the role of the fastigial nucleus in saccadic control and to evaluate activity in this region during vestibular stimulation in varying head-trunk positions. This work, which is documented in this volume, promises to give new insights into understanding the basis for cerebellar control of the oculomotor system. We anticipate that it will also be an important step in advancing our understanding of cerebellar control of movement in general. We and the participants at the 2003 meeting wish him much success in this important endeavor.

—THOMAS BRANDT
—BERNARD COHEN
—CHRISTOPH SIEBOLD

Acknowledgments

We also wish to thank all who helped with both the conference and the resulting volume, and in particular S. Langer, for her technical assistance at the conference, and K. Ogston, for preparing the manuscripts, as well as the *Annals* editorial department for seeing the book so quickly and skillfully through the press.

The Spa at Kreuth, or Why Did the Russian Czars Visit There?

WERNER GRAF

Laboratoire de Physiologie de la Perception et de l'Action, CNRS, Collège de France, 11, place Marcelin Berthelot, 75231 Paris Cedex 05, France

[EDITORS' NOTE: As a point of interest, we are including a brief history of the place where the conference was held.]

In the entrance of the former reception hall of Wildbad Kreuth, a plaque is found that commemorates the visits there of the Russian czars Alexander I and Nicholas I. Why would such illustrious monarchs have found their way into this lonely mountain valley above the lake of Tegernsee?

The area was more famous centuries ago than it is now. Its fame rests not only on the incomparable beauty of the surrounding area of the Tegernsee, the "Bavarian Garden of Eden," but also on the ancient "bad"—or spa—of Kreuth, whose healing powers had been known since medieval times. As legend goes, a huntsman had shot a deer, and following the blood trail, he found the animal bathing its wound in a spring. When word of the incident spread, shepherds and farmers from the area sought healing in the spring as well, all believing in small miracles. At the time, no one could have had an idea that the spring indeed was rich in minerals, especially sulfur. Thus, the spring of the "Holy Cross" and soon thereafter the spa of "St. Leonard" were officially established. The Benedictine monastery of Tegernsee owned the grounds around Kreuth, and the first mention of the spa appears in 1490, with its own water master established in 1498.

By that time, the Tegernsee monastery, founded in 746, about 200 years after the establishment of the Benedictine order by St. Benedict of Norcia, already had a long history. The dukes of the Agilolfing dynasty, whose last representative, Tassilo III, was deposed by Charlemagne in 788, then ruled Bavaria. The Tegernsee area is certainly one of the oldest post-Roman settlements in Germany—very old Europe, indeed! After the rule of the Agilolfing family, Bavaria fell to the Franks, that is, the House of Charlemagne, and then to the Saxons, whose most famous representative, Henry the Lion, founded the capital city of Munich. Finally, from 1180 to this day, the House of Wittelsbach holds avaria by decree of the Holy Roman Emperor and German King Frederic I Barbarossa.

Address for correspondence: Werner Graf, CNRS-LPPA, Collège de France, 11, place Marcelin Berthelot, 75231 Paris Cedex 05, France. Voice: +33-1-44 27 16 30; fax: +33-1-44 27 13 82.
werner.graf@college-de-france.fr

The Tegernsee monastery and its spa operation lasted until the year 1803, the year of the "secularization." Following the ideas of the French Revolution (1789), the government of Bavaria adopted a radical anticlerical policy, and, in this predominantly Catholic country, nationalized a great deal of church property. Thus, the property of the monks of Tegernsee was expropriated, and the spa was purchased by the then–water master, and became private property. Historically, Bavaria as a medium-sized power had always pursued a pro-French policy as a guarantee of survival against her larger neighbors, Austria and Prussia; during the early years of the Napoleonic Era, she had joined the Confederation of the Rhine, a conglomerate of pro-Napoleonic German states. Implementation of radical French-revolutionary ideas was thus no surprise.

In 1813, shortly before the "Battle of Nations" at Leipzig, Bavaria switched sides and joined the anti-Napoleonic coalition with Russia, Austria, and Prussia against France after 30,000 Bavarians perished in Napoleon's Russian campaign. The principal architect and driving force of this decisive anti-Napoleonic coalition was the Russian Czar Alexander I (1777–1825; ruled 1801–1825). He was also opposed to inflicting the final mortal blow against Napoleon at Leipzig, because he wanted no peace until he entered Paris, which he did in March 1814. To his credit, Alexander I was lenient toward defeated France, stressing that he had made war against Napoleon, not against the French people. As is well known, Napoleon met his final defeat in 1815 at Waterloo by Prussian and English forces under Marshall Blücher and the Duke of Wellington.

The peaceful setting of the spa at Kreuth, unfortunately, fell into disrepair under the private property management of the family of the water master. In 1818, however, the well and the surrounding buildings were bought by the royal house of Bavaria, namely, King Maximilian I Joseph (1756–1825; ruled 1799–1825). The king had the spa renovated and enlarged, and the early 19th century buildings, including the entrance hall where the commemorative plaque is located, are from this time. The king, furthermore, set up a trust fund to allow "stipends" to poor people in order to have them enjoy the pleasures of the spa. By this time, the spa had a certain reputation with wealthy Russians, and thus it comes as no surprise that the Russian czars, first Alexander and then his younger brother and successor, Nicholas I (1796–1855; ruled 1825–1855) took advantage of the setting in the Bavarian Garden of Eden. Presumably, ownership by the King of Bavaria himself gave additional prestige to the site. Besides the Russian czars, other members of European royalty frequented Wildbad Kreuth, notably the Hapsburg Emperor of Austria, Francis Joseph (1830–1916; ruled 1848–1916).

After the death of King Maximilian I Joseph in 1825, his widow, Queen Caroline, and the Prince Carl of Bavaria, younger brother of King Ludwig I of Bavaria (1786–1868; ruled 1825–1848) continued to manage the spa. Thus, the spa became the property of a side branch of the House of Wittelsbach, the dukes in Bavaria, who, however, were not in line for royal succession. Nevertheless, this ducal house of Bavaria produced a number of most marriageable princesses, the most famous being Elisabeth of Austria, Sissi (1837–1898; empress 1854–1898), wife of the Hapsburg Emperor Francis Joseph.

King Ludwig I had the ambition to make Munich and Bavaria a cultural and intellectual center in Germany, and initiated far-reaching city planning, architectural, construction, and museum-building programs, attracting scientists and artists to Munich, in addition to giving the country the most liberal constitution in Germany. However, King Ludwig had to abdicate following a public scandal over his infatuation with the Irish dancer and adventuress Lola Montez, and his son Maximilian II Joseph became king (1811–1864; ruled 1848–1864). After this monarch's premature death, his eldest son ascended the throne of Bavaria at the age of 18 as Ludwig II (1845–1886; ruled 1864–1886). There were rumors that the then-czar of Russia, Alexander II (1818–1881; ruled 1855–1881) would have liked to marry one of his daughters, the czarevna, to this young king of Bavaria. Perhaps the fame of the Bavarian Garden of Eden still lingered in the palaces of St. Petersburg and Moscow! At this point, it should be noted that the 19th century czars of Russia were essentially German by blood. The only Russian genetic material that had entered into their heritage was through Anna, a daughter of the Czar Peter I, the Great, and the mother of Peter III (1728–1762; ruled 6 months in 1762). Peter III's father was a duke of Holstein-Gottorp. Peter III's wife, of course, was Catherine II, the Great, originally the German princess Sophie Friederike of Anhalt-Zerbst (1729–1796; ruled 1762–1796). She had her feeble, unstable husband overthrown and deposed. Subsequently, all the future czars married German princesses, with the exception of Alexander III, who married Dagmar of Denmark.

Ludwig II of Bavaria had similar ambitions to those of his grandfather. One of his first actions after ascending the throne was to call the composer Richard Wagner to Munich, offering him his protection and generous financial support. Ludwig II abhorred war and detested the militaristic posturing and hegemonial ambitions of the Prussia of the "Iron Chancellor" Bismarck. The king's grandiose ideas and plans, such as his lifelong support for Richard Wagner and the construction of the Bayreuth Opera House, as well as his romantic palace projects at Linderhof, Neuschwanstein and Herrenchiemsee, together with a certain instability of character, finally led to his deposition. He found his death in the lake of Starnberg.

The spa at Kreuth flourished nevertheless under the dukes in Bavaria until the end of World War II, when the buildings were severely damaged by advancing American troops. After its postwar renovation, the spa experienced a short revival period, but evidently its time had passed, just as that of the absolute monarchies of Europe. There is no longer a spa at Kreuth, there are no more czars in Russia, no more emperors in Austria, and no more kings in Bavaria—but the Garden of Eden of Tegernsee remains.

Physiology of the Eyelid Motor System

JOSÉ M. DELGADO-GARCÍA, AGNÈS GRUART, AND JOSÉ A. TRIGO

División de Neurociencias, Laboratorio Andaluz de Biología, Universidad Pablo de Olavide, Sevilla 41013, Spain

> ABSTRACT: The eyelid motor system represents an excellent experimental model for the study of reflex and learned motor responses. Eyelid responses can be recorded quantitatively with the search coil in a magnetic-field technique. Stimuli able to evoke reflex blinks (air puffs, flashes of light, tones) can also be controlled quantitatively. Eyelid movements can be classified as spontaneous, passive (such as those following eye saccades), reflex, and acquired with classical conditioning procedures. Information is available regarding the firing activity of brainstem motoneuronal pools (abducens, accessory abducens, and facial motoneurons) involved in these types of eyelid response. In particular, facial motoneurons present different encoding properties for the generation of reflex against learned eyelid responses. In cats, accessory abducens motoneurons are involved only in reflex (but not in learned) blinks. The recent description of the complete organization of premotoneuronal pathways related to eyelid motorics opens new experimental possibilities for the study of this particular motor system.
>
> KEYWORDS: abducens nucleus; accessory abducens nucleus; blink; conditioned eyelid responses; eyelid; facial nucleus; proprioception

THE EYELID MOTOR SYSTEM AS A MODEL

The eyelid motor system represents an excellent experimental model for the *in vivo* study of how relatively simple movements (spontaneous, reflex, or acquired by learning) are generated and controlled by the central nervous system.[4,7,14] Nevertheless, and in spite of their apparent simplicity, eyelid responses present quite different profiles and kinematics and can be performed in relation to diverse behavioral situations. Moreover, eyelid responses result from the activity of up to three different motor systems—namely, the facial, oculomotor, and retractor bulbi systems.[4,7,11,14]

Essentially, a blink is a fast narrowing of the palpebral fissure mainly in response to mechanical activation of the corneal surface and/or the periorbital skin, or to electrical stimulation of the supraorbitary branch of the trigeminal nerve. Flashes of light or strong and potentially dangerous visual and acoustic stimuli can also evoke blinks. Spontaneous blinks are carried out in a repetitive manner and seem to be involved not only with corneal wetting and protection, but also with cognitive processing of visual percepts. Eyelid movements are also involved in the precise and timed

---

Address for correspondence: Prof. José M. Delgado-García, División de Neurociencias, Laboratorio Andaluz de Biología, Universidad Pablo de Olavide, Ctra. de Utrera, Km. 1, Sevilla 41013, Spain. Voice: +34-954-349374; fax: +34-954-349375.
  jmdelgar@dex.upo.es

motor displays characteristic of emotional expressions such as smiling, winking, and grimacing. Eyelids also accompany eye excursion in the orbit, mostly during vertical eye saccades and position of fixation. Finally, the classical conditioning of the nictitating membrane/eyelid response has become a procedure of choice for the study of brain mechanisms involved in motor learning.[1,6,16,17]

Available technical facilities for the presentation and recording of inputs (sensory stimulation) and outputs (muscle activity, eyelid or nictitating membrane displacement) of the eyelid motor system are fundamental for the appropriate understanding of its functional properties. Moreover, recent descriptions of the neural organization of premotor centers and pathways involved in the generation of eyelid responses,[2,13] as well as available information on the neural activity of nodal neural centers, such as brainstem motoneurons,[14] make this motor system very interesting for its detailed analysis, at both the anatomical and functional levels. Accordingly, we will briefly describe here the main types of eyelid responses, the biomechanical constraints involved in this motor system, and the functional properties of brainstem motoneuron pools governing reflex and learned blinks.

TECHNICAL DETAILS OF THE EXPERIMENTAL PREPARATION

This chronic preparation is illustrated in FIGURE 1. We have successfully recorded eyelid movements in alert behaving cats, rabbits, guinea pigs, and rats using the search coil in a magnetic-field technique.[9] For this, animals, under general anesthesia (Nembutal, 35 mg/kg and atropine sulfate, 0.5 mg/kg), are implanted in the upper eyelid with coils made from Teflon-coated multistranded stainless steel wire with an external diameter of 50 µm. The coil diameter ranges from 1 to 3 mm depending on the implanted species. The low weight of the coil (3–14 mg, i.e., about 2 to 10% of the animals' eyelid weight) precludes any noticeable eyelid drooping or impairment of movement when compared with non-implanted controls. Animals are also usually implanted with bipolar hook electrodes for recording the electromyographic (EMG) activity of the orbicularis oculi muscle and of other muscles (levator palpebrae, lateral rectus, and retractor bulbi) related to eyelid motorics. Bipolar stimulating electrodes are implanted in selected cerebral sites for the antidromic activation of recorded neurons.[14] Unitary recordings are carried out with glass micropipettes filled with a NaCl solution (1.5–2 M). Only antidromically identified neurons are further recorded and analyzed.

Reflex blinks are evoked by the random presentation of air puffs (1–3 kg/cm^2; 20–100 ms), flashes of light (xenon arc lamp; < 1 ms), or tones (600–6000 Hz, 90 dB, 20–350 ms). Classical conditioning of eyelid responses is achieved using both trace and delay paradigms. For trace conditioning, the conditioned stimulus (CS, a tone or an air puff) is presented for a brief time (usually 20 ms) and is followed about 250 ms later by the presentation of a strong (3 kg/cm^2), long (100 ms) air puff as unconditioned stimulus (US). For delay conditioning, the CS consists of a long (350 ms) tone (600 Hz, 90 dB); the US starts 250 ms after CS onset and also consists of a strong, long air puff. Up to 10 conditioning sessions are carried out per animal, preceded by 2–4 habituation sessions and followed by 4–5 extinction sessions. Further details of these conditioning paradigms and of basic procedures for *in vivo* recordings of eyelid movements and neuronal unitary activity can be found elsewhere.[7,9,14]

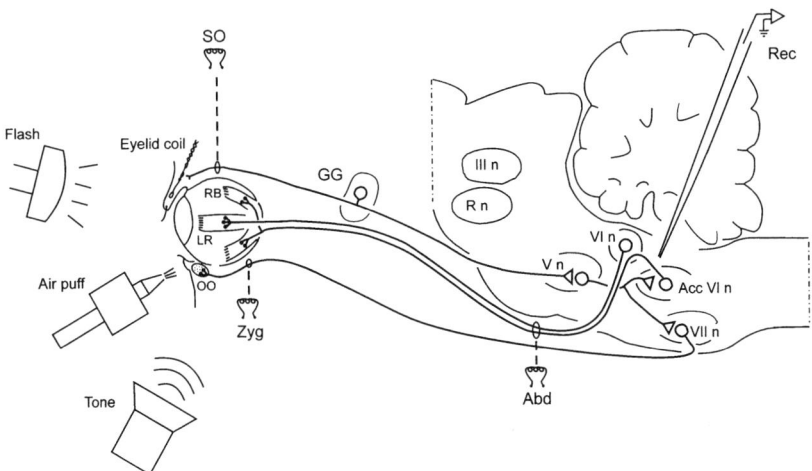

FIGURE 1. Experimental design. Cats were presented with flashes of light, air puffs, and tones to evoke eyelid reflex or classically conditioned responses. Eyelid movements were recorded with the search coil in a magnetic-field technique. The electromyographic activity of the orbicularis oculi muscle was recorded with bipolar stainless steel electrodes. Bipolar stimulating electrodes were also chronically implanted for the synaptic or antidromic activation of recorded motoneurons. Brainstem motoneurons were recorded with glass microelectrodes using a transcerebellar approach (Rec). *Abbreviations*: III n, oculomotor nucleus; V n, trigeminal nucleus; VI n, abducens nucleus; VII n, facial nucleus; Acc VI n, accessory abducens nucleus; GC, trigeminal ganglion of Gasser; LR, lateral rectus muscle; RB, retractor bulbi muscle; R n, red nucleus. (Modified from Trigo et al.[14])

TYPES OF EYELID RESPONSE

According to available information, eyelid movements can be classified into four different groups: spontaneous, reflex, passive, and learned.[3,7,9]

Spontaneous blinks consist of a fast downward displacement of the upper eyelid followed by a slower upward movement. The whole response lasts for 200–400 ms in the cat. Spontaneous blinks take place at quite different rates in rabbits (≪1/min), cats (1–2/min), and humans (10–20/min). Like other felines, cats commonly make a so-called *friendly eyelid display*, consisting of an incomplete closing of both eyelids. This eyelid response starts with a downward displacement of the upper lid, lasting for 30–40 ms, followed by a slower, wavy upward phase. Characteristically, the downward waves present in friendly eyelid displays (as well as in the active peering and grimacing of these animals) have a mean duration of ≈ 50 ms.

The latency, amplitude, peak velocity, and profiles of *reflex blinks* depend on the sensory modality used to evoke them, and on the intensity, duration, and side of presentation of the blink-evoking stimulus. *Air-puff–evoked blinks* consist of a fast downward displacement of the upper lid followed by a slower upward displacement. The latency of this reflex blink in cats is 11–12 ms for a 3 kg/cm^2 air puff. The initial downward phase of air-puff–evoked blinks has a constant duration (i.e., a rise time of 17–18 ms), independent of its amplitude. Thus, stimuli of increasing intensity increase the amplitude of the eyelid response by an increase in its velocity because the duration of this downward component cannot be modified. When the air puff lasts >20 ms, the initial downward movement is followed by a wavy (at ≈20 Hz, in the cat) profile. The final upward displacement does not usually present this wavy appearance. Blinks evoked by flashes of light in cats have a latency about four times longer than those evoked by a puff of air, and their amplitude is smaller. Interestingly, flash-evoked blinks consist of a single downward displacement, sometimes followed by a small downward sag, and a late upward displacement. In *tone-evoked blinks*, there are important species differences. Only 50% of cats produce a long-latency (≈50 ms), small (1–4 degrees against 15–20 degrees for air puffs) blink in response to a strong (90 dB) tone. Other species (rats) produce short-latency, large blinks in response to tone presentations, as part of a more complex startle reaction.

The upper eyelids *passively* follow eye saccades and fast phases of vestibular and optokinetic reflexes in the vertical plane. Although upward and downward lid saccades in the cat are similar in metric properties, the orbicularis oculi muscle is not active during these movements. This fact indicates that whereas upward lid saccades are produced by the activity of the levator palpebrae muscle, downward saccades are passive because no active muscle is moving the eyelid. These differences in active versus passive motor control are quantitatively noticeable when dealing with slow upper-eyelid responses, such as during the slow phase of vestibular and optokinetic reflexes. In this case, the gain of slow eyelid movements in the downward direction is 30–50% lower than the gain in the upward direction.[7,9]

The latency, amplitude, peak velocity and profile of *conditioned eyelid responses* depend on the sensory modality, intensity, and presentation side of the CS, and on the CS-US interval. Nevertheless, conditioned eyelid responses always have a ramp-like, wavy appearance, and their peak velocity never reaches > 1/10 of the peak eyelid velocity during reflexively evoked blinks. These important differences in eyelid kinematics suggest a different neural origin of (and/or mechanism involved in) reflex and learned eyelid responses. Moreover, since eyelid movement profiles characterizing conditioned responses (CRs) are not included in the usual motor repertoire of nonconditioned animals, it is difficult to envisage, from an evolutionary point of view, how those motor responses were acquired before the institutionalization of classical conditioning of nictitating membrane/eyelid responses in the 1960s.

SOME BIOMECHANICAL PROPERTIES OF EYELID RESPONSES

The eyelid motor system is peculiar for many different reasons. First, this motor system has an almost negligible mass and is load free. As a result, the system has a very low inertial damping. Furthermore, it has been demonstrated that eyelid motorics function in the absence of a stretch reflex.[15] In fact, facial motoneurons receive no proprioceptive information from the position of the eyelid, apart from that coming from cutaneous receptors. During alertness, the position of the eyelid is determined exclusively by the activity of the levator palpebrae muscle. As is known, levator palpebrae motoneurons share eye position information with extraocular motoneurons involved in eye movements in the vertical plane.[5] Finally, the activity of facial motoneurons is not under the regulatory control of axon collaterals projecting back into the facial nucleus. These described characteristics of the facial system, together with its special (visceral) origin, make it different (in control and performance) from the spinal motor system. For example, the voluntary control of eyelid position on the eye lacks the precision of voluntary movements carried out with the fingers, while facial movements of emotional origin (indicative of internal emotional states) cannot be easily controlled at will.[14,15]

Recent studies from our group indicate that eyelid movements are tuned at their frequency of resonance. Thus, both reflex and learned eyelid responses in cats present a dominant oscillation frequency at $\approx$ 20 Hz. This is not a passive property of the system, because the same oscillatory properties are present in innervating facial motoneurons, as shown by intracellular recordings both *in vitro*[12] and *in vivo*.[14] Interestingly, this neural oscillator governing eyelid responses is dependent (in an inverse logarithmic relationship, with slope of −0.25) on animal (or eyelid) weight.[9] Thus, the typical frequency of eyelid oscillation is $\approx$ 10 Hz for humans, but $\approx$ 20 Hz for cats (as indicated), and $\approx$ 35 for rats. Recent unpublished results indicate that the oscillation frequency goes up to $\approx$ 50 Hz in mice. Thus, eyelid biomechanics is tuned to the weight and viscoelastic properties of the eyelid; the firing of innervating motoneurons is also tuned to them. These adjustments in functional capabilities of a muscle and its innervating motoneuron pool take place early in development and cannot be modified when other brainstem motoneurons are forced to innervate *de novo* a given muscle.[8,10] For example, hypoglossal motoneurons obliged to innervate the orbicularis oculi muscle by means of a hypoglossal-facial anastomosis are unable, in cats, to accomplish the oscillatory needs of the reinnervated muscle (i.e., to fire at 20 Hz), but maintain their typical firing (with a dominant frequency of 4–7 Hz) for tongue movements.

GENESIS AND CONTROL OF EYELID RESPONSES BY BRAINSTEM MOTONEURONS

It is generally assumed that motor units of the orbicularis oculi muscle are rather small (1:25), although this contention has not been convincingly proved.[14,15] Indeed, a small motor unit size will secure better control during precise emotional expressions involving the eyelid. The orbicularis oculi muscle is innervated by motoneurons located at the dorsolateral subdivision of the facial motor nucleus. According to published information, orbicularis oculi motoneurons present a regional organization within their subdivision because the motoneurons innervating tarsal muscle fibers are located more dorsally and laterally than those innervating orbicularis oculi motor fibers located in septal and orbital areas.[2]

The kinematics and frequency-domain properties of eyelid responses depend directly on the firing properties of facial motoneurons innervating the orbicularis oculi muscle. In animals with a nictitating membrane, such as cats, abducens and accessory abducens motoneurons also contribute to eyelid displacement, because of the evoked eye retraction into the orbit. We have recently studied the firing properties of identified orbicularis oculi motoneurons recorded intracellularly in alert cats during evoked reflex and learned eyelid responses. For comparative purposes, we also recorded the activity of identified abducens and accessory abducens motoneurons. Data presented here have been described in detail elsewhere.[12,14]

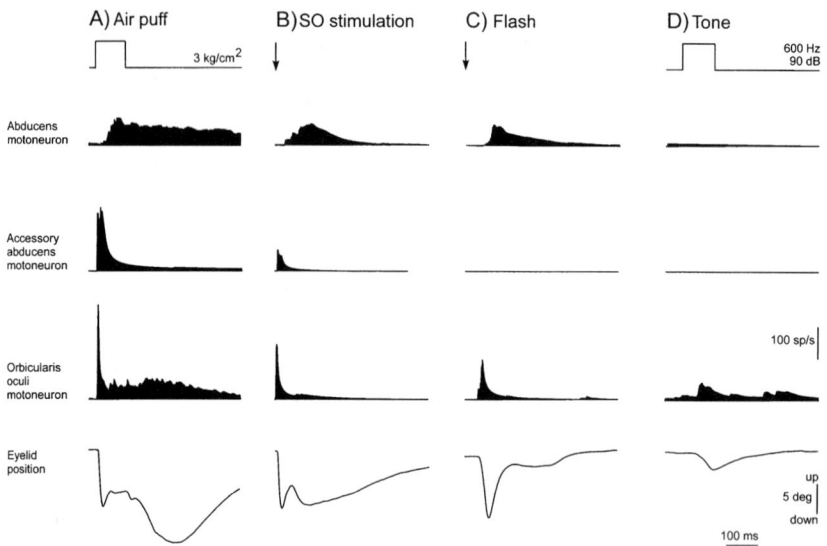

FIGURE 2. Characteristic firing of abducens, accessory abducens, and orbicularis oculi motoneurons during blinks evoked by air puffs (**A**), electrical stimulation of the supraorbitary branch of the trigeminal nerve (**B**), flashes of light (**C**), and tones (**D**) in alert cats. *Top to bottom*: Illustrated are the applied stimulus, the mean firing rate (in spikes/second) of three representative motoneurons recorded in each nucleus. The illustrated eyelid position was recorded at the same time as the activity of the orbicularis oculi motoneuron shown above. Each trace corresponds to the mean value of >10 single records of the unitary firing or of eyelid position. Calibrations in **D** are also for **A–C**. (Reprinted from Trigo *et al.*[14] with permission of the *Journal of Neurophysiology*.)

Orbicularis oculi and accessory abducens motoneurons fire an early, double burst of action potentials (at 4–6 ms and 10–16 ms) in response to air puffs and to electrical stimulation of the supraorbitary branch of the trigeminal nerve. Orbicularis oculi, but not accessory abducens, motoneurons fire to flash presentations, and are very weakly depolarized (i.e., the evoked excitatory postsynaptic potential is unable to induce a full spike) by tone presentations (see FIG. 2). In a study carried out in alert cats,[14] only 10–15% of recorded abducens motoneurons fired a late, weak burst of spikes following air-puff, supraorbital-nerve, or flash stimuli. The discharge rate of orbicularis oculi motoneurons is linearly related to eyelid velocity during reflex blinks, but as indicated above, these motoneurons do not seem to encode eyelid position.

The activation of orbicularis oculi motoneurons during the acquisition of classically conditioned eyelid responses takes place in a gradual and sequential manner. During the initial conditioning sessions, excitatory postsynaptic potentials increase their presence trial by trial in the CS-US time window. Starting around the 2nd–4th conditioning sessions, some single–action potentials are observed in the CS-US time window, increasing in number until some small movements are noticed in eyelid position traces. No abducens or accessory abducens motoneuron fires during the CS-US interval (see FIG. 3). Thus, and in opposition to what has been described in rab-

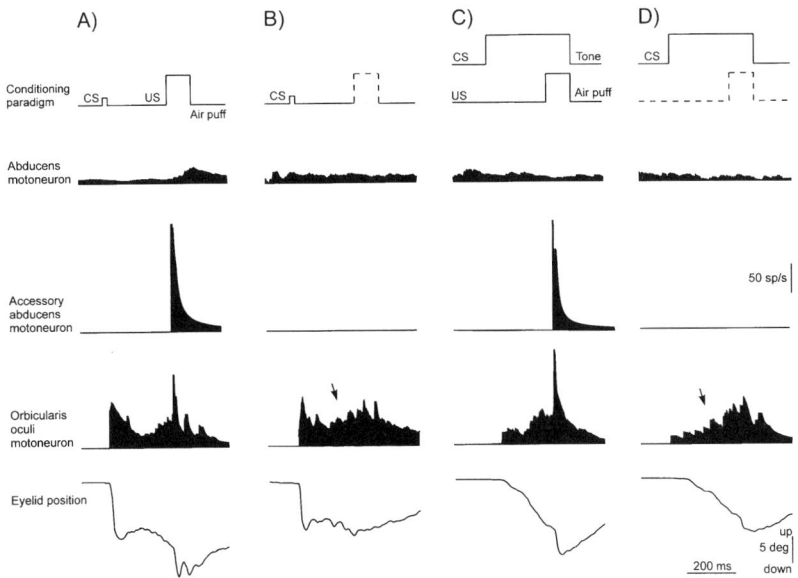

FIGURE 3. Characteristic firing of abducens, accessory abducens, and orbicularis oculi motoneurons during classically conditioned eyelid responses of alert cats. *Top to bottom*: Illustrated are the conditioning paradigm, the mean firing rate (in spikes/second) of 12 representative motoneurons from the abducens ($n = 4$), accessory abducens ($n = 4$), and orbicularis oculi ($n = 4$) nuclei, and the eyelid position traces (recorded simultaneously with the illustrated orbicularis oculi motoneurons). Each trace corresponds to the mean value of >10 single records of the unitary firing or of eyelid position. (**A,B**) For the trace conditioning paradigm, a 20 ms, 1 kg/cm^2 air puff was used as conditioned stimulus (CS), followed 250 ms later by a 100 ms, 3 kg/cm^2 air puff as unconditioned stimulus (US). The US was not presented during records illustrated in **B**. (**C,D**) For the delay conditioning paradigm, a 350 ms, 600 Hz, 90 dB tone was used as CS. The tone was followed 250 ms from its onset by a 100 ms, 3 kg/cm^2 air puff as US. The US was not presented during records illustrated in **D**. Note the absence of activity in accessory abducens motoneurons in relation to CS presentations. *Arrows* in **B** and **D** indicate the presence of repetitive peaks (at about 20 Hz) in the averaged profiles of orbicularis oculi motoneuron firing and in eyelid position traces. All recordings were carried out during the 6th conditioning session in two different animals. (Reprinted from Trigo et al.[14] with permission of the *Journal of Neurophysiology*.)

bits, accessory abducens motoneurons in cats are not involved in the generation of eyelid CRs.[9,14]

The firing of orbicularis oculi motoneurons during CRs is linearly related to eyelid position. The fact that facial motoneurons encode eyelid velocity during reflex blinks and eyelid position during learned responses suggests a different neural origin of the two types of response and/or a different location of the corresponding synaptic inputs (somatic for reflex and dendritic for learned responses). Moreover, cholinergic inputs to facial motoneurons seem capable of modifying the firing rate of the motoneuron from a phasic to a tonic manner.[12] Thus, it may be suggested that cholinergic neurons of reticular origin are able to adapt the firing of motoneurons and to prepare them to evoke learned responses.

According to recent studies from our laboratory,[12,14] the wavy appearance of reflex and learned eyelid responses is the result of the peculiar firing of facial motoneurons innervating the orbicularis oculi muscle. Orbicularis oculi motoneuron membrane potential oscillates at ≈ 20 Hz during reflex and conditioned eyelid responses. It should be pointed out that the oscillation in membrane potential of facial motoneurons is probably the result of both intrinsic (spike afterhyperpolarization lasting ≈ 50 ms and late depolarizations) and extrinsic (neural circuits involved in eyelid responses) properties of the motoneuronal pool.[12,14]

PREMOTONEURONAL CONTROL OF EYELID RESPONSES

A recent study using the attenuated rabies virus as a retrograde transsynaptic marker has furnished a rather complete picture of neural circuits underlying spontaneous, reflex, and learned blinks.[13] The virus was injected in selected sites of the upper eyelid of adult rats. Specific zones of brainstem sensory nuclei related to trigeminal, auditory, vestibular, and visual pathways were labeled at early stages following virus injection. During the successive stages, the dorsal and ventral reticular nuclei, the parvocellular and gigantocellular, rostral and caudal pontine nuclei, as well as the mesencephalic reticular formation, showed a specific and definite pattern of labeled neurons. Mesencephalic nuclei involved in eye–eyelid coordination (interstitial nucleus of Cajal, nucleus of Darkschewitsch, superior colliculus) were labeled at stages suggesting a monosynaptic input on orbicularis oculi motoneurons. Some brainstem relays of limbic pathways (parabrachial and Kölliker-Fuse nuclei) appeared labeled with the virus at late stages. The dorsolateral area of the contralateral red nucleus and the surrounding pararubral area and mesencephalic reticular formation were heavily labeled. Wide areas of the three deep cerebellar nuclei (mainly the lateral part of interpositus and the medial nucleus) were labeled as well as wide zones of the overlying vermal and paravermal Purkinje cells. Fifth layer pyramidal cells of the parietal cortex were labeled mostly contralaterally. As a whole, this study has given a more complete picture of the inverted pyramid of premotor networks controlling the different types of eyelid responses, in which the three main motor systems (motor cortex, red nucleus and pararubral area, and reticular formation) seem to be involved in precise correspondence with the correlated cerebellar structures.[13]

CONCLUSIONS AND PERSPECTIVES

The eyelid motor system is peculiar because of its intrinsic biomechanical properties, involvement in different types of eyelid response, and neuronal control at the motor and premotor levels. Moreover, it is widely used as an experimental model for the study of neuronal processes underlying associative learning. As reported here, the available information regarding its kinematics and frequency-domain properties, motoneuronal encoding of both reflex and learned responses, and hierarchical organization of its premotor circuits, represents a solid step toward further investigation of the neuronal coding controlling the generation and performance of those eyelid movements.

REFERENCES

1. DELGADO-GARCÍA, J.M. & A. GRUART. 2002. The role of interpositus nucleus in eyelid conditioned responses. Cerebellum **1:** 289–308.
2. DELGADO-GARCÍA, J.M., A. GRUART, J. A. TRIGO & S. MORCUENDE. 1998. Neuronal organization and functional properties of the eyelid motor system. *In* Brain Stem Reflexes and Functions. J. Valls-Sole & E. Tolosa, Eds. SmithKline Beecham. Madrid.
3. DOMINGO, J.A., A. GRUART & J.M. DELGADO-GARCÍA. 1997. Quantal organization of reflex and conditioned eyelid responses. J. Neurophysiol. **78:** 2518–2530.
4. EVINGER, C., K.A. MANNING & P.A. SIBONY. 1991. Eyelid movements. Mechanisms and normal data. Invest. Ophthalmol. Visual Sci. **32:** 387–400.
5. FUCHS, A.F., W. BECKER, L. LING, *et al.* 1992. Discharge patterns of levator palpebrae superioris motoneurons during vertical lid and eye movements in the monkey. J. Neurophysiol. **68:** 233–243.
6. GORMEZANO, I., E.J. KEHOE & B.S. MARSHALL. 1983. Twenty years of classical conditioning research with the rabbit. Prog. Psychobiol. Physiol. Psychol. **10:** 197–275.
7. GRUART, A., P. BLÁZQUEZ & J.M. DELGADO-GARCÍA. 1995. Kinematics of spontaneous, reflex, and conditioned eyelid movements in the alert cat. J. Neurophysiol. **74:** 226–248.
8. GRUART, A., A. GUNKEL, W.F. NEISS, *et al.* 1996. Changes in eye blink responses following hypoglossal-facial anastomosis in the cat: evidence of adult mammal motoneuron unadaptability to new motor tasks. Neuroscience **73:** 233–247.
9. GRUART, A., B.G. SCHREURS, E. DOMÍNGUEZ DEL TORO & J.M. DELGADO-GARCÍA. 2000. Kinetic and frequency-domain properties of reflex and conditioned eyelid responses in the rabbit. J. Neurophysiol. **83:** 836–852.
10. GRUART, A., M. STREPPEL, O. GUNTINAS-LICHIUS, *et al.* 2003. Motoneuron adaptability to new motor tasks following two types of facial-facial anastomosis in cats. Brain **126:** 115–133.
11. KUGELBERG, E. 1952. Facial reflexes. Brain **75:** 385–396.
12. MAGARIÑOS-ASCONE, C., A. NUÑEZ & J.M. DELGADO-GARCÍA. 1999. Different discharge properties of rat facial nucleus motoneurons. Neuroscience **94:** 879–886.
13. MORCUENDE, S., J.M. DELGADO-GARCÍA & G. UGOLINI. 2002. Neuronal premotor networks involved in eyelid responses: retrograde transneuronal tracing with rabies virus from the orbicularis oculi muscle in the rat. J. Neurosci. **22:** 8808–8818.
14. TRIGO, J.A., A. GRUART & J.M. DELGADO-GARCÍA. 1999. Discharge profiles of abducens, accessory abducens, and orbicularis oculi motoneurons during reflex and conditioned blinks in alert cats. J. Neurophysiol. **81:** 1666–1684.
15. TRIGO, J.A., A. GRUART & J.M. DELGADO-GARCÍA. 1999. Role of proprioception in the control of lid position during reflex and conditioned blink responses in the alert behaving cat. Neuroscience **90:** 1515–1528.
16. THOMPSON, R.F. & D.J. KRUPA. 1994. Organization of memory traces in the mammalian brain. Annu. Rev. Neurosci. **17:** 519–549.
17. WOODY, C.D. 1986. Understanding the cellular basis of memory and learning. Annu. Rev. Psychol. **37:** 433–493.

Development of the Optokinetic Response in Macaques

A Comparison with Cat and Man

C. DISTLER AND K.-P. HOFFMANN

Allgemeine Zoologie & Neurobiologie, Ruhr-Universität Bochum, D-44780 Bochum, Germany

ABSTRACT: In macaque monkeys, an optokinetic response (OKR) can be elicited monocularly both in temporonasal and, albeit weaker, in nasotemporal direction very early after birth. The further maturation of equal strengths of OKR in both directions depends on stimulus velocity: at low-stimulus velocities (10–20°/s) symmetry is reached at 3–4 weeks of age, at higher-stimulus velocities (40–80°/s) it is reached only at 4–5 months of age. Retinal slip neurons in the NOT-DTN are direction selective for ipsiversive stimulus movement shortly after birth. Most of these neurons receive input from both eyes; many are dominated by the contralateral eye. Electrophysiological and neuroanatomical evidence suggests that the cortical input to the NOT-DTN starts to become functional by postnatal day 14, at the latest. Based on these behavioral and physiological data, as well as on comparison with data from kittens and human infants, we hypothesize that the very early monocularly elicited bidirectional optokinetic response is due to the direct retinal input from both eyes to the NOT-DTN. As the cortical projection matures, it gains more and more influence upon the response properties of retinal slip neurons in the NOT-DTN, and the retinal influence gradually decreases.

KEYWORDS: optokinetic nystagmus; monkey; cat; man; cortical input; NOT-DTN

NEURONAL SUBSTRATE OF THE OPTOKINETIC REFLEX

In all mammals investigated thus far, the neuronal substrate underlying the optokinetic response is very similar (FIG. 1). The visuomotor interface for this stabilizing reflex is formed by neurons in the nucleus of the optic tract and the dorsal terminal nucleus of the accessory optic system, which form a functional entity, the NOT-DTN. These retinal slip neurons in the NOT-DTN code for the retinal velocity error signal, i.e., the difference between stimulus and eye velocity. The retinal slip neurons are characterized by their strong selectivity for ipsiversive stimulus movement; i.e., neurons in the left NOT-DTN prefer movement to the left and vice versa. In non-

---

Address for correspondence: C. Distler, Allgemeine Zoologie & Neurobiologie, Ruhr-Universität Bochum, Postfach 102148, D-44780 Bochum, Germany. Voice: 49-234-3224365; fax: 49-234-3214185.

distler@neurobiologie.ruhr-uni-bochum.de

Ann. N.Y. Acad. Sci. 1004: 10–18 (2003). © 2003 New York Academy of Sciences.
doi: 10.1196/annals.1303.002

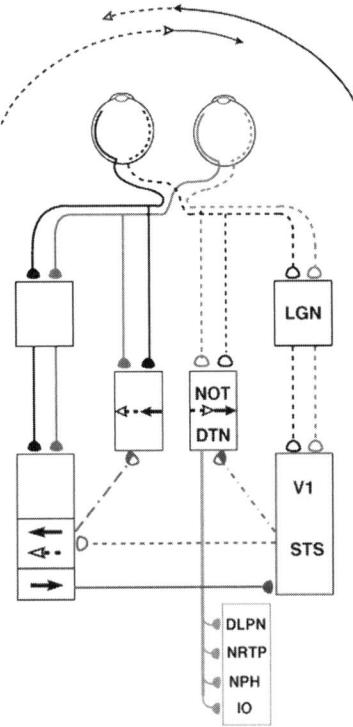

FIGURE 1. Depicted is the neuronal pathway underlying the horizontal optokinetic reaction in mammals, especially in primates. Projections of the left eye are shown in *black*; those of the right eye in *light grey*. Presumably binocular callosal and corticofugal projections are shown in *dark grey*. *Continuous lines* indicate the representation of the right, and *broken lines* the representation of the left visual hemifield. *Arrows* indicate the direction of stimulus movement represented in the various areas of the pathway. For further explanation see text. DLPN: dorsolateral pontine nucleus; IO: inferior olive; LGN: lateral geniculate nucleus; NOT-DTN: nucleus of the optic tract and dorsal terminal nucleus; NPH: nucleus prepositus hypoglossi; NRTP: nucleus reticularis tegmenti pontis; STS: motion sensitive areas in the superior temporal sulcus; V1: primary visual cortex.

primates, the NOT-DTN receives direct retinal input predominantly from the contralateral eye. Due to the distinct retinal decussation pattern, in primates this retinal projection is much more bilateral, the ipsilateral projection reaching about 40% of the contralateral projection.[1] This bilateral retinal projection is present at birth.[2] Experiments in wallabies strongly indicate that the retina imprints the behaviorally relevant direction selectivity on the retinal slip neurons: rotation of the anlage of the eye causes a corresponding rotation of the preferred direction of retinal slip neurons. Consequently, horizontal OKR can then best be elicited by the "old" temporonasal direction, i.e., downward stimulation after a 90° counterclockwise rotation of the anlage.[3] In all animals investigated (turtle,[4] rabbit,[5] cat[6]), it was shown that the retinal input to the accessory optic system is derived from direction-selective ganglion cells and, even though it has yet to be shown, it is assumed that this is also true for primates.

In addition to the retinal input, retinal slip neurons receive input from various cortical areas (e.g., rat,[7] guinea pig,[8] cat,[9] monkey[10,11]). In monkey, the main cortical input originates from area MT followed by V1, V2, and V3.[12] Lesion studies indicate that the cortical input to the NOT-DTN is responsible for the binocularity and response to high-stimulus velocities in retinal slip neurons at least in non-primates and for symmetry of OKR in both non-primates and primates (e.g., Refs. 13–17).

Retinal slip neurons project to the dorsal cap of the inferior olive, to the nucleus prepositus hypoglossi, the nucleus reticularis tegmenti pontis, and the dorsolateral pontine nucleus. The information is then transmitted to the vestibular nuclei and via climbing fibers to the flocculus of the cerebellum. Projections of the above structures to the nucleus oculomotorius, nucleus abducens, and nucleus trochlearis innervating the extraocular muscles close the loop.[18–21]

DEVELOPMENT OF THE OPTOKINETIC SYSTEM IN CAT

In cat, OKR can first be elicited reliably at around postnatal day P18 (FIG. 2). During monocular stimulation, only temporonasal stimulus movement is efficient in driving stabilizing eye movements. Only at about 4 weeks of age (P30) OKR can be elicited for the first time also in the nasotemporal direction. During further maturation, nasotemporal OKR becomes stronger so that in the adult cat OKR is almost symmetrical.[22,23]

Electrophysiological recordings in the NOT-DTN of kittens of various ages revealed that in 3-week-old animals retinal slip neurons are already direction selective for ipsiversive stimulus movement, but their stimulus-driven as well as their spontaneous activity is significantly lower than in adults. When tested at different stimulus velocities, the velocity-tuning curve is relatively flat with an optimum around 10°/s. Most important perhaps is the fact that almost all retinal slip neurons (83%) are ex-

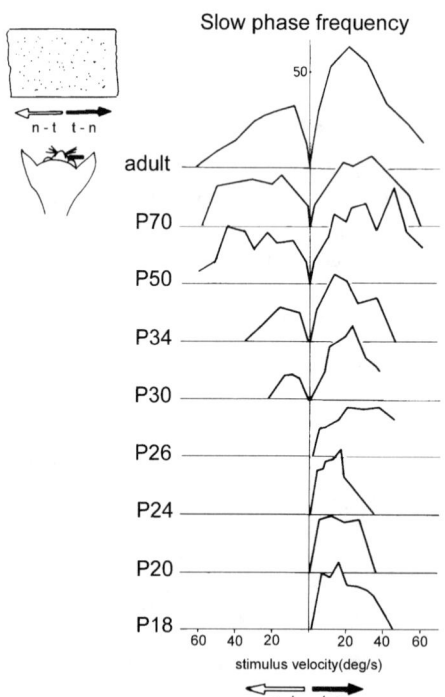

FIGURE 2. Slow-phase frequency of monocular horizontal OKR (*ordinate*) during stimulation in temporonasal (*right*) and nasotemporal (*left*) direction at various stimulus velocities (*abscissa*). The graphs represent the optokinetic reaction at various ages ranging from postnatal day 18 (P18) to adulthood (Meyer-Koll and Hoffmann, unpublished observation).

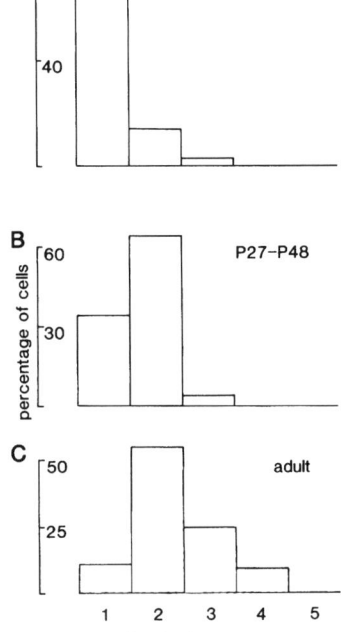

FIGURE 3. Ocular dominance distribution of retinal slip neurons in P18–P23 kittens (**A**), in P27–P48 kittens (**B**), and adult cats (**C**). *Ordinate*: percentage of cells; *abscissa*: ocular dominance groups. Neurons in group 1 (5) are exclusively activated by the contralateral (ipsilateral) eye; neurons in group 2 (4) are dominated by the contralateral (ipsilateral) eye but receive additional input from the ipsilateral (contralateral) eye; and neurons in group 3 are equally influenced by both eyes.

clusively activated by the contralateral eye; only few neurons receive an additional but weaker input from the ipsilateral eye (FIG. 3).

At 4 weeks of age, sudden changes occur in numerous response properties of retinal slip neurons. Stimulus-driven and spontaneous activity as well as neuronal modulation, that is, the difference in firing rate during stimulation in the preferred and non-preferred direction, become adultlike. The neurons begin to respond to a wider range of stimulus velocities, including also higher velocities. At this developmental stage, the influence of the ipsilateral eye suddenly increases significantly so that now most retinal slip cells receive an additional though weaker input from the ipsilateral eye, the proportion of neurons exclusively activated by the contralateral eye is reduced. During further maturation, the ipsilateral input becomes even stronger, and the velocity tuning of retinal slip neurons broadens toward lower-stimulus velocities.

In an attempt to reveal the cause for these developmental changes, we electrically stimulated the area 17/18 border representing the central visual field in order to elicit orthodromic potentials at retinal slip neurons in the NOT-DTN. At 3 weeks of age, no orthodromic potentials could be elicited at retinal slip cells, even though such responses could be elicited in the central visual field representation of the superior colliculus. At 4 weeks of age, orthodromic potentials could also be elicited at retinal slip cells confirming earlier results.[9] During further maturation, orthodromic latencies shorten significantly. These electrophysiological results are supported by anatomical studies in the literature, indicating that the cortico-subcortical projections to the superior colliculus (and the pretectum?) in neonatal cats consist mainly of fibers and growth cones but only few boutons. At around 4 weeks of age, this projection consists mainly of boutons, and only few growth cones are left (for references see Distler and Hoffmann[24]).

Thus, in the cat the beginning symmetry of monocular OKR can be linked to the increase of the input of the ipsilateral eye onto retinal slip cells. Because the direct retinal input in the cat comes almost exclusively from the contralateral retina, this ipsilateral influence most likely is transmitted via the cortical input becoming functional at the same developmental stage as the binocularity in the NOT-DTN, and bi-directionality of OKR is first observed.

DEVELOPMENT OF THE OPTOKINETIC SYSTEM IN MONKEY

In order to investigate whether a similar developmental sequence is present in monkeys, we undertook a longitudinal study using EOG recordings to measure horizontal optokinetic eye movements in infant monkeys ranging in age from 2 days to about 6 months.[25] In the 2-day-old animal, monocular OKR could already be elicited both in temporonasal and, albeit more weakly, in nasotemporal direction. During further maturation, especially the nasotemporal component grew stronger so that eventually symmetry was reached. The age when symmetry was reached depended on the velocity of the stimulus (FIG. 4). To quantify this we calculated an asymmetry

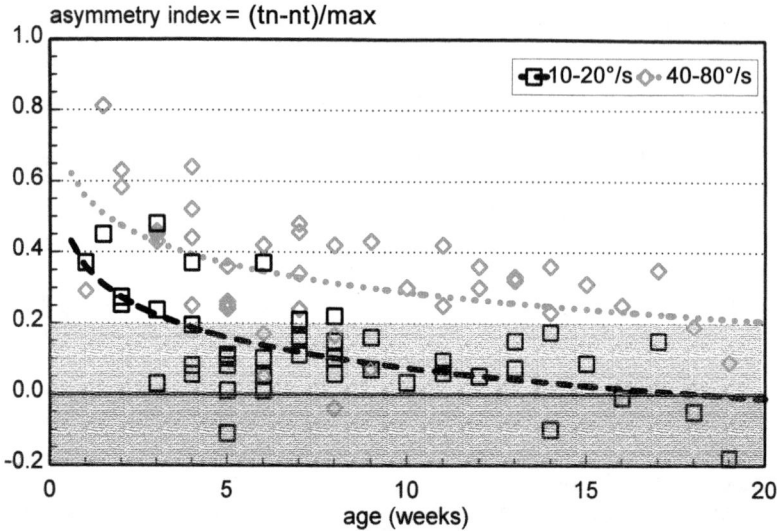

FIGURE 4. Development of monocular horizontal OKR in infant macaques. *Ordinate*: asymmetry index of OKR (difference between the OKR in temporonasal and nasotemporal direction, normalized to the larger of the two); *abscissa*: postnatal age in weeks. *Shaded area* indicates symmetry of OKR. *Black line and symbols*: asymmetry index during stimulation at low-stimulus velocities (10–20°/s); *grey line and symbols*: asymmetry index during stimulation at high-stimulus velocities (40–80°/s).

index, that is, the difference between the reaction to temporonasal and nasotemporal stimulation divided by the larger of the two. An index of ± 0.2 was regarded as symmetry. In FIGURE 3 we segregated the data according to stimulus velocity in a low-velocity (10–20°/s, black symbols and line) and in a high-velocity group (40–80°/s, grey symbols and line). For low-stimulus velocities, symmetry of monocular OKR was reached between 3 and 4 weeks of age; for higher-stimulus velocity OKR symmetry was reached only between 4 and 5 months of age. At the highest velocity tested (120°/s) symmetry was not reached during our period of observation.

Electrophysiological recordings were performed in a P9 and a P14 infant monkey under deep anesthesia and paralysis. As seen in kitten, retinal slip neurons were already strongly direction selective for ipsiversive stimulus movement in the P9 animal. When tested at various stimulus velocities, the resulting tuning curve was very narrow, with an optimal stimulus velocity around 10°/s. By contrast, in adults stimulus velocities yielding very good reactions range from about 1°/s to several 100°/s.[26] In contrast to cat, most retinal slip neurons in the NOT-DTN already received input from both eyes in the P9 animal (FIG. 5). In both infant monkeys, about half of the neurons received equal input from both eyes, and the other half was dominated by the contralateral eye. During further maturation, the influence of the ipsilateral eye strengthens so that in the adult the majority of neurons receives equal input from the contralateral and the ipsilateral eye.[26]

In order to find out whether the binocularity in the NOT-DTN can be attributed to the presence of a cortical input, we electrically stimulated the central visual field representation of V1. In the P9 infant, we were unable to elicit orthodromic responses in the NOT-DTN. In the P14 animal, however, orthodromic responses could be elicited after stimulation in V1 in the SC as well as in about 40% of the retinal slip

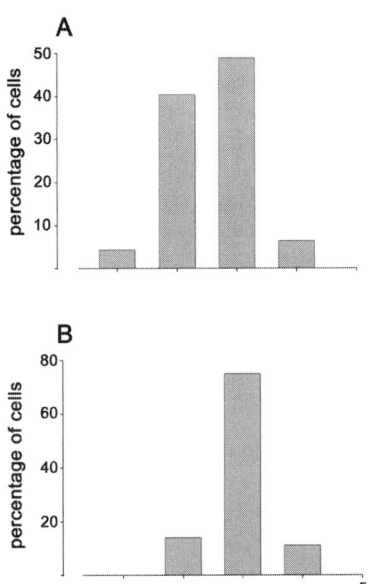

FIGURE 5. Ocular dominance distribution of retinal slip neurons in infant (P9 and P14, **A**) and adult (**B**) macaques. *Ordinate*: percentage of cells; *abscissa*: ocular dominance groups.

neurons tested. This is a considerably smaller proportion than in the adult where 97% of the neurons tested could be activated by electrical stimulation in V1.[27] In addition, the orthodromic latencies were significantly longer in the infant than in the adult.

Thus, bidirectionality of monocular OKR can be linked to binocularity in the NOT-DTN also in monkey. However, due to the bilateral direct retinal input to the NOT-DTN in primates, it is difficult to decide whether the binocularity present shortly after birth is caused by the bilateral retinal or by a cortical input. In the present study, we were unable to demonstrate a cortical input to the NOT-DTN prior to two weeks of age. Although we cannot completely rule out that a weak projection may be present even earlier, we propose that the early binocularity and the bidirectionality of monocular OKR at low-stimulus velocities shortly after birth is indeed mediated by the direct retinal input from both eyes to the NOT-DTN. As the cortical input starts to mature, it gradually dominates the NOT-DTN and the retinal input loses much of its influence so that after cortical lesion it is unable to maintain a normal performance of OKR.

COMPARISON TO MAN

Can these results be extrapolated to humans? Monocular OKR in human infants becomes symmetrical at around 4–5 months of age, thus closely resembling the monkey data.[28,29] Obviously, the optokinetic system seems to be an example where the "weeks to months" rule (one week in monkey development corresponds to one month in human) does not apply.

It can be safely assumed that the neuronal substrate for the optokinetic reflex in man corresponds to that found in other mammals. It has been shown that man has a complete accessory optic system,[30] and a nystagmogenic region, presumably the NOT-DTN, has been identified by electrical stimulation.[31] Further clues come from lesion studies in children.[32] Hemispherectomized infants younger than about 10 months of age perform bidirectional, albeit quite asymmetric, OKR during monocular and binocular viewing condition. However, toward the damaged side OKR gets weaker and finally is completely lost during further development, that is, the children are optokinetically blind during stimulation toward the lesioned hemisphere.

These data can be explained by assuming that in man as in other primate and subprimate species the retinal input to the NOT-DTN is responsible for imprinting the system and for the optokinetic response shortly after birth. As the cortex and/or the corticofugal projections during normal development become functional and mature, the system is taken over completely by the cortical input. The retina then loses its influence to a degree that it cannot drive the system at all, even if the cortical input is lost.

REFERENCES

1. TELKES, I., C. DISTLER & K.-P. HOFFMANN. 2000. Retinal ganglion cells projecting to the nucleus of the optic tract and the dorsal terminal nucleus of the accessory optic system in macaque monkeys. Eur. J. Neurosci. **12:** 2367–2375.
2. KOUROUYAN, H.D. & J.C. HORTON. 1997. Transneuronal retinal input to the primate Edinger-Westphal nucleus. J. Comp. Neurol. **381:** 68–80.

3. HOFFMANN, K.-P., C. DISTLER, R.F. MARK, et al. 1995. Neural and behavioral effects of early eye rotation on the optokinetic system in the wallaby, *Macropus eugenii*. J. Neurophysiol. **73:** 727–735.
4. ROSENBERG, A.F. & M. ARIEL. 1991. Electrophysiological evidence for a direct projection of direction selective retinal ganglion cells to the turtle's accessory optic system. J. Neurophysiol. **65:** 1022–1033.
5. OYSTER, C.W., E. TAKAHASHI & H. COLLEWIJN. 1972. Direction selective retinal ganglion cells and control of optokinetic nystagmus in the rabbit. Vision Res. **12:** 183–193.
6. HOFFMANN, K.-P. & J. STONE. 1985. Retinal input to the nucleus of the optic tract of the cat assessed by antidromic stimulation of ganglion cells. Exp. Brain Res. **59:** 395–403.
7. SCHMIDT, M., H.-Y. ZHANG & K.-P. HOFFMANN. 1993. OKN-related neurons in the rat nucleus of the optic tract and dorsal terminal nucleus of the accessory optic system receive a direct cortical input. J. Comp. Neurol. **330:** 147–157.
8. LUI, F., R.A. GIOLLI, R.H. BLANKS & E.M. TOM. 1994. Patterns of striate cortical projections to the pretectal complex in the guinea pig. J. Comp. Neurol. **344:** 598–609.
9. SCHOPPMANN, A. 1985. Functional and developmental analysis of visual corticopretectal pathway in the cat: a neuroanatomical and electrophysiological study. Exp. Brain Res. **60:** 363–374.
10. DISTLER, C. & K.-P. HOFFMANN. 2001. Cortical input to the nucleus of the optic tract and dorsal terminal nucleus (NOT-DTN) in macaques: a retrograde tracing study. Cereb. Cortex **11:** 572–580.
11. HOFFMANN, K.-P., F. BREMMER, A. THIELE & C. DISTLER. 2002. Directional asymmetry of neurons in cortical areas MT and MST projecting to the NOT-DTN in macaques. J. Neurophysiol. **87:** 2113–2123.
12. DISTLER, C., M.J. MUSTARI & K.-P. HOFFMANN. 2002. Cortical projections to the nucleus of the optic tract and dorsal terminal nucleus and to the dorsolateral pontine nucleus in macaques: a dual retrograde tracing study. J. Comp. Neurol. **444:** 144–158.
13. WOOD, C.C., P.D. SPEAR & J.J. BRAUN. 1973. Direction specific deficits in horizontal optokinetic nystagmus following removal of the visual cortex in the cat. Brain Res. **60:** 231–237.
14. LYNCH, J.C. & J.W. MCLAREN. 1983. Optokinetic nystagmus deficits following parieto-occipital cortex lesions in monkeys. Exp. Brain Res. **49:** 125–130.
15. GRASSE, K.L., M.S. CYNADER & R.M. DOUGLAS. 1984. Alterations in response properties in the lateral and dorsal terminal nucleus of the cat accessory optic system following visual cortex lesions. Exp. Brain Res. **55:** 69–80.
16. ZEE, D.S., R.J. TUSA, S.J. HERDMAN, et al. 1986. Effects of occipital lobectomy upon eye movements in primate. J. Neurophysiol. **58:** 883–907.
17. THURSTON, S.E., R.J. LEIGH, T. CRAWFORD, et al. 1988. Two distinct deficits of visual tracking caused by unilateral lesions of cerebral cortex in humans. Ann. Neurol. **23:** 266–273.
18. SIMPSON, J.I., R.A. GIOLLI & R.H.I. BLANKS. 1988. The pretectal nuclear complex and the accessory optic system. *In* Neuroanatomy of the Oculomotor System. J.A. Buettner-Ennever, Ed.: 335–364. Elsevier. Amsterdam.
19. AAS, J.-E. 1989. Subcortical projections to the pontine nuclei in the cat. J. Comp. Neurol. **282:** 331–354.
20. MUSTARI, M.J., A.F. FUCHS, C.R.S. KANEKO & F. R. ROBINSON. 1994. Anatomical connections of the primate pretectal nucleus of the optic tract. J. Comp. Neurol. **349:** 111–128.
21. BUETTNER-ENNEVER, J.A., B. COHEN, A.K.E. HORN & H. REISINE. 1996. Pretectal projections to the oculomotor complex of the monkey and their role in eye movements. J. Comp. Neurol. **366:** 348–359.
22. VAN HOF–VAN DUIN, J. 1978. Direction preference of optokinetic responses in monocularly tested normal kittens and light deprived cats. Arch. Ital. Biol. **116:** 471–477.
23. MALACH, R., N. STRONG & R.C. VAN SLUYTERS. 1981. Analysis of monocular optokinetic nystagmus in normal and visually deprived kittens. Brain Res. **210:** 367–372.

24. DISTLER, C. & K.-P. HOFFMANN. 1993. Visual receptive field properties in kitten pretectal nucleus of the optic tract and dorsal terminal nucleus of the accessory optic tract. J. Neurophysiol. **70:** 814–827.
25. DISTLER, C., F. VITAL-DURAND, R. KORTE, et al. 1999. Development of the optokinetic system in macaque monkeys. Vision Res. **39:** 3909–3919.
26. HOFFMANN, K.-P. & C. DISTLER. 1989. Quantitative analysis of visual receptive fields of neurons of the nucleus of the optic tract and the dorsal terminal nucleus of the accessory optic tract in macaque monkeys. J. Neurophysiol. **62:** 416–428.
27. HOFFMANN, K.-P., C. DISTLER & R. ERICKSON. 1991. Functional projections from striate cortex and superior temporal sulcus to the nucleus of the optic tract (NOT) and dorsal terminal nucleus of the accessory optic tract (DTN) of macaque monkeys. J. Comp. Neurol. **313:** 707–724.
28. NAEGELE, J.R. & R. HELD. 1982. The postnatal development of monocular optokinetic nystagmus in infants. Vision Res. **22:** 341–346.
29. ROY, M.-S., P. LACHAPELLE & F. LEPORÉ. 1989. Maturation of the optokinetic nystagmus as a function of the speed of stimulation in fullterm and preterm infants. Clin. Vis. Sci. **4:** 357–366.
30. FREDERICKS, C.A., R.A. GIOLLI, R.H.I. BLANKS & A.A. SADUM. 1988. The human accessory optic system. Brain Res. **454:** 116–122.
31. TAYLOR, R.B., R.A. WENNBERG, A.M. LOZANO & J.A. SHARPE. 2000. Central nystagmus induced by deep-brain stimulation for epilepsy. Epilepsia **41:** 1637–1641.
32. MORRONE, M.C., J. ATKINSON, G. CIONI, et al. 1999. Developmental changes in optokinetic mechanisms in the absence of unilateral cortical control. Neuroreport **10:** 2723–2729.

GABAergic Neurons in the Rostral Mesencephalon of the Macaque Monkey That Control Vertical Eye Movements

ANJA K.E. HORN,[a] CHRISTOPH HELMCHEN,[b] AND PETRA WAHLE[c]

[a]*Institute of Anatomy, Ludwig-Maximilians-University of Munich, D-80336 Munich, Germany*

[b]*Department of Neurology, University of Lübeck, Ratzeburger Allee 160, 23538 Lübeck, Germany*

[c]*AG Entwicklungsneurobiologie, Ruhr-Universität, Universitätsstr. 150, 44780 Bochum, Germany*

ABSTRACT: The mesencephalic reticular formation is important for the generation of vertical eye movements, but up until now the location of inhibitory premotor neurons is not known in primates. With tract-tracer methods combined with immunocytochemistry or *in situ* hybridization, we investigated the location of GABAergic premotor neurons in the rostral interstitial nucleus of the medial longitudinal fascicle (riMLF) and interstitial nucleus of Cajal (iC) in macaque monkeys. In the present work, only the premotor pathways of the downward pulling eye muscles, superior oblique (SO) and inferior rectus (IR), were studied. We found that very few, small GABAergic neurons are present in the riMLF, and none of them was found to project to the oculomotor nuclei, suggesting the presence of exclusively excitatory projections from the riMLF to the oculomotor neurons. However, in the iC, medium-sized and large GABAergic neurons were identified projecting contralaterally to the SO and IR motoneurons, and presumably the iC of the other side. These commissural GABAergic projections are well suited to inhibit the SO and IR motoneurons and possibly premotor down–burst-tonic neurons during upward eye movements.

KEYWORDS: interstitial nucleus of Cajal; rostral interstitial nucleus of the medial longitudinal fascicle; saccades

INTRODUCTION

In the primate, the interstitial nucleus of Cajal (iC) and the rostral interstitial nucleus of the medial longitudinal fascicle (riMLF) are essential for the generation of vertical eye movements.[1,2] Both nuclei contain premotor neurons that project exclusively to the motoneurons of vertical pulling eye muscles.[3–5] The riMLF and iC lie adjacent to each other, but can be easily delineated with immunostaining for the calcium-binding protein parvalbumin (PV).[1,5] Whereas two groups of premotor burst neurons, excitatory and inhibitory, were identified within the paramedian pontine reticular formation for the horizontal eye movement system,[6,7] the presence of premotor inhibitory neurons for vertical eye movements is unclear. GABAergic premotor neurons were reported within the riMLF in the cat,[8] but were not seen in the monkey with GABA-immunocytochemistry.[9] In the present work, we studied the presence of GABAergic neurons within the riMLF and iC of the monkey with immunocytochemistry, using GABA and glutamate decarboxylase (GAD) antibodies and *in situ* hybridization to visualize the mRNA encoding GAD.[10] The boundaries of the riMLF and iC were outlined by PV-immunoflourescence in the same sections.[5] In two monkeys the vertical premotor neurons mediating downward eye movements were also retrogradely labeled either by a tracer injection into the rostral oculomotor nucleus containing the motoneurons of the inferior rectus muscle (IR),[11] or into the trochlear nucleus containing superior oblique (SO) motoneurons.

MATERIALS AND METHODS

GABA- and GAD-Immunocytochemistry. Four macaque monkeys were killed with an overdose of pentobarbital (96 mg/kg) and transcardially perfused with saline (37°C) followed by either 1% paraformaldehyde (PFA)/2.5% glutaraldehyde (GA) or 4% PFA/0.3% GA in 0.1 M phosphate buffer (PB), pH 7.4 for GABA-immunohistochemistry or 4% PFA in 0.1 M PB for GAD-immunohistochemistry. The brains were blocked and equilibrated in increasing concentrations of sucrose in 0.1 M PB for freeze cutting. Free-floating transverse sections (40 µm) were processed for immunocytochemical detection of GABA (Incstar, Hamburg; 1:4000) or GAD (W.H. Oertel, Marburg; 1:2000), as described earlier.[12] One animal received a prior wheatgerm agglutinin horseradish peroxidase (WGA-HRP) injection (5% in saline) into the left trochlear nucleus (IV). The tracer was detected by the tetramethyl-benzidine method and stabilized with a DAB-Co reaction before being processed for the immunocytochemical detection of GAD.[13]

In situ hybridization for GAD-mRNA. Two monkeys were killed with an overdose of pentobarbital and transcardially perfused with saline followed by 4% PFA. One animal had received a prior tetramethylrhodamine-dextran injection (TMR-DA; Molecular Probes, 3000 MW; 0.5 µl; 15% in acetate buffer, pH 3) into the rostral oculomotor nucleus (III) and survived for 4 days.[14] The brains were blocked and equilibrated in increasing concentrations of RNAse-free sucrose, then cut transversely under sterile conditions using a cryostat and collected in $2 \times$ SSC (0.3M NaCl and 0.03M sodium citrate). Hybridization with an antisense digoxigenin-UTP–labeled GAD-cRNA probe and staining was carried out as described earlier.[12] Since the fluorescence signal of the TMR-DA was not detectable after the *in situ* hybridization, the sections were treated for the immunocytochemical detection of TMR-DA using rabbit anti-TMR-DA (Molecular Probes; 1:1000) for 3 days at 4°C followed by Cy3-conjugated goat anti-rabbit (Dianova, 20 µg/ml) for 2 hours.[14] Some sections were additionally reacted for the detection of PV using mouse anti-PV (Sigma; 1:250) and Cy2-tagged goat anti-mouse (Dianova, 20 µg/ml) for 2 h in order to delineate the riMLF and iC.[5] The slides were examined with a fluorescence microscope (Leica DMRB) equipped with appropriate filters for red fluorescence Cy3 (N2.1) and green fluorescence Cy2 (13). The images were digitalized with a 3-CCD videocamera (Hamamatsu; C5810) mounted on the microscope and captured on a computer with Adobe Photoshop 5.0 software and converted into black and white. The sharpness and contrast were adjusted to reflect the appearance of the labeling seen through the microscope. The pictures were arranged and labeled with drawing software (CorelDRAW 11.0; Corel).

RESULTS

Immunocytochemistry revealed very few small GABA- or GAD-positive neurons within the riMLF (FIG. 1A, arrow, inset). In the iC, similarly few GABA-positive neurons were present, in contrast to the adjacent nucleus of Bechterew (nB) that contains numerous GABA-immunoreactive neurons (FIG. 1B, arrow, inset). With *in situ* hybridization, a similar group of small-sized GAD-mRNA–expressing neurons was detected in the riMLF (FIG.1C). However, in contrast to the GABA-immunostaining, approximately 40% of the neurons in the iC express high levels of GAD-mRNA or GAD-immunoreactivity, whereby a population of smaller neurons in the dorsal iC could be distinguished from a group of more ventral, medium-sized neurons (FIGS. 1D and 3B). The PV-immunofluorescence in the same sections helped to outline exactly the riMLF and iC (FIG. 1C–F).

Double Labeling. The TMR-DA injection site in the one animal involved the dorsal part of the rostral oculomotor nucleus (III) containing the IR motoneurons,[11] but extended into the ipsilateral iC at its caudal part as well (FIG. 2A). Retrogradely labeled neurons were present predominantly in the ipsilateral riMLF and in the iC of both sides, but only the contralateral iC was analyzed. In addition, the medial part of the ipsilateral riMLF showed strong anterograde labeling, whereas less terminal labeling was seen in the contralateral riMLF. Inspection at high-power magnification revealed that none of the tracer-labeled neurons in the riMLF contain GAD-mRNA (FIG. 2B, C) but at least 20% of the GAD-mRNA–expressing neurons in the contralateral iC, involving only medium-sized neurons, were retrogradely labeled with TMR-DA (FIG. 2D, E). The small WGA-HRP injection site in the other animal was centered on the left trochlear nucleus (IV), with some involvement of the ventrally located medial longitudinal fascicle (MLF), which did not result in retrograde tracing via uptake by the MLF fibers as judged from the labeling pattern in the abducens and vestibular nuclei. The III and the contralateral IV were spared from the tracer (FIG. 3A). Retrogradely labeled neurons were found in the ipsilateral riMLF, and in the iC of both sides. As reported earlier, the populations of labeled premotor neurons in both iC differed: in the contralateral iC mainly medium-sized and large cells were labeled compared with the smaller-sized labeled cells in the ipsilateral iC[5] (FIG. 3C, D). The careful analysis of double-labeled sections at high-power magnification revealed that virtual all retrogradely labeled medium-sized neurons in the contralateral iC are GAD-immunoreactive (FIG. 3F), whereas the smaller neurons in the ipsilateral iC lack GAD-immunoreactivity (FIG. 3E). In addition, both sets of premotor neurons receive afferents from GAD-positive terminals (FIG. 3E, F, arrows).

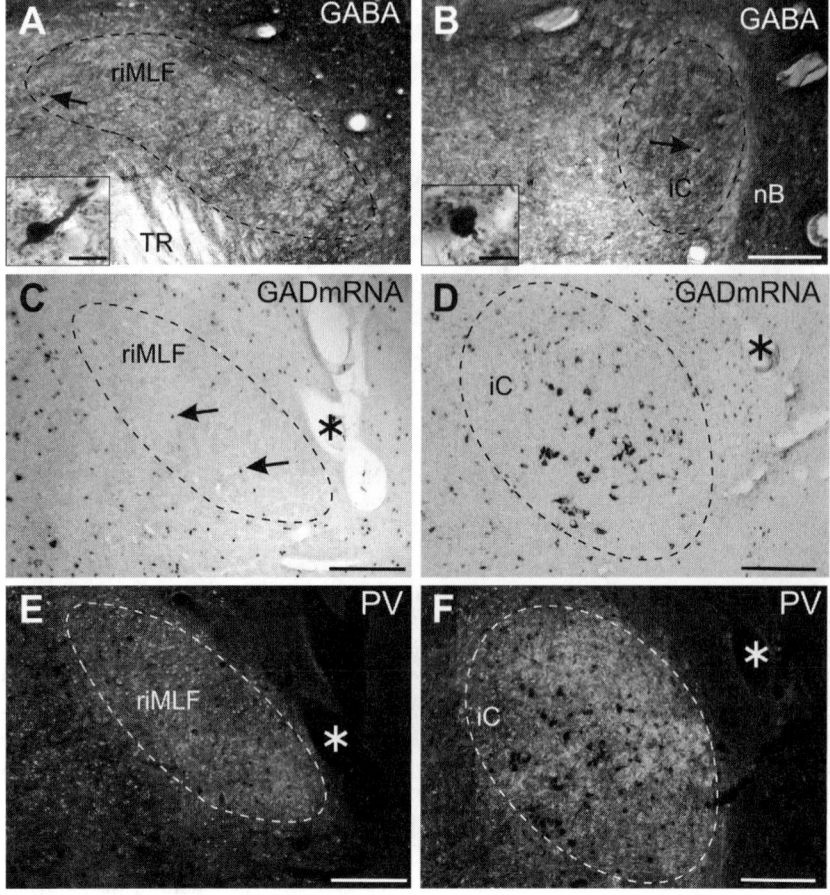

FIGURE 1. Transverse sections through the monkey rostral mesencephalon showing the rostral interstitial nucleus of the medial longitudinal fascicle (riMLF, *dashed lines*) in **A, C, E,** and the interstitial nucleus of Cajal (iC, *dashed lines*) in **B, D, F,** stained for different markers. (**A, B**) Only few small GABA-immunoreactive cells are present in riMLF and iC (*arrows and insets; scale bar* = 10 µm); (**C, D**) GAD-mRNA detection in the riMLF (*arrows*) and iC, which are outlined by parvalbumin (PV)-immunoflourescence in the same sections (**E, F**). The blood vessel (*asterisk*) serves as a guide in corresponding photographs of the same sections. Note that the iC contains numerous strongly GAD-mRNA–expressing neurons, smaller neurons dorsally and medium-sized neurons more ventrally (**D**). *Scale bar* = 250 µm in **A–F**.

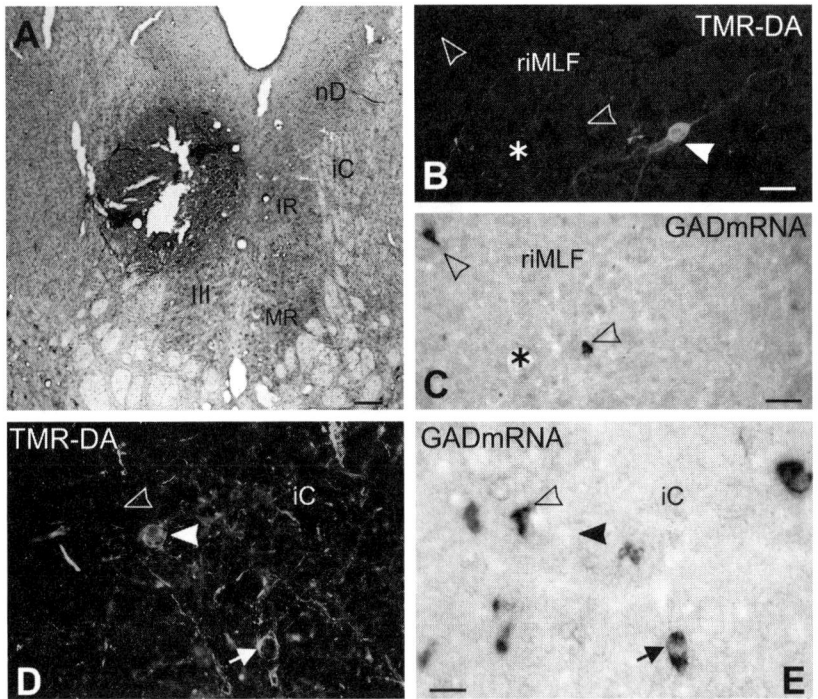

FIGURE 2. Transverse brainstem sections of a monkey that had received an injection of tetramethyl-rhodamine dextran (TMR-DA) into the dorsal oculomotor nucleus (III) and the caudal iC (**A**). (**B, C**) Retrogradely labeled neurons in the riMLF (**B,** *white, closed arrowhead*) seen at fluorescent illumination do not contain GAD-mRNA (**C,** *open arrowheads*). (**D, E**) Numerous medium-sized retrogradely labeled neurons in the contralateral iC contain GAD-mRNA (*arrow* in **D** and **E**), but not all tracer-labeled neurons express GAD mRNA and vice versa (**D, E,** *open and solid arrowheads*). Scale bar = 0.5 mm (**A**); 50 μm (**B–E**).

DISCUSSION

GABAergic Neurons in the riMLF

With different histochemical methods, we showed that in the monkey only few, small GABAergic neurons are present in the riMLF, whereas the iC contains numerous neurons that contain the messenger RNA of the GABA-synthesizing enzyme glutamate decarboxylase (GAD) and the protein itself, indicating a considerable population of GABAergic neurons. GABA-antibodies have failed to label larger GABAergic projection neurons in other studies,[15] presumably due to the fact that their cell bodies may not accumulate appreciable concentrations of GABA detect-

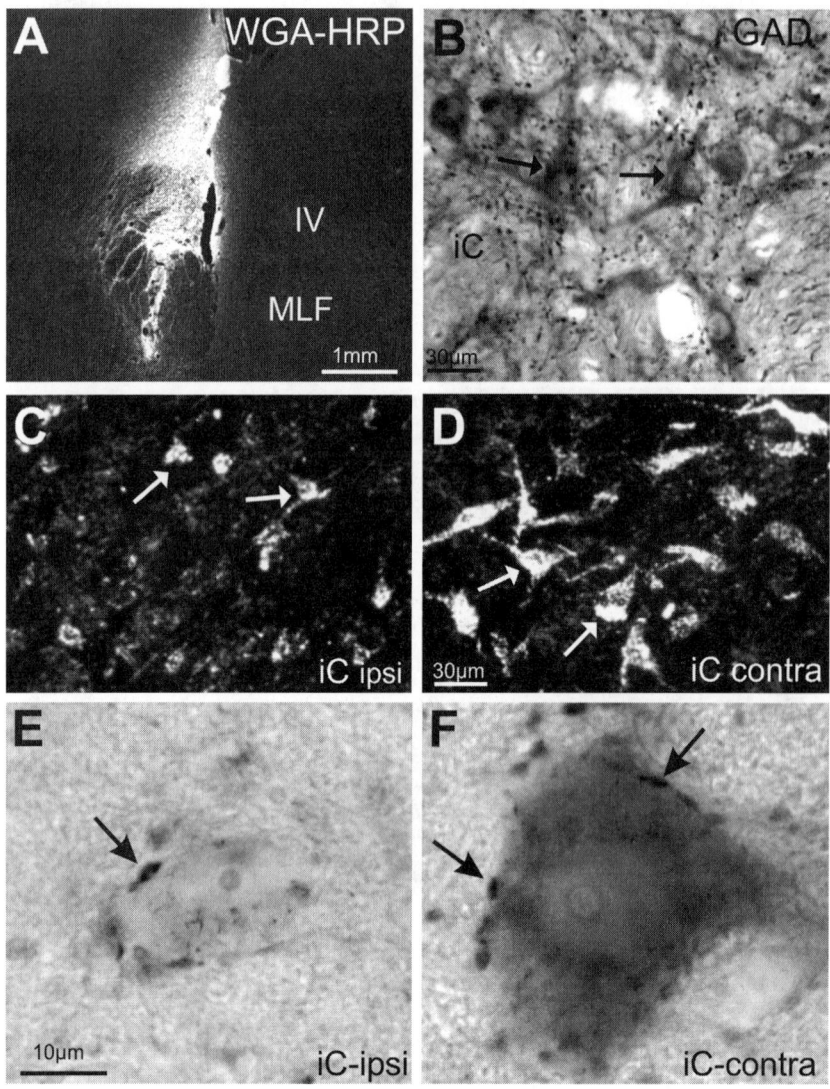

FIGURE 3. Dark- and brightfield photographs of transverse brainstem sections of a monkey that had received a WGA-HRP injection into the left trochlear nucleus (**A**; IV); (**B**) a similar medium-sized neuron population compared with contralateral projection neurons in the iC is GAD-immunoreactive (*arrows*; compare **B** and **D**); (**C, D**) retrogradely labeled neurons in the ipsilateral iC (**C**, *arrows*) are smaller and not GAD-immunoreactive (**E**), compared to the larger retrogradely labeled neurons in the contralateral iC (**D**, *arrows*) that contain GAD (**F**). Numerous GAD-positive punctuate profiles are present in the iC (**B**), which partly contact both neuron populations (**E, F**, *arrows*). *Scale bars* = 1 mm (**A**); 30 μm (**B–D**); 10 μm (**E, F**).

able by GABA-antibodies. This is particularly true in studies carried out without prior colchicine treatment.[16] We believe this is why GABA-immunoreactive neurons were not detected in the monkey iC.[9] The presence of GABAergic premotor neurons in the riMLF of the cat may reflect another species difference.[8] It is possible that the riMLF in monkey is highly specialized for eye movements only, whereas the riMLF in cat is involved in various other functions, such as head movements[17] or coordination of eyelid movements,[18] which is mediated by a separate nucleus in monkey.[19]

GABAergic Projections from the iC to the Vertical Eye Muscle Motoneurons

The retrograde labeling of neurons in the riMLF and bilateral iC are in accordance with earlier descriptions of monosynaptic inputs from riMLF and iC to the motoneurons of vertical pulling extraocular muscles in III and IV.[5,20] The present work confirms earlier observations that extraocular motoneurons are controlled by different populations of premotor neurons in the iC: from medium-sized and large neurons of the contralateral iC and from smaller neurons of the ipsilateral iC.[5] These observations are extended by our present demonstration that the contralateral iC projection to SO motoneurons in IV originates from GABAergic neurons, whereas the ipsilateral IV receives afferents from smaller non-GABAergic neurons in the iC, therefore presumably excitatory neurons, because glycinergic neurons are not present in the iC (Horn, personal observations) (FIG. 4). Electrical stimulation experiments in the iC region of cats were the first to demonstrate excitatory and inhibitory projections to IV,[21] although the authors could not exclude that traversing fibers had been stimulated. Because in the case of TMR-DA the iC was partly included in the tracer injection site, it cannot be ruled out that the GABAergic projection from the contralateral iC arises, at least additionally, from the ipsilateral iC[22]; hence this provides evidence for a GABAergic commissural iC projection. In a simplified diagram (FIG. 4), the new findings are added to the current scheme of proposed connections for the generation of vertical saccades by dashed lines[23]: premotor down-burst neurons in the riMLF monosynaptically activate the IR and SO motoneurons in the ipsilateral III and IV and, presumably via collaterals, premotor down–burst-tonic neurons in the ipsilateral iC,[4] both by excitatory projections, since no GABAergic or glycinergic premotor neurons are present in the riMLF of the monkey.[12] During upward saccades the IR and SO motoneurons would be inhibited by commissural fibers from our larger GABAergic premotor up-neurons in the contralateral iC, which in turn would be driven by premotor up-burst neurons in the contralateral riMLF. Our GABAergic commissural projection from presumably up–burst-tonic neurons in the case of WGA-HRP could also inhibit contralateral iC neurons with downward directions (FIG. 4, dashed line), as suggested earlier.[24,25] Based on our findings of GABAergic and non-GABAergic commissural iC neurons in the case of TMR-DA tracer, we cannot rule out that additional commissural projection neurons, excitatory and inhibitory, exist that do not project to oculomotor neurons, but which could activate or turn off their contralateral counterparts (FIG. 4, solid commissural line). Nonpremotor saccade-related up- and down-burst neurons have been identified in the iC.[3,4,26] They were proposed to be inhibitory, presumably forming a local feedback loop according to the eye displacement model,[3,4] and could therefore be part of our GABAergic neurons in iC that were not retrogradely labeled from motoneurons. Theoretically, these neurons could be the source of the anterograde labeling in

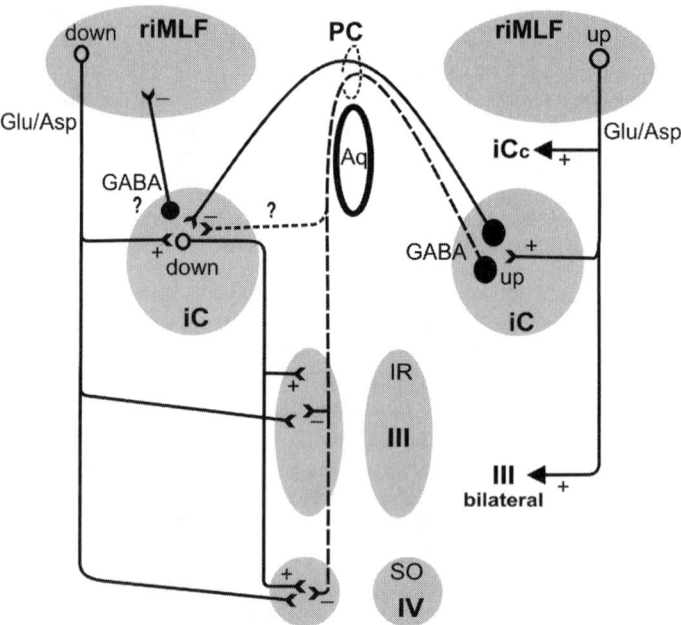

FIGURE 4. Simplified diagram summarizing the pathways for the generation of vertical saccades including the new findings of this study (*dashed lines*); "down"-neurons are shown on the *left side*, "up"-neurons on the *right side*. This study shows that the riMLF of the monkey does not contain inhibitory GABAergic premotor neurons, and therefore provides only excitatory projections to IR and SO motoneurons in the oculomotor (III) and trochlear nucleus (IV), and presumably to premotor down-burst–tonic neurons in the iC, which themselves excite (*open circle*) SO motoneurons of the same side. Further, the SO and IR motoneurons receive an inhibitory GABAergic input from the contralateral iC (*filled circle*). These GABAergic neurons could be activated by premotor up-burst neurons in the riMLF, thereby inhibiting the SO and IR motoneurons during upward saccades. From this study it is not clear whether the GABAergic projection via the posterior commissure (PC) is mediated via collaterals from premotor burst-tonic neurons in the contralateral iC (*question mark*) or by separate projections. It is possible that GABAergic neurons in the iC may include nonpremotor saccade-related up- and down-burst neurons in the iC (*question mark, left side*). Down-burst neurons were shown to project back to the ipsilateral riMLF, and there is some evidence that saccade-related up-burst neurons project to the contralateral iC. In addition, a parallel excitatory projection between both iC must be anticipated (not shown).

the riMLF. Although premotor up- and down-burst and burst-tonic neurons are intermingled in the riMLF and iC, differences are known for both systems, intracellular staining of identified burst neurons revealed that up-burst neurons in one riMLF appear to control the iC and oculomotor neurons of both sides, whereas down-burst neurons activate the iC and motoneurons only of the ipsilateral side[4,23] (FIG. 4). Here, we have only studied the premotor connections of downward-moving eye muscles; how far a mirror-like organization of premotor inhibitory and excitatory connections from the iC to the motoneurons of the upward-moving superior rectus and inferior oblique muscle can be anticipated remains unclear.

ACKNOWLEDGMENTS

We thank Dr. W.H. Oertel (University Hospital of Marburg) for the generous supply of the GAD antibody. This work was supported by the German Research Council (SFB 462, B3, B1) and the German-Israeli Foundation (Grant No. 1-0574-037.01/98).

REFERENCES

1. FUKUSHIMA, K. 1991. The interstitial nucleus of Cajal in the midbrain reticular formation and vertical eye movement. Neurosci. Res. **10:** 159–187.
2. BÜTTNER, U., J.A. BÜTTNER-ENNEVER & V. HENN. 1977. Vertical eye movement related activity in the rostral mesencephalic reticular formation of the alert monkey. Brain Res. **130:** 239–252.
3. MOSCHOVAKIS, A.K., C.A. SCUDDER & S.M. HIGHSTEIN. 1991. The structure of the primate oculomotor burst generator. I. Medium-lead burst neurons with upward on-directions. J. Neurophysiol. **65:** 203–217.
4. MOSCHOVAKIS, A.K., C.A. SCUDDER, S.M. HIGHSTEIN & J.D. WARREN. 1991. The structure of the primate oculomotor burst generator. II. Medium-lead neurons with downward on-directions. J. Neurophysiol. **65:** 218–229.
5. HORN, A.K.E. & J.A. BÜTTNER-ENNEVER. 1998. Premotor neurons for vertical eye-movements in the rostral mesencephalon of monkey and man: the histological identification by parvalbumin immunostaining. J. Comp. Neurol. **392:** 413–427.
6. STRASSMAN, A., S.M. HIGHSTEIN & R.A. MCCREA. 1986. Anatomy and physiology of saccadic burst neurons in the alert squirrel monkey. I. Excitatory burst neurons. J. Comp. Neurol. **249:** 337–357.
7. STRASSMAN, A., S.M. HIGHSTEIN & R.A. MCCREA. 1986. Anatomy and physiology of saccadic burst neurons in the alert squirrel monkey. II. Inhibitory burst neurons. J. Comp. Neurol. **249:** 358–380.
8. SPENCER, R.F. & S.F. WANG. 1996. Immunohistochemical localization of neurotransmitters utilized by neurons in the rostral interstitial nucleus of the medial longitudinal fasciculus (riMLF) that project to the oculomotor and trochlear nuclei in the cat. J. Comp. Neurol. **366:** 134–148.
9. CARPENTER, M.B., A.B. PERIERA & N. GUHA. 1992. Immunocytochemistry of oculomotor afferents in the squirrel monkey (*Saimiri sciureus*) J. Hirnforsch. **33:** 151–167.
10. WAHLE, P. & S. BECKH. 1992. A method of in situ hybridization combined with immunocytochemistry, histochemistry and tract tracing to characterize the mRNA expressing cell types in heterogeneous neuronal populations. J. Neurosci. Methods **41:** 153–166.
11. EVINGER, C. 1988. Extraocular motor nuclei: location, morphology and afferents. Rev. Oculomot. Res. **2:** 81–117.
12. HORN, A.K.E., J.A. BÜTTNER-ENNEVER, P. WAHLE & I. REICHENBERGER. 1994. Neurotransmitter profile of saccadic omnipause neurons in nucleus raphe interpositus. J. Neurosci. **14:** 2032–2046.
13. HORN, A.K.E. & K.P. HOFFMANN. 1987. Combined GABA-immunocytochemistry and TMB-HRP histochemistry of pretectal nuclei projecting to the inferior olive in rats, cats and monkeys. Brain Res. **409:** 133–138.
14. KANEKO, T., K. SAEKI, T. LEE & N. MIZUNO. 1996. Improved retrograde transport and subsequent visualization of tetramethylrhodamine (TMR)-dextran amine by means of an acidic injection vehicle and antibodies against TMR. J. Neurosci. Methods **65:** 157–165.
15. WAHLE, P., V. STUPHORN, M. SCHMIDT & K.P. HOFFMANN. 1994. LGN-projecting neurons of the cats pretectum express glutamic acid decarboxylase messenger RNA. Eur. J. Neurosci. **6:** 454–460.
16. STORM-MATHISEN, J. & O.P. OTTERSEN. 1986. Antibodies against amino acid neurotransmitters. *In* Neurohistochemistry: Modern Methods and Applications. P. Panula, H. Päivärinta & S. Soinila, Eds.: 107–136. Alan R. Liss, Inc. New York.

17. ISA, T. & S. SASAKI. 2002. Brainstem control of head movments during orienting; organization of the premotor circuits. Prog. Neurobiol. **66:** 205–241.
18. CHEN, B. & P.J. MAY. 2002. Premotor circuits controlling eyelid movements in conjunction with vertical saccades in the cat: I. The rostral interstitial nucleus of the medial longitudinal fasciculus. J. Comp. Neurol. **450:** 183–202.
19. HORN, A.K.E., J.A. BÜTTNER-ENNEVER, M. GAYDE & A. MESSOUDI. 2000. Neuroanatomical identification of mesencephalic premotor neurons coordinating eyelid with upgaze in the monkey and man. J. Comp. Neurol. **420:** 19–34.
20. MOSCHOVAKIS, A.K., C.A. SCUDDER & S.M. HIGHSTEIN. 1996. The microscopic anatomy and physiology of the mammalian saccadic system. Prog. Neurobiol. **50:** 133.
21. SCHWINDT, P.C., W. PRECHT & A. RICHTER. 1974. Monosynaptic excitatory and inhibitory pathways from medial midbrain nuclei to trochlear motoneurons. Exp. Brain Res. **20:** 223–238.
22. KOKKOROYANNIS, T., C.A. SCUDDER, C.D. BALABAN & S.M. HIGHSTEIN. 1996. Anatomy and physiology of the primate interstitial nucleus of Cajal. I. Efferent projections. J. Neurophysiol. **75:** 725–739.
23. BHIDAYASIRI, R., G.T. PLANT & R.H. LEIGH. 2000. A hypothetical scheme for the brainstem control of vertical gaze. Neurology **54:** 1985–1993.
24. FUKUSHIMA, K. & C.R. KANEKO. 1995. Vestibular integrators in the oculomotor system. Neurosci. Res. **22:** 249–258.
25. CHIMOTO, S., Y. IWAMOTO & K. YOSHIDA. 1999. Projections and firing properties of down eye-movement neurons in the interstitial nucleus of Cajal in the cat. J. Neurophysiol. **81:** 1199–1211.
26. HELMCHEN, C., H. RAMBOLD & U. BÜTTNER. 1996. Saccade-related burst neurons with torsional and vertical on-directions in the interstitial nucleus of Cajal of the alert monkey. Exp. Brain Res. **112:** 63–78.

Shared Brainstem Pathways for Saccades and Smooth-Pursuit Eye Movements

EDWARD L. KELLER[a] AND MARCUS MISSAL[a,b]

[a]*The Smith-Kettlewell Eye Research Institute, 2318 Fillmore Street, San Francisco, California 94115, USA*

[b]*Laboratoire de Neurophysiologie, Université Catholique de Louvain, Avenue Hippocrate 54 49, 1200 Brussels, Belgium*

ABSTRACT: A long-standing belief holds that the saccadic and smooth-pursuit eye movement systems are composed of largely separate premotor circuits, at least in the brainstem. One crucial prediction predicated on this belief is that the tonic discharge of omnipause neurons (OPNs), which are thought to be part of only the saccadic system, should not be modulated during pursuit eye movements. This report shows that the discharge of OPNs, in contradiction, is modulated downward during pursuit movements. In contrast to their behavior during saccades, where they pause completely for the duration of the movement, the downward modulation during pursuit did not totally silence OPNs. The depth of the downward modulation was correlated with the speed of the ongoing pursuit movement. Another type of cell, which we have named saccade/pursuit neurons, was recorded in the paramedian pontine reticular formation near the location of OPNs. This subpopulation of burst cells discharged a cascade of spikes for saccades in a preferred direction. They also displayed a lower-frequency sustained discharge of spikes for the duration of pursuit in the same preferred direction. These data suggest a new type of combined model for the organization of the brainstem saccade/pursuit system. In this new combined model, the OPNs form a common inhibitory mechanism for both types of movements, and the saccade/pursuit neurons participate in the eye-velocity modulation of OPN discharge or membrane polarization during either type of movement.

KEYWORDS: saccades; smooth pursuit; shared pathways; omnipause neurons; burst neurons

INTRODUCTION

The premotor pathways subserving saccades and smooth-pursuit eye movements are usually thought to be largely separate (see Refs. 1 and 2 for reviews). FIGURE 1 summarizes these hypothesized separate brainstem saccade and pursuit pathways for horizontal movements. For the saccadic network shown in the upper portion of the schematic, each of the types of neurons are found in or near the paramedian pontine

Address for correspondence: Edward L. Keller, Ph.D., Smith-Kettlewell Eye Research Institute, 2318 Fillmore Street, San Francisco, CA 94115. Voice: 415-345-2102; fax: 415-345-8455.
elk@ski.org

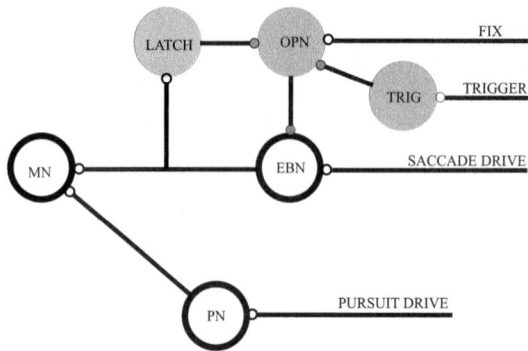

FIGURE 1. Schematic representation of separate brainstem premotor, saccade-generating (*upper*) and smooth-pursuit (*lower*) circuits. Excitatory neurons and synapses are shown with open circles while inhibitory neurons and synapses are shown with shaded circles. See text for an explanation of the circuits' operation.

reticular formation (PPRF). Among the burst neurons, only the excitatory burst neurons (EBNs) are shown. The inhibitory burst neurons, which also directly contact motoneurons (MNs), are left out for simplicity. The inhibitory gate for saccades formed by the omnipause neurons (OPNs) controls the timing of discharge in EBNs. The three saccadic control signals that input on the right come most importantly from the superior colliculus (SC), but other sources, for example, from the cerebellum are also significant. The saccadic drive signal excites EBNs and may be present before saccades are initiated. Before this drive can be translated into activity in MNs, the inhibitory gate from OPNs must be lifted. An inhibitory trigger signal into OPNs that briefly turns off OPNs and allows the EBNs to begin the saccade has been hypothesized to exist.[3] Recently, Yoshida and colleagues have demonstrated the existence of a powerful and abrupt inhibitory input into OPNs that completely turns off these cells just before saccade initiation.[4] They suggest that these inhibitory trigger cells are located close to the OPNs. Subsequent to this initial input, the level of membrane hyperpolarization in OPNs is very closely correlated with eye velocity, and this sustained hyperpolarization keeps OPNs turned off for the remainder of the saccade. Because the discharge of EBNs has been shown to be correlated with eye velocity during saccades, it seems likely that EBNs are the source of the sustaining OPN membrane hyperpolarization through local inhibitory neurons named latch neurons.[5] Some experimental evidence has been put forward for the existence of latch cells in the PPRF.[5] In contrast to the inhibition-gated, pulsatile circuit believed to control saccades, the lower portion of the schematic in FIGURE 1 shows the continuous brainstem throughput believed to exist in the smooth-pursuit system. The pursuit drive input on the right comes most importantly from the cerebellum.[6] This input excites pursuit neurons in the medial vestibular nucleus and the nucleus prepositus hypoglossi.[7] Pursuit neurons play a similar role in the generation of pursuit to that played by EBNs in the saccadic system in that they directly excite MNs with a signal correlated with eye velocity. In contrast, in the pursuit system this signal drives MNs whenever PNs are active, whereas in the saccadic system the EBN input to MNs is gated by the OPNs.

METHODS

Three monkeys were used in this study. All experimental protocols were approved by the Institutional Animal Care and Use Committee at the California Pacific Medical Center and complied with the guidelines of the Public Health Service policy on Humane Care and Use of Laboratory Animals.

To allow head-fixed eye movement recordings, a scleral eye coil and a head restraint system were implanted in each animal using dental cement and titanium orthopedic bone screws under isofluorane anesthesia and aseptic surgical conditions. A coil made of four turns of Teflon-coated stainless steel wire was implanted under the conjunctiva of one eye using the procedure described by Fuchs and Robinson[8] as modified by Judge and colleagues.[9] A stainless steel chamber was mounted stereotaxically on the skull, slanted laterally in a frontal plane at an angle of 25° and aligned on the OPN region.

Behavioral paradigms, visual displays, and data storage were under the control of a real-time program running on a laboratory PC system. The targets were presented via a computer-controlled, analogue oscilloscope, which backprojected light spots on the 90 × 90° translucent screen placed 40 cm in front of the monkey. The targets were 15-min arc in diameter and 2 cd/m² in intensity against a diffusely illuminated dim homogeneous background. Horizontal and vertical eye position and target position signals were sampled at 1 kHz and stored on computer disk for off-line analysis.

Animals were trained to follow the stepped motion of a visual spot or to pursue a smoothly moving target. Neural activity was recorded during separate blocks of saccades and pursuit trials. Within a block of saccade trials, each trial was initiated by the appearance of a stationary target for 400 ms during which the monkeys had to saccade to that initial position. After the animals had foveated the target, a fixation interval was initiated that lasted for 500 ms. During that period, animals had to maintain gaze within a square electronic window of $4 \times 4°$ centered on the target. At the end of the fixation period, the fixation point was turned off and simultaneously a target appeared at an eccentric position. The animal received a liquid reward for saccading to the location of the eccentric target. Blocks of pursuit trials were initiated by the same initial fixation sequence, but when the fixation point went off, the target then stepped to an eccentric position and simultaneously began to move toward the fixation position at constant speed. In order to obtain pursuit trajectories without catch-up saccades, the amplitude of the initial step was optimized.[10]

Eye velocity for data analysis was obtained by digital differentiation of the eye position signal. Eye velocity was filtered with a second-order digital filter (cutoff frequency = 50 Hz). Eye acceleration was obtained by digital differentiation of the eye velocity trace. The onset of the pursuit movement was determined by using an acceleration threshold (usually between 20 and $50°/s^2$). The offset of pursuit was the time when eye velocity returned to the value observed at the time of pursuit initiation. Saccade onset was determined using an acceleration threshold fixed at $250°/s^2$. The significance of response modulation during smooth pursuit was determined by comparing the firing rate during a 100-ms fixation period with the activity during a smooth-pursuit period of the same duration. The firing rate during fixation was estimated in each trial by computing the average activity from the spike density record during a 100-ms fixation epoch starting 150 ms before pursuit onset. Spike density records were obtained by smoothing the raw spike activity with a Gaussian filter with $\sigma = 10$ ms. The firing rate during pursuit was estimated in each trial by computing the average activity from the spike density record during a 100-ms smooth-pursuit epoch starting 50 ms after pursuit onset. The mean and 95% confidence interval of the estimated firing rate during fixation were also computed. The duration of the decreased OPN activity during pursuit was determined using a method based on the confidence interval. The onset of the activity decrease in an OPN was defined as the time when the spike density function exited the confidence interval of the estimated fixation firing rate for more than 50 ms on a trial by trial basis. The offset of the activity decrease was defined as the time when the spike density function reentered the confidence interval of the estimated fixation rate for more than 50 ms. In order to quantify the relationship between OPNs firing rate and pursuit eye velocity, the spike density and eye velocity were measured and averaged over a 20-ms interval centered 100 ms after pursuit onset, always during a saccade-free period.

RESULTS FOR OPNs

According to the hypothesis put forward in FIGURE 1, the discharge of OPNs should not be modulated during smooth pursuit because these neurons are supposedly gating inhibition on saccadic premotor neurons only. We have recently published a report that shows that this crucial prediction underlying the assumption of separate premotor paths for the pursuit and saccadic systems is not true.[11] Instead, we found that ~50% of the OPNs we recorded showed a significant downward modulation in their discharge rate during pursuit eye movements. FIGURE 2 shows an example of an OPN with this type of modulation during pursuit eye movements. The inset at the upper right shows the activity of the cell when the monkey made 10° horizontal saccades to the left in response to a target that stepped 10° to the left and then remained stationary. The discharge of the neuron pauses completely for the duration of the saccades. It also paused for saccades in all other directions (not shown). Thus, the saccade-related behavior of the neurons we recorded in our study appeared to be identical to that previously reported for OPNs—they discharged at a high tonic rate during fixation, but became quiescent before and during all saccades.

The remainder of FIGURE 2 shows the response of the same cell during a pursuit trial. Near the beginning of the trial the target stepped 4° to the right and simultaneously began a smooth movement at 20°/s to the left. This step/ramp motion causes the target to recross the fixation position at about the time the pursuit response began. We used the step/ramp paradigm to study the response of OPNs during pursuit with few, if any, catch-up saccades. When saccades did occur, they came late in the pursuit response as illustrated in the trial shown in FIGURE 2. The onset and time course of the pursuit response may be seen most clearly on the horizontal eye velocity trace (Ėh). The response of the OPN is shown below as an instantaneous spike density record and as a raw spike response in which the times of neural discharges are shown as upward tic marks. During fixation before the onset of the pursuit response, the cell discharges tonically at a rate of ~160 spikes/s, which is typical for OPNs during fixation. The OPN discharge is modulated downward at about the same time that the pursuit response begins. As the eyes accelerate to reach a speed a little less than the target speed, the discharge rate, as quantified by the spike density trace, decreases to a value about two-thirds of that present during fixation.

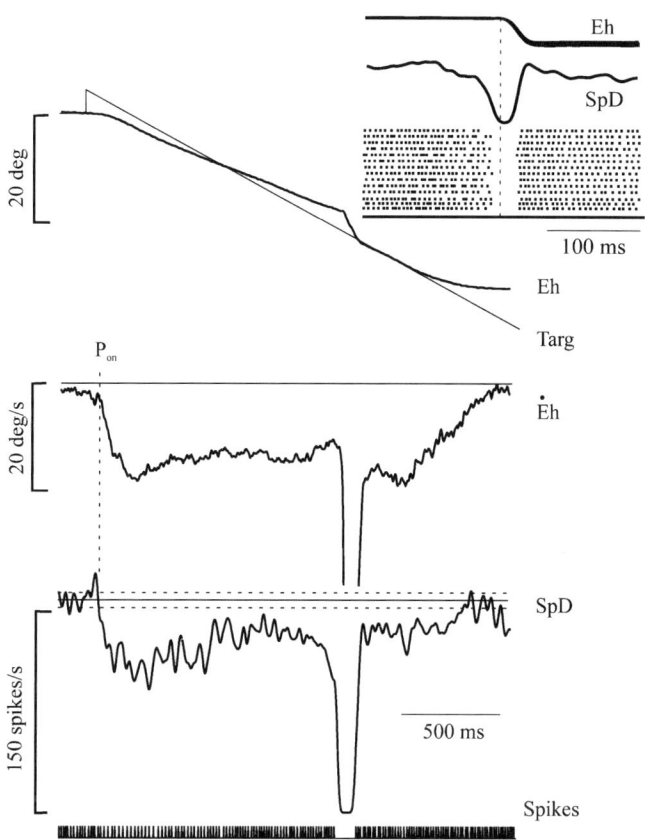

FIGURE 2. Behavior of an OPN whose discharge is modulated during pursuit eye movements. The inset at the upper right shows that this neuron is completely inhibited during saccadic movements to the left. For the single-trial pursuit response, horizontal eye position is shown by the trace labeled, Eh, and horizontal target position by Targ. Horizontal eye velocity ($\dot{E}h$) is shown in the middle trace. Because eye velocity lagged target velocity as the trial progressed, a catch-up saccade was made near the end of the trial. Eye velocity during this saccade is truncated for clarity. The *lower* set of traces show the raw spike discharge (Spikes) of the cell (only every other discharge shown for clarity) and the spike density (SpD) estimation of neuron activity. The *solid horizontal* line through the SpD trace shows the mean discharge rate of the cell during the period of fixation before pursuit onset. The *dashed* lines above and below the mean fixation rate are the 95% confidence limits of the estimate of fixation discharge. The vertical dotted line labeled, P_{on}, shows the estimated time of pursuit onset.

As the eyes continue to lag the target position during the pursuit response, a catch-up saccade is executed late in the trial. The discharge of the OPN pauses completely during this saccade. This pursuit/saccade response illustrates the difference between the modulation of OPNs during saccades and pursuit. All the OPNs we studied were completed turned off during any saccade either in response to stationary targets or during catch-up saccades made during pursuit. For the subpopulation of OPNs that showed a decrease in activity during pursuit, the pursuit-related modulation was never total, in contrast to the pause of activity that always accompanied saccades. Interestingly, by examining the behavior of OPNs during very small catch-up saccades during pursuit, we were able to show that these small saccades, which had velocities in the same range as the highest pursuit velocities we were able to generate, still were accompanied with a pause of activity. In contrast, the pursuit movements were always accompanied by a downward modulation of OPN discharge, but not complete pausings. This observation again emphasizes that a separate, more powerful inhibitory signal that is not present during pursuit seems to govern the behavior of OPNs just before the initiation of saccades. This signal may be responsible for the rapid triggering of OPN silence just before saccade onset.[4]

The depth of downward modulation in OPNs was correlated with eye velocity at the peak of pursuit responses, and the duration of this modulation was correlated with the duration of the pursuit movement.[11] Similar correlations between the level of OPN membrane hyperpolarization and saccadic eye velocity[4] and between the duration of the saccadic pause in OPN activity and movement duration have been reported.[12] Whereas the pause in OPN discharge for saccades occurred in all directions, the depth of the downward modulation in OPN discharge for pursuit was found to be sensitive to pursuit direction. Those OPNs that showed a significant reduction in activity during one direction of pursuit also showed some decrease in other directions, but more than half of the cells we studied showed different amounts of downward modulation during pursuit in different directions.[11]

The discharge pattern of OPNs during pursuit suggests that they may partially disinhibit the pursuit system, but to a lesser extent than during saccades. This suggestion is further confirmed by the results of electrical microstimulation delivered in the region of the OPNs. After we had recorded the activity of OPNs during saccades and pursuit, we had the monkeys initiate a series of step/ramp pursuit trials. On randomly selected trials after maximum pursuit velocity had been obtained, we delivered 200-ms pulse trains of high-frequency stimulation through the recording microelectrode. Electrical stimulation caused a strong deceleration in the ongoing pursuit movement in both horizontal directions of pursuit.[11] The quantitative amount of reduction in eye velocity was dependent on the direction of the pursuit movement. At one site the same level of microstimulation applied during saccades completely stopped the movements in midflight as has been previously reported for stimulation in the OPN region.

SACCADE/PURSUIT CELLS IN THE PPRF

In the remainder of this paper we briefly address the question of which neurons might be responsible for the partial inhibition of OPNs that occurs during pursuit. Missal and colleagues have recorded from a class of medium-lead burst neurons (MLBN) in the mesencephalic reticular formation or the interstitial nucleus of Cajal in the cat that burst during vertical saccades.[13] These neurons also displayed a weaker tonic level of activity during pursuit eye movements in either the up or down direction. The preferred direction associated with pursuit was the same preferred direction associated with saccadic activity. In order to determine whether similar cells exist for the horizontal eye movement systems, we recorded in the PPRF region

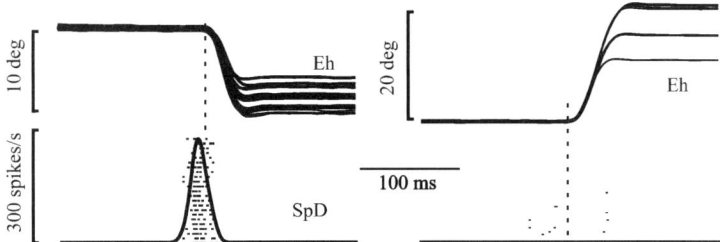

FIGURE 3. Saccade-related discharge of a saccade/pursuit neuron recorded in the PPRF. The plot on the *left* shows the burst discharge of the cell for leftward directed saccades. *Upper* set of traces shows horizontal eye position (Eh). *Lower* display is a raster of spike discharges. Each line in the raster shows the spike discharge during one of the saccades shown above. A mean spike density for all 23 saccade trials is superimposed on the raster. The plot on the *right* shows very little activity in the same cell for rightward saccades.

rostral to the abducens nucleus in the monkey. This region of the PPRF is known to contain the soma of the EBNs that discharge for saccades with an ipsilateral, horizontal component.[12] However, the area also contains a heterogeneous variety of other saccade-related burst neurons including MLBNs and LLBNs that have widely distributed preferred movement directions including horizontal and vertical. As we advanced microelectrodes into this region, we used a paradigm in which the animal executed saccades in different directions in response to the step movement of a visual target. Whenever a cell in this region was isolated that responded during saccadic eye movements, we determined its preferred direction and the onset time of its discharge prior to the onset of saccades in its preferred direction. We then had the animal perform a number of smooth-pursuit–related tasks to determine whether the neuron was also active for pursuit movements.

FIGURE 3 shows an example of one burst neuron recorded in the PPRF which was active for both saccades and pursuit. The plot on the left in this figure shows the activity of the neuron during a series of leftward saccades of different amplitudes. On average, for leftward saccades, the onset of discharge in this cell was 17.3 ms before saccade onset. It discharged only an occasional spike for rightward saccades as shown in the plot on the right.

FIGURE 4 shows the activity of this same saccadic burst neuron during step/ramp pursuit movements in both horizontal directions. The neuron discharges vigorously during leftward pursuit (FIG. 4A), but at a lower level during rightward pursuit (FIG. 4B). The initial discharge shown in FIGURE 4A does not appear to be associated with saccades. Moreover, the saccadic burst present for the small leftward catch-up saccade that occurs just as the pursuit response is ending in FIGURE 4A may be clearly differentiated from the pursuit-related response of this cell. In contrast, the two rightward saccades present during the trial shown in FIGURE 4B are not associated with saccade-related discharge.

The saccadic lead time of the neuron shown in FIGURES 3 and 4 straddles the lead times often used to differentiate between MLBNs and LLBNs.[5] In addition, the regularity and intensity of its saccade-related discharge is less than that usually associ-

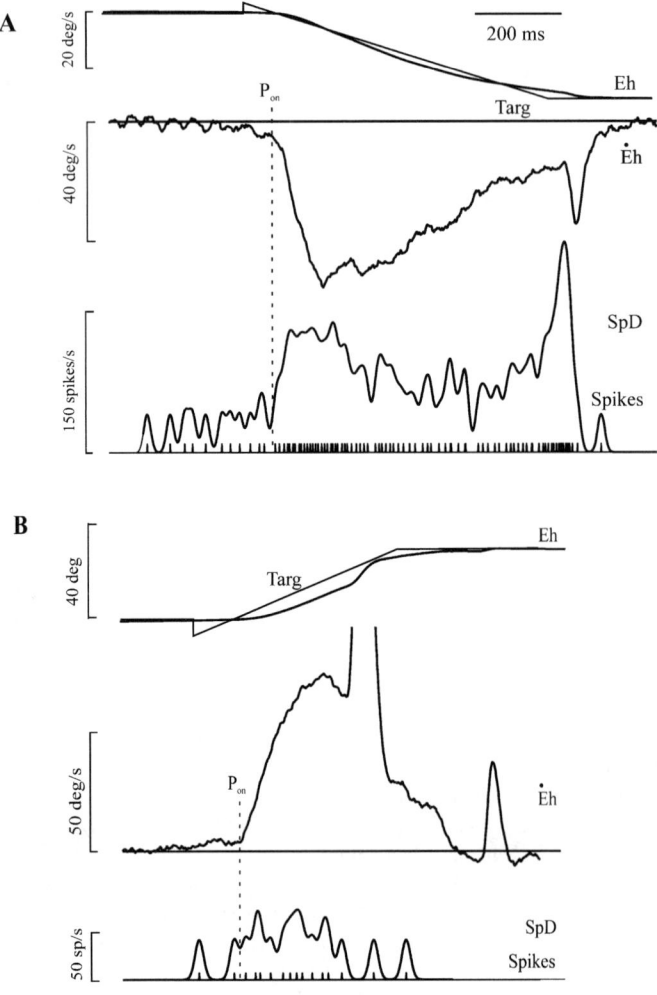

FIGURE 4. Activity of the same saccade/pursuit neuron shown in FIGURE 3, but now for pursuit movements to the left (**A**) and to the right (**B**). Arrangement of traces and labels the same as in FIGURE 2. (**A**) The eyes pursue the target accurately initially and then reduce their speed in anticipation of the end of the trial. A small catch-up saccade occurs just after target motion stops. A burst of higher-frequency discharge in association with this saccade is clearly seen on the spike density trace. (**B**) The pursuit-related activity in this cell for a rightward smooth movements is much less than in preferred leftward direction.

ated with EBNs. Thus, we hypothesize that this group of neurons may be a distinct class of PPRF neuron associated with both saccades and pursuit. Only a minority of the saccade-related burst cells (20/56) that we recorded in the PPRF were also active during pursuit movements.

Since the peak discharge rate of EBNs is correlated with maximum saccadic velocity,[12] we also conducted an analysis to determine whether the pursuit-related dis-

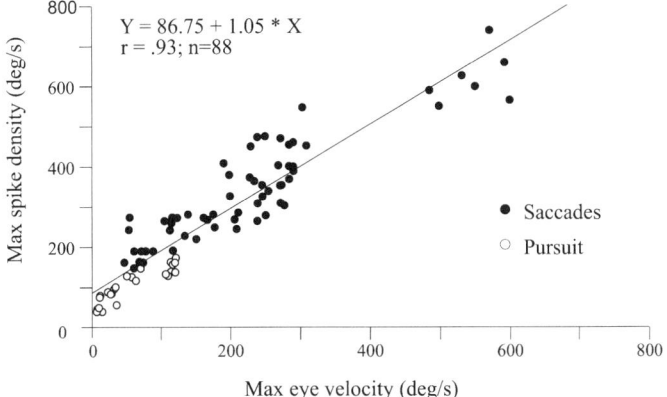

FIGURE 5. Relationship between maximum spike density and maximum eye velocity for the same saccade/pursuit neuron shown in FIGURES 3 and 4. Maximum discharge was well fit by a linear regression on maximum eye velocity both for pursuit and saccades to the left.

charge of our sample of saccade/pursuit neurons showed a similar correlation. For each trial in the preferred direction, we computed the mean level of discharge (from the spike density trace) in a 20-ms interval near the peak of the response as described in METHODS. We also computed the average pursuit speed in a similar time interval centered on the maximum pursuit speed. FIGURE 5 shows the result of such an analysis on one saccade/pursuit neuron. The filled circles on the right show that this neuron's discharge increased in proportion to peak saccadic velocity. The open circles on the left for pursuit show that this correlation extended into the range of lower velocities present during pursuit.

DISCUSSION

We have shown, in contrast to previous beliefs, that OPNs lower their high-frequency fixation-associated discharge during pursuit as well as saccades. Qualitatively, the inhibition present in OPNs for the two types of eye movement is different. During saccades the inhibition in OPNs is complete even for small movements. During pursuit the inhibition is a significant downward modulation, but never complete inhibition. Also in contrast to the inhibition shown in OPNs during saccades, which is total for any direction of movement, the quantitative amount of downward modulation during pursuit varies with the direction of the movement. We speculate that this directional effect may depend on the side of the brainstem on which the OPN is located, since the projections from the SC have different patterns of ipsi- and contralateral projections to OPNs.[14] However, we have been unable to confirm this speculation with our extracellular recording technique.

We have also shown that a class of burst cells exists in the PPRF that are active during both pursuit and saccades for a preferred horizontal movement direction. These cells appear to be similar in behavior to a class of cells recorded in the mesencephalon in the cat for vertical saccades and pursuit.[13] For saccades in the pre-

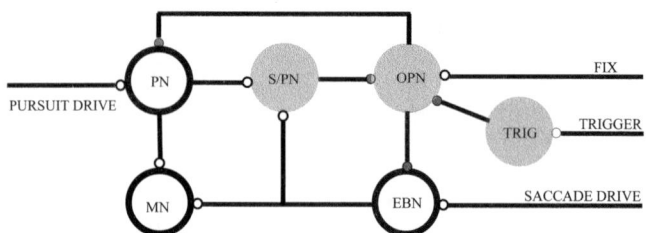

FIGURE 6. Hypothesized arrangement of the horizontal premotor saccade and pursuit circuits in the brainstem to account for the shared elements described in this paper. See text for an explanation of this combined circuit.

ferred direction, these cells discharge a discrete, medium frequency burst of spikes. The range of burst leads in the saccade/pursuit cells we recorded spanned the boundary between LLBNs and MLBNs (also EBNs which are a distinct subpopulation of MLBNs). Most of our saccade/pursuit cells did not display the extremely high and compact saccade-related burst that has been reported to occur in EBNs,[12] but further experiments will be required to determine whether our class of saccade/pursuit neurons is distinctly separate from EBNs.

Based on the discharge pattern we have recorded in OPNs and in saccade/pursuit neurons during saccades and pursuit the notion of completely separate premotor systems for these two types of movements (FIG. 1) may need to be modified. Instead the premotor portions of these two systems may be connected as shown by the schematic representation in FIGURE 6. Pursuit neurons (PN) in the vestibular and prepositus nuclei and saccadic excitatory burst neurons (EBN) in the PPRF project directly to ocular motoneurons (MN) and only discharge for pursuit and saccades, respectively. They receive separate drive signals from the cerebellum and elsewhere and from the SC and elsewhere, respectively. OPNs directly inhibit each of these neuronal populations, but modulate this inhibition to control the gain of smooth pursuit or to gate saccadic movements. The inhibition of OPNs is completely removed during saccades by the combined action of fixation neurons and inhibitory trigger neurons. The inhibition of OPNs on PN during pursuit is only partially removed. Saccade/pursuit neurons (S/PNs) receive eye velocity-related excitatory input from PN and EBN during pursuit and saccades, respectively, and connect with inhibitory inputs to OPNs.

ACKNOWLEDGMENTS

This research was supported by National Institutes of Health Grant No. EY08060. M.M. was supported by a long-term fellowship from the Human Frontier Science Program and an Atkinson Fellowship from the Smith-Kettlewell Eye Research Institute.

REFERENCES

1. LEIGH, R.J. & D.S. ZEE. 1999. The Neurology of Eye Movements. Oxford University Press. New York.

2. KELLER, E.L. & S.J. HEINEN. 1991. Generation of smooth-pursuit eye movements: neuronal mechanisms and pathways. Neurosci. Res. **11:** 79–107.
3. VAN GISBERGEN, J.A.M., D.A. ROBINSON & S. GIELEN. 1981. A quantitative analysis of generation of saccadic eye movements by burst neurons. J. Neurophysiol. **45:** 417–442.
4. YOSHIDA, K., Y. IWAMOTO, S. CHIMOTO & H. SHIMAZU. 1999. Saccade-related inhibitory input to pontine omnipause neurons: an intracellular study in alert cats. J. Neurophysiol. **82:** 1198–1208.
5. MOSCHOVAKIS, A.K., C.A. SCUDDER & S.M. HIGHSTEIN. 1996. The microscopic anatomy and physiology of the mammalian saccadic system. Prog. Neurobiol. **50:** 133–254.
6. HEINEN, S.J. & E.L. KELLER. 2003. Smooth pursuit eye movements: recent advances. *In* The Visual Neurosciences. L.M. Chalupa & J.S. Werner, Eds. MIT Press. Cambridge, MA. In press.
7. MCFARLAND, J.L. & A.F. FUCHS. 1992. Discharge pattern in nucleus prepositus hypoglossi and adjacent medial vestibular nucleus during horizontal eye movement in behaving macaques. J. Neurophysiol. **68:** 319–336.
8. FUCHS, A.F. & D.A. ROBINSON. 1966. A method for measuring horizontal and vertical eye movement chronically in the monkey. J. Appl. Physiol. **21:** 1068–1070.
9. JUDGE, S.J., B.J. RICHMOND & F.C. CHU. 1980. Implantation of magnetic search coils for measurement of eye position: an improved method. Vision Res. **20:** 535–538.
10. RASHBASS, C. 1961. The relationship between saccadic and smooth tracking eye movements. J. Physiol. (Lond.) **159:** 326–338.
11. MISSAL, M. & E.L. KELLER. 2002. Common inhibitory mechanism for saccades and smooth-pursuit eye movements. J. Neurophysiol. **88:** 1880–1892.
12. KELLER, E.L. 1991. The brainstem. *In* Eye Movements, Vol. 8. R.H.S. Carpenter, Ed.: 200–223. Macmillan Press. London.
13. MISSAL, M., S. DE BROWER, P. LEFÈVRE & E. OLIVIER. 2000. Activity of mesencephalic vertical burst neurons during saccades and smooth pursuit. J. Neurophysiol. **83:** 2080–2092.
14. BÜTTNER-ENNEVER, J.A., A.K.E. HORN, V. HENN & B. COHEN. 1999. Projections from the superior colliculus motor map to omnipause neurons in monkey. J. Comp. Neurol. **413:** 55–67.

Motor and Sensory Innervation of Extraocular Eye Muscles

J.A. BÜTTNER-ENNEVER, A. EBERHORN, AND A.K.E. HORN

Institute of Anatomy, Ludwig-Maximilians University of Munich, 80336 Munich, Germany

> ABSTRACT: Eye muscles are unusual in several ways; one is that they have up to three different layers—the inner global layer, the outer orbital layer, and in some species an external marginal layer has been described. In sheep this is called the "peripheral patch layer." Three different types of proprioceptors are found in eye muscles—muscle spindles, Golgi tendon organs, and palisade endings. A survey of the organization of their location leads us to the hypothesis that each receptor is confined to a separate layer of the eye muscle. The palisade endings are associated with the global layer, the muscle spindles lie predominantly in the orbital layer, and the Golgi tendon organs are found only in the peripheral patch layer. This well-organized scheme may help us to understand the proprioceptive system in eye muscles.
>
> KEYWORDS: non-twitch motoneurons; palisade endings; innervated myotendinous cylinders; global layer; orbital layer; pulleys; eye movements; Golgi tendon organs; muscle spindles; medial rectus C-group; final common pathway

MOTOR CONTROL

The increased interest in the motor control of eye muscles in the late 1960s was stimulated mainly by the vestibular studies of Bernard Cohen, and the recording-modelling approach of David A. Robinson and his colleagues. This has resulted in the development of a thorough understanding of many aspects of the oculomotor system.[1–4] Several relatively independent premotor circuits carrying vestibular, saccadic, smooth pursuit, or vergence signals have been discovered, modeled and shown to converge on the motoneurons in the oculomotor, trochlear, or abducens nuclei. The motoneurons generate motor responses, some with more tonic, others with a more phasic, properties; but all of the motoneurons respond with every type of eye movement.[5–7] This concept of a final common pathway has become widely accepted, but detailed studies show that it is not yet complete.[8,9]

Address for correspondence: Prof. J.A. Büttner-Ennever, Institute of Anatomy, Ludwig-Maximilians University, Pettenkoferstr. 11, D-80336 Munich, Germany. Voice: +49 89 5160 4851/4876; fax: +49 89 5160 4857.
buettner@anat.med.uni-muenchen.de

NON-TWITCH MUSCLE FIBERS

Eye muscles consist mainly of twitch fibers that undergo an all-or-nothing contraction on the activation of their centrally lying endplates. With the exception of levator palpebrae, they all contain 10–20% of non-twitch muscle fibers, a fiber type that is exceeding rare in mammal skeletal muscles.[10–12] These striated muscle fibers are multiply innervated along their whole length, and on activation they generate a local contraction that is *not* propagated throughout the muscle fiber, but remains local to the "en grappe" nerve endings.[13–16] The properties of non-twitch muscle fibers have not received much attention in oculomotor circles, probably because their function is unclear. They are a regular component of the skeletal muscles of amphibians, reptiles, and fish, where a spectrum of different types of non-twitch fiber can be found, with graduated properties.[17] The contraction of non-twitch muscle fibers is slower than in all other muscle types, but they can maintain the tension for long periods at less energy cost than a twitch fiber, due to the slow turnover of the myosin-actin bonding.

A recent study on the location of the motoneurons innervating non-twitch muscle fibers in the primate showed that the non-twitch motoneurons lie separate from the twitch motoneurons around the periphery of the classical oculomotor trochlear and abducens nuclei, and they receive different afferent inputs compared to the classical motoneuron subgroups.[18] In experiments on the primate lateral rectus rabies virus, a transsynaptic tract tracer was used to investigate the premotor innervation of non-twitch motoneurons with injections into the distal tip of the muscle where only non-twitch terminals exist.[19] In this way, only the non-twitch motoneurons were retrogradely labeled, and the virus was allowed to travel retrogradely over at least two synapses in these experiments. During this short survival period no clinical symptoms of rabies develop. The results revealed that the predominant inputs to the non-twitch motoneurons were *not* the fastest premotor networks generating saccades or the vestibulo-ocular reflex, but rather are driven by the networks subtending eye movements that depend on (visual) feedback circuits such as smooth pursuit, convergence, and gaze-holding.[20] The results fit well with the somewhat slower characteristics of the non-twitch muscle fibers.

The rabies experiments labeled the muscle tendon junction where the global layer of the eye muscle inserts on the sclera (see FIG. 2) and is hence an investigation confined to the global layer non-twitch muscle fibers and their motoneurons. The orbital layer contains only an intermediate form of non-twitch muscle fiber. These change their properties along their length so that at the distal and proximal ends of the orbital layer they have the characteristics and innervation of a non-twitch muscle fiber, but in the central region they have the characteristics and innervation of a twitch muscle fiber.[21] The intermediate form of non-twitch muscle fibers of the orbital layer will not be considered any further here.

SENSORY CONTROL

In contrast, the sensory control of eye muscles has been steadfastly ignored in terms of modeling or integration into the understanding of eye movements, in spite of the fact that there is a large body of information showing that eye muscle possess a proprioceptive system. For example, spatial localization in humans can be altered by either pulling eye muscles[22] or by strabismus surgery.[23] Stretching eye muscles in animals evokes responses in the superior colliculus,[24] cerebellum and the visual cortex.[25] Anatomical tracing studies have demonstrated projections through the trigeminal ganglion, and the spinal trigeminal nucleus.[26,27–29] And physiological evidence has been presented for the presence of proprioceptive signals in many areas of the central nervous system, including the superior colliculus, the lateral geniculate body, the vestibular nuclei, prepositus hypoglossi nucleus, the cerebellum as well as areas of the cerebral cortex.[25,30] Cutting the ophthalmic nerve (deafferentation) causes fixation instability in cat,[31] reduction in stereoacuity in cat,[32] and deviation of eye position in lambs.[33] Last and of most significance is that eye muscles contain proprioceptive end-organs—muscle spindles, Golgi tendon organs, and palisade endings.

Alongside the evidence for the existence of functional proprioception in eye muscles, a large body of counter evidence exists. No stretch reflex could be recorded in abducens motor units when the ipsi-eye was pulled.[34] Cutting ophthalmic nerves in monkey (assumed to achieve deafferentation) gave very little effect on saccades,[35] smooth pursuit, vestibular responses, conjugacy, adaptation, ocular alignment, etc.[36] Finally, the presence of eye muscle proprioceptors varies wildly between species, and often, as in rats, proprioceptors appear not to be present at all (Ruskell;[30] Donaldson[25]). For example humans, some species of monkey, giraffes, pigs, and all ungulates have muscle spindles, whereas other monkeys such as *Macaca fascicularis*, dogs, cats, rats, guinea pigs, and rabbits do not. These features do not correlate with any eye movement properties, and it has proved hard to find a clear concept. The purpose of this article is to present a simplified review of the evidence for proprioception in eye muscles by considering the orbital layer and the global layer of the eye muscle separately.

PROPRIOCEPTORS IN EYE MUSCLES

Muscle Spindles

It is well established that sensory information used for motor control of skeletal muscles is generated by muscle spindles, and Golgi tendon organs. Muscle spindles contain three types of intrafusal muscle fiber, termed nuclear chain, nuclear bag$_1$, and nuclear bag$_2$ fibers. Each receives an afferent innervation in its equatorial region, and the polar regions receive gamma-motor fibers to maintain the sensitivity of the muscle spindle during muscle shortening. Both intrafusal and extrafusal fiber muscle fibers develop by a similar process in the late gestational period whereby myoblasts fuse into myotubes; the intrafusal fibers, however, remain much shorter and thinner.[37] The occurrence of muscle spindles in muscles has been recently shown to be a highly dynamic process. For example, their occurrence is critically dependent on the timing of the sensory innervation of the developing spindles. If the sensory afferent is cut, then, depending on the developmental period, muscle spindles may fail to develop, or undergo degeneration and hypertrophy into a structure indistinguishable from an extrafusal fiber.[37,38] Furthermore, the application of nerve growth factor during the redevelopment of the cut sensory nerve leads to the formation of countless supernumery muscle spindles.[39] Similar changes in the occurrence of muscle spindles have been shown to be additionally dependent on specific genetic transcription factors.[37,39–41] In the light of this variability in the development of muscle spindles in skeletal muscles, it seems possible that the interplay of similar factors could lead to the wide variation in their presence in the extraocular eye muscles of different species.[11]

Eye muscles have a second unusual feature, apart from the presence of non-twitch, multiply innervated muscle fibers, that is, they have an inner "global" layer and an outer "orbital" layer. In sheep, a distinct third muscle layer was described by Harker.[42] It lies mainly distally in a C-shape around the outside of the orbital layer, and he called it the peripheral patch layer. A similar layer was described in human by Wasicky et al.[43] and was called the marginal layer. Its presence in other species is unclear. The two main eye muscle layers have several important differences: the orbital layer inserts onto the pulleys, whereas the global layer inserts on the sclera of the globe.[44,45] The layers do not appear to have a parallel development.[11] We would like to consider these two layers separately with respect to muscle spindles. An analysis of the literature shows that muscle spindles are always associated with the orbital layer or the transition zone of the orbital layer with the global layer, but they are not associated with the global layer (sheep;[46] monkey;[47] man[30,48–51]). This is shown in the drawing of sheep lateral rectus in FIGURE 1.

Palisade Endings

If the orbital layer uses muscle spindles to generate its sensory signals, what does the global layer use? The global layer possesses a third unusual feature, unique to eye muscles—the palisade endings at the myotendinous junctions.[30,51,52] Palisade endings form a cuff of fine vesicle-laden nerve terminals that insert only on the tip of the non-twitch muscle fibers of the global layer. In the majority of cases, terminals are also on the adjacent collagen fibers of the tendon.[53] The term "innervated myo-

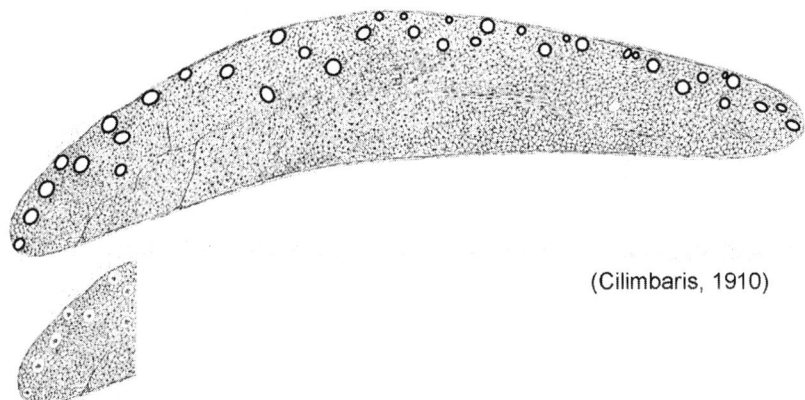

FIGURE 1. Drawings modified from the sketches of Cilimbaris (1910) from lateral rectus of the sheep. Note that all muscle spindles (*white dots*) are associated with the orbital layer.

tendinous cylinders" is used to describe the palisade endings along with their fibrous capsule. The palisade terminals arise from nerve fibers that enter the tendon from the central nerve entry zone, and then turn back 180°, to contact the tip of the muscle fibers.

Several authors have suggested that palisade endings could be the source of sensory afferent signals;[20,25,30,54] but there still are conflicting reports on the functional nature of palisade endings—whether they are sensory or motor structures, or both. The ultrastructural morphology of palisade endings in cat, rhesus monkey and sheep has been shown to be typical of a sensory structure, where the terminals *lack* a basal membrane.[55–57] Motor terminals, by contrast, typically *have* a basal membrane around their muscle endplates. In contrast, Lukas *et al.*[53] have shown that in humans only some palisade endings have a basal membrane around their contacts with the muscle, and in rabbit all palisade terminals have a continuous basal membrane. The problem is compounded by the conflicting evidence for the location of the cell soma of the palisade ending. If the palisade endings are sensory, their ganglion cell body should be in the trigeminal ganglion or in the mesencephalic trigeminal nucleus, whereas if the endings are of a motor origin then they would have cell bodies associated with the oculomotor nucleus. Tozer and Sherrington,[58] as well as Sas and Schab,[59] provided evidence for their location in the oculomotor nerve or nucleus, a result more compatible with a motor role for the palisade endings,[30,60] whereas the results of other studies point to the trigeminal ganglion as the location of palisade ending soma[61] and imply a sensory function. The function of palisade endings is at present not clearly understood.

Palisade endings have been found in almost all species that have been investigated, with the exception of the rat. Thus, at present, it is not possible to assume that all mammals have palisade endings in the global layer of their eye muscles. However, the scheme shown in FIGURE 2 represents the situation in all the species studied thus far, including monkey and man.

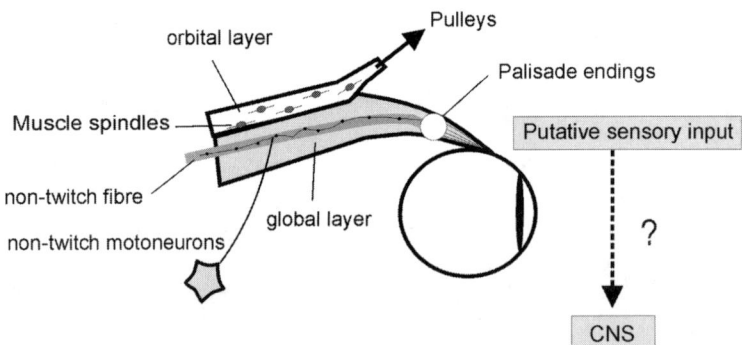

FIGURE 2. Non-twitch muscle fibers and palisade endings form a unit unique to the *global* layer of the extraocular muscles, whereas when muscle spindles occur in eye muscles they are associated with the orbital layer.

Golgi Tendon Organs

Golgi tendon organs have been reported in the tendons of extraocular eye muscles of some artidactyls such as sheep, camel, pig, and calf[30,62,63] and *Macaca mulatta*.[64] They exhibit structural features not seen in skeletal Golgi tendon organs. More specifically, they have an enlarged capsular space and are associated with one special type of eye muscle fiber—*the non-twitch multiply innervated muscle fiber*—which is exclusive to eye muscles, and in this case serves to adjust the sensitivity of the Golgi tendon organ.[63] Of particular interest in the context of this paper, is that all the Golgi tendon organs lie in one specific layer of the eye muscle, called the peripheral patch layer.[63] This "third" muscle layer surrounds the orbital side of the eye muscle and has been described in sheep eye muscles[42] and human.[43]

FINAL CONSIDERATIONS

The origin of palisade endings is unclear, but one exciting suggestion comes from the work of Zelena and Soukop.[65] In their study of the development of Golgi tendon organs in rat skeletal muscle, they found that at the embryological stage E21 a nerve inserts between the aponeurosis and the attaching muscle fibers. At the postnatal stage P5, the development of myelin around the nerve by Schwann cells is accompanied by the growth of a fibrous capsule; the nerve terminals withdraw from the muscle fibers into the tendon, and in addition the immature multiply innervated muscle fibers become singly innervated with a central endplate. The Golgi tendon organ is fully developed at the stage of P14. However, the immature Golgi tendon organ, at day P3 where the nerve is attached to the multiply innervated muscle fibers, is strikingly similar to the situation found morphologically in palisade endings. This led Zelena and Soukop[65] to suggest that palisade endings may represent immature Golgi tendon organs. This hypothesis is strengthened by the fact that both palisade endings and the Golgi tendon organs in eye muscles are associated only with multiply innervated, that is, *non-twitch muscle fibers*.[30,57,66,67]

It is odd that a common feature of the palisade endings and the Golgi tendon organs is *non-twitch muscle fibers,* and that it has long been known that non-twitch muscle fibers are also closely associated with muscle spindles; branches from the non-twitch muscle fibers enter the sheep muscle spindles and build nuclear bag fibers.[17,46,68] Non-twitch muscle fibers also have the same heavy-chain myosin as the nuclear bag$_1$ intrafusal fibers of muscle spindles.[69] It is hard to escape the feeling that the non-twitch muscle fibers and their sensory innervation play a crucial role in the proprioception of eye muscles. Non-twitch muscle fibers and palisade endings form a unit, unique to the global layer of the extraocular muscles in many mammals; at present several lines of evidence support the hypothesis that they subserve a sensory function. The premotor innervation of the non-twitch motoneurons imply a role in tension feedback, which could involve gaze-holding, eye alignment, and vergence (FIG. 3). The hypothesis presented here suggests that only the twitch fibers play a significant role in eye movement, whereas the global layer *non-twitch muscle fibers* adjust the tension on the palisade endings and modulate the afferent proprioceptive signal. The assumption that there is a lack of involvement of the non-twitch muscle fiber in eye movement is based on the absence of tension developed in a primate eye

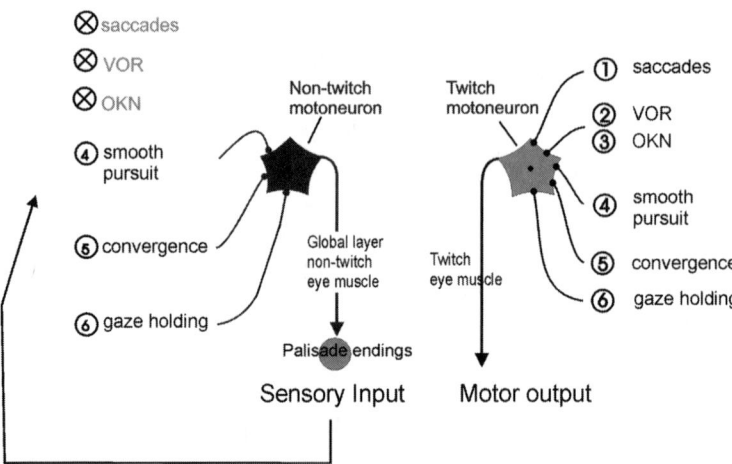

FIGURE 3. In eye muscles, twitch muscle fibers may generate the motor output, i.e., eye movement, while the (global layer) non-twitch muscle fibers together with palisade endings generate the sensory signal, assuming the sensory nature of palisade endings (*see text*), and the lack of contribution to muscle tension by non-twitch muscle fibers.[70]

muscle during tetanic activation of the non-twitch muscle fibers alone.[70] This system is associated with the global layer of the eye muscles which inserts onto the eyeball itself, and appears to be separate from the functioning of the pulleys which are contacted by the orbit layer. The orbital layer is associated with muscle spindles and modified non-twitch muscle fibers,[21] but at present we have no knowledge of the central connections of their sensory or motor innervation. Finally, the Golgi tendon organs in sheep are associated with a third separate eye muscle layer, the peripheral patch layer.

Therefore, it seems possible that each eye muscle layer has its own individual type of proprioceptor. If this hypothesis proves true, then it will certainly simplify the understanding of eye muscle proprioception. An important question to answer now is, what factors determine whether the proprioceptors occur and persist in each layer, or not?

ACKNOWLEDGMENT

This research was supported by the Deutsche Forschungsgemeinschaft SFB 462/B3.

REFERENCES

1. BÜTTNER, U. & J.A. BÜTTNER-ENNEVER. 1988. Present concepts of oculomotor organization. *In* Neuroanatomy of the oculomotor system. J.A. Büttner-Ennever, Ed.: 3–32. Elsevier. Amsterdam.

2. LEIGH, R.J. & D.S. ZEE. 1991. The neurology of eye movements. F.A. Davis Company. Philadelphia.
3. COHEN, B. 1974. The vestibulo-ocular reflex arc. *In* Handbook of Sensory Physiology. H.H. Kornhuber, Ed.: 477–540. Springer. New York.
4. LEIGH, R.J. & D.S. ZEE. 1999. The neurology of eye movements. Oxford University Press. New York.
5. KELLER, E.L. & D.A. ROBINSON. 1972. Abducens unit behavior in the monkey during vergence movements. Vision Res. **12:** 369–382.
6. DEAN, P. 1996. Motor unit recruitment in a distribution model of extraocular muscle. J. Neurophysiol. **76:** 727–742.
7. FUCHS, A.F., C.R. KANEKO & C.A. SCUDDER. 1985. Brainstem control of saccadic eye movements. Annu. Rev. Neurosci. **8:** 307–337.
8. LING, L., A.F. FUCHS, J.O. PHILLIPS & E.G. FREEDMAN. 1999. Apparent dissociation between saccadic eye movements and the firing patterns of premotor neurons and motoneurons. J. Neurophysiol. **82:** 2808–2811.
9. MILLER, J.M., C.J. BOCKISCH & D.S. PAVLOVSKI. 2001. Missing lateral rectus force and absence of medial rectus co-contraction in ocular convergence. J. Neurophysiol. **87:** 2421–2433.
10. PORTER, J.D. & R.S. BAKER. 1998. Anatomy and embryology of the ocular motor system. *In* Clinical Neuro-ophthalmology, Vol. 1. N.R. Miller & N.J. Newman, Eds.: 1043–1099. Williams & Wilkins. Baltimore.
11. PORTER, J.D., R.S. BAKER, R.J. RAGUSA & J.K. BRUECKNER. 1995. Extraocular muscles: basic and clinical aspects of structure and function. Surv. Ophthalmol. **39:** 451–484.
12. SPENCER, R.F. & J.D. PORTER. 1988. Structural organization of the extraocular muscles Rev. Oculomot. Res. **2:** 33–79.
13. NELSON, J.S., S.J. GOLDBERG & J.R. MCCLUNG. 1986. Motoneuron electrophysiological and muscle contractile properties of superior oblique motor units in cat. J. Neurophysiol. **55:** 715–726.
14. CHIARANDINI, D.J. & J. JACOBY. 1987. Dependence of tonic tension on extracellular calcium in rat extraocular muscle. Am. J. Physiol. **253:** C375–C383.
15. JACOBY, J., D.J. CHIARANDINI & E. STEFANI. 1989. Electrical properties and innervation of fibers in the orbital layer of rat extraocular muscles. J. Neurophysiol. **61:** 116–125.
16. Jacoby, J., K. ko, C. Weiss & J.I. Rushbrook. 1990. Systematic variation in myosin expression along extraocular muscle fibers of the adult rat. J. Muscle Res. Cell Motil. **11:** 25–40.
17. MORGAN, D.L. & U. PROSKE. 1984. Vertebrate slow muscle: its structure, pattern of innervation, and mechanical properties. Physiol. Rev. **64:** 103–138.
18. BÜTTNER-ENNEVER, J.A., A.K.E. HORN, H. SCHERBERGER & P. D'ASCANIO. 2001. Motoneurons of twitch and nontwitch extraocular muscle fibers in the abducens, trochlear, and oculomotor nuclei of monkeys. J. Comp. Neurol. **438:** 318–335.
19. UGOLINI, G., J.A. BÜTTNER-ENNEVER, M. DOLDAN, *et al.* 2001. Horizontal eye movement networks in primates: differences in monosynaptic input to slow and fast abducens motoneurons. Soc. Neurosci. Abstr. **27:** 403–413.
20. BÜTTNER-ENNEVER, J.A., A.K.E. HORN, W. GRAF & G. UGOLINI. 2002. Modern concepts of brainstem anatomy. Ann. N. Y. Acad. Sci. **956:** 75–84.
21. PACHTER, B.R. 1984. Rat extraocular muscle. 3. Histochemical variability along the length of multiply-innervated fibers of the orbital surface layer. Histochemistry **80:** 535–538.
22. LEWIS, R.F. & D.S. ZEE. 1993. Abnormal spatial localization with trigeminal-oculomotor synkinesis. Brain **116:** 1105–1118.
23. STEINBACH, M. & D. SMITH. 1981. Spatial localization after strabismus surgery: evidence for inflow. Science **213:** 1407–1409.
24. DONALDSON, I.M.L. & A.C. LONG. 1980. Interactions between extraocular proprioceptive and visual signals in the superior colliculus of the cat J. Physiol. **298:** 85–110.
25. DONALDSON, I.M.L. 2000. The functions of the proprioceptors of the eye muscles. Philos. Trans. R. Soc. Lond. [Biol.] **355:** 1685–1754.

26. PORTER, J.D. 1986. Brainstem terminations of extraocular muscle primary afferent neurons in the monkey. J. Comp. Neurol. **247:** 133–143.
27. BUISSERET, P. 1995. Influence of extraocular muscle proprioception on vision. Physiolog. Rev. **75:** 323–338.
28. BUISSERET-DELMAS, C. & P. BUISSERET. 1990. Central projections of extraocular muscle afferents in the cat. Neurosci. Lett. **109:** 48–53.
29. OGASAWARA, K., S. ONODERA, T. SHIWA, S. NINOMIYA & Y. TAZAWA. 1987. Projections of extraocular muscle primary afferent neurons to the trigeminal sensory complex in the cat as studied with the transganglionic transport of horseradish peroxidase. Neurosci. Lett. **73:** 242–246.
30. RUSKELL, G.L. 1999. Extraocular muscle proprioceptors and proprioception. Prog. Retinal Eye Res. **18:** 269–291.
31. MAFFEI, L. & A. FIORENTINI. 1976. Asymmetry of motility of the eyes and change of binocular properties of cortical cells in adult cats. Brain Res. **105:** 73–78.
32. FIORENTINI, A. & L. MAFFEI. 1977. Instability of the eye in the dark and proprioception. Nature **269:** 330–331.
33. PETTOROSSI, V.E., A. FERRARESI, F. DRAICCHIO, et al. 1995. Extraocular muscle proprioception and eye position. Acta Otolaryngol. (Stockh.) **115:** 137–140.
34. KELLER, E.L. & D.A. ROBINSON. 1971. Absence of a stretch reflex in extraocular muscles of the monkey. J. Neurophysiol. **34:** 908–919.
35. GUTHRIE, B.L., J.D. PORTER & D.L. SPARKS. 1983. Corollary discharge provides accurate eye position information to the oculomotor system. Science **221:** 1193–1195.
36. LEWIS, R.F., D. ZEE, M.R. HAYMAN & R.J. TAMARGO. 2001. Oculomotor function in the rhesus monkey after deafferentation of the extraocular muscles. Exp. Brain Res. **141:** 349–358.
37. WALRO, J.M. & J. KUCERA. 1999. Why adult mammalian intrafusal and extrafusal fibers contain different myosin heavy-chain isoforms. TINS **22:** 180–184.
38. KUCERA, J., J.M. WALRO & J. REICHLER. 1993. Differential effects of neonatal denervation on intrafusal muscle fibers in the rat. Anat. Embryol. **187:** 397–408.
39. SEKIYA, S., S. HOMMA, Y. MIYATA & M. KUNO. 1986. Effects of nerve growth factor on differentiation of muscle spindles following nerve lesion in neonatal rats. J. Neurosci. **6:** 2019–2025.
40. KUCERA, J., W. COONEY, A. QUE, et al. 1999. Formation of supernumerary muscle spindles at the expense of Golgi tendon organs in ER81-deficient mice. Dev. Dynamics **223:** 389–401.
41. KUCERA, J., W. COONEY, A. QUE, et al. 2002. Formation of supernumerary muscle spindles at the expense of Golgi tendon organs in ER81-deficient mice. Dev. Dynamics 223: 389–401.
42. HARKER, D.W. 1972. The structure and innervation of sheep superior rectus and levator palpebrae extraocular eye muscles. II: Muscle spindles. Invest. Ophthalmol. Visual Sci. **11:** 970–979.
43. WASICKY, R., F. ZHYA-GHAZVINI, R. BLUMER, et al. 2000. Muscle fiber types of human extraocular muscles: a histochemical and immunohistochemical study. Invest. Ophthalmol. Visual Sci. **41:** 980–990.
44. DEMER, J.L., S. YEUL OH & V. POUKENS. 2000. Evidence for active control of rectus extrocular muscle pulleys Invest. Ophthalmol. Visual Sci. **41:** 1280–1290.
45. PORTER, J.D., V. POUKENS, R.S. BAKER & J.L. DEMER. 1996. Structure-function correlations in the human medial rectus extraocular muscle pulleys. Invest. Ophthalmol. **37:** 468–472.
46. HARKER, D.W. 1972. The structure and innervation of sheep superior rectus and levator palpebrae extraocular muscles. Invest. Ophthalmol. **11:** 970–979.
47. GREENE, T. & R. JAMPEL. 1966. Muscle spindles in the extraocular muscles of the macaque. J. Comp. Neurol. **126:** 547–550.
48. BLUMER, R., J.R. LUKAS, M. AIGNER, et al. 1999. Fine structural analysis of extraocular muscle spindles of a two-year-old human infant Invest. Ophthalmol. **40:** 55–64.
49. LUKAS, J.R., M. AIGNER, R. BLUMER, et al. 1994. Number and distribution of neuromuscular spindles in human extraocular muscles. Invest. Ophthalmol. **35:** 4317–4327.

50. RUSKELL, G.L. 1989. The fine structure of human extraocular muscle spindles and their potential proprioceptive capacity. J. Anat. **167**: 199–214.
51. CILIMBARIS, P.A. 1910. Histologische Untersuchungen über die Muskelspindeln der Augenmuskeln. Archiv für mikroskopische Anatomie und Entwicklungsgeschichte **75**: 692–747.
52. DOGIEL, A.S. 1906. Die Endigungen der sensiblen Nerven in den Augenmuskeln und deren Sehnen beim Menschen und den Säugetieren. Archiv. für Mikroskopische Anatomie **68**: 501–526.
53. LUKAS, J.R., R. BLUMER, M. DENK, et al. 2000. Innervated myotendinous cylinders in human extraocular muscles. Invest. Ophthalmol. Visual Sci. **41**: 2422–2431.
54. WEIR, C.R., P.C. KNOX & G.N. DUTTON. 2000. Does extraocular muscle proprioception influence oculomotor control? Br. J. Ophthalmol. **84**: 1071–1074.
55. RUSKELL, G.L. 1978. The fine structure of innervated myotendinous cylinders in extraocular muscles in rhesus monkey. J. Neurocytol. **7**: 693–708.
56. BLUMER, R., J.R. LUKAS, R. WASICKY & R. MAYR. 1998. Presence and structure of innervated myotendinous cylinders in sheep extraocular muscle. Neurosci. Lett. **248**: 49–52.
57. ALVARADO-MALLART, R.M. & M. PINCON RAYMOND. 1979. The palisade endings of cat extraocular muscles: a light and electron microscope study. Tissue Cell **11**: 567–584.
58. TOZER, F.M. & C.S. SHERRINGTON. 1970. Receptors and afferents of the third, fourth and sixth cranial nerves. Proc. R. Soc. Lond. Ser. **82**: 451–457.
59. SAS, J. & R. SCHAB. 1952. Die sogenannten "Palisaden-Endigungen" der Augenmuskeln Acta Morph. Acad. Sci. (Hungary) **2**: 259–266.
60. GENTLE, A. & G.L. RUSKELL. 1997. Pathway of the primary afferent nerve fibers serving proprioception in monkey extaocular muscles. Ophthalmic Physiol. Opt. **17**: 225–231.
61. BILLIG, I., C. BUISSERET-DELMAS & P. BUISSERET. 1997. Identification of nerve endings in cat extraocular muscles. Anat. Rec. **248**: 566–575.
62. RUSKELL, G.L. 1990. Golgi tendon organs in the proximal tendon of sheep extraocular muscles. Anat. Rec. **227**: 25–31.
63. BLUMER, R., J.R. LUKAS, R. WASICKY & R. MAYR. 2000. Presence and morphological variability of Golgi tendon organs in the distal portion of sheep extraocular muscle. Anat. Rec. **258**: 359–368.
64. RUSKELL, G.L. 1979. The incidence and variety of Golgi tendon organs in extraocular muscles of the rhesus monkey. J. Neurocytol. **8**: 639–653.
65. ZELENÁ, J. & T. SOUKUP. 1977. The development of Golgi tendon organs. J. Neurocytol. **6**: 171–194.
66. MAYR, R. 1977. Funktionelle Morphologie Der Augenmuskeln. G. Kommerell, Ed.: 1–15. J.F. Bergmann Verlag. München.
67. RICHMOND, F.J.R. et al. 1984. Palisade endings in human extraocular muscle. Invest. Ophthalmol. Visual Sci. **25**: 471–476.
68. BAKER, D. 1974. The morphology of muscle receptors. *In* Handbook of Sensory Physiology. C.C. Hunt, Ed.: 1–190.
69. PEDROSA-DOMELLOF, F., T. SOUKUP & L.E. THORNELL. 1991. Rat muscle spindle immunocytochemistry revisited. Histochemistry **96**: 327–338.
70. FUCHS, A.F. & E.S. LUSCHEI. 1971. Development of isometric tension in simian extraocular muscle. J. Physiol. **219**: 155–166.

Activity-Related Postlesional Vestibular Reorganization

NORBERT DIERINGER

Physiologisches Institut der LMU München, 80336 München, Germany

ABSTRACT: The synaptic convergence patterns of semicircular canal and macular afferent nerve inputs onto second-order vestibular neurons reorganize in adult frogs after a change in the activity of vestibular nerve afferent fibers. Axotomized afferent nerve fibers become silent after a vestibular nerve lesion, and second-order vestibular target neurons become disfacilitated. These changes initiate an activity-related process that was studied in detail *in vitro* two months after a section of the ramus anterior (RA) of N. VIII. The postlesional reaction results in an expansion of signals, preferentially from intact, remaining afferent nerve fibers, but also from excitatory commissural and spinal ascending fibers. This process of expansion takes weeks, is graded in its extent, and reversible in case of a nerve regeneration, but is not competitive, i.e., the synaptic contacts from axotomized afferent nerve fibers are maintained without a change in their efficacy.

Postlesional synaptic reorganization in the brainstem is restricted to the operated side, underlies the improved responsiveness of disfacilitated second-order vestibular neurons, but also their altered spatial response tuning. The functional consequences of this reorganization were studied *in vivo* two months after RA nerve section by recording abducens nerve responses during linear or angular accelerations. The vector orientations of best responses of the abducens nerve of chronic RA frogs evoked by linear or angular acceleration differed from the vector orientations of controls. In chronic RA frogs, linear acceleration evoked contralesional abducens nerve responses that originated from the utricle on the intact side and from the lagena, a vertical macular organ in frogs. Such an inadequate lagenar response component was absent in controls and in the ipsilesional abducens nerve of chronic RA frogs. Similar differences were detected in the direction of abducens nerve responses of chronic RA frogs during angular acceleration. Thus, compensatory vestibulo-ocular reflexes of chronic RA frogs became more symmetric in gain, but less precise in direction.

KEYWORDS: compensation; synaptic plasticity; signal expansion; spatial tuning; response vectors

INTRODUCTION

Some of the most severe acute behavioral deficits like ocular nystagmus and static head tilt normalize to a large extent spontaneously after unilateral labyrinthectomy (UL). The central process underlying this spontaneous recovery—"vestibular com-

---

Address for correspondence: Dr. N. Dieringer, Physiologisches Institut der LMU, Pettenkoferstr. 12, 80336 München, Germany. Voice: + 49 89 5996253; fax: + 49 89 5996216.
dieringer@phyl.med.uni-muenchen.de

pensation"—is considered by some investigators to represent a goal-directed recovery process (organized either in a bottom-up or in a top-down fashion). As a logical consequence of this basic assumption, all neural changes encountered after UL (during the period of behavioral compensation) are then considered to be adaptive, to contribute to behavioral recovery, and to represent in essence neural mechanisms of compensation. Proponents of this view argue, for example, that the recovery of a normal head posture after UL cannot be a random process. Alternative viewpoints question the presence of a goal-directed recovery process[1,2] and explain the normalization of static and dynamic behavioral deficits as an emerging property of central reactions that are not directed toward behavioral recovery.

The above question is directly related to the next, more clinically related question: is there a need for rehabilitative activities after UL or not? In the presence of a goal-directed, autonomous central process of functional recovery, if UL patients were to benefit from rehabilitation, it would be in terms of a more rapid onset and progress of recovery, but not in terms of an improved functional outcome. If, however, rehabilitative treatment is considered to be necessary for UL patients, it is important to know how it can support behavioral normalization. Obviously, it is of great importance in this context to know precisely the mechanisms that are activated by UL and how these mechanisms can be influenced after UL.

Cellular mechanisms are best studied in animal models, and some of these models are better suited than others; unfortunately, none of them is ideal. We exploited in frogs the favorable anatomical location of the labyrinthine organs in a bony bulla. This allowed us to section *in vivo* individual vestibular nerve branches under visual control and to isolate at a later stage the brain with the branches of the VIIIth nerves attached for *in vitro* experiments. We used the results from *in vitro* and *in vivo* control experiments for a comparison with results obtained from frogs that had undergone UL or a section of the ramus anterior (RA) of N. VIII two months earlier (chronic UL or RA frogs).

VESTIBULAR NERVE SECTION ACTIVATES AN ACTIVITY-RELATED PROCESS OF PLASTICITY

The synaptic efficacy of excitatory commissural inputs in the ipsilesional vestibular nuclei of frogs is significantly increased two months after unilateral labyrinthectomy (UL). These postlesional changes were first observed *in vivo*[3,4] and were later confirmed in a number of *in vitro* studies.[5–7] The alterations in the amplitudes of evoked field potentials reflected the changes in the amplitudes of excitatory postsynaptic potentials of recorded second-order vestibular neurons (2°VN) on the operated side of the brainstem. Therefore, Kunkel and Dieringer[6] used evoked commissural field potentials on the operated side to study the time course of changes and to compare the alterations after a pre- and postganglionic vestibular nerve section, respectively.

After a proximal, *postganglionic* section of N. VIII, the central part of the vestibular nerve degenerated rapidly (within 2–4 days; FIG. 1B). However, such a degeneration was absent even two months after a more peripheral, *preganglionic* nerve section (FIG. 1A). In spite of these dramatic anatomically different consequences, electric stimulation of N. VIII on the intact side evoked commissural field potentials

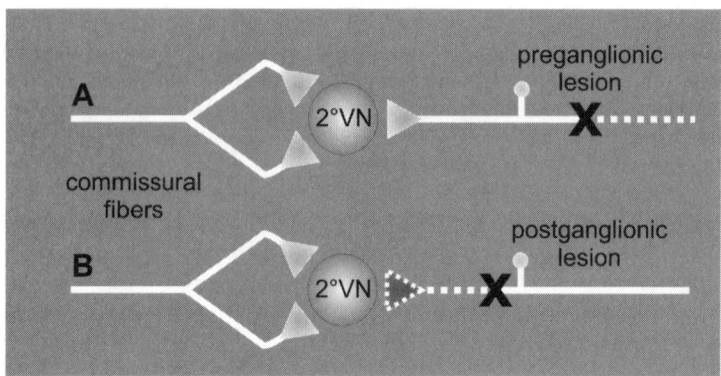

FIGURE 1. The VIIIth nerve was sectioned *in vivo* either preganglionically (**A**) or postganglionically (**B**). The axotomized nerve fibers were silenced in either case. However, after a preganglionic section the axotomized nerve fibers did not degenerate within the next two months, whereas all afferent nerve fibers degenerated within a few days after a postganglionic nerve section. The differential effects of these two conditions on the time course and on the extent of postlesional reactions of commissural synaptic inputs onto second-order vestibular neurons (2°VN) were analyzed.

on the operated side of chronic UL frogs (i.e., two months after UL) that had increased in amplitude to an almost identical extent of about 90% after preganglionic, as after postganglionic, nerve section. Even more surprising, the onset and the time course of this increase were practically the same in both groups of frogs. Obviously, degeneration and its metabolic products or reactions of glial cells were not instrumental in the activation of this postlesional reaction. However, a common consequence of both types of nerve lesions was the silencing of vestibular nerve afferent fibers (due to axotomy) that resulted in a disfacilitation of 2°VN (due to the loss of excitatory inputs from afferent nerve fibers). Apparently, the loss of electrical activity in afferent nerve fibers was instrumental in the activation of an increase in the synaptic efficacy of commissural inputs (for more direct evidence see below).

The increase in the synaptic efficacy after UL could have resulted, for example, from the development of a postsynaptic supersensitivity of disfacilitated 2°VN. This possibility, however, can be ruled out because excitatory commissural inputs use glutamate as a transmitter as do afferent nerve inputs, and only the commissural but not the afferent nerve evoked field potentials increased in amplitude. Changes in synaptic transmission could have resulted from a strengthening of already-existing commissural connections, or from the additional activation of new ones. This alternative and the hypothesis of an activity-related process were investigated in depth in a series of *in vitro* studies by Goto, Straka, and Dieringer.[8–10] A prerequisite for these experiments was a detailed and precise knowledge of the convergence patterns of afferent canal and macular signals onto 2°VN[11] (see also Straka and Dieringer, this volume) and of 2°VN onto extraocular motoneurons.[12] The consistency and predictability of the spatial convergence patterns of macular and canal-related signals in each of the extraocular motor pools allow the detection of alterations in the spatial organization due to postlesional reorganization.

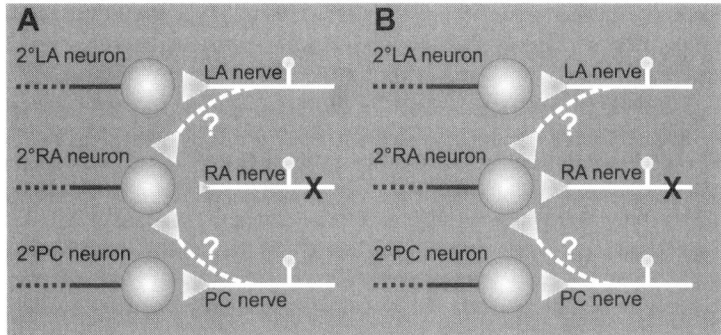

FIGURE 2. The ramus anterior (RA) of the VIIIth nerve was sectioned to investigate a possible expansion of synaptic signals from intact afferent nerve fibers onto those second vestibular neurons that had lost an excitation from their vestibular nerve afferent fibers (i.e., 2°RA neurons) due to axotomy. Two possible postlesional reaction patterns were conceivable: (**A**) repression of silenced RA nerve afferent synapses and compensatory expansion of signals from intact afferent nerve fibers (e.g., from lagenar to LA to, or posterior vertical canal to PC to nerve) or (**B**) expansion of LA and PC nerve signals even though silenced RA nerve synapses are maintained. The relative number of 2°LA and 2°PC was expected to remain unaltered in either case.

The ramus anterior (RA) of N. VIII was selectively sectioned *in vivo* in a first series of experiments (FIG. 2). Two months later the brain was isolated with the nerve branches of N. VIII attached. In this experiment, the afferent nerve fibers of the RA (from the horizontal and anterior vertical canal and from the utricle) were axotomized and thus silenced, whereas the nerve branches of the ramus posterior (posterior vertical canal, lagena, and saccule) remained intact. Therefore, this restricted nerve section created a competitive situation between axotomized RA nerve fibers and intact ramus posterior afferent nerve fibers within their common projection areas on the operated side, for example, in the vestibular nuclei. If an activity-related process were generated by the inactivation of RA nerve fibers, one should expect a reorganization of the remaining, intact afferent nerve inputs, similar to the situation in the somatosensory system after the amputation of an arm, a hand, or a digit.[13–15] In the course of this reorganization, the presynaptic terminals of axotomized and silenced RA afferent fibers might either become repressed (FIG. 2A) or maintained (FIG. 2B). Field potentials evoked by electric stimulation of the sectioned N. VIII on the operated side (after a preganglionic nerve section) were similar in amplitude to those recorded in controls or on the intact side of chronic UL frogs,[6] suggesting that the synaptic contacts between axotomized afferent nerve fibers and 2°VN were maintained.

An expansion of afferent input signals from intact afferent nerve fibers onto those 2°VN that had lost their afferent nerve activation (i.e., disfacilitated 2°VN) was expected and was in fact also demonstrated.[8] Two months after RA nerve section, the brain together with the attached N. VIII was isolated for *in vitro* experiments. On the operated side, the sectioned RA nerve branch was stimulated electrically in order to

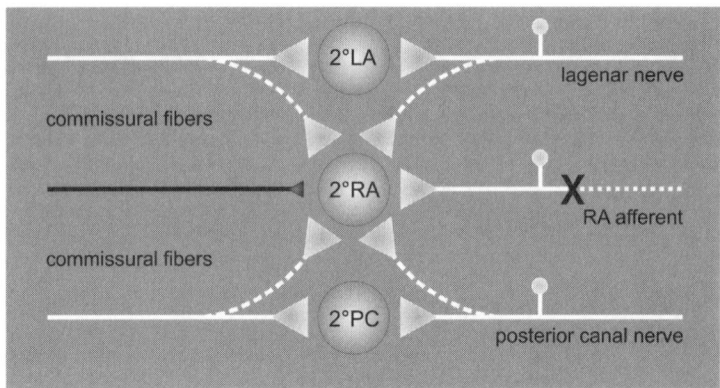

FIGURE 3. Summary of known synaptic changes encountered in the ipsilesional vestibular nuclei two months after a section of the ramus anterior (RA) of the VIIIth nerve. RA nerve stimulation evoked normal field potentials and monosynaptic excitatory postsynaptic potentials in 2°RA. In addition, many more of these neurons were monosynaptically excited by the posterior vertical canal nerve than on the intact side of the same individuals or in controls. Coplanar commissural inhibition was masked by strongly enhanced commissural excitation, in part from the coplanar canal and in part from other canals on the intact side. Postlesional reorganization in the vestibular nuclei was restricted to disfacilitated 2°RA neurons.

identify 2°VN on the basis of a monosynaptic input from the RA nerve. The intact posterior vertical canal nerve branch was stimulated to investigate a possible expansion of these input signals. From the results of control experiments, we expected that about 15% of the encountered 2°VN in chronic RA frogs receive a monosynaptic input exclusively from the posterior vertical canal nerve (2°PC neurons), about 56% a monosynaptic input only from the RA nerve (2°RA neurons), and only about 27% a monosynaptic input from the RA nerve, as well as from the posterior vertical canal nerve (2°RA + PC neurons). Indeed, a very similar distribution of classified 2°VN was found in the vestibular nuclei of the intact side. On the operated side, however, many more 2°VN responded to posterior vertical canal nerve stimulation than on the intact side of the same individual or in controls.[8] Interestingly, the percentage of 2°RA neurons had dropped significantly (from about 57% to about 34%) and the percentage of 2°RA + PC neurons had increased by a similar amount (from about 30% to about 53%), whereas the percentage of 2°PC neurons was practically the same on the intact (about 10%) and on the operated side (about 13%). In essence, the signals from intact afferent nerve fibers expanded on the operated side of RA frogs and contacted significantly more 2°RA neurons than in controls. The synapses from silenced RA nerve fibers were maintained and the synaptic efficacy of these connections remained unaltered.

Reorganization of commissural inputs on the operated side of the brainstem was investigated in the same *in vitro* preparations by separate electric stimulation of the three semicircular canal nerves on the intact side. In controls, most 2° canal neurons receive a commissural inhibition from the coplanar semicircular canal on the contralateral side and commissural excitatory inputs from one or two remaining contralateral semicircular canals.[16] In chronic RA frogs, the amplitudes of commissural field potentials evoked by separate electric stimulation of each of the three semicircular canal nerves on the intact side were increased. This increase resulted from an expansion of commissural excitatory inputs onto disfacilitated 2°RA and 2°RA + PC neurons and a weakening of coplanar commissural inhibition. An inhibitory commissural input from the coplanar semicircular canal on the intact side was encountered in significantly fewer disfacilitated 2°RA and 2°RA + PC neurons than in controls. Furthermore, many of these disfacilitated neurons received excitatory commissural inputs from all three contralesional semicircular canals. The inputs of 2°PC neurons on the operated side served as an internal control. Most of them received an inhibitory commissural input from the contralateral anterior vertical canal in addition to excitatory commissural inputs as in control animals.

Postlesional vestibular reorganization is a selective and graded reaction. After UL the signals from the axotomized N. VIII afferent fibers did not expand. Consistent with this negative result was the absence of an expansion of axotomized RA afferent nerve signals in the presence of an expansion of the signals from those afferent nerve fibers that were spared by the RA nerve section. However, after UL as after RA nerve section, the signals from excitatory commissural fibers terminating in the vestibular nuclei on the operated side expanded with a very similar time course onto those 2°VN that had lost their afferent nerve activation (i.e., became disfacilitated) due to axotomy.[10] These results strongly support the hypothesis that a vestibular nerve lesion activates an activity-related central process with disfacilitated 2°VN playing a dominant role. Thus far, the question as to whether signals from intact afferent nerve fibers expand in addition to excitatory commissural fibers (provided some afferent nerve fibers were spared by the lesion) or whether excitatory commissural fibers expand only if the number of intact afferent nerve fibers became too small was unsolved. This question was studied with vestibular nerve lesions that were limited either to the utricular or to the horizontal plus anterior vertical canal nerve branches. Two months after a section of the utricular nerve branch, no expansion of excitatory commissural inputs was found, but an expansion of signals from each of the three ipsilesional afferent canal nerve fibers was observed. However, after the combined horizontal and anterior vertical canal nerve section, neither excitatory commissural nor afferent RA nerve or posterior vertical canal nerve signals had expanded. Thus, the expansion of signals from intact afferent and excitatory commissural fibers is not an all-or-nothing response but a graded reaction. Either a minimum of afferent nerve fibers has to be silenced to activate this reaction or the reaction, after a combined horizontal and anterior vertical canal nerve section, was not strong enough to be detected with the rather crude method of evoked field potential recordings. As a result of the expansion of signals from excitatory inputs, the reduced excitation of disfacilitated 2°VN was replaced. As an alternative, a change in the intrinsic membrane properties of disfacilitated 2°VN could make these neurons spontaneously active again, as reported for some medial vestibular neurons in rat and guinea pig.[17,18] However, as far as there was a choice, disfacilitated 2°VN preferred not only excitatory to inhibitory inputs, but more importantly, afferent nerve to excitatory commissural inputs. These preferences indicate that electrical reactivation of 2°VN was not one of the top criteria for this selection. More likely, but still speculative, it was the composition of trophic factors that made some excitatory inputs more attractive than others.

FUNCTIONAL CONSEQUENCES OF POSTLESIONAL VESTIBULAR REORGANIZATION

The consequences of a postlesional synaptic reorganization were studied *in vivo* by recording the abducens nerve activity on the intact side of chronic RA frogs in response to linear acceleration on a sled. Horizontal linear acceleration evoked abducens nerve responses with an amplitude that depended on the orientation of the frog with respect to the direction of acceleration (FIG. 4A). From the null points of these responses (minimal response amplitude), we calculated the maximal activation direction (MAD) in the horizontal plane. Horizontal linear acceleration evoked no response in RA frogs acutely after the lesion, but did so in each of the tested chronic RA frogs. Differences in response sensitivity and onset latency allowed a separation of chronic RA frogs into those with and those without a functional RA nerve regeneration (i.e., reinnervation of vestibular sense organs). Here, only results from chronic RA frogs without a peripheral reinnervation will be reported.

Minimal abducens nerve responses were evoked on the intact side during longitudinal (about 0° in FIG. 4A) and maximal responses during rightward/leftward accelerations (about 90° in FIG. 4A). These responses must have originated in the utricle on the intact side, because abducens nerve responses are no longer acutely

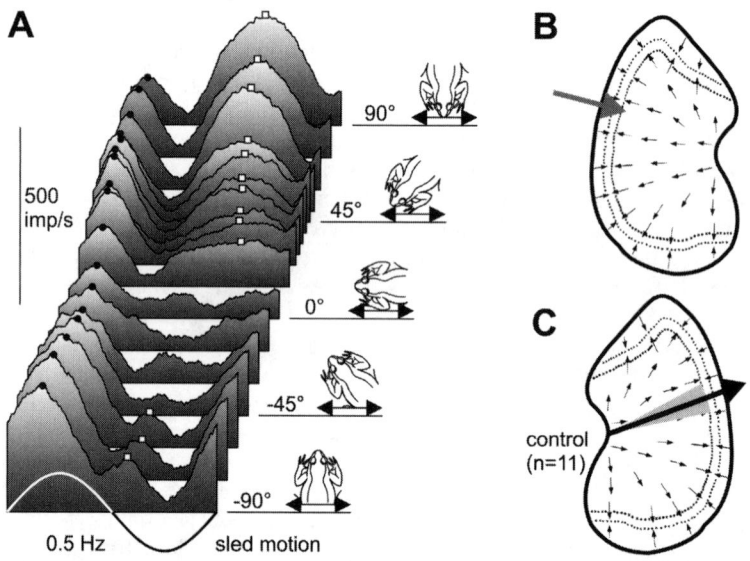

FIGURE 4. The instantaneous abducens nerve discharge rate in response to horizontal linear acceleration depends in its magnitude on the orientation of the static head position on the sled (**A**). The head orientation for maximal abducens nerve responses represents in control frogs the axis of a sector of hair cells on the contralateral utricle (**C**) from which these responses originated. The responses shown in **A** were recorded from the abducens nerve on the intact side of a chronic RA frog. Since the utricle on the operated side was disconnected, the responses must have originated in the utricle on the intact side (**B**). These signals were then mediated by excitatory commissural fibers to the operated side and by some of the second-order vestibular neurons to abducens motoneurons on the intact side.

present after contralateral RA nerve section[12] and because the utricle on the operated side was disconnected from ipsilateral 2°VN. The sector of hair cells that gave rise to these responses was either located laterally or medially with respect to the utricular striola. Since only excitatory but not inhibitory commissural fibers expanded their signals on the operated side (see above), the sector of hair cells is assumed to be located lateral with respect to the striola (FIG. 4B). Signals from this sector are then further assumed to be mediated by 2°VN sending a commissural axon across the midline to contact disfacilitated 2°VN on the operated side, some of which project then to the contralateral abducens motor pool. The orientation of the MAD in control frogs (FIG. 4C) is rather similar, even though less scattered than that in chronic RA frogs.

Linear vertical acceleration evoked abducens nerve responses on the intact side that differed more strongly from those in controls. In FIGURE 5A a chronic RA frog was accelerated first horizontally along the MAD of the recorded abducens nerve (0°), then in a ramp-like fashion and finally in vertical direction (± 90° in FIG. 5A). As in control frogs, the response magnitude declined with the angle of sled inclination, but contrary to the situation in control frogs responses were present during vertical linear acceleration (FIG. 5B, C). In chronic RA frogs, a response component originating from a vertical macular organ (lagena) was superimposed on the utricular response component (dotted curve in FIG. 5B). Such a lagenar component was absent in controls and was also absent in the ipsilesional abducens nerve of chronic RA frogs.[19]

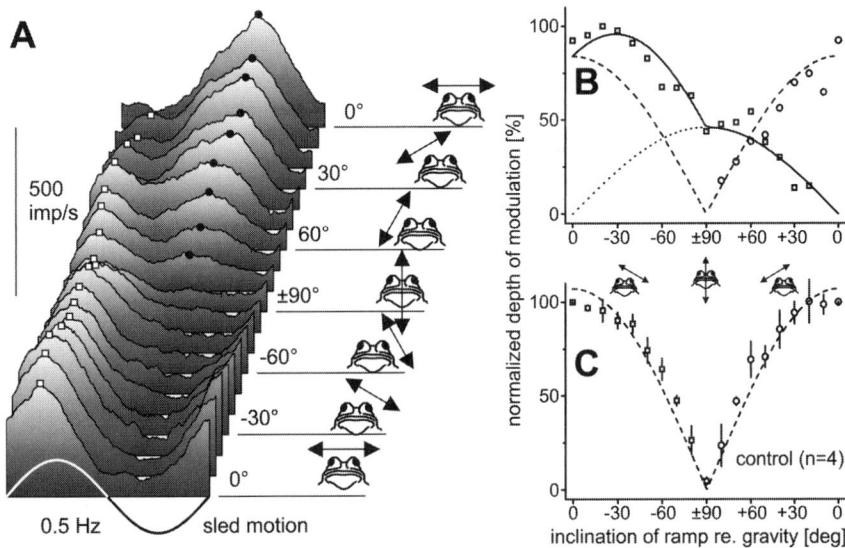

FIGURE 5. The instantaneous abducens nerve discharge rate in response to ramp-like oscillations on a sled depends in its magnitude on the inclination of the sled motion with respect to the gravity vector (**A**). Vertical linear acceleration (± 90°) evoked a response in chronic RA frogs (**A, B**), but not in controls (**C**). Therefore, utricular responses similar to those of controls (**C**) were superimposed in chronic RA frogs by a response component from the lagena (a vertical macular organ in frogs) as indicated in **B** by the dotted fit curve.

NERVE INJURY ACTIVATES A FUNDAMENTAL NEURAL REACTION PATTERN

The synaptic reorganization described here after vestibular nerve section was studied in frog and one might wonder if similar results would be obtained also from other species after a vestibular nerve lesion. So far this is the first study that investigated the consequences of synaptic reorganization after a vestibular nerve lesion for the spatial response tuning of the vestibulo-ocular reflex. However, plasticity after sensory loss in adult mammals including man was studied on the somatosensory system, the visual and the auditory systems.[20] Here we compare the features known from our plasticity studies after vestibular nerve lesions in frogs with studies on the postlesional plasticity of the somatosensory system in primates.

Even though most of these studies investigated postlesional alterations in the organization of sensory representations in primary sensory cortices, the reorganization of these sensory maps occurs at multiple anatomical sites that include thalamus and brainstem.[21] Reactivation of disfacilitated neurons after a nerve lesion by the expansion of signals from nearby intact excitatory neurons is one of the common features in these studies. Reversibility of the reorganized maps to the original map in case of nerve regeneration is another common feature. Sensory map reorganization is associated with the emergence of undesired sensations such as phantom sensations or even phantom pain[15] and tinnitus.[22] Similarly inadequate is the substitution of silenced vestibular nerve afferent inputs by spatially inappropriate active vestibular nerve afferent or commissural inputs as evidenced by the emergence of vestibulo-ocular reflex responses with directional abnormalities.

Results from our *in vitro* experiments clearly demonstrated that disfacilitated 2°VN did not recruit the expansion of excitatory inputs in general, but only that of particular inputs. The purpose of this selective activation could have been reflex repair, substitution of reduced excitation, or reduced trophic input. However, from a behavioral point of view, the preference of 2°VN was less than optimal. After a selective utricular nerve branch section, excitatory commissural fibers from the contralesional utricle were available and inputs from sectors located laterally with respect to the striola would have contributed the spatially appropriate excitatory signals for 2° utricular neurons on the operated side. However, not these spatially appropriate commissural inputs, but rather afferent nerve fibers from the three ipsilesional canal nerve branches with inappropriate signals had expanded and were accepted. As a consequence, the spatial response tuning of abducens motoneurons on the intact side but not on the operated side was altered as exemplified by the emergence of an inappropriate lagenar response component. Obviously, the selection of additional excitatory inputs by disfacilitated 2°VN is not made with respect to a repair of network properties or a behavioral recovery, but rather with respect to metabolic needs of these neurons.

Synaptic reorganization after a sensory loss is neither a goal-directed process (in the sense of behavioral repair) nor should it be considered as a model for conditioned (motor) learning. In fact, the vestibulo-ocular reflex of cats was asymmetric even months after unilateral labyrinthectomy in spite of the fact that these cats could readily alter their reflex gain during a motor-learning paradigm.[23] However, it should be remembered in this context that recovery of these experimental animals progressed spontaneously, i.e., without assistance in a dull environment. Given that the underlying process is activity related, rehabilitative training can shape the selection of active excitatory inputs and thereby improve the final outcome.

CONCLUSION

The central nervous system of adult vertebrates is highly plastic in different ways. Silencing of vestibular nerve inputs due to axotomy provokes an activity-related process of central reorganization. Extensive similarities exist between the synaptic reorganization in the vestibular nuclei of frogs (after a vestibular nerve lesion) and the cortical and subcortical reorganization of the somatosensory system in mammals (e.g., after the amputation of a digit, hand, or arm). These similarities include the expansion of excitatory inputs onto disfacilitated neighboring neurons on the sensory side and the emergence of undesired consequences on the motor side. Therefore, we suggest that silencing of sensory inputs due to nerve injury activates a fundamental neural reaction pattern that is common between sensory modalities and vertebrate species, but differs from conditioned motor learning. The emergence of undesired functional consequences during the spontaneous, unassisted period of vestibular compensation is of clinical relevance. The activity-related nature of the underlying postlesional process can be exploited by rehabilitative training to shape the subsequent reorganization after vestibular nerve lesion.

ACKNOWLEDGMENT

The support of Sonderforschungsbereich 462 of Deutsche Forschungsgemeinschaft (Teilprojekt B2) is gratefully acknowledged.

REFERENCES

1. LLINÁS, R. & K. WALTON. 1979. Vestibular compensation, a distributed property of the central nervous system. *In* Integration in the Nervous System. H. Asanuma & V. J. Wilson, Eds.: 145–166. Igaku Shoin. Tokyo.
2. DIERINGER, N. & W. PRECHT. 1986. Functional recovery following peripheral vestibular lesions: due to–in spite of–in parallel with–or without synaptic reorganization? *In* Adaptive Processes in Visual and Oculomotor Systems. E.L. Keller & D.S. Zee, Eds.: 383–390, Pergamon Press. Oxford.
3. DIERINGER, N. & W. PRECHT. 1977. Modified synaptic input in chronically deafferented vestibular neurons. Nature **269:** 431–433.
4. DIERINGER, N. & W. PRECHT. 1979. Mechanisms of compensation for vestibular deficits in the frog. I. Modification of the excitatory commissural system. Exp. Brain Res. **36:** 311–328.
5. KNÖPFEL, T. & N. DIERINGER. 1988. Lesion-induced vestibular plasticity in the frog: Are N-methyl-D-aspartate receptors involved? Exp. Brain Res. **72:** 129–134.
6. KUNKEL, A.W. & N. DIERINGER. 1994. Morphological and electrophysiological consequences of unilateral pre- versus postganglionic vestibular lesions in the frog. J. Comp. Physiol. **174:** 621–632.
7. DIERINGER, N. 1995. "Vestibular compensation": Neural plasticity and its relations to functional recovery after labyrinthine lesions in frogs and other vertebrates. Prog. Neurobiol. **46:** 97–129.

8. GOTO, F., H. STRAKA & N. DIERINGER. 2000. Expansion of afferent vestibular signals after the section of one of the vestibular nerve branches. J. Neurophysiol. **84:** 581–584.
9. GOTO, F., H. STRAKA & N. DIERINGER. 2001 Postlesional vestibular reorganization in frogs: evidence for a basic reaction pattern after nerve injury. J. Neurophysiol. **85:** 2643–2646.
10. GOTO, F., H. STRAKA & N. DIERINGER. 2002. Gradual and reversible central vestibular reorganization in frog after selective labyrinthine nerve branch lesions. Exp. Brain Res. **147:** 374–386.
11. STRAKA, H., S. HOLLER & F. GOTO. 2002. Patterns of canal and otolith afferent input convergence in frog second order vestibular neurons. J. Neurophysiol. **88:** 2287–2301.
12. ROHREGGER, M. & N. DIERINGER. 2002. Principles of linear and angular vestibuloocular reflex organization in the frog. J. Neurophysiol. **87:** 385–398.
13. MERZENICH, M.M. et al. 1984. Somatosensory cortical map changes following digit amputation in adult monkeys. J. Comp. Neurol. **224:** 591–605.
14. PONS, T.P. et al. 1991. Massive cortical reorganization after sensory deafferentation in adult macaques. Science **252:** 1857-1860.
15. FLOR, H. et al. 1998. Cortical reorganization and phantom phenomena in congenital and traumatic upper-extremity amputees. Exp. Brain Res. **119:** 205–212.
16. HOLLER, S. & H. STRAKA. 2001. Plane-specific brainstem commissural inhibition in frog second order semicircular canal neurons. Exp. Brain Res. **137:** 190–196.
17. VIBERT, N. et al. 1999. Plastic changes underlying vestibular compensation in the guinea-pig persist in isolated, in vitro whole brain preparations. Neuroscience **93:** 413–432.
18. CAMERON, S. & M.B. DUTIA. 1997. Cellular basis of vestibular compensation: changes in intrinsic excitability of MVN neurons. Neuroreport **8:** 2595–2599.
19. ROHREGGER, M. & N. DIERINGER. 2003. Postlesional vestibular reorganization improves the gain but impairs the spatial tuning of the maculo-ocular reflex in frogs. J. Neurophysiol. In press.
20. KAAS, J. 2002. Sensory loss and cortical reorganization in mature primates. In Progress in Brain Research, Vol. 138. M.A. Hofman, G.J. Boer, A.J.G.D. Holtmaat, E.J.W. van Someren, J. Verhaagen & D.F.S. Swaab, Eds.: 167–176. Elsevier Science Publishers. Amsterdam.
21. FLORENCE, S.L. & J.H. KAAS. 1995. Large-scale reorganization at multiple levels of the somatosensory pathway follows therapeutic amputation of the hand in monkeys. J. Neurosci. **15:** 8083–8095.
22. MÜHLNICKEL, W. et al. 1998. Reorganization of auditory cortex in tinnitus. Proc. Natl. Acad. Sci. USA **95:** 10340–10343.
23. MAIOLI, C., W. PRECHT & S. RIED. 1985. On the role of the vestibulo-ocular reflex plasticity in recovery after unilateral peripheral vestibular lesions. Exp. Brain Res. **50:** 259–274.

Discharge Patterns of Cerebellar Output Neurons in the Caudal Fastigial Nucleus during Head-Free Gaze Shifts in Primates

SANDRA C. BRETTLER, ALBERT F. FUCHS, AND LEO LING

Department of Physiology & Biophysics and Regional Primate Research Center, University of Washington, Seattle, Washington 98195, USA

ABSTRACT: Lesion studies in both human and non-human primates indicate that the cerebellum is important for accurate and stereotyped saccadic eye movements. Based on single-unit recordings and pharmacological inactivations in head-fixed monkeys, we suggested that the caudal fastigial nucleus (CFN) provides the brainstem saccade generator with a burst that helps accelerate contraversive saccades and decelerate ipsiversive ones. Here we examine this suggestion during head-free gaze shifts where there can be a 10-fold difference in saccade duration. First, the timing of the burst does not depend on whether the gaze shift has a head component. When a family of either ipsiversive or contraversive gaze shifts with a variety of saccadic durations is aligned on gaze onset, the high-frequency burst in the associated rasters occurs progressively later as saccade duration increases. Realignment of the same rasters with the end of the saccade reveals a tight timing of burst end with saccade end for all 10 CFN burst neurons studied. The delayed bursts for contraversive saccades were unexpected based on the early burst illustrated in the published head-fixed data. One hypothesis is that the late activity helps terminate contraversive as well as ipsiversive gaze shifts. An alternative explanation is that the late CFN burst could still be used as an excitatory drive to promote the late reacceleration or prolonged velocity plateau that is present during large gaze shifts.

KEYWORDS: cerebellum; saccades; discharge patterns; fastigial nucleus; saccade burst generator

INTRODUCTION

Experiments involving both naturally occurring lesions in humans and more deliberate lesions in monkeys have made it clear that the cerebellum is indispensable for the generation of accurate saccadic eye movements. In particular, the midline cerebellum, both the oculomotor vermis (lobules 6 and 7) and the fastigial nucleus (FN), the output nucleus to which it projects, seem to be the crucial elements.[4–8] In experiments begun in 1988, the lab of our honoree, Ulrich Büttner, revealed that only

---

Address for correspondence: Sandra Brettler, Department of Physiology & Biophysics and Regional Primate Research Center, University of Washington, Seattle, WA 98195. Voice: 206-543-0849.
brettler@u.washington.edu

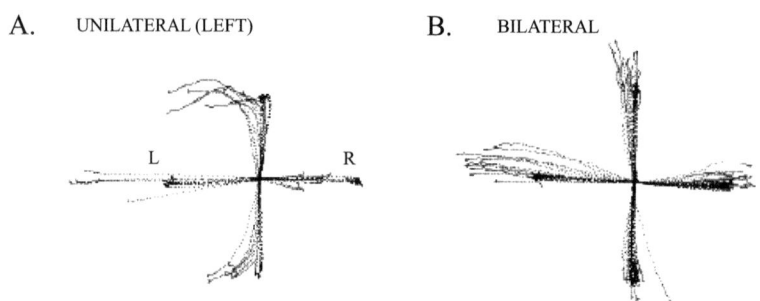

FIGURE 1. Effects of unilateral (**A**) and bilateral (**B**) pharmacological inactivations of the CFN on saccades in the head-fixed monkey. Saccadic trajectories are shown in two-dimensional space in response to targets jumping from the primary direction of gaze to loci at 10° eccentricities on the four cardinal axes. *Darker traces* are control trials and *lighter traces* are post-injection trials.

the caudal FN (CFN) contained neurons that discharged with voluntary eye movements, both saccades and smooth pursuit, whereas the neurons of the rostral FN responded best during vestibular yaw rotation and full-field optokinetic stimulation.[1] In subsequent years, Dr. Büttner concentrated on the vestibular zone, and his colleagues in Seattle pursued the role of the caudal zone in the control of saccades.

With the head fixed, most saccade-related neurons in the CFN discharge a burst of spikes for saccades in all directions, unlike the directionally specific burst neurons in the brainstem saccade generator. However, CFN neurons do have a preferred direction in that they discharge an early burst that usually leads contraversive saccades and a later burst that lags the onset of ipsiversive saccades. This difference in burst timing with saccade direction led us to suggest that the role of the CFN is to help the brainstem saccade generator accelerate contraversive saccades and help decelerate ipsiversive ones.[3] This suggestion was supported by the results of a study by Robinson *et al.*[10] in which one CFN was inactivated by the $GABA_A$ agonist, muscimol (FIG. 1A). Prior to inactivation, saccades from the primary direction of gaze to targets located at 10° eccentricities along the horizontal and vertical meridians exhibited essentially linear trajectories. Furthermore, their landing loci were tightly clustered, confirming that normal saccades are very stereotyped. After the left CFN was inactivated, rightward (contraversive) saccades were hypometric and leftward (ipsiversive) saccades were hypermetric. Also, saccades to targets on the vertical meridian veered off their control trajectories in the direction of the inactivated CFN. Note that in the absence of the oculomotor signals from the cerebellum, the brainstem saccade generator, which now presumably is driven predominantly by its other input from the superior colliculus, produces extremely inaccurate and very variable saccades. These data are consistent with our previous model in which unilateral inactivation is eliminating a contraversive acceleratory drive and an ipsiversive deceleratory drive.

The results of bilateral inactivation of both CFNs, however, appear to be at odds with the model. After inactivation of both CFNs, saccades in both horizontal directions are hypermetric (FIG. 1B), suggesting that the CFN may actually be required to decelerate saccades in all horizontal directions. If this were true, we might expect to see that the timing of the burst is well aligned not only with the end of ipsiversive saccades, but with the end of contraversive saccades as well. Such a timing relation is best examined when elicited saccades exhibit a range of durations. With the head held, the variation in saccade duration is relatively modest. With the head free, however, the duration of gaze saccades can vary from as little as 20 ms to over 200 ms. In this paper, we have used this 10-fold variation in head-free gaze durations to reveal a heretofore unexpected tight relation between the end of the burst and the end of *contraversive* saccades.

METHODS

Juvenile rhesus monkeys ($n = 2$) were trained to fixate small light-emitting diodes (LEDs) arrayed at 1° intervals on a hemispheric array located at a distance of 24 inches from the eye. The LEDs were positioned along the horizontal and vertical meridians and along arcs located halfway between, that is, every 45°. Shifts in the direction of gaze were elicited by extinguishing one LED and immediately lighting another. The monkey sat in a primate chair with shoulder or hip restraints to impair upper-body movement, but was otherwise completely free to move both its eyes and head to acquire the lighted LED. Eye position in space (gaze, G) and head position in space (H) were each measured by the rotating magnetic field–coil technique.[2,9]

Extracelluar single-unit activity was recorded with homemade iron-plated tungsten microelectrodes (~1MΩ) that were introduced hydraulically into the cerebellum through a chronic chamber placed vertically over a craniotomy centered on the midline at P. 9. Unit activity (10 μs resolution) and horizontal and vertical gaze, head, and target position were digitized online at 1 kHz or recorded to tape (Vetter 4000A) to be digitized off-line. Eye position was reconstructed off-line by subtracting head position from gaze position.

The digitized data were individually displayed and analyzed manually off-line using customized computer programs. These programs allowed us to measure the salient features of the saccade (e.g., amplitude, duration, and peak velocity) and the associated spike trains (burst onset, offset, duration, and peak and average firing rate). These data were then exported into another customized program and Microsoft Excel to perform linear regression analyses on burst characteristics (e.g., burst end time) and any saccadic parameter (e.g., gaze end time).

RESULTS

FIGURE 2 documents the behavior of a representative CFN neuron while a monkey tracks horizontal target steps of 20° and 60° with its head free to rotate. For both small and large gaze shifts, the CFN activity for saccades with similar metrics is somewhat variable as previously reported.[3] For small gaze shifts of 20°, the average burst for the 8 essentially identical gaze shifts illustrated began near the onset of ipsiversive saccades, but slightly led the onset of contraversive saccades. This timing pattern is similar to data obtained with the head held,[3,7] suggesting that the timing of the burst is not influenced by the head movement, per se. For large gaze shifts,

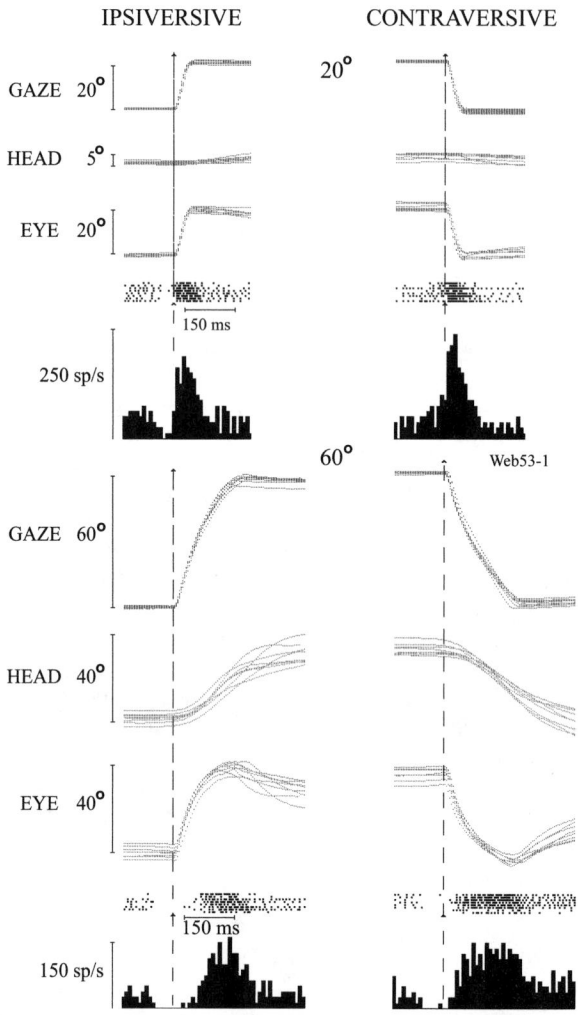

FIGURE 2. Burst timing of a representative CFN neuron during small (20°) and large (60°) horizontal gaze shifts with the head free. For each of the four sets of movements, the three components of a gaze shift (GAZE, gaze position in space; HEAD, head position in space; and EYE, eye position in head; GAZE-HEAD) are shown for 8 nearly identical gaze shifts together with their associated rasters and an average histogram. Note that for the 20° gaze shifts there is essentially no head contribution to the gaze shift.

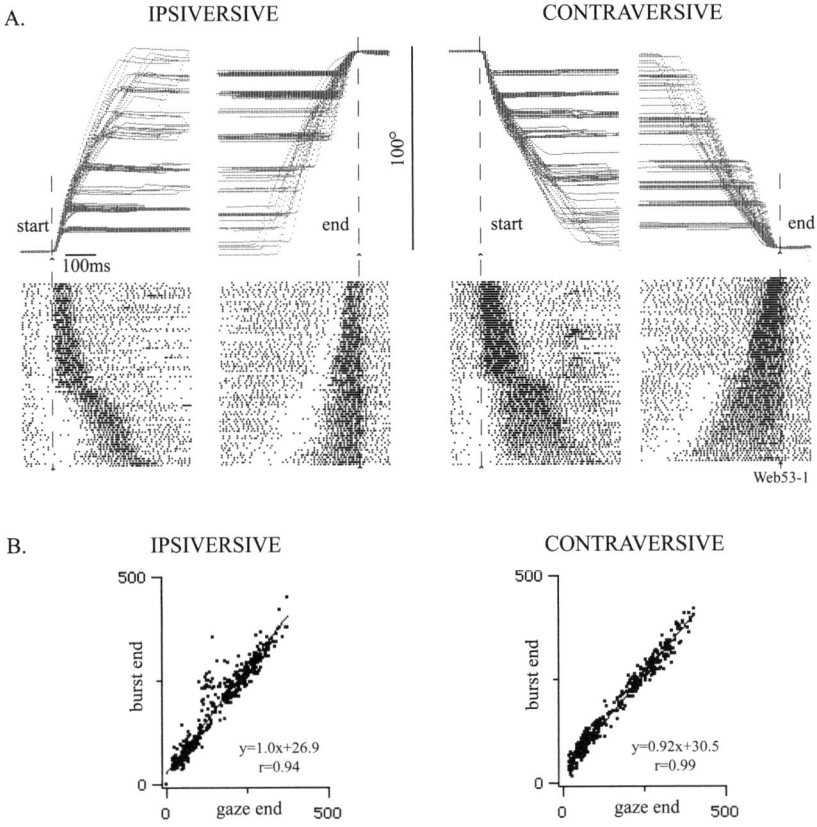

FIGURE 3. Timing of CFN bursts relative to saccade onset and end during head-free gaze shifts. (**A**) Families of head-free ipsiversive and contraversive gaze shifts of different sizes and hence durations aligned on saccade start time (*left-hand* columns) and saccade end time (*right-hand* columns). The associated rasters are ordered from *top to bottom* in terms of increasing saccade duration. (**B**) Plots of burst end time as a function of ipsiversive and contraversive gaze end time.

where there is a substantial head movement component, the burst for ipsiversive saccades is delayed relative to saccade onset with the peak discharge for this neuron occurring near the end of the gaze/eye movement. This shift in burst timing is consistent with our view based on head-fixed data that the CFN helps to terminate ipsiversive saccades. Unexpectedly, the burst associated with large contraversive saccades also is delayed relative to saccade onset so it occurs closer to saccade end. This late burst would appear to be inconsistent with our previous view that the CFN burst helps to accelerate contraversive saccades.

The increasing burst lag relative to saccade onset can be appreciated by considering the activity associated with a family of horizontal saccades with varying durations. In FIGURE 3A, such a family of representative rasters for the unit of FIGURE 2 are aligned on saccade onset and ordered, top to bottom, according to increasing saccade duration. It is clear that the delay of burst onset relative to saccade onset increases as the ipsiversive saccades become longer in duration. Similar increasing delays in burst timing relative to saccade onset as saccade duration increases also are present for contraversive saccades. In addition to the delayed burst, the illustrated unit has a clear pause before the burst. In other CFN units, the contraversive preburst pause was observed less frequently than the ipsiversive preburst pause.

The high-frequency burst is well timed with the end of the saccade. This can be appreciated by aligning the same data with the end of the saccade (right-hand columns, FIG. 3A). For this unit, the burst ends consistently with saccade end for both ipsiversive and contraversive saccades of all durations (and hence sizes), including those without (uppermost rasters) and with (lowermost rasters) an associated head movement. To quantify the timing of the burst relative to the saccade, we plot in FIGURE 3B the burst end time versus saccade end time for the entire data set of the unit illustrated in FIGURE 3A. The data are nicely captured by linear relations with regression coefficients for ipsiversive and contraversive saccades of 0.94 and 0.99 and with slopes of 1.0 and 0.92, respectively, indicating that the end of the burst is well correlated with the end of the saccade.

As a preliminary analysis, we constructed similar plots of burst end versus saccade end for 10 CFN burst neurons. For ipsiversive saccades, the correlation coefficient averaged 0.91 ± 0.09 (range: 0.72–0.98); the slopes averaged 0.97 ± 0.11 (range: 0.72–1.16); and the intercepts averaged 36.9 ms $\pm$ 45.3 (range: −8.2–147.6 ms). For contraversive saccades the correlation coefficient averaged 0.94 ± 0.06 (range: 0.8–0.99); the slopes averaged 0.95 ± 0.12 (range: 0.73–1.14), and the intercepts averaged 32.3 m $\pm$ 38.1 (range: 2.57–136.5). Therefore, the burst of our population of CFN neurons ends nicely with the end of the saccade.

In addition, we examined the timing of the peak firing rate of the burst relative to saccade end time for the same 10 neurons. These relationships were also strong (ipsiversive average slope: 0.84 ± 0.15, contraversive: 0.80 ± 0.14; ipsiversive average intercept: -7.13 ± 28.15, contraversive: -17.17 ± 14.78; and ipsiversive average correlation coefficient: 0.92 ± 0.08, contraversive: 0.91 ± 0.07). The early occurrence of peak firing relative to saccade end (7 ms and 17 ms before saccade end for ipsiversive and contraversive movements, respectively) is necessary if the CFN activity helps terminate the saccade. The relatively early time of the peak of the contraversive burst is necessary if the CFN activity is used to reaccelerate or sustain the gaze velocity plateau commonly seen in large gaze movements.

DISCUSSION

Do these head-free data force us to change our view about the role of the CFN in the control of saccades? In our earlier model based on head-fixed data, a late burst helps to brake ipsiversive saccades. Here we have shown that for the longer-duration saccades of head-free gaze shifts, the end of the burst is still well timed with saccade end. Furthermore, the peak burst rate occurs an average of 7 ms before saccade end. Therefore, the timing of the burst still is appropriate to help terminate the largest ipsiversive saccades.

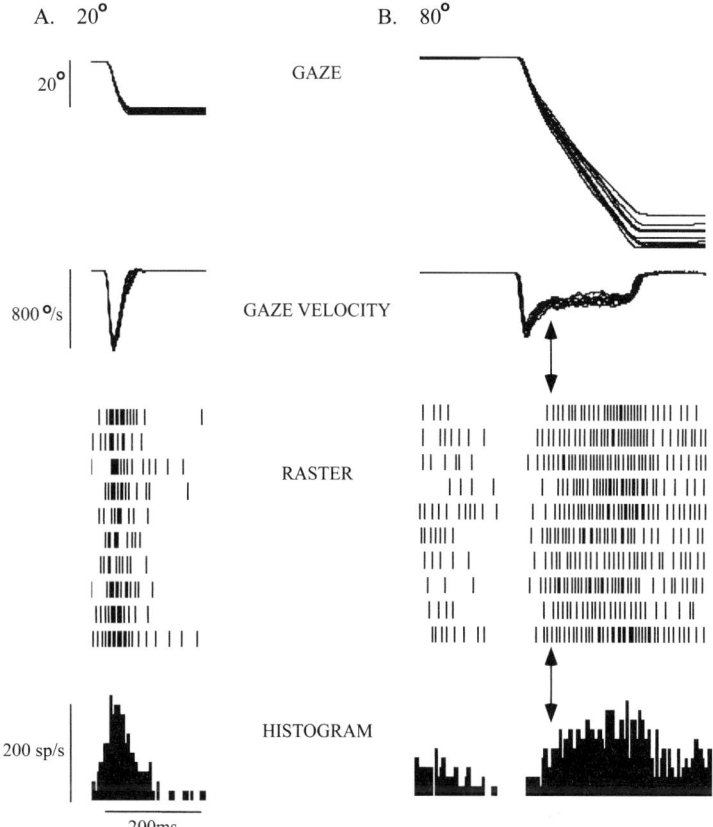

FIGURE 4. Examples of representative velocity profiles with associated spike trains and histograms for ten 20° (no head movement) and ten 80° (with head movement) contraversive gaze shifts. The larger gaze shifts exhibit a prolonged gaze velocity plateau, whose onset time is indicated by the *double arrow*. Note that the averaged activity increases before the occurrence of the velocity plateau.

The new revelation in our present study is that during head-free *contraversive* gaze shifts, the burst also is best timed with saccade end. This observation appears to suggest that the burst may also be involved with terminating rather than accelerating the contraversive saccade.

However, this delayed high-frequency portion of the contraversive CFN burst could also be used as a late excitatory drive to help reaccelerate or prolong the velocity plateau of large saccades. This latter view is supported by a closer consideration of the trajectories of head-free gaze shifts. FIGURE 4 compares the velocity profiles and the associated discharge patterns of representative large and small contraversive gaze shifts with the head free to rotate (of course, similar profiles are seen for ipsiversive gaze shifts). The velocity profiles of large gaze shifts, which usually have substantial head contributions, display an initial peak followed by a sustained plateau or a second reacceleration that culminates in a second velocity peak. We suggest that the late burst for contraversive saccades helps to sustain the late plateau and/or contribute to the second velocity peak. For this to occur, the bursting activity should start before the beginning of the plateau phase (see double pointed arrow in FIG. 4B). The precise timing of the end of the CFN burst with saccade end then serves to terminate the contraversive drive when the eye is on target.

If the late CFN activity serves to prolong contraversive saccades, then pharmacological inactivation of one CFN should eliminate the late plateau and/or the second hump (reacceleration) in the velocity profile. If this were true, the modified velocity profile after inactivation might be more bell-shaped and therefore would tend to resemble that of a smaller gaze shift (FIG. 4A). Therefore, inactivation would produce a hypometric contraversive gaze shift, just as it does with the head fixed. Inactivation studies are currently under way to test this prediction.

REFERENCES

1. BÜTTNER, U., A. FUCHS, G. MARKERT-SCHWAB & P. BUCKMASTER. 1991. Fastigial nucleus activity in the alert monkey during slow eye movements and head movements. J. Neurophysiol. **65:** 1360–1371.
2. COLLEWIJN, H. 1977. Eye and head movements in freely moving rabbits. J. Physiol. (Lond.) **266:** 471–498.
3. FUCHS, A., F. ROBINSON & A. STRAUBE. 1993. Role of the caudal fastigial nucleus in saccade generation. I. Neuronal discharge patterns. J. Neurophysiol. **70:** 1723–1740.
4. NODA, H. & T. FUJIKADO. 1987. Involvement of Purkinje cells in evoking saccadic eye movements by microstimulation of the posterior cerebellar vermis of monkeys. J. Neurophysiol. **57:** 1247–1261.
5. NODA, H., S. MURAKAMI, J. YAMADA, et al. 1988. Saccadic eye movements evoked by microstimulation of the fastigial nucleus of macaque monkeys. J. Neurophysiol. **60:** 1036–1052.
6. NODA, H., S. SUGITA & Y. IKEDA. 1990. Afferent and efferent connections of the oculomotor region of the fastigial nucleus in the macaque monkey. J. Comp. Neurol. **302:** 330–348.
7. OHTSUKA, K. & H. NODA. 1991. Saccadic burst neurons in the oculomotor region of the fastigial nucleus of macaque monkeys. J. Neurophysiol. **65:** 1422–1434.
8. OPTICAN, L. & D. ROBINSON. 1980. Cerebellar-dependent adaptive control of primate saccadic system. J. Neurophysiol. **44:** 1058–1076.
9. ROBINSON, D. 1963. A method of measuring eye movement using a scleral search coil in a magnetic field. IEEE Trans. Bio-Med. Electron. BME **10:** 137–145.
10. ROBINSON, F., A. STRAUBE & A. FUCHS. 1993. Role of the caudal fastigial nucleus in saccade generation. II. Effects of muscimol inactivation. J. Neurophysiol. **70:** 1741–1758.

Adaptation of Saccadic Eye Movements: Transfer and Specificity

NADIA ALAHYANE AND DENIS PÉLISSON

"Espace et Action" INSERM U534, IFR19 Institut Fédératif des Neurosciences de Lyon,16 avenue du doyen Lépine, 69500 Bron, France

> ABSTRACT: The present study was designed to test whether the adaptation of saccadic eye movements depends only on the eye displacement vector of the trained saccade or also on eye position information. Using the double-step target paradigm in eight human subjects, we first induced in a single session two "opposite directions adaptations" (ODA) of horizontal saccades of the same vector. Each ODA (backward or forward) was linked to one vertical eye position (12.5° up or 25° down) and alternated from trial to trial. The results showed that opposite changes of saccade amplitude can develop simultaneously, indicating that saccadic adaptation depends on orbital eye position. This finding has important functional implications because in everyday life our eyes saccade from constantly changing orbital positions. A comparison of these data to two control conditions in which training trials of a single type (backward or forward) were presented at both 12.5° and −25° eye elevations further indicated that eye position specificity is complete for backward, but not for forward, adaptation. Finally, the control conditions also indicated that the adaptation of a single saccade fully transferred to untrained saccades of the same vector, but initiated from different vertical eye positions. In conclusion, our study indicates that saccadic adaptation mechanisms use vectorial eye displacement signals, but can also take eye position signals into account as a contextual cue when the training involves conflicting saccade amplitude changes.
>
> KEYWORDS: eye movement; human; adaptation; eye displacement vector; context

INTRODUCTION

Saccades are quick and accurate eye movements that constitute a good model for the study of sensorimotor plasticity. By using the double-step target paradigm pioneered by McLaughlin,[1] both saccade amplitude increases or decreases can be elicited when the second, intrasaccadic, target step is directed in the direction of the first target step (forward adaptation) or opposite to it (backward adaptation), respectively. With this paradigm, a number of studies have analyzed the properties of saccadic adaptation. On the one hand, it was found that saccadic adaptation is specific to the am-

---

Address for correspondence: Dr. Denis Pélisson," Espace et Action" INSERM U534, 16 avenue du doyen Lépine, 69500 Bron, France. Voice: 33 (0)472 91 34 14; fax: 33 (0)472 91 34 01.

pelisson@lyon.inserm.fr; alahyane@lyon.inserm.fr

plitude and the direction of the trained saccade (vector-specific adaptation) because all saccades of the same vector as the adapted saccade—regardless of their starting orbital position—show a similar adaptive modification.[2-5] On the other hand, Shelhamer and Clendaniel[6] have suggested that eye position can serve as a contextual cue for saccadic adaptation. Indeed, they showed that two different adaptative states can develop concurrently in a single training session when forward and backward adaptation trials are associated with two different vertical eye positions. However, the conclusions of these authors are limited because (1) the number of tested subjects (four) is small given the known intersubject variability of saccadic adaptation, (2) the effectiveness of context-specific adaptations was evaluated indirectly and in only one of the four subjects, and (3) the two different types of adaptations were not presented randomly in interleaved trials but in alternating blocks of 20 identical trials. For these reasons, we designed a study measuring in the same group of 8 subjects both the simultaneous acquisition of two conflicting adaptations and the transfer of a single saccade adaptation to saccades initiated from untrained locations. In the main condition ("opposite directions adaptations," ODA), both backward and forward adaptations of horizontal saccades were elicited in a single training session, each direction of adaptation being related to a different eye elevation. This was compared with two control conditions ("same direction adaptations"), in which the same training (backward or forward) was performed with the eyes deviated up and down.

MATERIALS AND METHODS

Experimental Device

Subjects sat in a dimly illuminated room, with their head immobilized by a biteboard. They looked at red light-emitting diodes (LEDs) located on a concave spherical target board (distance 1.1 m) along four horizontal meridians (meridians 1 to 4: elevation of $12.5°$, $0°$, $-12.5°$, and $-25°$, respectively).

Experimental Protocol

The three experimental conditions each comprised a pretest session (40 trials), an adaptation session (240 trials), and a posttest session (40 trials). The ODA condition was always performed first. It was followed by the same direction backward adaptation (SDBA) and the same direction forward adaptation (SDFA) conditions carried out in a random order according to subjects. Each condition was done on a separate day.

Adaptation session. At the beginning of a trial, the subject looked at a fixation point (FP) located in the left hemifield at a distance of $12.5°$ from the center. After a 1200 ms delay, FP was turned off while a target (T1) was simultaneously illuminated in the right hemifield at a $18.75°$ location (step 1 = $31.25°$). During the saccade to step 1 (primary saccade), T1 was replaced by another target (T2) located $6.25°$ away (step 2 = 20% of step 1). Step 2 was leftward (backward relative to step 1) in backward adaptation and rightward in forward adaptation. In the ODA condition, for four subjects (see FIG. 1A), target T2 stepped forward when the subject's eyes were directed at meridian 1 and stepped backward when the subject's eyes were directed at meridian 4, according to a random sequence; this pattern was reversed for the other

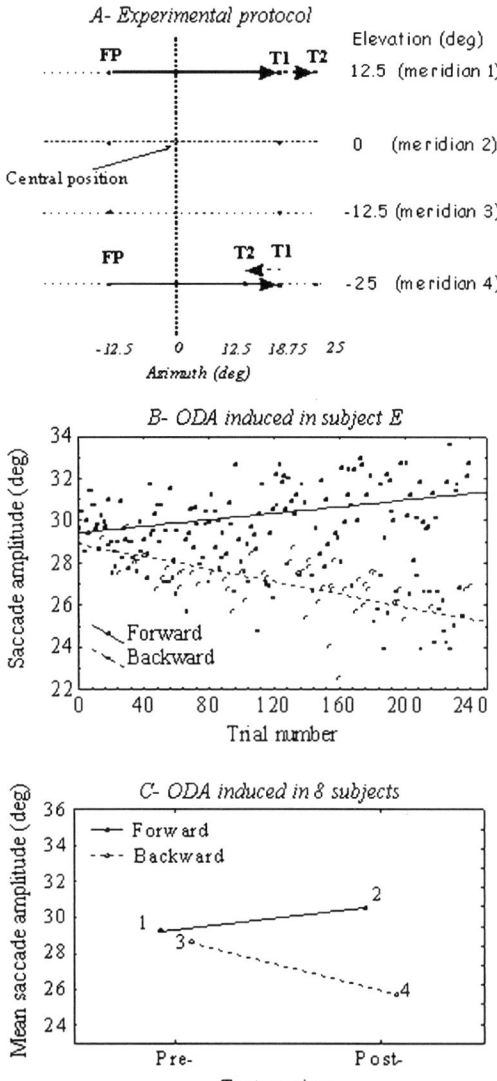

FIGURE 1. Opposite directions adaptation (ODA). (**A**) Experimental protocol showing the double target stimulations along meridians 1 and 4 used in four subjects to simultaneously produce forward and backward adaptations with the eyes deviated 12.5° up or 25° down, respectively. The reverse pattern was used in the other four subjects. FP: fixation point; T1: target 1; T2: target 2; step 1: FP→T1 (31.25°); step 2: T1→T2 (6.25°). (**B**) Plots of saccade amplitude versus trial number during the adaptation session for backward (*open circles*) and forward (*filled circles*) saccadic adaptation induced in subject E. Linear regressions shown by a broken (backward; R = –0.68, $P < 0.001$) or a continuous line (forward; R = 0.38, $P < 0.001$). (**C**) Mean saccade amplitude recorded during pre- and posttest sessions for forward and backward adaptations (results of the two-way repeated measures ANOVA in text) (8 subjects).

four subjects. In the two SDA conditions, step 2 was the same regardless of the meridian (1 or 4) and was directed to the left in the SDBA condition or to the right in the SDFA condition.

Pretest and posttest sessions. The target made a single step from FP (−12.5°) to T1 (18.75°), which was extinguished at the beginning of the saccadic response. This single step occurred along meridians 1 and 4 as in the adaptation sessions, but also along meridians 2 and 3 to test the existence of transfer of adaptation to these two "untrained" meridians in SDBA and SDFA conditions.

Eye Movement Recording and Data Analysis

Horizontal and vertical eye movements were recorded by an eye-link system (SMI, Berlin). A PC program (DataWave, Longmont, CO) controlled the experiment and recorded to disk eye-position signals. An electronic circuit fed by the left-eye position signal triggered the computer routine during the primary saccade to displace target T1 to T2 (step 2) during adaptation sessions and to switch it off during test sessions. The start and end of each saccade were detected off-line on the basis of a velocity threshold of 40°/s and corrected manually if necessary. The horizontal amplitude of each primary saccade of the left eye was calculated as the difference between initial and final eye positions. The time course of adaptation was evaluated by fitting a linear regression to the relationship between primary saccade amplitude and trial number. The percent saccade amplitude change between the posttest and the pretest sessions was calculated as follows: 100 * [(mean posttest amplitude − mean pretest amplitude) / mean pretest amplitude]. Finally, in both SDBA and SDFA conditions, the mean rate of adaptation transfer was computed separately for meridians 2 and 3 as follows: 100 * [mean amplitude change of untrained saccades (meridian 2 or 3)/mean amplitude change of all trained saccades (meridians 1 and 4)].

Statistical Analyses

These analyses were performed on the mean saccade amplitude recorded during test sessions. First, in the ODA condition, a two-way repeated measures ANOVA was designed with adaptation direction (backward vs. forward) and type of test session (pre vs. post) as within-subject factors, and vertical eye position (meridian 1 vs. meridian 4) as between-subject factor. Second, the data of the ODA and of the SDA protocols were compared by performing, for each direction (backward and forward) separately, a two-way repeated measures ANOVA with type of adaptation (ODA vs. SDA) and type of test session (pre vs. post) as within-subject factors and vertical eye position as between-subject factor.

RESULTS

Opposite Directions Adaptation (ODA) Condition

Adaptation session. FIGURE 1B illustrates representative relationships between saccade amplitude and number of trials for subject E who underwent a forward adaptation when her eyes were directed upward (meridian 1) and a backward adaptation when her eyes were directed downward (meridian 4). The statistically significant linear regressions show that saccade amplitude decreased for the backward down-looking trials and simultaneously increased for the forward up-looking condition. These data of subject E were representative of the group of subjects since the 16 regressions (forward or backward × 8 subjects) all showed a slope consistent with the direction of the adaptation and only two failed to reach statistical significance ($P = 0.05$).

Statistical analysis of amplitude changes in test sessions. The results of the two-way ANOVA (adaptation direction × type of test session) on the mean primary saccade amplitude indicated a significant difference between backward adaptation and forward adaptation ($P < 0.01$), but no significant difference between the two types of test session ($P = 0.2$). The "vertical eye position" independent factor had no significant effect ($P = 0.6$). There was a significant ($P < 0.001$) interaction between the adaptation direction and the type of test session, as illustrated in FIGURE 1C. Post-hoc Fisher LSD tests showed that saccades made after backward adaptation (FIG. 1C, 4) were significantly smaller in amplitude than saccades made in the other three cases ($P < 0.001$). Similarly, saccades performed after forward adaptation (FIG. 1C, 2) were significantly larger in amplitude than those performed in the other three cases ($P < 0.05$). In conclusion, ODA induced simultaneously led to significant modifications of saccade amplitude in the direction specified by step 2, and irrespective of vertical eye position. Note that backward adaptation ($-9.6 \pm 6.9\%$) was stronger than forward adaptation ($4.6 \pm 4.6\%$).

Opposite Directions Adaptation vs. Same Direction Adaptation Conditions

We then compared the ODA and control (SDA) conditions for backward and forward adaptations separately. For backward adaptation (FIG. 2A), the two conditions induced a similar change of saccade amplitude of about 12%. The two-way ANOVA (type of adaptation × type of test session) revealed a significant difference between the two types of test sessions ($P < 0.01$), but not between the two types of backward adaptations ($P = 0.2$). Moreover, no significant interaction between the two factors ($P = 0.8$) was found. For forward adaptation (FIG. 2B), the adaptation was more effective when induced in the SDA condition than in the ODA situation (mean amplitude changes: $13 \pm 5.6\%$ vs. $4.6 \pm 4.6\%$, respectively). The ANOVA indeed revealed a significant difference between the two types of test session ($P < 0.01$), no significant difference between the two types of forward adaptations ($P = 0.09$), but a significant interaction between the two factors ($P < 0.01$). Post-hoc Fisher LSD tests indicated that the mean saccade amplitude in the posttest SDA condition (FIG. 2B, 4) was significantly larger than in the other three cases ($P < 0.01$). Similarly, the saccade amplitude in the posttest ODA condition (FIG. 2B, 2) was significantly different from the other three values ($P < 0.05$). Last, for both backward and forward adaptations, the vertical eye position independent factor had no significant effect ($P = 0.3$ and $P = 0.5$, respectively). This suggests that the pattern of results described above was independent of the meridian along which subjects actually experienced backward or forward adaptation in the ODA condition. In conclusion, the analyses of the present section indicate that when performed simultaneously in a single session, backward and forward adaptations interacted asymmetrically at the expense of forward adaptation.

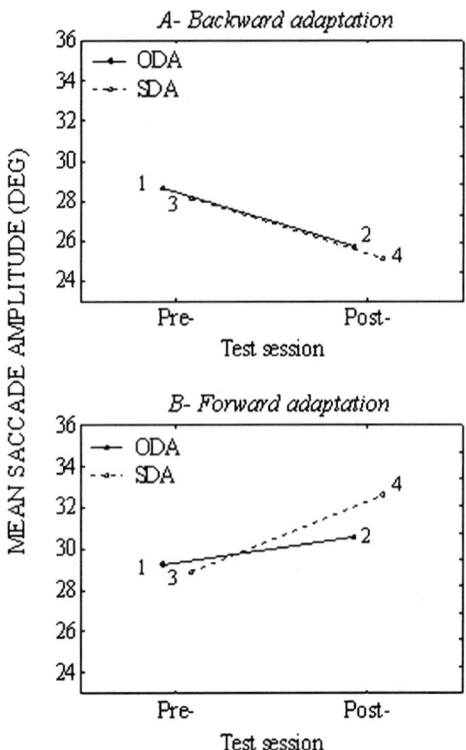

FIGURE 2. Comparison of opposite directions adaptation (ODA) to same direction adaptation (SDA) conditions (8 subjects). Plots of mean saccade amplitude recorded during the test sessions (pre vs. post) for ODA and SDA (results of the two-way repeated measures ANOVAs in text). (**A**) Backward adaptation. (**B**) Forward adaptation.

Adaptation Transfer in Same Direction Adaptation Conditions

In SDA conditions, the adaptation achieved along meridians 1 and 4 transferred to untrained saccades made along the two intermediate meridians (see FIG. 3). In addition, both for backward and forward adaptations, the transfer to these two untrained meridians was similar. Indeed, for backward adaptation, the transfer rate to meridian 2 (102 ± 21%) was not statistically different from the transfer rate to meridian 3 (91 ± 27%; paired t test, $P = 0.2$). Similarly, for forward adaptation, the transfer rates were again statistically indistinguishable (104 ± 25% vs. 100 ± 32%; paired t test, $P = 0.8$). These results indicate a complete adaptation transfer from saccades made along trained meridians (1 and 4) to untrained saccades (meridians 2 and 3).

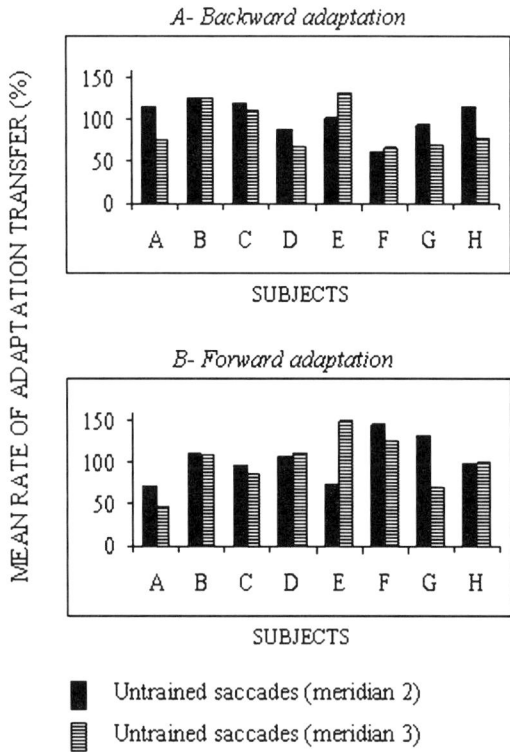

FIGURE 3. Transfer of adaptation from trained saccades to untrained saccades in the same direction adaptation (SDA) conditions (8 subjects). The rate of adaptation transfer from trained saccades performed along meridians 1 and 4 to untrained saccades elicited on intermediate meridians 2 (*black bars*) or 3 (*striped bars*) is plotted in all subjects (A–H). (**A**) Backward adaptation. (**B**) Forward adaptation.

DISCUSSION

Our study shows that saccadic adaptation is eye position–specific. Indeed, subjects were able to switch from an amplitude increase adaptation to an amplitude decrease adaptation when varying vertical eye position. Importantly, this switch operates on the short term, i.e., every time vertical eye position changed between successive trials. On the other hand, and in agreement with previous studies,[2–5] saccadic adaptation is vector-specific. Indeed, we observed, in SDA conditions, a complete transfer of adaptation to untrained saccades of the same vector (same amplitude and direction) as the two trained saccades, but initiated from intermediate vertical eye positions. In fact, these two experimental situations test different phenomena. The second situation, demonstrating the vector specificity of saccadic adaptation, is unnatural as far as a single adaptation occurs. Instead, the first situation provides a more stringent test of eye-position dependency based on conflicting adaptations as encountered in everyday life. We thus conclude that saccadic adaptation (1) is specific to the trained eye-saccade vector and (2) transfers to other eye positions when there is no competing training. Eye position is, however, taken into account when competing trainings are performed at different orbital eye positions. Therefore, both eye position and eye displacement signals are used by the saccade-adaptive mechanisms under natural conditions.

Our results also indicate that the eye-position dependency of forward saccadic adaptation is not complete. Indeed, forward adaptation was weakened when paired with backward adaptation as compared to when it was induced alone in the control session (saccade amplitude changes: 23% vs. 65%, respectively). This illustrates the effect of a conflict with backward adaptation. This conflict is partial and asymmetrical because the backward adaptation was as efficient as when induced alone in the control session (saccade amplitude changes: 48% vs. 52%, respectively). This conflict in favor of the backward adaptation is consistent with the differences found in the speed of adaptation (data not shown), and suggests that forward adaptation shows less eye-position specificity. This agrees with the hypothesis of a differential control of these two opposite types of adaptation (e.g., Ref. 7).

Shelhamer and Clendaniel[6] have recently investigated the effect of vertical eye position on horizontal saccadic adaptation, and their conclusions are somewhat consistent with ours. However, contrary to us, they observed a slight saccade amplitude *decrease* with forward adaptation. Because it was not compared to a SDA condition, this result casts some doubt as to the eye-position specificity of forward adaptation. This difference between the two studies can be explained by the fact that in the Shelhamer and Clendaniel study the two opposite types of adaptation were performed at vertical eye positions closer to each other than in our study (20° vs. 37.5° vertical separation), leading to a stronger conflict. Furthermore, 760 training trials were used as compared to only 240 in the present study, revealing a possible trade-off for saccadic adaptation between training duration and eye-position selectivity. Another difference between our study and the previous one[6] is that in our study forward and backward adaptation double-step stimuli alternated randomly across successive trials, whereas in the previous study[6] stimuli were presented in blocks of 20 identical trials. Thus, our study directly demonstrates that eye position interacts with saccadic adaptation over the short term, a situation closer to that experienced in everyday life. Since vertical eye position alternated randomly during the training as well as the test phases, our results also indicate that eye-position information is necessary both during the acquisition of adaptation and the retention of the modified behavior.

The behavioral properties discussed in this paper should be taken into account to try to understand the neurophysiological processes underlying saccadic adaptation. It is now quite clear that the medial part of the cerebellum is involved in saccadic adaptation (e.g., Refs. 8–10). In addition, the cerebellum receives afferent input from extraocular muscles and oculomotor commands from the brainstem (see Ref.[11] for references), which possibly provide both eye position and eye displacement signals. The cerebellum is therefore well situated to change adaptively saccade amplitude in an eye position–dependent manner. Future studies will have to determine which dynamic selection processes are used by the cerebellum to switch between different adapted states according to different contexts, such as eye position.

ACKNOWLEDGMENTS

We thank the subjects for their participation in this study. We also thank Marcia Riley and Christian Urquizar for designing the data replay/parameter extraction software. Research was supported by INSERM U534.

REFERENCES

1. McLaughlin, S.C. 1967. Parametric adjustment in saccadic eye movements. Percept. Psychophys. **2:** 359–362.
2. Miller, J.M., T. Anstis, et al. 1981. Saccadic plasticity: parametric adaptive control by retinal feedback. J. Exp. Psychol. Hum. Percept. Perform. **7:** 356–366.
3. Deubel, H. 1987. Adaptivity of gain and direction in oblique saccades. In Eye Movements: From Physiology to Cognition. J.K. O'Regan & A. Levy-Schoen, Eds.: 181–190. Elsevier/North-Holland. New York.
4. Frens, M.A. & A.J. Van Opstal. 1994. Transfer of short term adaptation in human saccadic eye movements. Exp. Brain Res. **100:** 293–306.
5. Albano, J.E. 1996. Adaptive changes in saccade amplitude: oculocentric or orbitocentric mapping? Vision Res. **36:** 2087–2098.
6. Shelhamer, M. & R.A. Clendaniel. 2002. Context-specific adaptation of saccade gain. Exp. Brain Res. **146:** 441–450.
7. Deubel, H., W. Wolf, et al. 1986. Adaptive gain control of saccadic eye movements. Hum. Neurobiol. **5:** 245–253.
8. Desmurget, M., D. Pélisson, et al. 1998. Functional anatomy of saccadic adaptation in humans. Nat. Neurosci. **1:** 524–528.
9. Takagi, M., D.S. Zee, et al. 1998. Effects of lesions of the oculomotor vermis on eye movements in primate: saccades. J. Neurophysiol. **80:** 1911–1931.
10. Barash, S., A. Melikyan, et al. 1999. Saccadic dysmetria and adaptation after lesions of the cerebellar cortex. J. Neurosci. **19:** 10931–10939.
11. Pélisson, D., L. Goffart, et al. 2003. Control of saccadic eye movements and combined eye/head gaze shifts by the medio-posterior cerebellum. In Progress in Brain Research: Neural Control of Space Coding and Action Production. C. Prablanc, D. Pélisson, et al., Eds.: 69–89. Elsevier. Amsterdam.

Adaptive Changes in the Angular VOR: Duration of Gain Changes and Lack of Effect of Nodulo-Uvulectomy

SERGEI B. YAKUSHIN,[a] SVETLANA E. BUKHARINA,[a] THEODORE RAPHAN,[a,c] JEAN BÜTTNER-ENNEVER,[d] AND BERNARD COHEN[a,b]

Departments of Neurology[a] and Physiology and Biophysics,[b] Mount Sinai School of Medicine, New York, New York 10029, USA

[c]*Department of Computer and Information Science, Brooklyn College of the City University of New York, Brooklyn, New York 11210, USA*

[d]*Institute of Anatomy, University of München, 80366 München, Germany*

ABSTRACT: Alterations in the gain of the vertical angular vestibulo-ocular reflex (VOR) are dependent on the head position in which the gain changes were produced. We determined how long gravity-dependent gain changes last in monkeys after four hours of adaptation, and whether the adaptation is mediated through the nodulus and uvula of the vestibulocerebellum. Vertical VOR gains were adaptively modified by rotation about an interaural axis, in phase or out of phase with the visual surround. Vertical VOR gains were modified with the animals in one of three orientations: upright, left-side down, or right-side down. Monkeys were tested in darkness for up to four days after adaptation using sinusoidal rotation about an interaural axis that was incrementally tilted in 10° steps from vertical to side down positions. Animals were unrestrained in their cages in normal light conditions between tests. Gravity-dependent gain changes lasted for a day or less after adaptation while upright, but persisted for two days or more after on-side adaptation. These data show that gravity-dependent gain changes can last for prolonged periods after only four hours of adaptation in monkeys, as in humans. They also demonstrate that natural head movements made while upright do not provide an adequate stimulus for rapid recovery of vertical VOR gains that were induced on side. In two animals, the nodulus and uvula were surgically ablated. Vertical gravity-dependent gain changes were not significantly different before and after surgery, indicating that the nodulus and uvula do not have a critical role in producing them.

KEYWORDS: monkey; vestibulo-ocular reflex; adaptation; gravity; cerebellum

Address for correspondence: Sergei B. Yakushin, Ph.D., Department of Neurology, Box 1135, Mount Sinai School of Medicine, 1 East 100th Street, New York, NY 10029. Voice: 212-241-7068; fax: 212-831-1610.
sergei.yakushin@mssm.edu

INTRODUCTION

The angular vestibulo-ocular reflex (VOR) causes the eyes to counter-rotate during head movement to stabilize vision. If ocular counterrotation is not adequate, slip of retinal images provides a stimulus that, over time, will change or adapt the gain of the VOR so that eye velocity more closely equals head velocity (see Ref. 3 for review). In both monkeys and humans, the first significant gain changes occur as early as 20–40 min after onset of the conditioning procedure,[4–7] and two hours of adaptation will produce gain changes in the monkey of more then 20–25%.[6–8] If adaptation is continued for an additional two hours, there is only a slight additional gain change (about 5%). At that point, the gain stabilizes and is unchanged even if stimulation is prolonged for up to 8 h.[8–13]

In several studies, it has been demonstrated that the VOR gain can be modified in relation to particular contexts such as eye position[14,15] and orientation of the head with regard to gravity.[16–19] If vertical VOR gain changes are adapted in a particular head orientation, the gain changes are maximal when animals or humans are tested in the head orientation in which the VOR gain was adapted, and the changes gradually decrease as the head is oriented away from this position.[1,2] In humans, the gain changes can persist for two to three days after on-side adaptation.[2] We questioned whether the persistence of the gain changes was due to limited head movements in side-down position in normal daily behavior. If so, then the gain changes induced while upright should not last as long as gain changes induced on side. A determination of the comparative persistence of the vertical VOR gain changes after upright or on-side adaptation was the first objective of this study.

The finding that the gravity-dependent changes occur almost immediately after assuming the head position in which the gains were adapted, and that the extent of gain change decreases as the head is positioned away from the adapted orientation, suggests that the otoliths, which code information about head position provide an important input to central canal units to determine angular VOR gains. Whether other brain structures also convey head orientation information to central VOR-related units is unknown. The nodulus and uvula of the vestibulocerebellum are involved in orienting the axis of eye velocity generated through the VOR toward the spatial vertical.[20–25] A second goal of this study was to determine whether the nodulus and uvula are also involved in processing head orientation signals to implement the gravity-dependent gain changes.

METHODS

Two cynomolgus (*Macaca fascicularis*, M9358 and M0102) and one rhesus (*Macaca mulatta*, M98065) monkeys were used in this study. The experiments conformed to the Guide for the Care and Use of Laboratory Animals[26] and were approved by the Institutional Animal Care and Use Committee. Experimental techniques have been described in detail in previous publications, and only essential details will be provided here. Under anesthesia, a head mount was implanted on the skull to provide painless head fixation in stereotaxic coordinates.[8,27] Two scleral search coils were implanted on the left eye. One measured the horizontal and vertical components of eye position.[28] Another coil, placed approximately orthogonal to the frontal coil, was used to measure the torsional component of eye position. Nodulo-uvulectomy was performed in two animals after pretesting.[20] The extent of lesions was determined in histological sections.

During testing, the monkey's head was fixed to a plastic frame, which held two sets of field coils that generated orthogonal oscillating magnetic fields at the same frequency. The primate chair was centered in a four-axis vestibular stimulator surrounded by an optokinetic drum with black and white vertical stripes. To calibrate eye movements, the animals were rotated in light at 30°/s about a spatial vertical axis. Animals were upright for calibration of yaw eye movements, left-side down (LSD) for pitch movements, and prone for roll movements. It was assumed that horizontal and vertical gains were close to unity when upright or side down,[28,29] and torsional gains were assumed to be 0.6 when the rotation was performed around a naso-occipital axis aligned with the spatial vertical.[30,31] Positive directions of eye movement were leftward for yaw, downward for pitch, and clockwise (from the animal's point of view) for roll components.

Vertical VOR gains were adapted by oscillating the monkeys in light for four hours about an interaural axis in one of three positions: upright, LSD, or right-side down (RSD). Gains were decreased by rotating the animal and visual surround in the same direction and increased by rotating the animal and visual surround in opposite directions. Sinusoids of 0.25 Hz and 0.5 Hz as well as steps of velocity[1] were used for gain adaptation.

To measure gravity-dependent effects on vertical VOR gain adaptation [(eye velocity)/(head velocity)], animals were oscillated sinusoidally at 0.5 Hz (60°/s peak velocity) in darkness about a pitch (interaural) axis that was either upright or tilted toward side-down positions in roll in 10° increments up to 90°. Ten cycles of data were obtained in each head orientation. Because the animals were always rotating in pitch, canal activation was the same in every head orientation. Eye position voltages and voltages related to the velocity of the chair oscillation and the tilt of the axis of rotation were recorded with amplifiers having a bandpass of DC to 40 Hz. Data were acquired by computer and analyzed off-line. Voltages were digitized at 1000 Hz/channel with 16-bit resolution. Voltages related to eye position were digitally differentiated by finding the slope of the least squares linear fit over 25-ms time period. This corresponds to a filter, which has a 3-dB cutoff above 40 Hz, the cutoff frequency of the filters used for data acquisition. Saccades were eliminated using a maximum likelihood ratio criterion.[32]

The gain of the VOR was tested sequentially for 2–4 days after adaptation. Desaccaded eye velocity was fitted with sinusoids to estimate the gain and phase of the response in each head orientation (temporal gain and phase). Changes in gain were expressed as a percentage relative to the preadapted level for each head orientation and plotted as a function of head tilt. To analyze the magnitude of the gravity-dependent VOR gain adaptation, we applied a sine approximation with a bias (C) to the data

$$y = A^* \cos(x + B) + C \qquad (1)$$

where A is a half of the magnitude of the gravity specific effect and B is the angle of the head tilt where the maximal gain changes occurred, i.e., the spatial phase. C is the bias of the sinusoid, which gives a measure of the gravity-independent gain changes.

Standard t tests and ANOVA were used to analyze pairs or sets of data, respectively. A generally accepted statistical approach for data-model comparison, the χ^2 test, provided a robust statistical analysis if there were several hundred data points.[33] This assumption failed if the sample size was small. An analysis of variance (ANOVA) is less sensitive to any non-normality in the data distribution.[34] To avoid possible complications in the statistical analysis, we utilized a reduced case of the analysis of variance (F-statistic).[35]

RESULTS

Gravity-Dependent and Gravity-Independent Gain Changes of Normal Animals

When animals were sinusoidally oscillated about an interaural axis in darkness before adaptation, the induced vertical eye velocities were about the same in all tested head orientations (FIG. 1A). After the vertical VOR gain was decreased with the animal in the LSD position, modulation of the eye velocities induced by interaural rotation was reduced maximally when the animal was LSD in darkness (FIG. 1B, top trace), and peak eye velocity increased toward the original value as the animal was tilted toward the right-side down (RSD) position (FIG. 1B, middle and low traces). As previously shown,[1] there was an up-down asymmetry in the velocity decreases, and the gain changes were larger for downward (+) than upward (–) slow-phase velocities (FIG. 1B). The induced eye velocity and retinal slip were minimal, and visual suppression was complete when head was pitched up (FIG. 1C, positive eye velocity), but not when the head was pitched down (FIG. 1C, negative velocities). This asymmetry is likely related to a difference in visual suppression, which could result in a difference in upward and downward gain adaptation.[8] Since we were concerned with the overall vertical VOR performance in this study, these differences will not be considered further.

The gain of the vertical VOR was calculated for each head orientation in the unadapted state and plotted as a function of head tilt to obtain the spatial responses. Before adaptation, vertical VOR gains were independent of the angle of head tilt (FIG. 1D, dashed line, ± 1 SD, dotted lines), and the average gains were approximately the same over all head orientations. After the pitch VOR gain was decreased for four hours with animal LSD; the measured gain was minimal when the animal was tested LSD; and gain values progressively increased as the monkey was reoriented toward the contralateral side down (FIG. 1D, filled symbols).

Two types of VOR gain changes are induced when the VOR is adapted: one is dependent on the head orientation re position in which gain was changed, while the other is independent of head position.[1] When the gain changes were fit with a sine function (Eq. 1; FIG. 1E), the bias of the sinusoid represented the gravity-independent gain change, and the peak-to-peak amplitude, the gravity-dependent changes. Gravity-independent gain changes in FIGURE 1E were –21%, and the amplitude of the fitted sine was ≈14%. Therefore, the peak-to-peak gravity-dependent gain changes were 28%, that is, twice the amplitude.

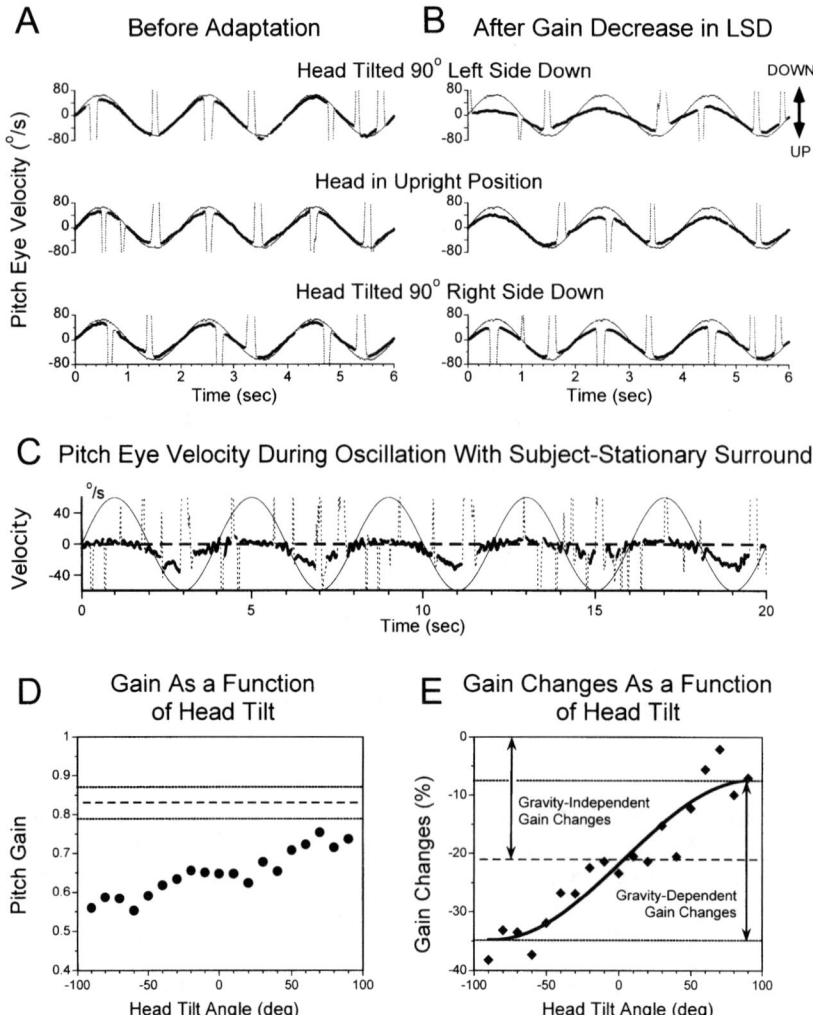

FIGURE 1. (**A, B**) Eye velocities induced by sinusoidal oscillation around an interaural axis with the animal left-side down (*top trace*), upright (*middle trace*) and right-side down (*bottom trace*), before (**A**) and after (**B**) the VOR gain was decreased while LSD. The *heavy lines* are slow-phase velocity, and saccadic velocities, which were removed for the analysis, are shown by the *thin vertical dotted lines*. The *thin solid lines* show head velocity, inverted to facilitate comparison. (**C**) Suppression of eye velocities induced by sinusoidal rotation in a subject-stationary visual surround. Downward (+) eye velocities were suppressed more completely than upward eye velocities (−). (**D**) Vertical VOR gains were not dependent on head orientation before adaptation (*dashed line; dotted lines* around the dashed line represent ± 1 SD). After the gain was decreased in the LSD position (*solid symbols*), gain values varied as a function of head tilt, and were smallest when the head was close to the position of adaptation (−90°). (**E**) Gain changes as a function of head tilt re gravity from the data in **D** are shown by the *solid symbols*. The *heavy line* shows a sinusoidal fit to these data. The *dashed line* is the bias of the sinusoidal fit, which is the gravity-independent gain change. The peak-to-peak amplitude of the sinusoid (*dotted lines*) represents the magnitude of the gravity-dependent gain changes.

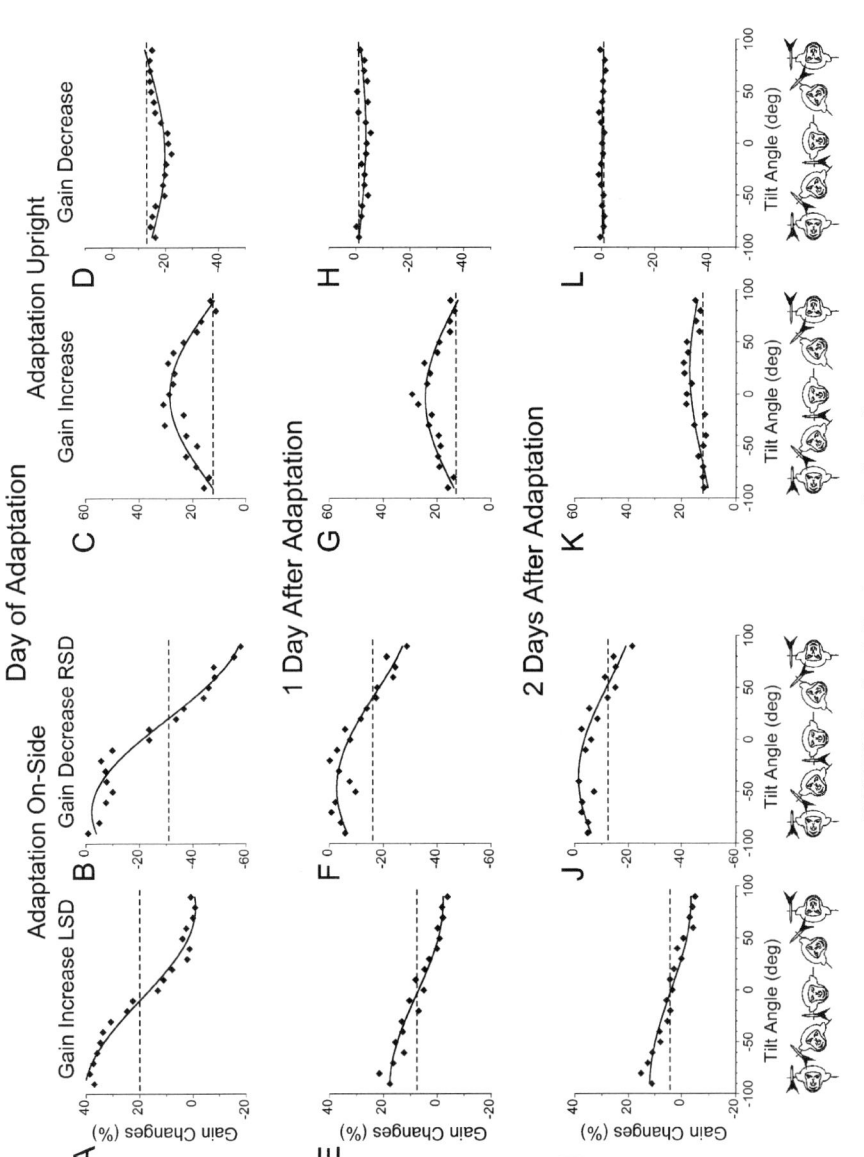

FIGURE 2. See following page for legend.

Prolonged Effects of Gravity-Dependent VOR Gain Changes

In two animals, the pitch component of the VOR gain was adaptively increased and decreased in each of the three positions, and the animals were tested sequentially for up to four days after adaptation. Between tests, animals were caged, but were otherwise unrestricted in their daily activity. After the VOR gain was increased in animal M98065 while in LSD position, the gravity-dependent gain changes were 42% when tested on the same day (FIG. 2A). One and two days after adaptation, the gravity-dependent gain changes were 20% (FIG. 2E) and 15% (FIG. 2I), respectively. Gravity-independent gain changes were 20% on the day of adaptation, but only 8% and 4% on the first and second days. When the VOR gain was decreased in the RSD head position in the same animal, the gravity-dependent gain changes were −57% on the day of adaptation (FIG. 2B), and decreased to 28% (FIG. 2F) and 22% (FIG. 2J), when tested one and two days afterward. The gravity-independent gain changes were −31% on the day of adaptation, and −17% and −13% on the two following days. Thus, four hours of on-side adaptation produced gravity-dependent gain changes in the monkeys that were present for at least two days after adaptation (F-statistic, $P < 0.05$).

When the vertical VOR gain was adaptively increased with the animal M0102 in the upright position, the peak-to-peak gravity-dependent changes were 33% on the day of adaptation (FIG. 2C), but rapidly decreased to 23% (FIG. 2G) and 9% (FIG. 2K) in the following two days. These gain changes were only significant on the day of adaptation and one day afterward (F-statistic, $P < 0.05$). Gravity-independent changes were $\approx 12\%$ on the day of adaptation and on both subsequent days. Gain decreases with the animal adapted in the upright position were smaller, although significant ($P < 0.05$), than when the gains were modified on-side (FIG. 2D). In one experiment, the gravity-dependent gain changes were 12% and gravity-independent changes were −14% in the day of adaptation. Changes observed in the two days following adaptation were not significant (FIG. 2H, L).

The gravity-dependent gain changes at different times after adaptation are summarized in FIGURE 3. The gravity-dependent gain increases and decreases were significant in all instances just after adaptation varying from 15–55% and were approximately the same for gain increases and decreases for all positions (FIG. 3A). When adaptation was done in the on-side position, gain changes were significant within the first two days after adaptation or longer (FIG. 3A, filled symbols). After upright adaptation, however, significant gain changes were observed only in one case and only on the first day after adaptation (FIG. 3B).

FIGURE 2. Gain changes of the vertical VOR in two animals after adaptation in on-side (1st and 2nd columns) and upright (3rd and 4th columns) positions. Data are show for the day of adaptation (**A–D**), one day after adaptation (**E–H**) and two days after adaptation (**I–L**). The *dashed line* represents the bias of the sinusoidal fits to the gain changes in the different positions. The inserts below show approximate head positions and axes of rotation during testing and can be related to the data in the graphs above.

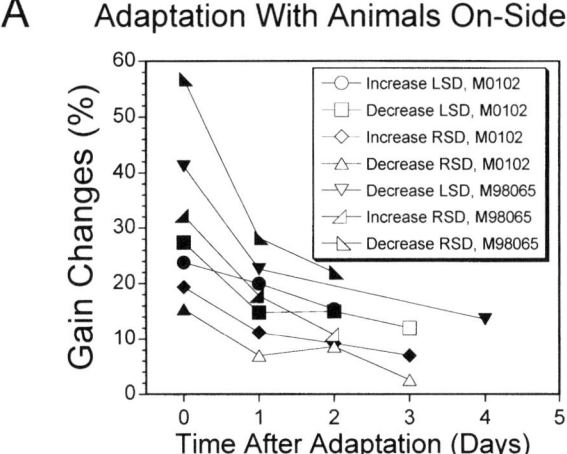

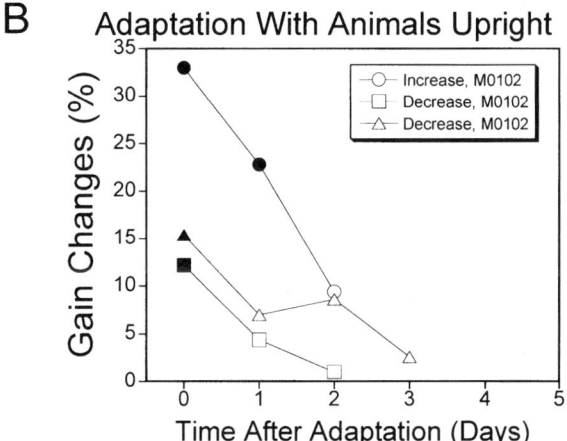

FIGURE 3. Average changes of the vertical VOR gain (%) in two animals at different times after adaptation on side (**A**) and upright (**B**). The *filled symbols* represent significant values.

Gravity-Dependent VOR Gain Adaptation after Nodulo-Uvulectomy

Two animals were tested for their ability to generate gravity-dependent VOR gain adaptation before and after surgical ablation of the nodulus and uvula. One animal was M98065, whose data are described in the previous section. The second animal was M9358, which had been used in single-unit experiments from the nodulus and uvula that are described elsewhere.[21] The previous experiments in M9358 were completed about one year before the control data for the present experiments were taken.

When M98065 was rotated in darkness with the steps of velocity (60°/s), the velocity storage time constant had symmetrical responses for leftward and rightward

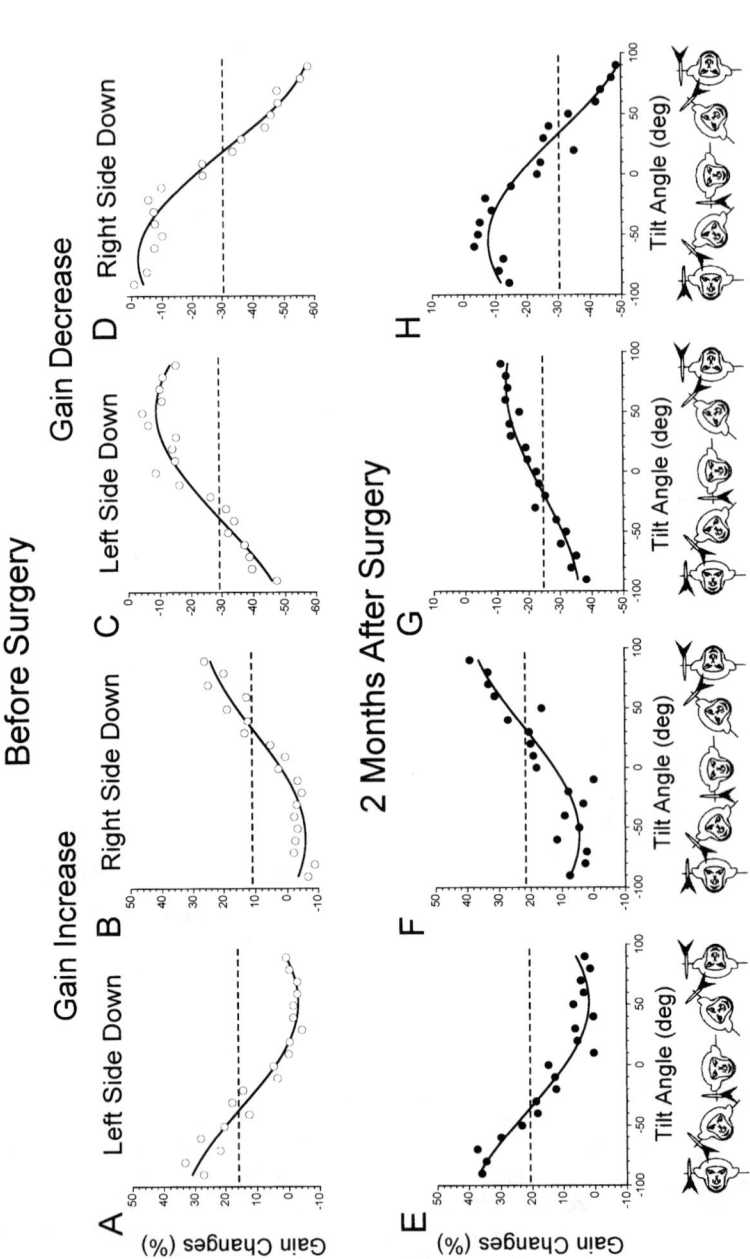

FIGURE 4. Gain increases (1st and 2nd columns) and decreases (3rd and 4th columns) in M98065. The gain changes were similar before (A–D) and two months after (E–H) nodulo-uvulectomy.

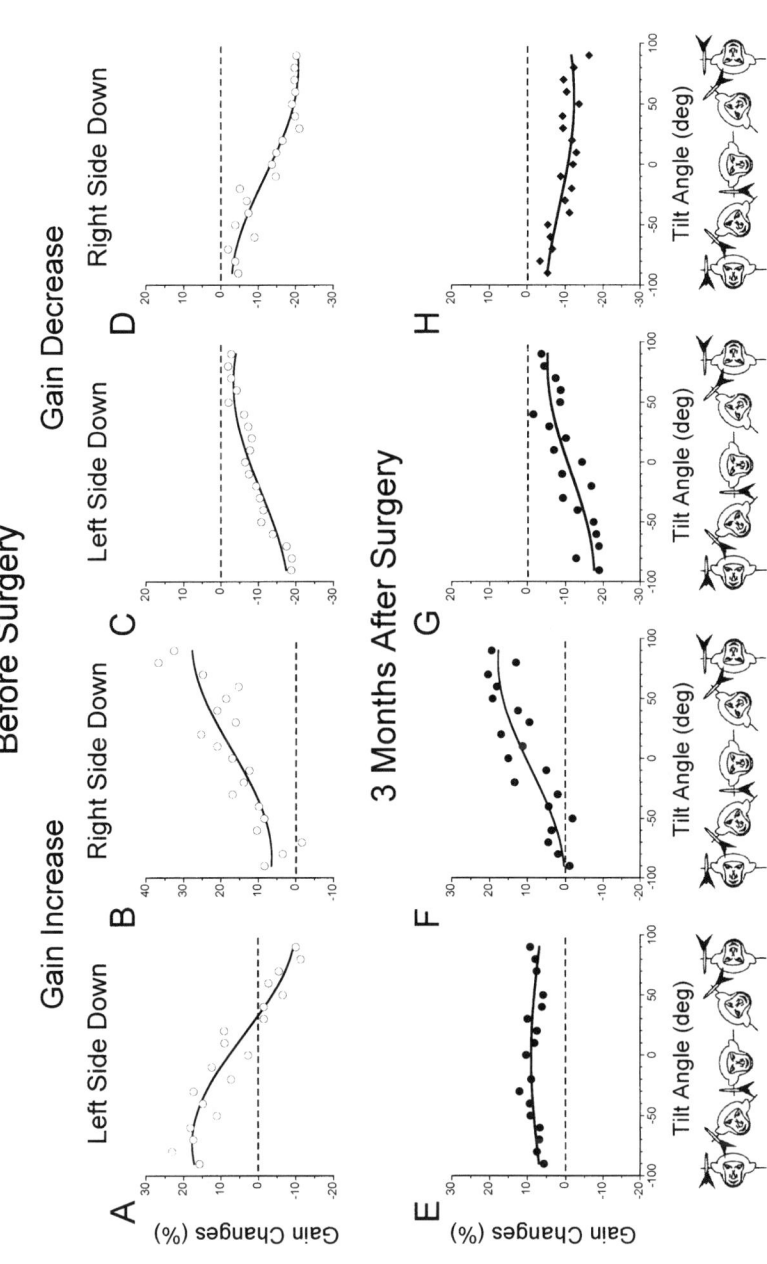

FIGURE 5. Gain increases (1st and 2nd columns) and decreases (3rd and 4th columns) in M9358. The gain changes were significant before surgery (**A–D**). Three months after surgery (**E–H**), the gains could not be increased in the LSD position (**E**), but the changes were close to the presurgical values in all other conditions (**F–H**).

TABLE 1. Parameters of gain changes obtained from M98065 before and two months after the nodulo-uvulectomy

Gain changes	Head tilt	Gain parameters	Before surgery	Two months after surgery
Increase	LSD	Gravity-dependent gain	38%	39%
		Phase	−127°	−128°
		Gravity-independent gain	16%	21%
	RSD	Gravity-dependent gain	32%	34%
		Phase	122°	123°
		Gravity-independent gain	10%	22%
Decrease	LSD	Gravity-dependent gain	42%	23%
		Phase	−128°	−108°
		Gravity-independent gain	−30%	−25%
	RSD	Gravity-dependent gain	56%	46%
		Phase	110°	124°
		Gravity-independent gain	−31%	−30%

Gain changes were all significant ($P < 0.05$) and were not substantially different before and after operation.

rotations before and after ablation, but the time constants were reduced from ≈40 s before to ≈20 s one month after surgery. Since isolated removal of the nodulus and uvula prolongs the horizontal time constant of velocity storage and causes a loss of habituation (see Ref. 36 for review), this suggested that the lesion had extended beyond the nodulus and uvula in this animal. On histological analysis, the vermis of lobules VIIa– X were ablated, but the lesion extended into the fastigial nucleus and the caudal interpositus nucleus on the right. There was also a residual tag of nodulus tissue just above the choroids plexus, but there were no Purkinje cells in the remaining tissue. Since the nodulus and uvula were almost completely removed in this animal, we considered that it could be used to determine whether gravity-dependent adaptation could be induced after nodulo-uvulectomy.

When the vertical VOR gain was increased in the LSD position before ablation (FIG. 4A), the peak-to-peak gravity-dependent and gravity-independent gain changes in animal M98065 were 38% and 16%, respectively. Two months after the surgery, there were both gravity-dependent and -independent gain changes of 39% and 21%, respectively, in response to the same stimulus (FIG. 4E). The head orientations in which peak gravity-dependent changes occurred were also the same before and after (−127° and −128°). Similar results were obtained when gain was increased in RSD (FIG. 4B, F), or decreased in LSD (FIG. 4C, G), or RSD positions (FIG. 4D, H). The averages for all conditions were 42 ± 10% for the gravity-dependent changes before and 36 ± 10% after surgery, and the gravity-independent changes were 22 ± 10% and 25 ± 4% before and after surgery (TABLE 1).

The time constant of the second animal (M9358), which was initially about 30–40 s before operation, was reduced to 8–9 s as a result of repeated testing. One week after nodulo-uvulectomy, central control of the VOR time constant was lost, and the

TABLE 2. Parameters of gain changes obtained from M9358 before and one and two months after the nodulo-uvulectomy

Gain changes	Head tilt	Gain parameters	Before surgery	One month after surgery	Three months after surgery
Increase	LSD	Gravity-dependent gain	28%	5%*	4%*
		Phase	−74°	−136°	−2°
		Gravity-independent gain	4%	5%*	7%*
	RSD	Gravity-dependent gain	22%	15%	18%
		Phase	97°	65°	81°
		Gravity-independent gain	17%	3%	9%
Decrease	LSD	Gravity-dependent gain	15%	8%*	14%
		Phase	−115°	−135°*	−143°
		Gravity-independent gain	−11%	−9%*	−15%
	RSD	Gravity-dependent gain	18%	8%*	8%
		Phase	80°	69°*	51°
		Gravity-independent gain	−12%	−6%*	−9%

*Indicates non-significant changes in gain and/or phase.

evoked per-rotatory nystagmus did not diminish even after 5 min of constant velocity rotation in darkness. Two months after surgery, the time constants of the per- and post-rotatory nystagmus were ≈500 and ≈300 s for rotations to the left and right, respectively. Periodic alternating nystagmus in darkness was also present in this animal. Histological analysis demonstrated that the nodulus and uvula were completely ablated. Thus, the behavioral data obtained after ablation correlated with the histological analysis in this animal[20] and with previous results.[22,37–41]

The gravity-dependent gain changes also persisted after nodulo-uvulectomy in this animal (FIG. 5A–D). Before operation, they were about 20 ± 6% (TABLE 2). In the first month after surgery, significant gravity-dependent gain changes were only present for gain increase while RSD (TABLE 2). Three months after surgery, however, there were significant gravity-dependent gain changes in three of the four conditions (FIG. 5F, G, H). In two of these conditions (FIG. 5F, G), the gravity-dependent gain increases in RSD and decreases in LSD changes were comparable to prelesion data (22% vs. 18% and 14% vs. 14%, respectively; TABLE 2). Thus, data obtained from both animals demonstrate that complete removal of the nodulus and uvula did not abolish the gravity-dependent gain changes.

DISCUSSION

This study confirms previous findings that gain adaptation of the vertical VOR is dependent on head orientation re gravity, that modifications in gain are largest in the head orientation in which vertical gain was adapted, and that the changes in gain gradually decrease as animals are reoriented away from this position.[1,2] Additionally, we show here that the gravity-dependent gain changes that were induced by only four hours of adaptation persisted for several days in the monkey, similar to the persistence of the changes in vertical VOR gain in humans after one hour of adaptation.[2]

Horizontal VOR gains will normalize within an hour in humans[42] and animals[43] if the subjects are allowed to move their heads freely in light. However, adaptive changes in the horizontal VOR were maintained for over a week if the monkeys' heads were immobilized.[13] This implies that adaptive gain changes of the VOR will decay at a very slow rate spontaneously unless these changes are actively reversed. Based on the data presented in this study, we further suggest that the same conditions that had led to adaptation of the VOR must be present to readapt the VOR back to its original state, and that the orientation of the head relative to gravity is an important context for readaptation as for adaptation. The gravity-dependent gain changes of the vertical VOR induced in the upright position returned to normal faster than gains adapted on side. A likely explanation for this is that monkeys predominantly assume an upright position, so that changes related to movements that activate the vertical VOR about this position are detected and corrected more readily than for similar movements made in animals that were adapted on side.

The finding that a specific amount of gain change is induced in every head orientation after the VOR has been adapted in a particular position suggests that central neurons responsible for gain modification of the VOR receive both semicircular canal and otolith related inputs. The canal input sets the direction of the movement relative to the head and provides a measure that can be compared to the visual input, while the otolith input alters the gain of the VOR as a function of the orientation of the head re gravity. There are several places where this interaction could occur. One is in the nodulus and uvula. This portion of the vestibulocerebellum does not have a significant role in VOR gain adaptation,[6] but does receive direct canal and otolith input,[44,45] as well as visual input,[46] and is important for gravity-dependent spatial orientation of the VOR. Data in this study rule out significant nodulus and uvular participation in the gravity-dependent gain changes, however. The flocculus, which is known to control VOR adaptation,[47] or the vestibular and/or cerebellar nuclei that receive convergent canal and otolith inputs,[48–52] are other likely sites that could contribute to the implementation of the gravity-dependent gain changes.

ACKNOWLEDGMENTS

We thank Dmitri Ogorodnikov for developing programs used in processing the data and Victor Rodriguez for technical assistance. This study was supported by National Institutes of Health grants DC03787, DC04996, DC05204, EY11812, EY04148, and EY01867.

REFERENCES

1. YAKUSHIN, S.B., T. RAPHAN & B. COHEN. 2003. Gravity specific adaptation of the vertical angular vestibulo-ocular reflex; dependence on head orientation with regard to gravity. J. Neurophysiol. **89:** 571–586.
2. YAKUSHIN, S.B., A. PALLA, T. HASLWANTER, *et al.* 2003. Dependence of adaptation of the human vertical angular vestibulo-ocular reflex on gravity. Exp. Brain Res. **152:** 137–142.
3. ITO, M. 1984. The Cerebellum and Neural Control. Raven Press. New York.
4. GONSHOR, A. & G. MELVILL JONES. 1976. Short-term adaptive changes in the human vestibulo-ocular reflex arc. J. Physiol. (Lond.) **256:** 361–379.

5. COLLEWIJN, H., A.J. MARTINS & R.M. STEINMAN. 1983. Compensatory eye movements during active and passive head movements: fast adaptation to changes in visual magnification. J. Physiol. (Lond.). **340:** 259–286.
6. COHEN, H., B. COHEN, T. RAPHAN & W. WAESPE. 1992. Habituation and adaptation of the vestibuloocular reflex: a model of differential control by the vestibulocerebellum. Exp. Brain Res. **90:** 526–538.
7. PARTSALIS, A.M., Y. ZHANG & S.M. HIGHSTEIN. 1995. Dorsal Y group in the squirrel monkey. I. Neuronal responses during rapid and long-term modifications of the vertical VOR. J. Neurophysiol. **73:** 615–631.
8. YAKUSHIN, S.B., H. REISINE, J. BÜTTNER-ENNEVER, et al. 2000. Functions of the nucleus of the optic tract (NOT). I. Adaptation of the gain of the horizontal vestibulo-ocular reflex. Exp. Brain Res. **131:** 416–432.
9. GODAUX, E., J. HALLEUX & C. GOBERT. 1983. Adaptive change of the vestibulo-ocular reflex in the cat: the effects of a long-term frequency-selective procedure. Exp. Brain Res. **49:** 28–34.
10. BELLO, S., G.D. PAIGE & S.M. HIGHSTEIN. 1991. The squirrel monkey vestibulo-ocular reflex and adaptive plasticity in yaw, pitch, and roll. Exp. Brain Res. **87:** 57–66.
11. NAGAO, S. 1989. Behavior of floccular Purkinje cells correlated with adaptation of vestibulo-ocular reflex in pigmented rabbits. Exp. Brain Res. **77:** 531–540.
12. LISBERGER, S.G., F.A. MILES & D.S. ZEE. 1984. Signals used to compute errors in monkey vestibuloocular reflex: possible role of flocculus. J. Neurophysiol. **52:** 1140–1153.
13. MILES, F.A. & B.B. EIGHMY. 1980. Long term adaptive changes in primate vestibuloocular reflex. I. Behavioral observations. J. Neurophysiol. **43:** 1406–1425.
14. SHELHAMER, M., D.A. ROBINSON & H.S. TAN. 1992. Context-specific adaptation of the gain of the vestibulo-ocular reflex in humans. J. Vestib. Res. **2:** 89–96.
15. TILIKET, C., M. SHELHAMER, D. ROBERTS & D.S. ZEE. 1994. Short-term vestibuloocular reflex adaptation in humans. I. Effect on the ocular motor velocity-to-position neural integrator. Exp. Brain Res. **100:** 316–327.
16. BAKER, J., C. WICKLAND & B. PETERSON. 1987. Dependence of cat vestibulo-ocular reflex direction adaptation on animal orientation during adaptation and rotation in darkness. Brain Res. **408:** 339–343.
17. BAKER, J.F., S.I. PERLMUTTER, B.W. PETERSON, et al. 1987. Simultaneous opposing adaptive changes in cat vestibulo-ocular reflex direction for two body orientations. Exp. Brain Res. **69:** 220–224.
18. TILIKET, C., M. SHELHAMER, H.S. TAN & D.S. ZEE. 1993. Adaptation of the vestibuloocular reflex with the head in different orientations and positions relative to the axis of body rotation. J. Vestib. Res. **3:** 181–195.
19. YAKUSHIN, S.B., T. RAPHAN & B. COHEN. 2000. Context-specific adaptation of the vertical vestibuloocular reflex with regard to gravity. J. Neurophysiol. **84:** 3067–3071.
20. COHEN, B., P. JOHN, S.B. YAKUSHIN, et al. 2002. The nodulus and uvula: source of cerebellar control of spatial orientation of the angular vestibulo-ocular reflex. Ann. N. Y. Acad. Sci. **978:** 28–45.
21. SHELIGA, B.M., S.B. YAKUSHIN, A. SILVERS, et al. 1999. Control of spatial orientation of the angular vestibuloocular reflex by the nodulus and uvula of the vestibulocerebellum. Ann. N. Y. Acad. Sci. **871:** 94–122.
22. WEARNE, S., T. RAPHAN & B. COHEN. 1998. Control of spatial orientation of the angular vestibuloocular reflex by the nodulus and uvula. J. Neurophysiol. **79:** 2690–2715.
23. ANGELAKI, D.E. & B.J. HESS. 1994. The cerebellar nodulus and ventral uvula control the torsional vestibulo-ocular reflex. J. Neurophysiol. **72:** 1443–1447.
24. ANGELAKI, D.E. & B.J. HESS. 1995. Lesion of the nodulus and ventral uvula abolish steady-state off-vertical axis otolith response. J. Neurophysiol. **73:** 1716–1720.
25. SOLOMON, D. & B. COHEN. 1994. Stimulation of the nodulus and uvula discharges velocity storage in the vestibulo-ocular reflex. Exp. Brain Res. **102:** 57–68.
26. NATIONAL RESEARCH COUNCIL. 1996. Guide for the care and use of laboratory animals. National Academy Press. Washington, DC.
27. SIROTA, M.G., B.M. BABAEV, I.N. BELOOZEROVA, et al. 1988. Neuronal activity of nucleus vestibularis during coordinated movement of eyes and head in microgravitation. Physiologist **31:** 8–9.

28. ROBINSON, D.A. 1963. A method of measuring eye movement using a scleral search coil in a magnetic field. IEEE Trans. Bio-Med. Electron. **10:** 137–145.
29. RAPHAN, T., V. MATSUO & B. COHEN. 1979. Velocity storage in the vestibulo-ocular reflex arc (VOR). Exp. Brain Res. **35:** 229–248.
30. CRAWFORD, J.D. & T. VILIS. 1991. Axes of eye rotation and Listing's law during rotations of the head. J. Neurophysiol. **65:** 407–423.
31. HENN, V., D. STRAUMANN, B.J.M. HESS, et al. 1992. Three-dimensional transformations from vestibular and visual input to oculomotor output. Ann. N.Y. Acad. Sci. **656:** 166–180.
32. SINGH, A., G.E. THAU, T. RAPHAN & B. COHEN. 1981. Detection of saccades by a maximum likelihood ratio criterion. Proceedings of the 34th Annual Conference on Engineering in Medicine and Biology. Houston, TX. p136.
33. SNEDECOR, G.W. & W.G. COCHRAN. 1967. Statistical methods. The Iowa State University Press. Ames, IA.
34. KEPPEL, G. 1991. Design and Analysis: A Researcher's Handbook. Prentice Hall. Englewood Cliffs, NJ.
35. YAKUSHIN, S.B., M. DAI, J.-I. SUZUKI, et al. 1995. Semicircular canal contributions to the three-dimensional vestibuloocular reflex: a model-based approach. J. Neurophysiol. **74:** 2722–2738.
36. COHEN, B., S. WEARNE, M. DAI & T. RAPHAN. 1999. Spatial orientation of the angular vestibulo-ocular reflex. J. Vestib. Res. **9:** 163–172.
37. WAESPE, W., B. COHEN & T. RAPHAN. 1985. Dynamic modification of the vestibuloocular reflex by the nodulus and uvula. Science **228:** 199–202.
38. HASEGAWA, T., K. HARADA, T. IKARASHI, et al. 1991. Effect of uvulonodular lesions on optokinetic nystagmus and optokinetic after-nystagmus in cats. Acta Otolaryngol. Suppl. (Stockh.) **481:** 251–253.
39. HASEGAWA, T., I. KATO, K. HARADA, et al. 1994. The effect of uvulonodular lesions on horizontal optokinetic nystagmus and optokinetic after-nystagmus in cats. Acta Otolaryngol. Suppl. (Stockh.) **511:** 126–130.
40. ANGELAKI, D.E. & B.J. HESS. 1995. Inertial representation of angular motion in the vestibular system of rhesus monkeys. II. Otolith-controlled transformation that depends on an intact cerebellar nodulus. J. Neurophysiol. **73:** 1729–1751.
41. WEARNE, S., T. RAPHAN & B. COHEN. 1996. Nodulo-uvular control of the central vestibular dynamics determines spatial orientation of the angular vestibulo-ocular reflex. Ann. N. Y. Acad. Sci. **781:** 364–384.
42. ISTL-LENZ, Y., D. HYDEN & D.W. SCHWARZ. 1985. Response of the human vestibulo-ocular reflex following long-term 2× magnified visual input. Exp. Brain Res. **57:** 448–455.
43. PAIGE, G.D. & E.W. SARGENT. 1991. Visually-induced adaptive plasticity in the human vestibulo-ocular reflex. Exp. Brain Res. **84:** 25–34.
44. MUGNAINI, E. & W.H. OERTEL. 1985. An atlas of the distribution of GABAergic neurons and terminals in the rat CNS as revealed by GAD immunohistochemistry. *In* GABA and Neuropeptides in the CNS. Handbook of Chemical Neuroanatomy. A. Björklund & H.T. Hökte, Eds. Vol. **4:** 436–608. Elsevier. Amsterdam.
45. FRITZSCH, B. 1981. Transneuronal vestibular afferent influence on the nodular molecular layer synaptogenesis. Anat. Embryol. Berl. **162:** 199–208.
46. KANO, M., M. KANO & K. MAEKAWA. 1991. Binocular interaction and signal component of optokinetic responses of climbing fiber afferents in the cerebellar flocculus and nodulus of the pigmented rabbits. Neurosci. Res. **12:** 151–159.
47. ZEE, D.S., A. YAMAZAKI, P.H. BUTLER & G. GÜCER. 1981. Effects of ablation of flocculus and paraflocculus on eye movements in primate. J. Neurophysiol. **46:** 878–899.
48. WILSON, V.J., Y. YAMAGATA, B.J. YATES, et al. 1990. Response of vestibular neurons to head rotations in vertical planes. III. Response of vestibulocollic neurons to vestibular and neck stimulation. J. Neurophysiol. **64:** 1695–1703.
49. ANGELAKI, D.E., G.A. BUSH & A.A. PERACHIO. 1993. Two-dimensional spatiotemporal coding of linear acceleration in vestibular nuclei neurons. J. Neurosci. **13:** 1403–1417.
50. ZAKIR, M., K. KUSHIRO, Y. OGAWA, et al. 2000. Convergence patterns of the posterior semicircular canal and utricular inputs in single vestibular neurons in cats. Exp. Brain Res. **132:** 139–148.

51. UCHINO, Y., H. SATO, K. KUSHIRO, *et al.* 2000. Canal and otolith inputs to single vestibular neurons in cats. Arch. Ital. Biol. **138:** 3–13.
52. SATO, H., M. IMAGAWA, K. KUSHIRO, *et al.* 2000. Convergence of posterior semicircular canal and saccular inputs in single vestibular nuclei neurons in cats. Exp. Brain Res. **131:** 253–261.

Short-Term Adaptation of the VOR: Non-Retinal-Slip Error Signals and Saccade Substitution

SCOTT D.Z. EGGERS,[a] NICK DE PENNINGTON,[a] MARK F. WALKER,[a] MARK SHELHAMER,[b] AND DAVID S. ZEE[a,b]

[a]*Department of Neurology, The Johns Hopkins University School of Medicine, Baltimore, Maryland 21287, USA*

[b]*Department of Otolaryngology–Head & Neck Surgery, The Johns Hopkins University School of Medicine, Baltimore, Maryland 21287, USA*

ABSTRACT: We studied short-term (30 min) adaptation of the vestibulo-ocular reflex (VOR) in five normal humans using a "position error" stimulus without retinal image motion. Both before and after adaptation a velocity gain (peak slow-phase eye velocity/peak head velocity) and a position gain (total eye movement during chair rotation/amplitude of chair motion) were measured in darkness using search coils. The vestibular stimulus was a brief (~700 ms), 15° chair rotation in darkness (peak velocity 43°/s). To elicit adaptation, a straight-ahead fixation target disappeared during chair movement and when the chair stopped the target reappeared at a new location in front of the subject for gain-decrease (×0) adaptation, or 10° *opposite* to chair motion for gain-increase (×1.67) adaptation. This position-error stimulus was effective at inducing VOR adaptation, though for gain-increase adaptation the primary strategy was to substitute augmenting saccades during rotation while for gain-decrease adaptation both corrective saccades and a decrease in slow-phase velocity occurred. Finally, the presence of the position-error signal alone, at the end of head rotation, without any attempt to fix upon it, was not sufficient to induce adaptation. Adaptation did occur, however, if the subject did make a saccade to the target after head rotation, or even if the subject paid attention to the new location of the target without actually looking at it.

KEYWORDS: vestibulo-ocular reflex; adaptation; saccades; cognition

INTRODUCTION

An abnormal vestibulo-ocular reflex (VOR) leads to a motion of images on the retina during movement of the head which degrades vision. To maintain clear vision, the brain must compensate for lesions that alter the VOR. Typically, we think of VOR compensation as being accomplished by detection of an error signal such as movement of images across the retina, or "slip," during movement of the head, with

Address for correspondence: David S. Zee, M.D., Pathology 2-210, The Johns Hopkins Hospital, Baltimore, MD 21287. Voice: 410-955-3319; fax: 410-614-1746.
dzee@dizzy.med.jhu.edu

a subsequent adaptive readjustment in the slow-phase response.[1] Most VOR adaptation experiments artificially superimpose retinal slip during head rotation (visual-vestibular mismatch) and then look for a change in the measured VOR gain in darkness as an index of VOR adaptive capability. But retinal slip may not be the only error signal for adaptation, and adjustment of the slow phase may not be the only adaptive response. Other stimuli, such as retinal position errors, and other responses, such as saccades, may be critical to the adaptive process.[2–12]

The use of non-retinal-slip error signals to drive VOR adaptation is not surprising. During head motion, the demands of a fovea necessitate more than simply stabilizing the image of the visual environment on the entire retina. The brain needs to *point* the eyes at particularly important locations in the environment—both across the visual field and in depth—so that it can receive and then analyze the necessary information from the fovea. Because translation of the orbits invariably accompanies all natural head rotation, the VOR also must be adjusted for the location of the target of interest relative to the two orbits. The necessary adjustment—which may even require that the two eyes rotate by different amounts—depends upon the exact pattern of head rotation and translation and the particular depth and eccentricity of the target of interest. Thus, ocular motor responses specifically driven by the presence of a fovea—saccades, pursuit, and vergence—are reasonable candidates to assist the slow-phase response of the VOR during head motion, and might also be expected to play a role in adaptive adjustments of the VOR. Furthermore, stimuli that typically drive such eye movements, such as retinal position errors, might then serve as error signals to drive VOR adaptation.

One further consequence of having a fovea is that there must be mechanisms to *choose* which part of the image of the visual environment is placed and stabilized on the fovea. Hence, cognitive factors related to directing the focus of attention might also be expected to play a role in ocular motor performance during head motion and in VOR adaptation. To investigate these issues further, we studied short-term (30 min) VOR adaptation in normal human subjects using error signals without retinal image motion.

METHODS

Subjects

Five normal subjects, ages 21–58, participated in these experiments. They had no known vestibular or neurological disorders. Informed consent was obtained from all subjects, and all procedures were approved by the local institutional review board.

Vestibular Stimulus

The vestibular stimulus for both training and test trials was a 15° chair rotation, with a duration of ~ 700 ms that reached a peak velocity of 43°/s (see FIG. 1). From the starting position, the chair moved either to the right or left, with the direction randomly chosen. In the next trial, however, the chair motion was always back to the center. The time of onset of chair motion was randomly varied so the subjects could not predict when the chair would begin moving. The head of the subject was immobilized in the chair using a bite bar made of dental impression material.

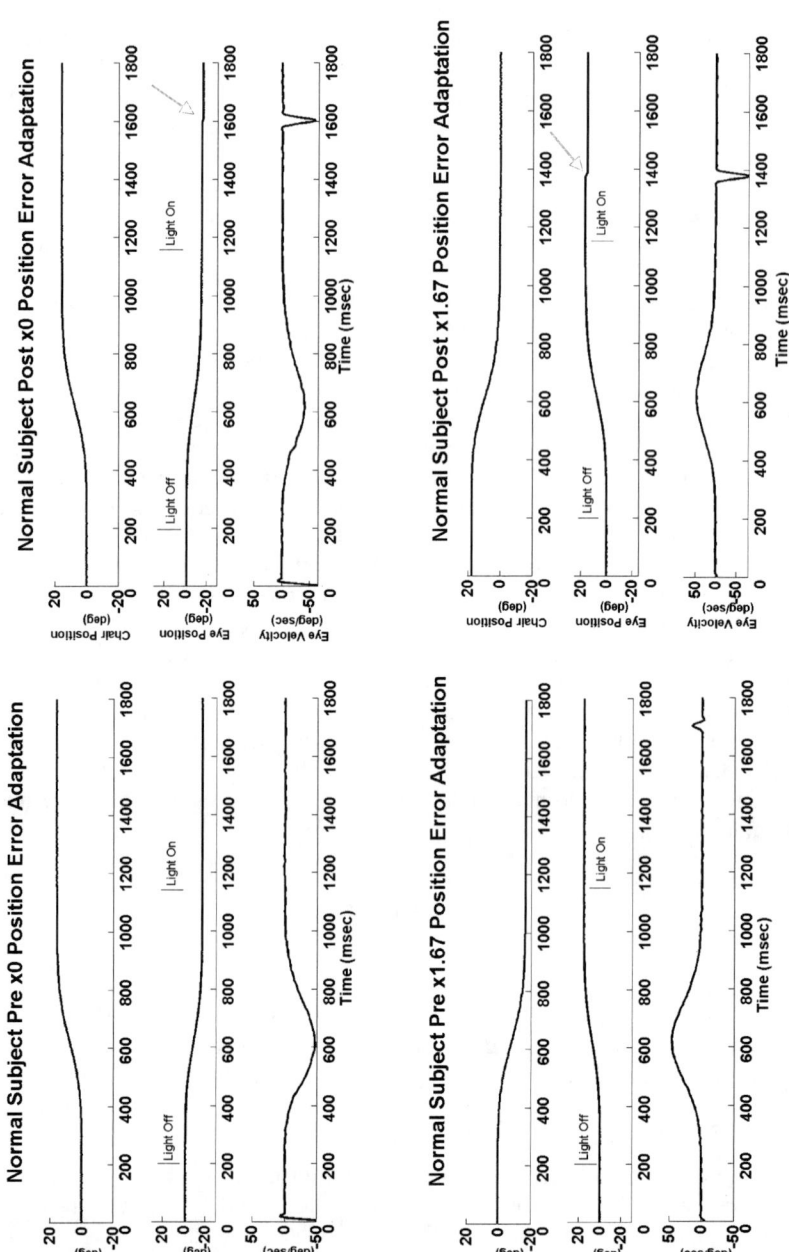

FIGURE 1. *See following page for legend.*

Test Trial Paradigm

The test trials to assess adaptation were the same for all training paradigms: 40 trials before and 40 trials after 30 min of training. The room was completely dark except for a small target (<1.0°), either an LED or a rear-projected laser dot. The trial began with the target located straight ahead of the subject; the target was turned off when the chair began moving. The same target reappeared when the chair stopped. The target was then extinguished for several seconds and then reappeared in front of the subject for the start of the next trial. In this way all test trials began with the target directly in front of the subject. During test trials, subjects were instructed to "maintain gaze on the location of the previously seen target and when it reappears look at it."

Training Paradigms

All adaptation paradigms consisted of 350 trials lasting 30 min. For the "position error" adaptation paradigm, each trial began with the target located straight ahead of the subject; it was turned off when the chair began moving. When the chair stopped moving, the target reappeared but in a different location. For ×0 adaptation (gain-decrease paradigm), the target reappeared directly in front of the subject, asking for a VOR gain of 0. For ×1.67 adaptation (gain-increase paradigm), the target reappeared 10° from its original location in the direction *opposite* to chair motion, asking for a VOR gain of 1.67.

Four different sets of instructions were used in the position error training paradigms. The instruction for the primary experiment was, "Smoothly move your eyes during the head rotation so they are at the new target position when it appears." In two secondary experiments the instructions were either (1) "During rotation attempt to maintain gaze on the location of the previously seen target (attempt to maintain a VOR gain of 1.0), and at the end of the rotation *look* at the target wherever it reappears" (late-saccade paradigm) or (2) "During rotation attempt to maintain gaze on the location of the previously seen target (attempt to maintain a VOR gain of 1.0), and at the end of the rotation *do not* look at the target when it appears" (no-saccade paradigm). With these last sets of instructions, the subjects were given a signal (target off, then on again) to indicate the start of the next trial with fixation of the straight-ahead target. The late-saccade paradigm induces a position error that is corrected by a saccade after head rotation (visual-motor error signal), while the no-saccade paradigm induces a position error only; it is specifically not corrected by a saccade after head rotation (visual error only).

In the final position error training paradigm (no saccade, visual error, attention), the target appeared in its new location but flashed on and off a variable number of times (1–3). The subject was instructed "during rotation attempt to maintain gaze on the location of the previously seen target" (i.e., attempt to maintain a VOR gain of

---

FIGURE 1. Adaptive changes following position-error training. For the ×0 paradigm (*top*), note the small *forward* corrective saccade (*arrow*) postadaptation, indicating an adaptive *decrease* in the VOR during head rotation in darkness. For the ×1.67 paradigm (*bottom*), note the small *backward* corrective saccade (*arrow*) postadaptation, indicating an adaptive *increase* in the VOR during head rotation in darkness.

1.0), and "at the end of the rotation *do not* look at the flashing target when it appears, but pay attention to it," and "after the target stops flashing, press the button the number of times you saw the target flash."

For the "velocity error" training paradigm, each trial began with the target located directly ahead of the subject. The target stayed on throughout the chair movement and remained on after the chair stopped. The target was moved using mirror galvanometers in the path of a rear-projected laser. For ×0 adaptation (gain-decrease), the target moved in the same direction, at the same speed, as the chair, asking for a VOR gain of 0. For ×1.67 adaptation (gain-increase), the target moved in the opposite direction as the chair, at 0.67 its speed, arriving 10° in the opposite direction from the original location, asking for a VOR gain of 1.67. Subjects were asked to "always maintain fixation on the target." Just before the beginning of each trial the target was presented directly in front of the subject.

Eye Movement Recordings

Eye movements were recorded using the magnetic search-coil technique with a directional scleral annulus placed in one eye after application of topical anesthesia. Analogue coil signals were filtered in hardware with a single pole RC analogue filter (bandwidth 0–90 Hz) and then sampled at 1000 Hz and analyzed offline.

Data Analysis

Two measures of VOR gain were used. A *position* gain was defined as the ratio of total eye movement during chair motion to amplitude of chair motion. A *velocity* gain was defined as the ratio of slow-phase eye velocity to chair velocity at the time of peak chair velocity. Preadaptation and postadaptation gains from test trials were compared using a two-sample t test assuming unequal variance, with a significance level of $P < 0.01$ unless otherwise noted.

RESULTS

Adaptive Changes following Position and Velocity Error Training

Sample eye-movement records before and after adaptation in the main position error paradigm are shown in FIGURE 1 for gain-decrease (×0) and gain-increase (×1.67) training. Unless explicitly stated, all results from position-error paradigms are from primary experiment trials, in which the subject was instructed to "Smoothly move your eyes during the head rotation so they are at the new target position when it appears." For the ×0 paradigm (top), note the small *forward* corrective saccade (arrow) after adaptation, indicating an adaptive *decrease* in the VOR during head rotation in darkness. For the ×1.67 paradigm (bottom), note the small *backward* corrective saccade (arrow) after adaptation, indicating an adaptive *increase* in the VOR during head rotation in darkness.

Quantitative results for this position-error paradigm from all subjects and a comparison to VOR changes from the velocity-error paradigm are shown in FIGURES 2 and 3. For ×0 adaptation (FIG. 2), both position-error and velocity-error paradigms led to a decrease in VOR gain as assessed by both position and velocity measures.

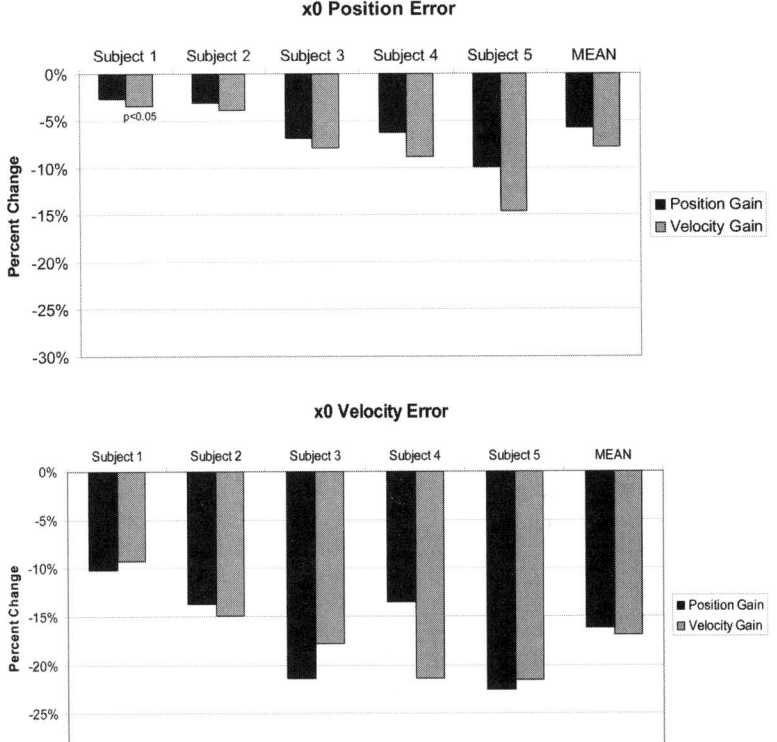

FIGURE 2. Summary of gain-decrease adaptation. For ×0 adaptation both position error (*top*) and velocity error (*bottom*) training led to a decrease in both the position and velocity VOR gain. Velocity-error training, however, was a more robust stimulus. Unless otherwise indicated, here and in all subsequent figures, pre- and postchanges were significant at a level of 0.01.

Velocity-error training, however, was a more robust stimulus. For ×1.67 adaptation (FIG. 3), velocity-error adaptation (bottom) caused a robust increase in both VOR velocity and position gains. Position-error adaptation (top) generally led to an increase in VOR position gain but not in VOR velocity gain. The increase in VOR position gain occurred by virtue of embedded saccades during rotation in darkness (see FIG. 4, right, lower panel). In one subject (No. 5), velocity gain even paradoxically *decreased*.

Adaptive Changes during Position Error Training

FIGURE 4 shows some of the adaptive changes that were apparent *during* ×1.67 position-error adaptation. Note that early in training the VOR was quite hypometric for the new requirement of increased gain and a single saccade brought the eye to the new target location after it appeared (arrow, top left panel). Later in training, in some trials multiple sequential saccades augmented and almost replaced the VOR slow

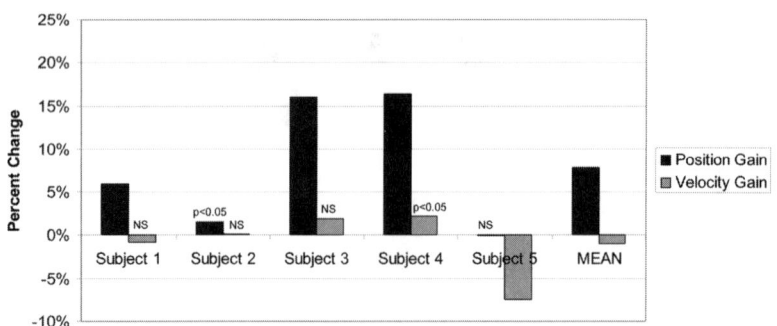

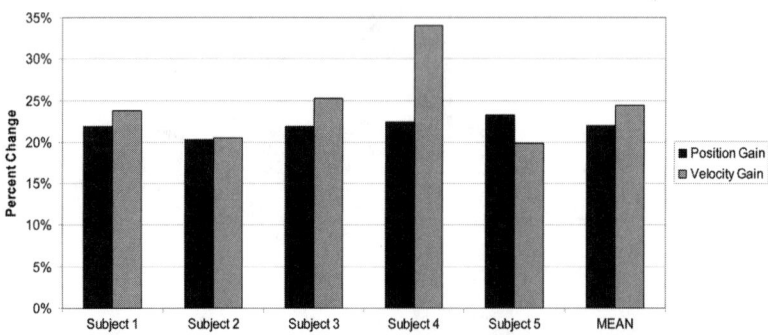

FIGURE 3. Summary of gain-increase adaptation. For ×1.67 adaptation, a velocity error (*bottom*) caused a robust increase in both VOR velocity and position gain. A position-error (*top*) generally led to an increase in position but not in VOR velocity gain. Same statistical analysis as in FIGURE 2.

phase (top right panel). On other trials, one or two large saccades were used to augment the VOR position gain. In the postadaptation test trials (bottom right panel), an augmenting saccade persisted (left arrow) and created an increased VOR position gain, reflected in the corrective saccade after the light reappeared (right arrow).

A similar pattern, but with oppositely directed saccades, was seen with downward ×0 position-error training (FIG. 5). Early in training (left panel) a single saccade occurred during head rotation to "cancel" the VOR slow phase. Later in training (right panel), multiple sequential saccades could occur, again almost replacing the VOR slow phase.

The changes of VOR gain during adaptation were compared by extracting sets of 10 consecutive trials early and late in the training session for each subject. FIGURE 6 shows that slow-phase gain changed little during ×1.67 position-error training, but clearly decreased during ×0 training. In the ×0 position-error paradigm with the first set of secondary instructions to make no corrective saccade until target appeared at the end of the head movement (late-saccade paradigm), there was still some decrease

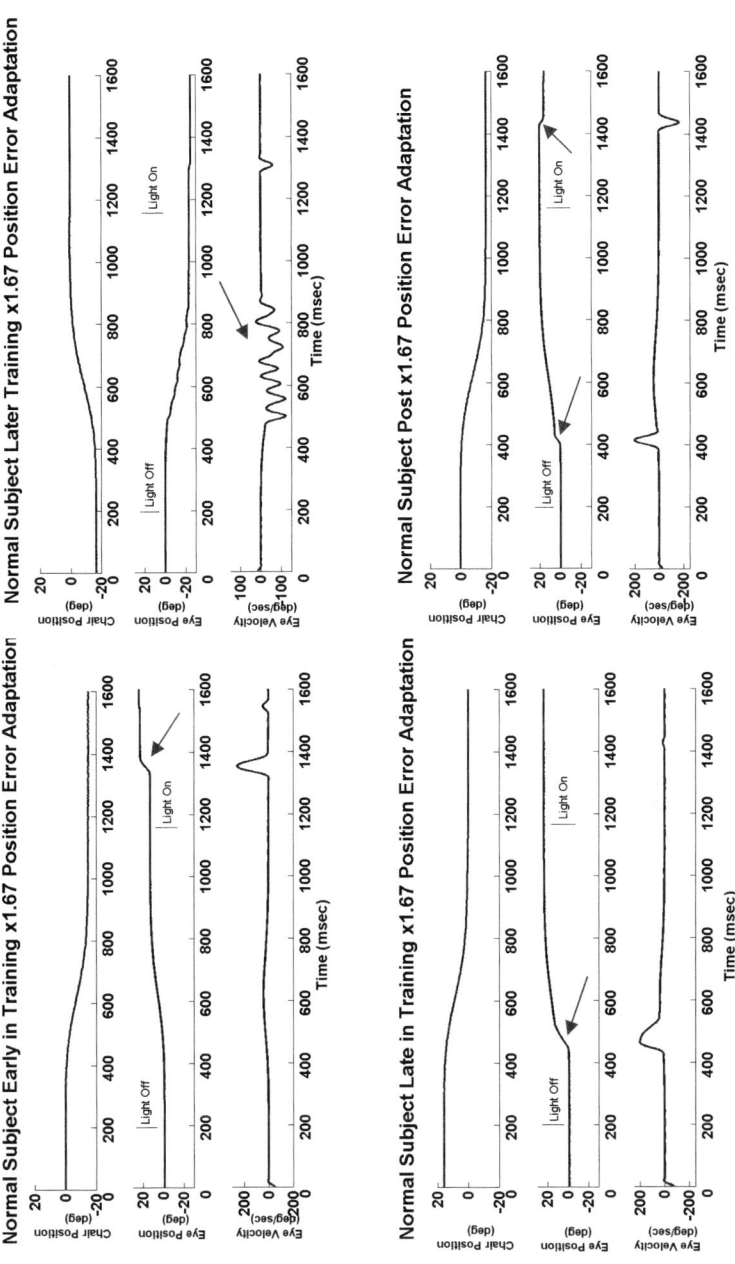

FIGURE 4. Adaptive changes during gain-increase position-error training. During ×1.67 adaptation, embedded saccades increased the VOR position gain. See text for details.

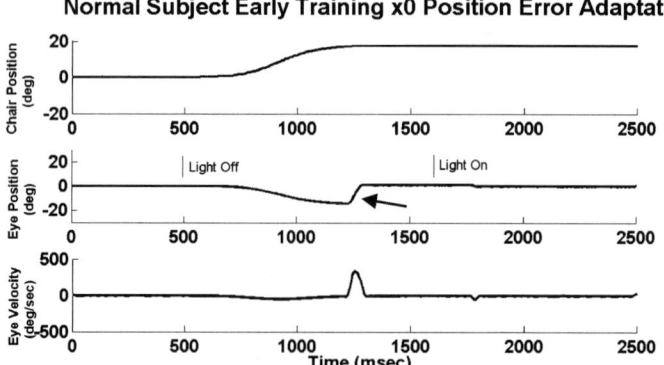

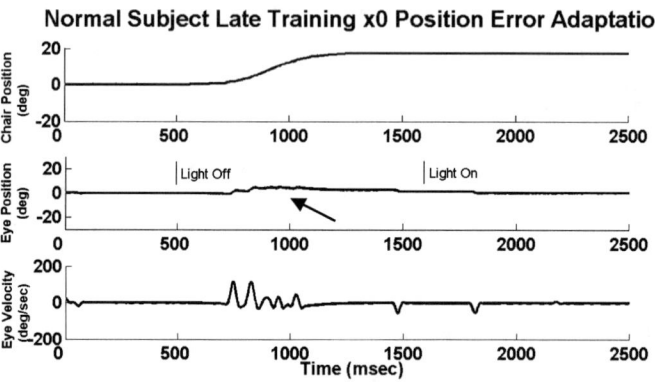

FIGURE 5. Adaptive changes during gain-decrease position-error training. Later in ×0 position-error training, multiple, sequential saccades could occur, effectively canceling the VOR slow phase (*right panel*).

in slow-phase velocity during adaptation. FIGURE 7 shows changes in the amplitude of the corrective saccade required when the target reappears after rotation (top) and of the latency of the first saccade during rotation (bottom) during the ×0 position-error paradigm. Especially for ×1.67 adaptation, the size of the corrective saccade diminished (top panel), though the values for corrective saccades for ×1.67 adaptation were larger to begin with. The latency to the first corrective saccade during rotation decreased (bottom panel). Even in the late-saccade ×0 position-error paradigm, there was a decrease in corrective saccade amplitude indicating an adaptive change during rotation.

Finally, "readaptation" could sometimes be seen even during the postadaptation test trials (FIG. 8). After ×0 velocity-error adaptation, early in postadaptation trials, there was a corrective saccade when the target reappeared (left panel, arrow). Later during this same testing period, the subject began to add augmenting saccades *during* rotation in order to compensate for the hypoactive VOR slow-phase gain (right panel, arrow).

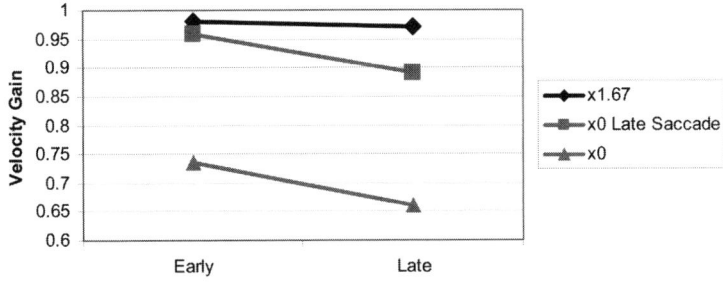

FIGURE 6. Changes in velocity gain *during* position-error adaptation. Slow-phase gain showed little change during ×1.67 position-error training, but did decrease during ×0 position-error training. Even in the ×0 paradigm when subjects were instructed to maintain gaze on the location of the previously seen straight-ahead target until the chair stopped and then look at the new target (late-saccade paradigm) velocity gain decreased.

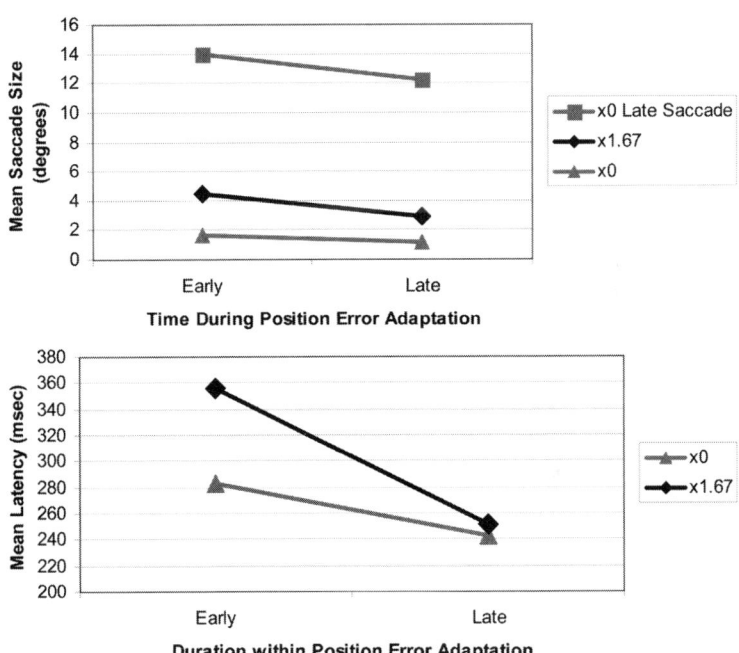

FIGURE 7. Changes in saccade behavior *during* position-error adaptation. The amplitude of the required corrective saccade when the target reappeared decreased during training, particularly with the ×1.67 position-error paradigm, indicating an adaptation in position gain (*top panel*). The latency from onset of chair movement to the first saccade also decreased during training, indicating an adaptive response (*bottom panel*).

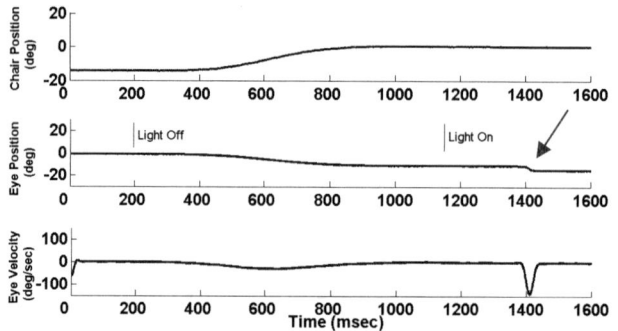
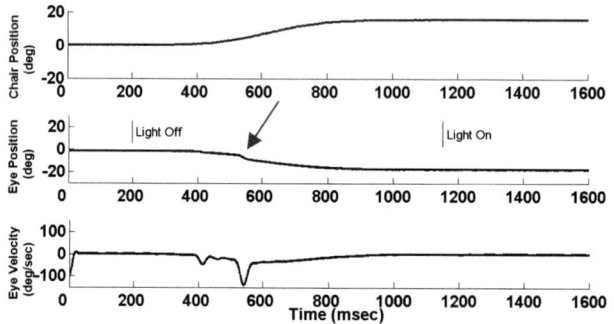

FIGURE 8. Readaptation during postadaptation testing. 'Readaptation' could sometimes be seen even during the post-training test trials. After ×0 velocity-error adaptation, early in postadaptation testing there was a corrective saccade when the light reappeared (*left panel, arrow*). Later during the same postadaptation testing, the subject begins to add augmenting saccades *during* rotation to compensate for the hypoactive VOR slow-phase gain (*right panel, arrow*).

Effect of Instructions on Position-Error Adaptation

Most of the results shown thus far with the position-error stimulus were obtained when the subjects were instructed to move their eyes *during* the course of the head movement so that their eyes would already be in a new location when the head stopped moving. On the other hand, when the subjects were instructed in the first secondary experiment *not* to alter their eye movement response during the head rotation itself (i.e., to make an effort to hold gaze on the imagined location of the previously visible straight-ahead target, but then to make a saccade to the new location of the target at the end of head rotation [late-saccade paradigm]), there was VOR adaptation comparable to that with the primary position-error paradigm, though perhaps relying more on saccades than a change in slow-phase velocity (compare FIG. 9, top, with FIG. 2). In a further experiment, we showed there was a comparable de-

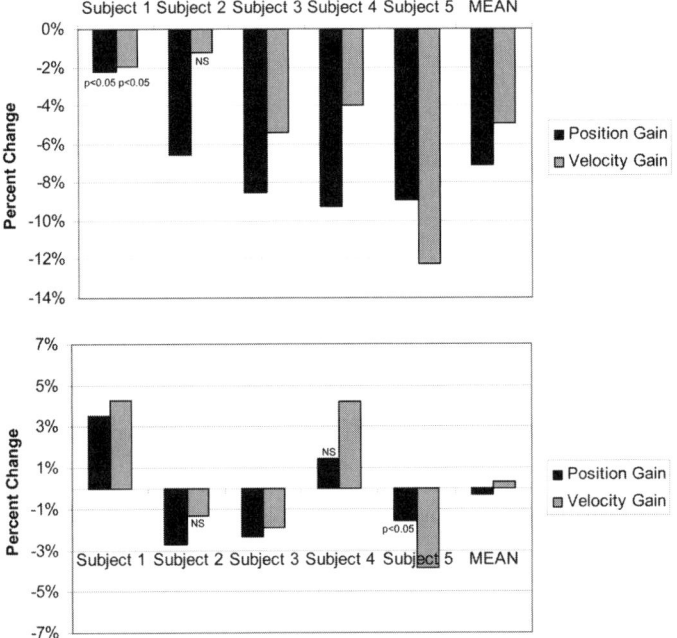

FIGURE 9. Effect of instructions on position-error adaptation. When the subjects were instructed to hold gaze on the imagined location of the previously visible straight-ahead target, and then to make a saccade to the new location of the target at the end of head rotation (late-saccade paradigm), there was still considerable VOR adaptation (*top panel*). In contrast, when subjects were further instructed *not* to make the corrective saccade to the target when it appeared in its new location at the end of head rotation (no-saccade paradigm), there was little adaptation (*bottom panel*).

gree of adaptation when the saccade after head rotation was made to the "imagined" location of the target in its new position (FIG. 10, top). In contrast, when subjects were further instructed in the second secondary experiment *not* to make the corrective saccade to the target when it appeared in its new location at the end of head rotation (no saccade paradigm), there was little adaptation and in a few cases a slight *increase* in VOR gain (FIG. 9, bottom). In contrast, in the no-saccade, visual error, attention paradigm (FIG. 10) a considerable degree of adaptation occurred similar to that when the eyes actually moved to the new target location (compare FIG. 9, top and FIG. 10, bottom).

DISCUSSION

Four main results emerged from this study. First, training with a position-error stimulus—in which a target appears in a new location *after* head rotation in darkness—elicited an adaptive readjustment in VOR gain as measured in darkness even though there was no retinal slip during head rotation. Second, the pattern of VOR

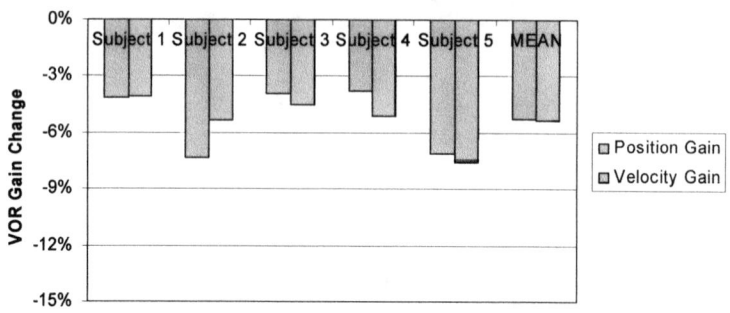

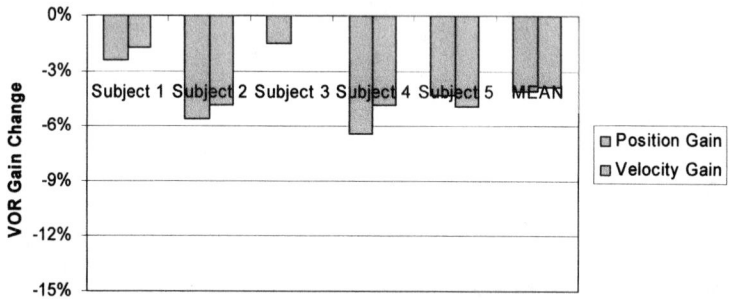

FIGURE 10. Effect of imagination and of attetnion on VOR adaptation. When subjects were instructed to move their eyes to the imagined location of the new target after head movement, there was considerable adaptation (*top*), similar to that in the late-saccade paradigm (compare with FIG. 9, *top panel*). When subjects were instructed to pay attention to a blinking target that appeared in a new location after head rotation but not to look at it, VOR adaptation still occurred (*bottom*).

adaptation depended upon whether an increase or a decrease in the VOR had been requested. For a gain decrease, the adjustment of the VOR consisted of a decrease in slow-phase velocity *and* the use of saccades in the *same* direction as head motion. For a gain increase, the adjustment of the VOR consisted primarily of the use of saccades in the *opposite* direction to head motion. Third, saccades were an integral part of the adaptive process, occurring during rotation in darkness to augment or diminish the overall VOR response as requested. And fourth, the presence of a visual error signal alone, at the end of head rotation (without either a visual refixation or attention to the target) was not sufficient to induce substantial VOR adaptation. For adaptation to occur, subjects had (1) to make a corrective saccade to the new location of the target when the head stopped moving, (2) to attempt to move the eyes toward the new target location during head rotation, or (3) to pay attention to the target in its new location, even though not directly looking at it.

Error Signals That Drive VOR Adaptation

Much evidence exists that both retinal slip and the attempt to overcome it during head rotation can drive VOR adaptation, at least during the more conventional retinal-slip training paradigms.[13] What might be the error signals that drive VOR adaptation when the stimulus is a position error as in the present study? Possibilities include (1) the presence of a position-error signal at the end of the head movement (the new target location relative to the initial straight-ahead position just before the beginning of the head movement), (2) the presence of a position-error signal at the end of the head movement *and* the corrective saccade that brings the eye there, and (3) the effort to move the eyes during the head movement so that the eyes would point at the new target location when the head stops moving. With respect to the third possibility, it has already been shown that VOR adaptation can be driven without any visual error signals at all. Simply fixing upon an imagined location of a target moving with the head (×0 viewing), without any targets visible before, during or after rotation, can lead to an adaptive decrease in the VOR measured in darkness.[6]

Our experiments with the no-saccade paradigm seem to exclude the first possibility that a post-rotation position-error signal alone, without an attempt to correct it, can drive VOR adaptation. This result appears at odds with recent studies of short-term saccade amplitude adaptation in which a visual error signal alone, occurring at or just after the primary saccade is finished, was thought to be the critical factor for producing saccade adaptation. The occurrence of corrective saccades in response to the new visual information does not seem needed to induce saccade adaptation.[14–20] Perhaps a way to resolve this seeming discrepancy is to consider that the error signal in both saccade adaptation and position-error VOR adaptation is based upon a perceived demand to change the relationship between where the fovea would normally point after a movement and the new place to which it must point based upon the adaptation stimulus.

A visual error signal at the end of a movement could be one source of information used by the brain to appreciate the mismatch between actual and desired eye movement.[20] Thus, in saccade-amplitude training paradigms, even if the need for a corrective saccade is eliminated by a subsequent readjustment in target position or by extinguishing the target, there would still have been an initial error signal informing the brain that it should have programmed a saccade to move the eyes to a different location in the environment. In contrast, there was little adaptation in our no-saccade VOR paradigm in which a target was presented at a new location at the end of the head movement, but there was a specific instruction *not* to look at it. Thus, even though there was a visual "error" signal at the end of head movement to decrease VOR gain, the brain never had to program a corrective saccade or adjust its slow-phase velocity in anticipation that its gaze would need to be redirected at the end of the head movement.

Further evidence for this idea comes from the finding that in the no-saccade paradigm not only was there was no decrease in gain, but in two subjects there was a slight *increase*. Perhaps, to avoid automatically making a saccade to the target as it reappeared at the head-fixed (×0) location, subjects had to concentrate more so than usual on maintaining a ×1.0 (normal) VOR gain and holding the final eye position after head motion. In fact, these findings raise the possibility that the critical error signal driving adaptation may depend not so much upon where the eyes actually point, but where the focus of visual attention is directed. McFadden et al.[19] have shown that one can induce saccade adaptation by adapting shifts of visual attention without any saccades actually being made during training. And, as indicated above, Melvill Jones et al.[6] have shown that an "effort of spatial localization" during rotation in total darkness can lead to a subsequent adaptive change in the VOR. Compatible with this idea were the results from our last experiment (no-saccade visual error attention paradigm), in which we found that VOR adaptation occurred with a shift of attention alone, without any associated eye movement toward the new location of the target. Thus, the brain can create a new internal model of the perceived relationship of its head and eyes to the external environment, and use error signals based on that model to drive adaptive processes. These considerations, of course, suggest that many higher-level cognitive processes such as effort, choice, imagination, attention, and saliency which are presumably related to activity within the cerebral cortex, may modulate and drive adaptation of naturally occurring, "subconscious" sensory-motor responses mediated by "low-level" cerebellar and brainstem circuits.[12,21]

Saccade Substitution during Rotation in the Dark

A prominent finding was the use of saccades during rotation in darkness to augment or diminish the VOR response as required by the training paradigm. It has been long recognized that "saccadic substitution" is a common adaptive strategy to improve VOR performance both in humans with labyrinthine disease and in normal subjects, both during natural behavior and in response to artificially imposed adaptive requirements.[2,3,8,10,22–28] In our study, on some trials during adaptation, there was a series of saccades made in darkness—one immediately following the other—that closely mimicked the new desired eye movement trajectory during head rotation. The latency to the first saccade during rotation in darkness also decreased with training, though there was an asymmetry in increase vs. decrease gain adaptation. Exactly how corrective saccades are generated during head rotation in darkness is not known, though the brainstem saccadic generating structures have ample access to information from the vestibular system that could be used to trigger saccades during head rotation.[29]

Differences between Gain-Increase and Gain-Decrease VOR Adaptation

One striking finding was the difference in the responses to upward (×1.67) versus downward (×0) adapting stimuli when using position but not velocity errors. Position-error stimuli were not effective at driving VOR slow-phase velocity gain upward, though overall adaptation combining saccades and slow phases, as reflected in the mean position gain combining all subjects, was similar for upward and downward adaptation. In some individual subjects, however, there were often striking asymmetries in the pattern of response to upward versus downward adapting stimuli. These idiosyncrasies in vestibular adaptive strategies remain unexplained. It has been suggested that the mechanisms underlying saccade adaptation might be closely linked to VOR adaptation because saccades and VOR slow phases are commonly linked during changes of gaze with the head free.[20] It would be interesting to compare the patterns of response of individual subjects in VOR and saccade adaptation paradigms.

ACKNOWLEDGMENTS

This work was supported by National Institutes of Health grants RO1-EY01849, RO1 DC02849, and K23-EY00400, and NASA through cooperative agreement NCC 9-58 with the National Space Biomedical Research Institute.

REFERENCES

1. ITO, M. 2000. Mechanisms of motor learning in the cerebellum. Brain Res. **886:** 237–245.
2. SEGAL, B.N. & A. KATSARKAS. 1988. Goal-directed vestibulo-ocular function in man: gaze stabilization by slow-phase and saccadic eye movements. Exp. Brain Res. **70:** 26–32.
3. BERTHOZ, A. 1988. The role of gaze in compensation of vestibular dysfunction: the gaze substitution hypothesis. Prog. Brain Res. **76:** 411–420.
4. BERTHOZ, A. 1985. Adaptive mechanisms in eye-head coordination. *In* Adaptive Mechanisms in Gaze Control. A. Berthoz & G. Melvill Jones, Eds.: 177–201. Elsevier. Amsterdam.
5. ZHOU,W., P. WELDON, B. TANG & W.M. KING. 2001. Retinal slip not required for rapid adaptation of the translational vestibulo-ocular reflex. Soc. Neurosci. Abstr. **27**.
6. MELVILL JONES, G., A. BERTHOZ & B. SEGAL. 1984. Adaptive modification of the vestibulo-ocular reflex by mental effort in darkness. Exp. Brain Res. **56:** 149–153.
7. SHELHAMER, M., B. RAVINA & P.D. KRAMER. 1995. Adaptation of the gain of the angular vestibulo-ocular reflex when retinal slip is zero [Abstr.]. Soc. Neurosci. Abstr. **21:** 518.
8. MELVILL JONES, G., D. GUITTON & A. BERTHOZ. 1988. Changing patterns of eye-head coordination during 6 h of optically reversed vision. Exp. Brain Res. **69:** 531–544.
9. JONES, G.M. & G. MANDL. 1979. Effects of strobe light on adaptation of vestibulo-ocular reflex (VOR) to vision reversal. Brain Res. **164:** 300–303.
10. KASAI, T. & D.S. ZEE. 1978. Eye-head coordination in labyrinthine-defective human beings. Brain Res. **144:** 123–141.
11. BLOOMBERG, J., G. MELVILL JONES & B. SEGAL. 1991. Adaptive plasticity in the gaze stabilizing synergy of slow and saccadic eye movements. Exp. Brain Res. **84:** 35–46.
12. MELVILL JONES, G. & H. FADLALLAH. 1996. Modulation of compensatory VOR-saccade synergy by post-test cognitive feedback [abstract]. J Vestib Res **6:** S91.
13. SHELHAMER, M., C. TILIKET, D. ROBERTS, *et al.* 1994. Short-term vestibulo-ocular reflex adaptation in humans. II. Error signals. Exp. Brain Res. **100:** 328–336.
14. NOTO, C.T. & F.R. ROBINSON. 2001. Visual error is the stimulus for saccade gain adaptation. Brain Res. Cogn. Brain Res. **12:** 301–305.
15. ROBINSON, F., C. NOTO & S. WATANABE. 2000. Effect of visual background on saccade adaptation in monkeys. Vision Res. **40:** 2359–2367.
16. SEEBERGER, T., C. NOTO & F. ROBINSON. 2002. Non-visual information does not drive saccade gain adaptation in monkeys. Brain Res. **956:** 374–379.
17. WALLMAN, J. & A.F. FUCHS. 1998. Saccadic gain modification: visual error drives motor adaptation. J. Neurophysiol. **80:** 2405–2416.
18. FUJITA, M., A. AMAGAI, F. MINAKAWA & M. AOKI. 2002. Selective and delay adaptation of human saccades. Brain Res. Cogn. Brain Res. **13:** 41–52.
19. MCFADDEN, S.A., A. KHAN & J. WALLMAN. 2002. Gain adaptation of exogenous shifts of visual attention. Vision Res. **42:** 2709–2726.
20. BAHCALL, D.O. & E. KOWLER. 2000. The control of saccadic adaptation: implications for the scanning of natural visual scenes. Vision Res. **40:** 2779–2796.
21. ISRAEL, I., S. RIVAUD, B. GAYMARD, A. BERTHOZ & C. PIERROT-DESEILLIGNY. 1995. Cortical control of vestibular-guided saccades in man. Brain **118:** 1169–1183.
22. BLOOMBERG, J., G. MELVILL JONES & B. SEGAL. 1991. Adaptive plasticity in the gaze stabilizing synergy of slow and saccadic eye movements. Exp. Brain Res. **84:** 35–46.

23. SEGAL, B.N. & A. KATSARKAS. 1988. Long-term deficits of goal-directed vestibulo-ocular function following total unilateral loss of peripheral vestibular function. Acta Otolaryngol. (Stockh.) **106:** 102–110.
24. TIAN, J.-R., B.T. CRANE & J.L. DEMER. 2000. Vestibular catch-up saccades in labyrinthine deficiency. Exp. Brain Res. **131:** 448–457.
25. TIAN, J.-R., B.T. CRANE, G. WIEST & J.L. DEMER. 2002. Effect of aging on the human initial interaural linear vestibulo-ocular reflex. Exp. Brain Res. **145:**142–149.
26. RAMAT, S. & D.S. ZEE. 2002. TVOR responses to abrupt interaural accelerations in normal humans. Ann. N. Y. Acad. Sci. **956:** 551–554.
27. BERTHOZ, A., I. ISRAEL, T. VIEVILLE & D.S. ZEE. 1987. Linear head displacement measured by the otoliths can be reproduced through the saccadic system. Neurosci. Lett. **82:** 285–290.
28. RAMAT, S. & D.S. ZEE. 2003. Ocular motor responses to abrupt interaural head translation in normal humans. J. Neurophysiol. **90:** 887–902.
29. CARTWRIGHT, A.D., D.P. GILCHRIST, A.M. BURGESS & I.S. CURTHOYS. 2003. A realistic neural-network simulation of both slow and quick phase components of the guinea pig VOR. Exp. Brain Res. **149:** 299–311.

Adaptations and Deficits in the Vestibulo-Ocular Reflex after Peripheral Ocular Motor Palsies

JAMES A. SHARPE,[a,b] DOUGLAS TWEED,[a,c] AND AGNES M.F. WONG[a,b]

[a]Division of Neurology, and Departments of [b]Ophthalmology, and [c]Physiology, University Health Network, University of Toronto, Toronto, Ontario, Canada

ABSTRACT: Palsy of a nerve might be expected to lower vestibulo-ocular reflex (VOR) responses in its fields of motion, but effects of peripheral neuromuscular disease were unknown. We recorded the VOR during sinusoidal head rotations in yaw, pitch, and roll at 0.5–2 Hz and static torsional gain in 43 patients with unilateral nerve palsies. Sixth nerve palsy ($n = 21$) reduced both abduction and adduction VOR gains in darkness. In light, horizontal visually enhanced VOR (VVOR) gains were normal in moderate and mild palsy. In severe palsy, horizontal VVOR gains remained low in the paretic eye when it was fixating, whereas gains in the nonparetic eye became higher than normal. Third nerve palsy ($n = 10$) decreased VOR and VVOR gains during abduction, adduction, elevation, depression, extorsion, and intorsion. Fourth nerve palsy ($n = 13$) reduced VOR gains of the paretic eye during intorsion, extorsion, elevation, depression, abduction, and adduction, but in light vertical and horizontal VVOR gains were normal. In the nonparetic eye, all gains were normal. Reduced VOR gains in the direction of paretic muscles and also in the direction of their antagonists, together with normal gains in the nonparetic eye, indicate a selective adjustment to the antagonists of paretic muscles. Increase of VVOR gains to normal in the paretic eye, when used for fixation, without conjugate increase in gains in the occluded nonparetic eye, provides further evidence of selective adaptation for the paretic eye. Motions of the eyes after nerve palsies indicate monocular VOR adaptation in three dimensions.

KEYWORDS: adaptation; nerve palsies; sixth nerve palsy; third nerve palsy; fourth nerve palsy; static torsional vestibulo-ocular reflex; angular vestibulo-ocular reflex; torsional vestibulo-ocular reflex; vertical vestibulo-ocular reflex; horizontal vestibulo-ocular reflex; Hering's law; diplopia

INTRODUCTION

Assessment of strabismus emphasizes static deviations and little information is available about the effects of paralytic strabismus on eye-movement dynamics such as during the vestibulo-ocular reflex (VOR). Adaptive changes in the VOR occur in

---

Address for correspondence: Dr. James A. Sharpe, Division of Neurology, University Health Network TWH, WW 5-440, 399 Bathurst Street, Toronto, Ontario M5T 2S8, Canada. Fax: 416-603-5596.

sharpej@uhnres.utoronto.ca

response to different visual stimuli.[1,2] Disconjugate VOR adaptation has been elicited in monkeys in response to anisometropic prisms[3] and experimental weakening of the horizontal rectus muscles.[4,5] We examined the angular VOR in patients with unilateral peripheral sixth, third, and fourth nerve palsies to determine effects of palsies in different directions on the VOR and its adaptation, if any, in each eye to monocular palsies. We identified changes in the actions of antagonists to paretic muscles that indicate monocular adaptations to peripheral neuromuscular deficits.

METHODS

Patients with unilateral peripheral palsy of the sixth ($n = 21$), third ($n = 10$), or fourth ($n = 13$) ocular motor nerves were recruited from the Neuroophthalmology Center at the University Health Network.[6-8] The duration and age of onset of diplopia, the presence or absence of risk factors for ischemia (diabetes mellitus and hypertension), and associated neurologic symptoms and signs were determined. The magnitude of strabismus was measured objectively using the prism and cover test and subjectively using the Maddox rod and prism test. Appropriate tests were performed to rule out myasthenia gravis, thyroid ophthalmopathy, other orbital diseases, or intracranial lesions. Ranges of duction were estimated as the estimated percentage of the normal abduction in the other eye. On the basis of the duction defect, patients with sixth nerve palsies were classified into three groups: mild (81–95% of normal range of abduction), moderate (51–80%), and severe ($\leq 50\%$). Fifteen normal subjects of similar ages served as controls (mean age, 52 years; SD, 15 years; median age, 58 years; age range 19–69; 8 women).

The angular dynamic VOR was measured in darkness while patients made active sinusoidal head on body rotations in yaw and pitch at approximately 0.5 and 2 Hz, and in roll at approximately 0.5, 1, and 2 Hz at amplitudes of approximately $\pm 10°$ from orbital midposition. The dynamic visually enhanced VOR (VVOR) was measured while they fixated on a stationary laser target 1 M from the naision, with one eye occluded, fixating in turn with the paretic and nonparetic eye. To measure the static torsional VVOR, we had patients fixate on the center target with one eye occluded as we measured their ocular responses to static head rolls of approximately 30° toward each shoulder, as measured with a head search coil. Static torsional gain is defined as change in torsional eye position divided by change in head position during maintained head roll. The test then was repeated with the other eye fixating and the fellow eye occluded, and also in total darkness (VOR).

Eye movements were recorded by three-dimensional binocular magnetic scleral search coils (Skalar Instrumentation, Delft, the Netherlands) using 1.83-m-diameter field coils arranged in a cube (CNC Engineering, Seattle, WA). There was minimal cross talk; large horizontal and vertical movements produced deflections in the torsional channel of less than 4% of the amplitude of the horizontal and vertical movement. Any coil slippage was assessed by offsets in torsional eye position signal during testing. Consistency of calibrated positions after each eye movement provided evidence that the coil did not slip on the eye. Eye and head position signals were filtered with a bandwidth of 0 to 90 Hz, and digitized at 200 Hz.

Fast phases of vestibular nystagmus were identified[9] and positions between 80 ms before and after fast phases were removed, the gaps being replaced with quadratic fits. The offset due to the fast phase then was removed, and the ongoing slow phase was interpolated to yield a cumulative trace of eye position.

Using a least squares sinusoidal fit,[10] we fitted eye and head positions with one cycle, and phases and amplitudes and amplitude gains were computed. We also plotted head velocity against eye velocity and performed a linear regression for each direction. The slopes of the fitted lines were the gains, and the results were comparable to those computed by the least squares sinusoidal fit technique.

RESULTS

Of 21 patients with sixth nerve palsy, six had severe, seven had moderate, and eight had mild palsy; the duration of symptoms ranged from 2 weeks to 96 months (mean, 16 months). For 10 patients with third nerve palsies, the duration of symptoms ranged from 1 week to 50 months (mean, 18 months). In 13 patients with fourth nerve palsies, duration of symptoms ranged from 1 week to 132 months (mean, 35 months). VOR function was tested at one point in the course of their palsies and expressed as changes from normal, rather than serial intrasubject changes. Any recovery toward normal values was not assessed. Abnormalities are interpreted as deficits or adaptation to those deficits.

Horizontal VOR

Sixth nerve palsy. In all patients, horizontal VOR gains in darkness were decreased in the paretic eye in both abduction and adduction and remained normal in the nonparetic eye in both directions (FIG. 1). In light, horizontal VVOR gains were normal in both eyes in moderate and mild palsy. During active head movement, normal persons have both VOR (in darkness) and the VVOR gains approximating unity.[11] In severe palsy, horizontal VVOR gains were low in the paretic eye in both directions, during viewing with either eye, whereas those in the nonparetic eye were higher than normal (>1.0) when the paretic eye viewed (FIG. 1). In light and darkness, mean phase differences between the eye and head positions approximated 180°, designated as zero phase shift.

Third nerve palsy. Horizontal VOR and VVOR gains of the paretic eye were decreased during both abduction and adduction.

Fourth nerve palsy. In darkness, horizontal VOR gains of the paretic eye were reduced symmetrically during both abduction and adduction ($P < 0.01$), whereas gains of the nonparetic eye were normal. In light, during paretic or nonparetic eye viewing, horizontal VVOR gains of both the paretic and the nonparetic eyes were normal ($P < 0.05$). Neither eye showed any significant phase shift from zero in light or in darkness.

Vertical VOR

Sixth nerve palsy. Vertical VOR and VVOR gains were normal in severe and mild palsies.

Third nerve palsy. In darkness (FIG. 2, top graph), vertical VOR gains of the paretic eye were reduced ($P < 0.01$) symmetrically during both elevation and depression, whereas gains of the nonparetic eye were normal. In light, during paretic eye or nonparetic eye viewing (FIG. 2, middle and bottom graphs), vertical VVOR gains of the

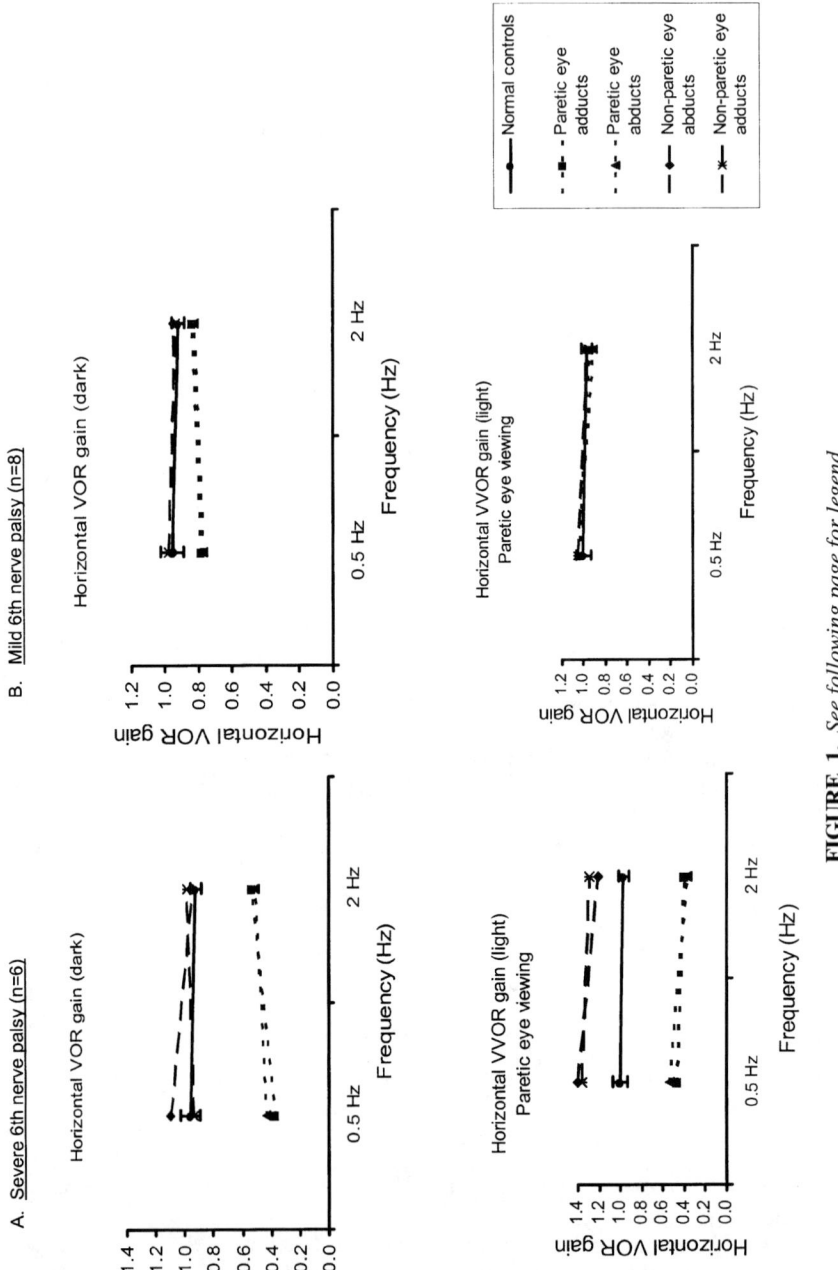

FIGURE 1. *See following page for legend.*

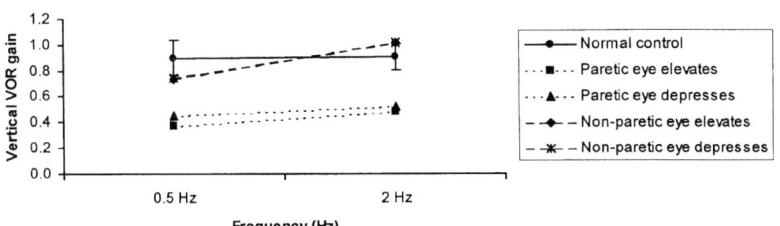
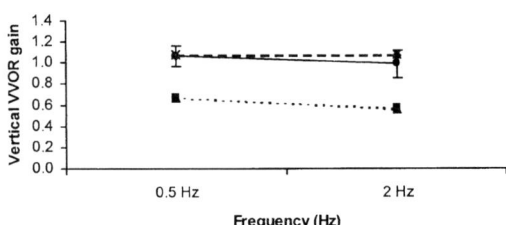
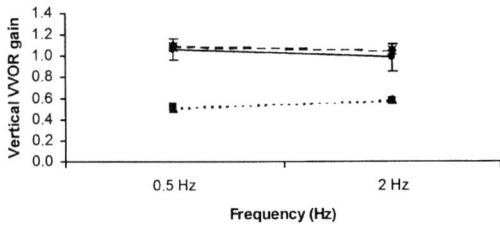

FIGURE 2. Vertical VOR and VVOR in 10 patients with third nerve palsy. The VOR gain of the paretic eye is severely reduced in elevation and depression (*top*). The VVOR gain remains low during fixation with the paretic eye or with the normal eye occluded. *Error bars* are 1 SD above and below group mean.

FIGURE 1. Horizontal VOR and VVOR gains during active head rotation at approximately 0.5 and 2 Hz in sixth nerve palsy. (**A**) Group mean VOR gains in severe palsy are reduced symmetrically in the paretic eye (*top*). VVOR gains with the paretic eye fixating and the normal eye occluded (*bottom*) become well above unity in the normal eye, but VVOR gains in the paretic eye remain reduced. (**B**) In mild palsy VOR gains for the patient group are reduced also in the paretic eye during abduction and adduction (*top*), but VVOR gains increase to normal values (*bottom*). *Error bars* indicate 1 SD. *Insets* in FIGURES 1, 2, and 4 show lines keys for paretic eye and normal eye and directions of movement.

paretic eye remained reduced ($P < 0.05$), whereas gains in the nonparetic eye were normal. Neither eye showed any significant phase shift from zero in light or in darkness.

Fourth nerve palsy. In darkness, vertical VOR gains of the paretic eye were symmetrically reduced during both depression and elevation ($P < 0.05$), whereas gains of the nonparetic eye were normal. In light, during paretic eye and nonparetic eye viewing, vertical VVOR gains of both the paretic and the nonparetic eyes were normal ($P < 0.05$). Neither eye showed any significant phase shift from zero in light or in darkness.

Torsional VOR, Dynamic and Static

Sixth nerve palsy. Dynamic torsional VOR and VVOR gains were significantly reduced during head roll in both the paretic and nonparetic eyes when compared with normal controls ($P < 0.05$). Neither eye showed any significant phase shift from zero during vertical or torsional rotation. Static torsional gains were reduced in 19 (90%) of the 21 patients in light and in dark (Z-tests, $P < 0.05$). Static torsional VOR and VVOR gains of each eye were conjugate between the two eyes in all patients and did not differ during right eye or left eye viewing.

Third nerve palsy. In darkness dynamic torsional VOR gains of the paretic eye were reduced during both intorsion and extorsion ($P < 0.01$), whereas gains of the nonparetic eye were normal. In light, and during viewing with either eye, torsional VVOR gains of the paretic eye remained reduced ($P < 0.01$), whereas gains in the

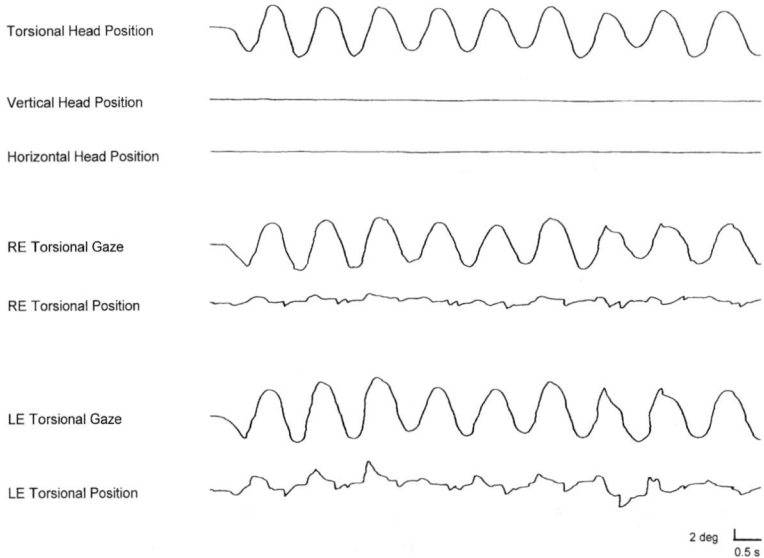

FIGURE 3. Torsional VOR in darkness during 2-Hz head roll in a patient with a right fourth nerve palsy. Responses are low in the right eye during both extortion and intorsion and normal in the left eye. Gaze is summed head and eye motion as recorded by a search coil. Upward movements in torsional traces are clockwise with reference to the patient (i.e., toward her right shoulder), and downward movements are counterclockwise.

nonparetic eye were normal.[7] In normal persons, viewing a foveal target does not appreciably raise torsional VVOR gains of above torsional gains in darkness.[12] Neither eye showed any significant phase shift from zero in light or in darkness. Static torsional VOR and VVOR gains of the paretic eye were reduced during intorsion and extorsion ($P < 0.05$) but were normal in the nonparetic eye.

Fourth nerve palsy. In darkness, dynamic torsional VOR gains of the paretic eye were reduced symmetrically during intorsion and extorsion (FIG. 3) in each of 13 patients ($P < 0.01$), whereas gains of the nonparetic eye were normal (FIG. 4, top graph). In light, during either paretic or nonparetic eye viewing (FIG. 4, middle and bottom graphs), torsional VVOR gains of the paretic eye were also low in both di-

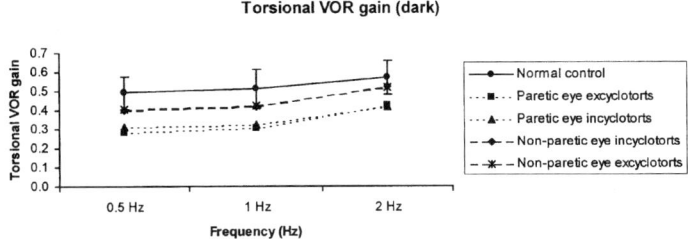

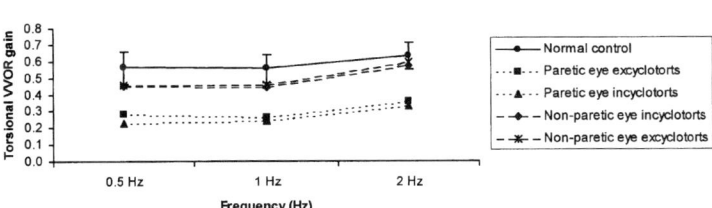

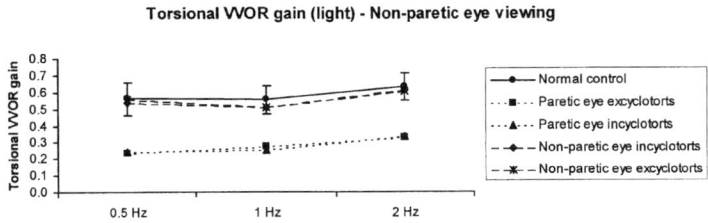

FIGURE 4. Torsional VOR and VVOR gains in 13 patients with trochlear nerve palsy. Intorsion and extortion gains are symmetrically reduced in the paretic eye in darkness (*top*) and during fixation with either eye. A foveal target has no appreciable effect on torsional gain. *Error bars* are 1 SD.

rections ($P < 0.05$), whereas those of the nonparetic eye remained normal.[8] In light and in darkness, the mean phase was zero. Static torsional VOR and VVOR gains of the paretic eye were reduced during intorsion ($P < 0.05$) and normal during extorsion of the paretic eye. In the nonparetic eye, static torsional VOR and VVOR gains were normal.

DISCUSSION

During head rotation in darkness, angular VOR gains are reduced during movement in the directions of actions of paretic muscles as anticipated from their palsy. However, dynamic gains are also reduced in the fields of actions of their antagonist muscles. VOR gains in the nonparetic eye remain normal, indicating a selective adjustment of the paretic eye, specifically to the antagonists of paretic muscles. In light, visual input increases gain of the paretic eye when it is used for fixation, providing further evidence of selective adaptation in the paretic eye. Torsional dynamic VOR and VVOR gains of the paretic eye are reduced for both extortion and intorsion in third and fourth nerve palsies. Motion of the eyes after nerve palsies exemplifies monocular adaptation of the VOR in three dimensions.

Sixth Nerve Palsy

In darkness, horizontal VOR gains are reduced during *abduction* of the paretic eye in all patients, as anticipated in sixth nerve palsy. Gains are also reduced during *adduction* of the paretic eye (FIG. 1), suggesting that innervation to the medial rectus has changed. After severe palsy, vision does not increase abducting or adducting horizontal VVOR gains to normal in the paretic eye but causes secondary increase in VVOR gains to values above unity in the nonparetic eye, when the paretic eye fixates. To adopt a conventional term from strabismology, this is a secondary change in the VOR, occurring when the paretic eye fixates. In mild and moderate palsy, vision enhances the VOR in the paretic eye but causes no change in the nonparetic eye, suggesting a monocular readjustment of innervation selectively to the paretic eye. Vertical VOR and VVOR gains are normal, indicating that the lateral rectus does not have significant vertical actions through the ±10° excursions that we tested.

Reduced torsional VOR gains in the paretic eye can be explained by the esotropia in sixth nerve palsy. Torsional VOR gain normally varies with vergence.[13,14] We attribute the reduced torsional gains in the paretic eye to the mechanism that normally lowers it during convergence.[6] The low torsional gains in the nonparetic eye may be an adaptation to reduce torsional disparity between the two eyes.

Third Nerve Palsy

Adducting VOR gains are reduced, as anticipated from medial rectus palsy. Abducting gains are also reduced; the reduction is attributed to an adaptive decrease in innervation to the lateral rectus, to achieve symmetry of the horizontal VOR. Torsional VOR gains are reduced during extorsion from palsy of the inferior oblique muscle. Gains are also reduced during intorsion,[7] which may be explained by an adaptive decrease in innervation to the superior oblique, to restore symmetry of the torsional VOR.

Fourth Nerve Palsy

During head rotation in darkness, VOR gains are reduced during intorsion, depression, and abduction of the paretic eye, as anticipated from paresis of the superior oblique muscle. VOR gains during extorsion (FIG. 3), elevation, and adduction of the paretic eye also are reduced, whereas VOR gains in the nonparetic eye remain normal, indicating a selective central adjustment of innervation to the paretic eye. In light, torsional VVOR gains in the paretic eye remained reduced (FIG. 4). Visual input increases vertical and horizontal VVOR gains to normal in the paretic eye, without a conjugate increase in VVOR gains in the nonparetic eye,[8] providing further evidence of selective adaptation in the paretic eye.

Patients selected a preferred eye for viewing during the course of their palsies. We did not control the eye of habitual fixation, which was probably the nonparetic eye in most cases, although they may have switched from one eye to the other at their whim or subconscious choice. The adaptation might have differed if patients predominantly used the paretic eye for fixation.

Changes in Antagonists of Paretic Agonist Muscles

Without the decreased VOR gains in the direction of action of antagonists of paretic muscles, the VOR would be asymmetric in the paretic eye. The asymmetry would drive the paretic eye further into direction of action of the antagonist with each cycle of head rotation, resulting in increasing position disparity between the two eyes and more diplopia (FIG. 5). The brain might adopt any one of four strategies to prevent this disparity. First, it might increase its innervation to the paretic agonist to increase VOR gain of the paretic eye, but this strategy is limited by the palsy itself. Second, the brain might generate saccades in direction of paresis to correct for the low agonist VOR gains. However, during activation of the paretic agonist, if common premotor signals are sent to motoneurons of the yolked agonist in the other eye, unwanted saccades would appear conjugately in the nonparetic eye, driving its fovea off its target. Third, the brain might attempt to prevent asymmetry of the VOR by

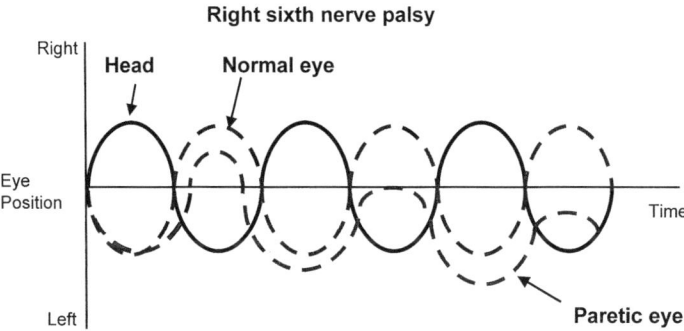

FIGURE 5. Schematic of consequence of asymmetry of VOR in unilateral sixth nerve palsy. Without adaptation to achieve symmetry, the paretic eye would move further into adduction with each cycle of head motion.

decreasing antagonist gains in the paretic eye. Hering[15] suggested that the brain controls gaze by two systems, one for conjugate movements and the other for vergence. However, if common and conjugate premotor signals were sent to motoneurons to both eyes, the yolked antagonist gain in the other (normal) eye would be reduced as well. For example, in the case of a left lateral rectus weakness from a left sixth nerve palsy, any adaptive reduction in innervation to the left medial rectus muscle would be accompanied by reduced innervation to the right lateral rectus muscle, in accord with Hering's proposal or "law." It was not. Fourth, the brain could selectively reduce VOR gains during action of the antagonist of the paretic muscle by reducing its innervation. This is apparently the strategy that the brain uses, in violation of Hering's law.

Changes in normal orbital plant mechanics might contribute to the decreased VOR gains of the paretic eye in the direction of the antagonists to paretic muscles. The relative contribution of agonist contraction and antagonist relaxation varies with orbital position,[16] and it may be altered when one muscle of an agonist–antagonist pair is palsied. Contracture is characterized by muscle shortening and stiffening as a result of decreased number of sarcomeres.[17] If the reduction of VOR gains in both directions were caused by changes in extraocular muscle mechanics, one would expect VOR gains to be subnormal during rotation or in light (VVOR) as well as in darkness, and that the peak velocities of nystagmus quick phases would be reduced in each direction. However, our results indicate that although VOR gains were decreased, VVOR gains could increase to normal values in light. In addition, although VOR gains were reduced in each direction, peak velocities of saccades in the antagonist's direction of action were normal (data not shown here). Our results provide evidence that decrease in VOR gains is not the result of changes in mechanical properties of the orbital plant but is caused by a functional central adaptation to the palsy.

Proprioceptive signals from extraocular muscles[18] might contribute to VOR adaptation. Proprioceptive afferent fibers project via the ophthalmic branch of the trigeminal nerve to the spinal trigeminal nucleus, but a portion also may enter via the ocular motor nerves.[19] Although visual information plays a massively dominant role in the control of VOR, altered proprioceptive inflow from a shortened (slack) antagonist or a palsied muscle might participate in the monocular adaptations that we identified after peripheral nerve palsies. Binocular disparity of retinal images that increases during head motion and asymmetry of retinal image slip when the VOR is imbalanced by palsy of a muscle appears to be the visual drive for monocular adaptation to reduce image slip and diplopia.

ACKNOWLEDGMENTS

This work was supported by Canadian Institutes of Health Research grants MT 15362 and ME 5504.

REFERENCES

1. GONSHOR, A. & G. MELVILL JONES. 1976. Extreme vestibulo-ocular adaptation induced by prolonged optical reversal of vision. J. Physiol. (Lond.) **256:** 381–414.

2. YAGI, T., M. SHIMIZU, S. SEKINE & T. KAMIO. 1981. New neurootological test for detecting cerebellar dysfunction. Vestibulo-ocular reflex changes with horizontal vision-reversal prisms. Ann. Otol. Rhinol. Laryngol. **90:** 276–280.
3. OOHIRA, A. & D.S. ZEE. 1992. Disconjugate ocular motor adaptation in rhesus monkey. Vision Res. **32:** 489–497.
4. SNOW, R., J. HORE & T. VILIS. 1985. Adaptation of saccadic and vestibulo-ocular systems after extraocular muscle tenectomy. Invest. Ophthalmol. Visual Sci. **26:** 924–931.
5. VIRRE, E., C. WERNER & T. VILIS. 1988. Monocular adaptation of the saccadic system and vestibulo-ocular reflex. Invest. Ophthalmol. Visual Sci. **29:** 1339–1347.
6. WONG, A.M.F., D. TWEED & J.A. SHARPE. 2002. Adaptations and deficits in the vestibulo-ocular reflex after sixth nerve palsy. Invest. Ophthalmol. Visual Sci. **43:** 99–111.
7. WONG, A.M.F. & J.A. SHARPE. 2002. Adaptations and deficits in the vestibulo-ocular reflex after third nerve palsy. Arch. Ophthalmol. **120:** 360–368.
8. WONG, A.M.F., J.A. SHARPE & D. TWEED. 2002. The vestibulo-ocular reflex in fourth nerve palsy: deficits and adaptations. Vision Res. **42:** 2205–2218.
9. RANALLI, P.J. & J.A. SHARPE. 1988. Vertical vestibulo-ocular reflex, smooth pursuit and eye-head tracking dysfunction in internuclear ophthalmoplegia. Brain **111:** 1299–1317.
10. SOKOLNIKOFF, I.S. & E.S. SOKOLNIKOFF. 1941. Higher Mathematics for Engineers and Physicists. McGraw Hill. New York.
11. KIM, J.S. & J.A. SHARPE. 2001. The vertical vestibulo-ocular reflex and its interaction with vision during active head motion: effects of aging. J. Vestib. Res. **11:** 3–12.
12. MORROW, M.J. & J.A. SHARPE. 1993. The effects of head and trunk position on torsional vestibular and optokinetic eye movements in humans. Exp. Brain Res. **95:** 144–150.
13. TWEED, D., M. FETTER, D. SIEVERING, et al. 1994. Rotational kinematics of the human vestibuloocular reflex. II. Velocity steps. J. Neurophysiol. **72:** 2480–2489.
14. MISSLISCH, H., D. TWEED & B.J.M. HESS. 2001. Stereopsis outweighs gravity in the control of the eyes. J. Neurosci. **21:** RC126.
15. HERING, E. 1868. Die Lehre vom binokularen Sehen. Wilhelm Englemann. Leipzig.
16. COLLINS, C.C. 1975. The human ocular system. *In* Basic Mechanisms of Ocular Motility and their Clinical Implications. G. Lennerstrand & P. Bach-y-Rita, Eds.: 145–180. Pergamon Press, New York.
17. SCOTT, A.B. 1994. Change of eye muscle sarcomeres according to eye position. J. Pediatr. Ophthalmol. Strabismus **31:** 85–88.
18. HAYMAN, M.R., J.P. DONALDSON & I.M. DONALDSON. 1995. The primary afferent pathway of extraocular muscle proprioception in the pigeon. Neuroscience **69:** 671–683.
19. GENTLE, A. & G. RUSKELL. 1997. Pathway of the primary afferent nerve fibers serving proprioception in monkey extraocular muscles. Ophthalmic Physiol. Opt. **17:** 225–231.

Neural Control of Three-Dimensional Eye and Head Posture

ELIANA M. KLIER AND J. DOUGLAS CRAWFORD

Canadian Institute of Health Research Group for Action and Perception, York Centre for Vision Research and Departments of Psychology, Biology and Kinesiology & Health Sciences, York University, Toronto, Ontario, Canada

ABSTRACT: The neural commands for gaze control include not only signals that drive the eyes and head from one point to the next, but also those that hold the eyes and head steady at the end of each movement. Studies using microstimulation and chemical inactivation techniques, in head-fixed and head-free macaques, were used to investigate the role of the interstitial nucleus of Cajal (INC) in the production of the latter, tonic signals. The right INC was found to control clockwise-up and clockwise-down components of both eye and head orientation, whereas the left INC was found to control the counterclockwise-up and counterclockwise-down components. Temporary inactivation of the INC left the eyes and head unable to hold their final torsional and vertical positions after each gaze shift. Thus, the INC is strongly implicated in the production of the tonic, step-like commands that maintain eye and head orientations between gaze shifts. In addition, these studies also found that the INC represents the torsional and vertical commands for eye and head orientation using different coordinate coding strategies, optimally matched to the different three-dimensional postural constraints observed in the eye and head.

KEYWORDS: interstitial nucleus of Cajal (INC); three-dimensional; eye; head; stimulation; inactivation; Listing plane; Fick surface

The gaze control system has long attracted the attention of those interested in sensory and motor systems and sensorimotor transformations. And although the eyes have been the major focus of this research, with new technologies for performing gaze control experiments with the head unrestrained, it is becoming clear that the eyes do not work alone. Sensory visual inputs as well as gaze motor outputs depend on the positions of both the eyes and head. This article highlights the contributions of the interstitial nucleus of Cajal (INC) to the control of three-dimensional eye and head posture in the macaque monkey.

Address for correspondence: J. Douglas Crawford, CIHR Group for Action and Perception, York Centre for Vision Research and Departments of Psychology, Biology and Kinesiology & Health Sciences, York University, 4700 Keele Street, Toronto, Ontario, Canada. Voice: 416-736-2100, ext. 88621; fax: 416-736-5814.

jdc@yorku.ca

NEURAL COMMANDS FOR MOVEMENT

Movements of the eyes from one position to another require two distinct signals. The first is a "velocity" command that overcomes the inertia of the eyes and drives them at a certain speed, in a specified direction. This signal is sufficient to bring the eyes to a new location but will not hold them there against the elastic restoring forces of the eye muscles. Therefore, a second "position" command is necessary to hold the eyes in their new position. Both these types of signals exist in the oculomotor neurons that exhibit characteristic "burst-tonic" firing patterns, where the burst of activity provides the eye with a velocity signal and the subsequent tonic input acts as the position command.[1]

The theoretical basis for generating these two types of signals was provided by David A. Robinson.[2] Robinson proposed that the two commands do not arise separately, but rather that the position signal is derived from the velocity signal (in a process equivalent to mathematical integration). Indeed, Robinson's theory was verified for the horizontal eye movement system. Burst neurons producing horizontal eye velocity signals were identified in the paramedian pontine reticular formation,[3] whereas the horizontal neural integrator was identified in the nucleus prepossitus hypoglossi.[4]

In the brainstem, as in the eye muscles and semicircular canals, horizontal components are found separately from vertical and torsional components. This idea was reinforced with the discovery of a separate vertical burst generator located in the rostral interstitial nucleus of the medial longitudinal fasciculus (riMLF).[5] But the location of torsional burst neurons and the vertical/torsional integrator remained unknown. This was partly because torsional rotations were not yet readily measurable and, in retrospect, because of how the vertical burst neurons are distributed anatomically. As it turns out, the torsional burst generator is also found in the riMLF, simultaneously represented in the vertical burst neurons so that those on the left also control counterclockwise (CCW) torsion (from the subject's point of view) and those on the right also control clockwise (CW) torsion.[6,7] At about the same time, the adjacent midbrain nucleus, the INC, was implicated in the control of vertical and torsional eye movements,[8–10] but its role as an integrator would not be examined until the 1980s.[11]

DONDERS' AND LISTING'S LAWS

Before one can completely appreciate the role of the INC in eye and head control, it is first necessary to be familiar with the kinematic laws that govern three-dimensional eye and head movements. Both the eyes and head can rotate in three unique directions (that is, horizontally, vertically, and torsionally). However, to direct gaze (that is, the direction of current regard) toward any object within the visual field, one only requires two of these components to be specified (that is, horizontal and vertical). The last variable, torsion, is free to assume any value without affecting the direction of gaze. Thus, the brain must find a solution to this classical "degrees of freedom" problem.

For both the eyes and head, the solution to this problem is known as Donders' law.[12] It states that for any one gaze direction, the eyes and head always assume the same, unique, torsional orientation, regardless of how they reach that position. For the eyes, the amount of torsion permitted at each eye orientation is strictly held at zero, and this is known as Listing's law.[12] If one were to measure eye orientations during random eye movements, torsional eye positions would all lie in a single plane, which is referred to as Listing's plane.[13] For the head, the amount of torsion, although fixed at each head orientation, can assume nonzero values. If one were to measure head positions during random head fixations, one would observe a pattern of head movements that resembles rotations made by a Fick gimbal (a setup in which the torsional axis of rotation is nested in the horizontal axis of rotation, while both are nested in the vertical axis). Thus, movements of the head resemble movements of a camera mounted on a tripod, where torsion increases as the head assumes progressively more tertiary positions (for example, up-right, up-left, down-right, and down-left).[14] These behavioral constraints will become important when the coordinate systems employed by the INC are examined.

THE INC AS A NEURAL INTEGRATOR FOR THREE-DIMENSIONAL EYE ORIENTATION

Because the INC receives input from both the vertical/torsional burst neurons in the riMLF[15] and the vertical semicircular canals,[16] and because it projects to the oculomotor nuclei that drive the vertical/torsional eye muscles,[17] it would seem logical to propose that the INC may function as the neural integrator for vertical/torsional eye movements. This hypothesis was tested using a combination of microstimulation and chemical inactivation techniques.

Using the former approach, Crawford and colleagues[18] first showed that unilateral microstimulation of the INC in head-fixed macaques produces constant velocity, binocular rotations of the eyes in both torsional and vertical directions (little or no horizontal components were elicited) (FIG. 1A, B). At the end of these stimulation-induced movements, the final torsional and vertical eye positions were maintained (for example, eye position held steady at the end of the rotation). This maintenance of final eye position confirms that the velocity commands were successfully integrated into position signals, but does not necessarily show that this integration is occurring in the INC (that is, it could be taking place downstream from the INC).

However, this unilateral stimulation study did reveal a functional difference between the INC nuclei on either side of the midline. Right INC stimulation consistently produced CW eye rotations, whereas left INC stimulation produced only CCW eye rotations (FIG. 1A, B). In contrast, upward and downward eye rotations were smaller and more variable, consistent with previous findings that up and down signals were intermingled on each side of the INC.[19] Thus, it appeared that upward and downward components were canceling each others' effects during stimulation. It follows that, in normal physiology, the torsional effects could only cancel each other if both sides of the INC were activated simultaneously.

This study then went on to unilaterally inactivate neurons in the INC. This was done by injecting 0.3 μL of a 0.05% muscimol (a GABA agonist) solution into the region and observing the resultant deficits. Although saccades themselves were not affected, the eyes could no longer hold their final torsional or vertical positions. Vertical eye positions drifted toward some null vertical value in a direction opposite to

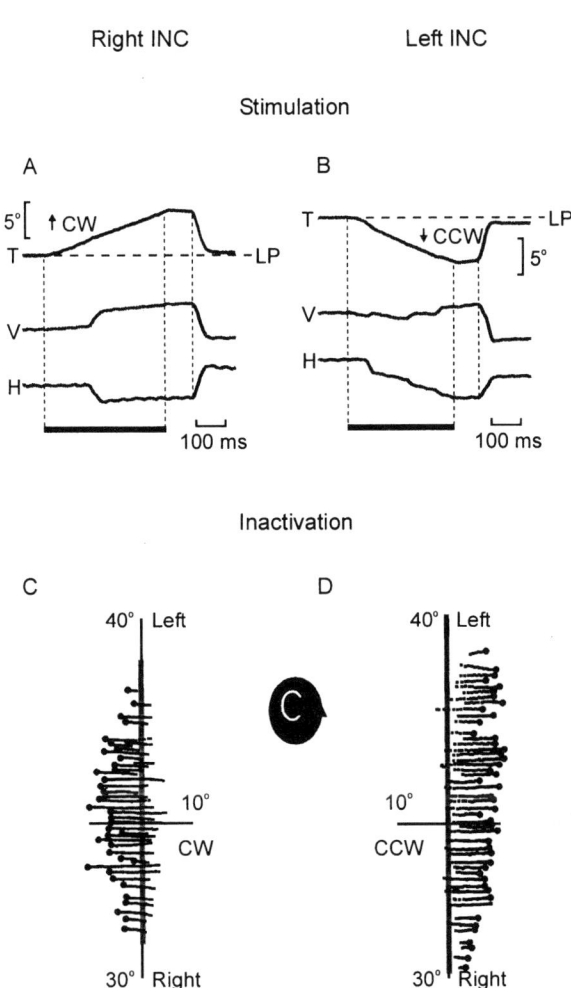

FIGURE 1. INC control of eye movements. *Top row:* INC head-fixed stimulation. Torsional (T), vertical (V), and horizontal (H) traces of eye position are plotted as a function of time. The stimulation train is indicated by the horizontal black bar lying between the first two vertical dashed lines. LP denotes the location of Listing's plane. Right INC stimulation (**A**) caused mainly CW eye rotations, whereas left INC stimulation (**B**) caused mainly CCW eye rotations. Smaller, more variable vertical components (and even smaller horizontal components) were also observed. Note how eye positions ramp smoothly during the stimulation train and how final eye positions are maintained steadily at the end of the stimulation train. The third vertical *dashed line* indicates the subsequent saccade that reversed the stimulation-induced position effects. *Bottom row:* INC head-fixed inactivation. Side views of horizontal eye position (ordinate) are plotted against torsional eye position (abscissa). Right INC inactivation (**C**) caused the eyes to drift in a CCW direction, whereas left INC inactivation (**D**) caused CW eye drifts. The *black circles* represent the endpoints of drift. Modified from Crawford.[32]

initial eye position (that is, initial upward eye positions drifted downward, while initial downward eye positions drifted upward). In the torsional dimension, the eyes drifted in a systematic manner. Right INC inactivation caused CCW eye drift, whereas left INC inactivation produced CW eye drift (FIG. 1C, D). More recently, Helmchen and colleagues[20] performed a similar series of experiments and obtained similar results.

The resultant drift was quantified by measuring its time constant of decay (that is, the time it took the eye to drift two-thirds of the way to its new null position). This procedure, often used to indicate the stability of eye position, indicates to what extent the neural integrator has been damaged. For example, complete integrator failure would result in a time constant of drift equal to the time it would take the eye to naturally drift back to its resting position if it lacked any neural innervation (previously measured by Robinson[21] at ~200 ms). Here, on average, both the vertical and torsional time constants reached values close to 200 ms, again indicating that the neural integrators in these two dimensions were nearly completely damaged.[18]

Taken together with the stimulation data, the inactivation results can be understood in the following way: CW eye position signals are controlled on the right side of the brain, and when these neurons are incapacitated, the eyes can no longer maintain eccentric CW eye orientations. Thus, the eye drifts in a CCW direction. Conversely, CCW eye position commands are processed on the left side of the brain, and damage to this side results in CW ocular drift because the CCW eye orientations can no longer be held.

ROLE OF THE INC IN HEAD POSTURE

As mentioned previously, the eyes and head often work together to perform a change in gaze. Therefore, could the INC also function as the neural integrator for head posture? From an anatomical standpoint, the INC has efferent connections to the cervical spine via the interstitiospinal tract.[22,23] Also, several investigators have previously examined the role of the INC in head control. The most prolific of these was Fukushima,[10] who examined the role of the INC in head-free cats. He and his colleagues showed that unilateral INC lesions cause contralateral head tilts,[24] while bilateral INC inactivation causes dorsiflexion of the head.[25] However, their explanation of these phenomena focused the pattern of innervation from the INC to the neck muscles and not on the specific neural role played by the INC.

Other researchers have implicated the INC in clinical conditions such as torticollis, where patients cannot maintain their heads upright but rather hold their heads in unnatural, twisted, and often painful orientations,[26] and progressive supranuclear palsy, where patients show characteristic upturned head postures.[27] But none of these studies evaluated the INC as a possible neural integrator for head posture and whether its role as an integrator could produce the observed deficits. However, some investigators (such as Crawford) of INC oculomotor function in head-fixed monkeys had anecdotally noticed that, upon freeing the head at the end of INC inactivation experiments, the head sometimes showed deficits quite similar to those that had been observed in the eye, perhaps suggesting that it also contains a head integrator.

To investigate whether the INC functions as a neural integrator for vertical/torsional head positions, the stimulation and muscimol inactivation experiments, which

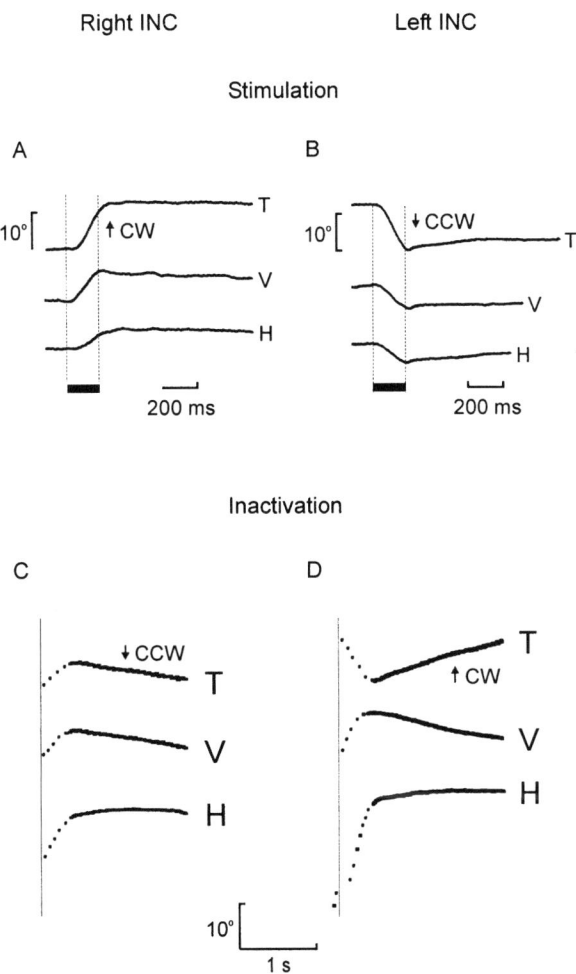

FIGURE 2. INC control of head movements. *Top row:* INC head-free stimulation. Torsional (T), vertical (V), and horizontal (H) traces of head position are plotted as a function of time. Right INC stimulation (**A**) caused mainly CW head rotations, whereas left INC stimulation (**B**) caused mainly CCW head rotations. Smaller, more variable vertical components (and even smaller horizontal components) were also observed. The stimulation train is indicated by the horizontal *black bar*. Again, head positions ramp smoothly until the end of the stimulation train, and final head positions are maintained steadily at the end of each stimulation train. Although not shown, subsequent gaze shifts reversed the stimulation-induced position effects. *Bottom row:* INC head-free inactivation. Torsional (T), vertical (V), and horizontal (H) traces of head position are plotted as a function of time. INC inactivation left the head unable to maintain final torsional and vertical head positions after gaze shifts (horizontal head positions were much less affected). Right INC inactivation (**C**) caused the head to drift in a CCW direction, whereas left INC inactivation (**D**) caused CW head drift. Modified from Klier *et al.*[28]

had previously been performed on the head-fixed monkeys, were repeated in head-free macaques (measuring head-in-space orientations).[28] As with the eyes, unilateral stimulation of the right INC resulted in CW deviations of the head, whereas left INC stimulation produced CCW head rotations (FIG. 2A, B). Vertical and horizontal head movements were also elicited bilaterally, but again they were smaller and more variable than the torsional components. A closer analysis of the time course of these movements revealed that the head moved with constant velocity for the entire stimulation duration and then held nearly all of its induced torsion at the end of the movement. This abnormal torsion was corrected during the subsequent self-generated head movement. Thus, the INC seemed to be actively controlling movements of the head in a similar way to which it controls the eyes.

If this latter statement is true, then inactivating the INC should lead to deficits similar to those observed in the eyes. Indeed, when muscimol was injected into the right INC, the head drifted in a CCW direction, whereas the head drifted CW when the left INC was inactivated (FIG. 2C, D). Again, the animals were still able to generate torsional, vertical, and horizontal movements during gaze shifts; however, they could no longer maintain their final vertical and torsional head postures at the end of the gaze shifts (FIG. 2C, D). This time, the resultant drift was quantified by measuring the time constant of decay of head positions after the muscimol injection and comparing this value to head time constants measured prior to the injection. This comparison resulted in a dramatic 20-fold drop in the vertical and torsional time constants. Thus, the vertical and torsional head integrators were essentially destroyed.

Head orientations were typically recorded up to 1 h following the initial injection. As the muscimol spread across the INC, the torsional head deviations became progressively larger, and ultimately the animal stopped producing the quick corrective movements to counteract the drift. This caused the head to settle in abnormal torsional orientations that were reminiscent of the head postures found in torticollis patients. In fact, comparing head movement strategies between our INC-inactivated monkeys and those previously collected from torticollis patients,[29] indicated that the two were indistinguishable from one another. Both our monkeys and the torticollis patients used a normal Fick strategy to move their heads, although their resultant Fick surfaces were shifted along the torsional dimension (a CCW shift with right INC inactivation and CW shift with left INC inactivation). Thus, the INC not only appeared to be the vertical/torsional head integrator, but damage to it pointed toward one possible etiology of torticollis.

COORDINATE SYSTEMS IN THE INC

The INC neurons described above, for both the eye and head, appear to have clearly defined directions of action. Cells in the right INC encode CW-up and CW-down rotations, whereas cells in the left INC encode CCW-up and CCW-down rotations. Along with the horizontal gaze system that encodes and rightward and leftward movements separately on either side of the midline, these six directions can be paired into three groups that become the basis vectors for a functional coordinate system. The three push-pull axes of this coordinate system are as follows: (1) left-right, (2) CW-up/CCW-down, and (3) CW-down/CCW-up. But why did this organization arise, and what reference frame contains this coordinate system?

Although these three effective perpendicular axes are not as simple as one might have anticipated (that is, distinct torsional, vertical, and horizontal axes), as mentioned previously, this framework does agree with the anatomy of the eye muscles and the semicircular canals that formed the basis of the earliest eye movement—the vestibuloocular reflex. And in this way, these canal-like coordinates (or eye muscle-like coordinates) are three-dimensional, orthogonal, and symmetrical across the sagittal plane.[30–32]

However, although the axes looked canal-like, they do not appear to be aligned with any head-fixed anatomical landmarks such as stereotaxic coordinates. Instead, a head-fixed INC inactivation study by Crawford[32] showed that these axes actually align with Listing's plane. In this study, the INC was unilaterally inactivated, and the resultant eye drift (CCW with right INC inactivation and CW with left INC inactivation) was observed to consistently drift in a direction perpendicular to Listing's plane. And perhaps it is not surprising that eye-related nuclei operate in Listing's plane because Listing's law is a fundamental behavioral constraint of several eye movements including saccades, smooth pursuit, and vergence.[33–35] For example, if equal CW and CCW components are to cancel out and produce zero torsion, they must be expressed in Listing's coordinates. What this result portends for anatomic projections from the INC to ocular motoneurons is not clear because we do not yet know enough about the physiology of eye muscle pulling directions to know how well they coincide with either gross muscle anatomy or Listing's plane (that is, it could turn out that Listing's coordinate *are* muscle coordinates).

Could the INC be using a similar, but head-specific, strategy to control head posture? Because normal head movements (and even those performed after INC inactivation) obey a Fick rule,[14,28] it is possible that INC head-related neurons are aligning their coordinate axes with this behavioral strategy. If one is to show that this is the case, INC stimulation-induced head movements must be analyzed to see if they obey the fundamentals rules of a Fick system. For example, because in a Fick set-up the horizontal axis (used for making vertical head rotations) is fixed inside the vertical axis (for horizontal head rotations), this vertical axis must be dependent on, and must move with, the horizontal orientation of the head. Also, because the torsional axis is fixed inside both the horizontal and vertical axes, it must therefore move with both vertical and horizontal positions of the head. Preliminary results show that this is in fact the case.[36] Thus, although INC neurons seem to encode similar directions for both the eyes and head, they orient the resultant movement axes with modality-specific behavioral constraints.

CONCLUSION

Although much is still unknown about gaze control and eye-head coordination, a strong picture is emerging about the brain center responsible for three-dimensional eye and head posture. For both the eyes and head, INC neurons encode directions of movement in a similar and systematic way on both sides of the midline. We do not yet know if individual neurons within the INC contribute to both the eye and head integrators, or if these are subserved by completely different neuronal populations. Generally, eye and head position are not just scaled versions of each other, so the latter possibility seems more likely. Moreover, the INC is flexible enough such that its outputs are aligned with behaviorally relevant strategies that differ for eye and head movements, so one suspects that at least some, if not most, of the INC neurons are either eye or head neurons. If so, the coexistence of eye and head integrators in the INC can probably be traced to evolutionary factors and the sharing of local biological resources such as input anatomy and the cellular characteristics required for neural integration.

REFERENCES

1. HENN, V., J.A. BUTTNER-ENNEVER & K. HEPP. 1982. The primate oculomotor system. I. Motoneurons: a synthesis of anatomical, physiological, and clinical data. Hum. Neurobiol. **1:** 77–85.
2. ROBINSON, D.A. 1968. Eye movement control in primates. Science **161:** 1219–1224.
3. LUSCHEI, E.S. & A.F. FUCHS. 1972. Activity of brain stem neurons during eye movements of alert monkeys. J. Neurophysiol. **35:** 445–461.
4. CANNON, S.C. & D.A. ROBINSON. 1987. Loss of the neural integrator of the oculomotor system from brain stem lesions in monkey. J. Neurophysiol. **57:** 1383–1409.
5. BUTTNER, U., J.A. BUTTNER-ENNEVER & V. HENN. 1977. Vertical eye movement related unit activity in the rostral mesencephalic reticular formation of the alert monkey. Brain Res. **130:** 239–252.
6. VILIS, T., K. HEPP, U. SCHWARZ & V. HENN. 1989. On the generation of vertical and torsional rapid eye movements in the monkey. Exp. Brain Res. **77:** 1–11.
7. CRAWFORD, J.D. & T. VILIS. 1992. Symmetry of oculomotor burst neuron coordinates about Listing's plane. J. Neurophysiol. **68:** 432–448.
8. SZENTAGOTHAI, J. 1943. Die zentrale Innervation der Augenbewegungen. Arch. Psychiatr. Nervenkr. **116:** 721–760.
9. KING, W.M., A.F. FUCHS & M. MAGNIN. 1981. Vertical eye movement-related responses of neurons in midbrain near interstitial nucleus of Cajal. J. Neurophysiol. **46:** 549–562.
10. FUKUSHIMA, K. 1987. The interstitial nucleus of Cajal and its role in the control of movements of head and eyes. Prog. Neurobiol. **29:** 107–192.
11. RANALLI, P.J., J.A. SHARPE & W.A. FLETCHER. 1988. Palsy of upward and downward saccadic, pursuit, and vestibular movements with a unilateral midbrain lesion: pathophysiologic correlations. Neurology **38:** 114–122.
12. HELMHOLTZ, H. 1867. Treatise on Physiological Optics. Optical Society of America. Rochester, NY.
13. TWEED, D. & T. VILIS. 1987. Implications of rotational kinematics for the oculomotor system in three dimensions. J. Neurophysiol. **58:** 832–849.
14. CRAWFORD, J.D., M.Z. CEYLAN, E.M. KLIER & D. GUITTON. 1999. Three-dimensional eye-head coordination during gaze saccades in the primate. J. Neurophysiol. **81:** 1760–1782.
15. BUTTNER-ENNEVER, J.A. & U. BUTTNER. 1992. Neuroanatomy of the ocular motor pathways. Baillieres Clin. Neurol. **1:** 263–287.
16. MARKHAM, C.H., W. PRECHT & H. SHIMAZU. 1966. Effect of stimulation of interstitial nucleus of Cajal on vestibular unit activity in the cat. J. Neurophysiol. **29:** 493–507.
17. STEIGER, H.J. & J.A. BUTTNER-ENNEVER. 1979. Oculomotor nucleus afferents in the monkey demonstrated with horseradish peroxidase. Brain Res. **160:** 1–15.
18. CRAWFORD, J.D., W. CADERA & T. VILIS. 1991. Generation of torsional and vertical eye position signals by the interstitial nucleus of Cajal. Science **252:** 1551–1553.
19. FUKUSHIMA, K., J. FUKUSHIMA, C. HARADA, *et al.* 1990. Neuronal activity related to vertical eye movement in the region of the interstitial nucleus of Cajal in alert cats. Exp. Brain Res. **79:** 43–64.
20. HELMCHEN, C., H. RAMBOLD, L. FUHRY & U. BUTTNER. 1998. Deficits in vertical and torsional eye movements after uni- and bilateral muscimol inactivation of the interstitial nucleus of Cajal of the alert monkey. Exp. Brain. Res. **119:** 436–452.

21. ROBINSON, D.A. 1970. Oculomotor unit behavior in the monkey. J. Neurophysiol. **33:** 393–403.
22. NYBERG-HANSEN, R. 1966. Sites of termination of interstitiospinal fibers in the cat: an experimental study with silver impregnation methods. Arch. Ital. Biol. **104:** 98–111.
23. FUKUSHIMA, K., S. MURAKAMI, J. MATSUSHIMA & M. KATO. 1980. Vestibular responses and branching of interstitiospinal neurons. Exp. Brain Res. **40:** 131–145.
24. FUKUSHIMA, K., K. TAKAHASHI, J. KUDO & M. KATO. 1985. Interstitial-vestibular interaction in the control of head posture. Exp. Brain Res. **57:** 264–270.
25. FUKUSHIMA, K., J. FUKUSHIMA & T. TERASHIMA. 1987. The pathways responsible for the characteristic head posture produced by lesions of the interstitial nucleus of Cajal in the cat. Exp. Brain Res. **68:** 88–102.
26. SANO, K., H. SEKINO, Y. TSUKAMOTO, N. YOSHIMASU & B. ISHIJIMA. 1972. Stimulation and destruction of the region of the interstitial nucleus in cases of torticollis and see-saw nystagmus. Confinia Neurologica **34:** 331–338.
27. FUKUSHIMA, J., K. FUKUSHIMA, M. KATO & K. TASHIRO. 1986. Rigidity and dorsiflexion of the neck in progressive supranuclear palsy and the interstitial nucleus of Cajal. J. Neurol. Neurosurg. Psych. **50:** 1197–1203.
28. KLIER, E.M., H. WANG, A.G. CONSTANTIN & J.D. CRAWFORD. 2002. Midbrain control of three-dimensional head orientation. Science **295:** 1314–1316.
29. MEDENDORP, W.P., J.A.M. VAN GISBERGEN, M.W.I.M. HORSTINK & C.C.A.M. GIELEN. 1999. Donders' law in torticollis. J. Neurophysiol. **82:** 2833–2838.
30. ROBINSON, D.A. 1985. The coordinates of neurons in the vestibulo-ocular reflex. *In* Adaptive Mechanisms in Gaze Control: Facts and Theories. A. Berthoz & G. Melvill Jones, Eds.: 297–311. Elsevier. Amsterdam.
31. SIMPSON, J.I. & W. GRAF. 1985. The selection of reference frames by nature and its investigators. Rev. Oculomotor Res. **1:** 3–16.
32. CRAWFORD, J.D. 1994. The oculomotor neural integrator uses a behavior-related coordinate system. J. Neurosci. **14:** 6911–6923.
33. FERMAN, L., H. COLLEWIJN & A.V. VAN DEN BERG. 1987. A direct test of Listing's law. I. Human ocular torsion measured in static tertiary positions. Vision Res. **27:** 929–938.
34. HASLWANTER, T., D. STRAUMANN, K. HEPP, *et al.* 1991. Smooth pursuit eye movements obey Listing's law in the monkey. Exp. Brain Res. **87:** 470–472.
35. MOK, D., A. RO, W. CADERA, *et al.* 1992. Rotation of Listing's plane during vergence. Vision Res. **32:** 2055–2064.
36. KLIER, E.M., H. WANG & J.D. CRAWFORD. 1999. Stimulation of the interstitial nucleus of Cajal (INC) produces torsional and vertical head rotations in Fick coordinates [abstract]. Soc. Neurosci. **25:** 50.

Dynamic Modulation of Ocular Orientation during Visually Guided Saccades and Smooth-Pursuit Eye Movements

BERNHARD J.M. HESS[a] AND DORA E. ANGELAKI[b]

[a]*Department of Neurology, Zürich University Hospital, Switzerland*
[b]*Department of Neurobiology, Washington University School of Medicine, St. Louis, Missouri, USA*

ABSTRACT: Rotational disturbances of the head about an off-vertical yaw axis induce a complex vestibuloocular reflex pattern that reflects the brain's estimate of head angular velocity as well as its estimate of instantaneous head orientation (at a reduced scale) in space coordinates. We show that semicircular canal and otolith inputs modulate torsional and, to a certain extent, also vertical ocular orientation of visually guided saccades and smooth-pursuit eye movements in a similar manner as during off-vertical axis rotations in complete darkness. It is suggested that this graviceptive control of eye orientation facilitates rapid visual spatial orientation during motion.

KEYWORDS: eye movements; vestibular; vestibuloocular; Listing's plane; oculomotor; monkey; counterroll

INTRODUCTION

Disturbances of head position challenge not only visual acuity during exploration of the physical surround but may interfere also with updating visual spatial orientation. Visual updating of spatial orientation is bound to be a relatively slow process because of the long delays in visual information processing. Vestibular reflexes that maintain ocular orientation constant in space could support spatial orientation by bridging the delayed processing of visual signals. One way to optimize visual spatial processing would be to interleave visual processing with vestibular-driven saccades that anticipate the direction of rapid changes in head orientation relative to the physical environment. Such an orientation mechanism might underlie the peculiar characteristics of vestibuloocular reflexes that become apparent when head disturbances occur in the yaw plane while head orientation relative to gravity simultaneously changes.[1–6] In fact, the characteristics of the vestibuloocular reflex (VOR) dramatically change when rotational disturbances occur about an off-vertical axis. Under these circumstances, it becomes apparent that canal-ocular signals alone provide in-

Address for correspondence: Bernhard J.M. Hess, Department of Neurology, Zurich University Hospital, Frauenklinikstrasse 26, CH-8091, Zürich, Switzerland. Voice: (+411) 255-5500; fax: (+411) 255-4507.
bhess@neurol.unizh.ch

sufficient information for generating compensatory ocular reflexes that keep the orientation of the visual field invariant in space. The reason for this shortcoming is that in general orientation information cannot be derived from integration of angular velocity signals alone.[7]

Here we first briefly describe the three-dimensional characteristics of the VOR to off-axis rotations in the yaw plane. One hallmark of these characteristics is that they suggest the existence of a mechanism that modulates quick phases as a function of head orientation relative to gravity.[5,8–13] Then we address more specifically the hypothesis that fast disturbances in head orientation generate slow- and/or quick-phase movements that rotate and shift the visual field systematically in an orientation-compensatory manner, although at a reduced gain, thereby helping to maintain and update visual spatial orientation. We say that a reflex keeps the *visual field orientation invariant relative to gravity* if (and only if) it does not change the orientation of the horizontal retinal meridian relative to gravity. This concept of orientation constancy is explained in more detail in FIGURE 1. Then we describe qualitatively the results of some recent experiments in which we studied the effects of in-phase rotations of a subject and its visual background about an off-vertical axis on saccades and visual tracking movements. The goal of these experiments was to further elucidate the influence of a dynamically changing head orientation on the ocular orientation of visually guided eye movements.

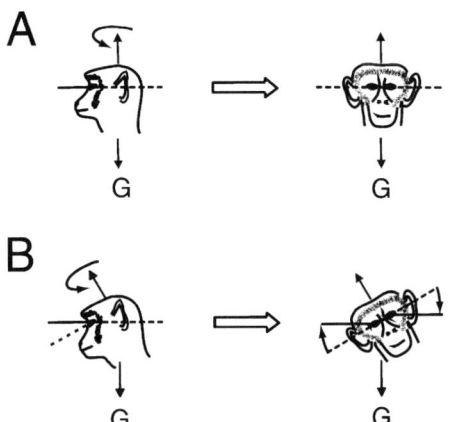

FIGURE 1. Spatial constancy of the visual field relative to the horizon. (**A**) During a head movement through 90° about an earth-vertical axis, the VOR would normally maintain the orientation of the visual field constant relative to gravity by keeping the vertical eye position (*left panel, solid/dashed line*) and torsional eye position (*right panel, dashed line*) parallel to the horizon throughout the movement. (**B**) During an off-vertical axis movement, the same reflex must change a given vertical eye position (relative to gravity; *solid line in left panel*) into a corresponding torsional eye position (relative to gravity; *solid lines in right panel*) to maintain the orientation of the visual field constant relative to gravity.

METHODS

Data were obtained from two juvenile rhesus monkeys (*Macaca mulatta*) that were chronically prepared with scleral dual-search coils, for three-dimensional eye movement recordings, and skull bolts, for restraining head motion during the experiments. Details of fabrication and implantation of the dual-search coil have been reported elsewhere.[14] All surgical and animal handling procedures were in accordance with the National Institute of Health's Guide for the Care and Use of Laboratory Animals and approved by the Veterinary Office of the Canton of Zurich.

Three-dimensional eye position was measured with a two-field search coil system (Eye Position Meter 3000, Skalar, Delft). The search coil signals were calibrated as described by Hess and colleagues.[15] Horizontal, vertical, and torsional eye positions were digitized at a sampling rate of 833 Hz and stored on a computer for off-line data analysis. Eye positions were expressed as rotation vectors, $\mathbf{E} = \tan(\rho/2)\,\mathbf{u}$, where $\mathbf{u}$ is a unit vector pointing along the axis of rotation that brings the eye from the reference position to current position, and ρ is the angle of rotation about $\mathbf{u}$.[16] Rotation vectors were expressed relative to a right-handed coordinate system, where the y-axis was aligned with the interaural axis (positive direction leftward as seen from the monkey), and the x–y plane was rotated upward by 15° relative to stereotactic horizontal. A positive torsional, vertical, or horizontal eye position component (E_{tor}, E_{ver}, E_{hor}) corresponded to a clockwise, downward, or leftward rotation of the eye (from the subjective viewpoint). The eye angular velocity vector $\mathbf{\Omega} = (\Omega_{tor}, \Omega_{ver}, \Omega_{hor})$ was computed from the eye position vector, $\mathbf{E}$, according to the equation $\mathbf{\Omega} = 2\,(d\mathbf{E}/dt + \mathbf{E} \times d\mathbf{E}/dt)\,/\,(1 + |\mathbf{E}|^2)$. Listing's plane and primary eye position were determined from spontaneous eye movements in the light with the head upright and stationary. All rotation vectors in tilted head orientations were expressed relative to primary position that was calculated in upright position as the unique eye orientation with gaze direction normal to Listing's plane.

Animals were seated in a primate chair and placed inside the inner frame of a superstructure consisting of three motor-driven gimbaled axes that were surrounded by a motor-driven, light-proved optokinetic sphere. Dynamic changes in head orientation were induced by rotating the animal in synchrony with the optokinetic sphere (inner diameter: 80 cm) while either performing visually guided saccades or smooth-pursuit eye movements. The inner wall of the sphere was covered with a random dot pattern. When the outmost manual gimbaled axis of the superstructure was used, the animal and the optokinetic sphere could be tilted relative to an earth-vertical axis without changing the animal's orientation relative to its visual surround.

The experimental protocols consisted of the following visual-vestibular stimulation protocols that were each tested with the animal in upright or 30° (90°) tilted nose-up positions: (a) Projection of a laser spot at random locations on the inner wall of the sphere to elicit visually guided saccades while both the animal and its visual surround were rotated in synchrony with steps of constant-velocity rotation of 180°/s (180°/s^2 acceleration). (b) Projection of a horizontally or vertically moving laser spot oscillating at a frequency of 0.1 Hz (±15°, corresponding to ±9.4°/s). Trained animals maintained their eye position on the target within a 2° behavioral window for fluid reward. (c) Steps of constant-velocity rotation of 180°/s (180°/s^2 acceleration) of the animal in complete darkness. Data were also collected during spontaneous saccades in upright position to determine Listing's plane.

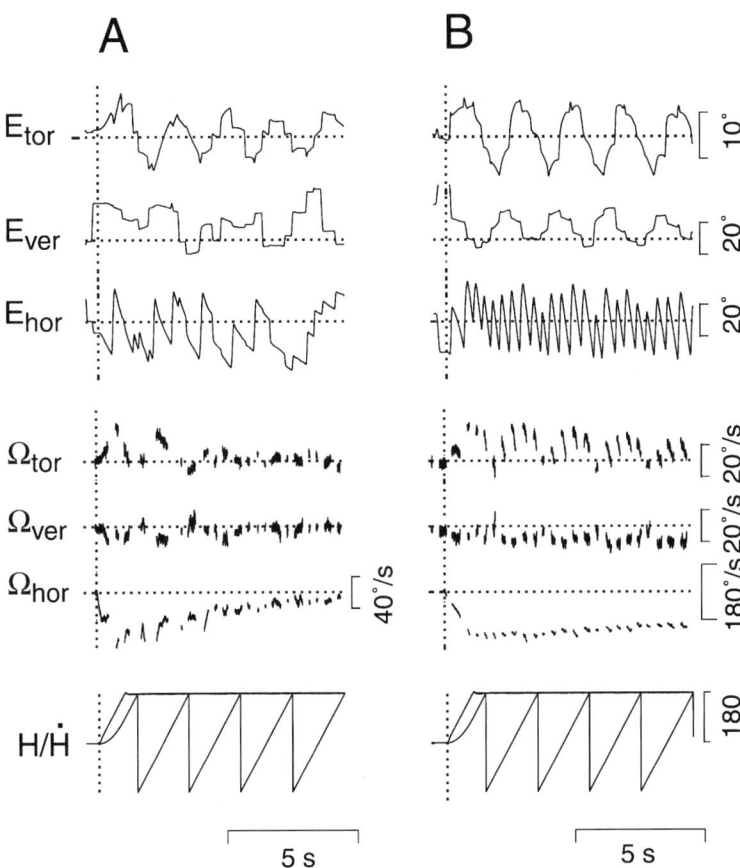

FIGURE 2. Modulation of ocular orientation by visually guided saccades and quick phases of the vestibulo-ocular reflex during off-vertical motion. (**A**) Visually-guided saccades: Modulation of torsional (and to a lesser extend vertical) eye position when both the observer and the visual surround move about an earth-horizontal axis (180°/s). Note the initially large torsional modulation of eye position. Although initially it is generated by a combination of slow and quick phases, it is later almost exclusively maintained through quick phases. (**B**) VOR: Modulation of torsional and vertical eye position, phase-locked to head orientation relative to gravity, during constant-velocity rotation (180°/s) about an earth-horizontal axis in total darkness. Note synergistic effect of slow- and quick-phase modulation on torsion and vertical eye position. E_{tor}, E_{ver}, E_{hor}: torsional, vertical, and horizontal eye position; Ω_{tor}, Ω_{ver}, Ω_{hor}: torsional, vertical, and horizontal angular velocity; H: head position (0°: nose up, +90°: left ear down, +180°: nose down, −90°: right ear down); H-dot: head velocity (in °/s).

RESULTS

Dynamic Modulation of Ocular Orientation during Saccades

In these experiments, the axis of the optokinetic sphere and the animal were oriented in 90° nose-up position. While scanning the visual surround, both the animal and its visual surround started to rotate together about an earth-horizontal axis, accelerating at 180°/s^2 up to a constant velocity of 180°/s (FIG. 2). The rotation induced a horizontal VOR whose amplitude was attenuated because of the suppressing effect of the visual field that remained stable relative to the animal (FIG. 2A). In addition to the horizontal nystagmus, both the torsional eye orientation and torsional slow-phase eye velocity exhibited a clear modulation that was phase-locked with respect to head orientation relative to gravity. Interestingly, torsional slow-phase velocity modulation was large for only a few seconds after the start of rotation but was greatly reduced with the time course of decay of the horizontal nystagmus. In contrast, the torsional eye position modulation persisted throughout the rotation, but it was maintained almost exclusively by quick-phase modulation. Vertical eye movements comprised only quick-phase modulation.

Other than the lack of a persistent horizontal nystagmus, this particular oculomotor response pattern is similar to the VOR elicited during constant-velocity rotation about an earth-horizontal axis in complete darkness (FIG. 2B). As shown earlier,[5,8–10] yaw rotation in darkness elicits an otolith-driven constant horizontal nystagmus (so-called bias velocity) proportional to head angular velocity. Superimposed to this nystagmus there are also modulations of torsional and vertical eye position that reflect head orientation in space. These modulations in eye orientation only partly consist of slow-phase eye movements. We have previously shown that the higher the frequency (that is, during high-speed rotations) the larger the contribution of quick phases to the torsional and vertical eye position modulation.[5,8,9]

The finding of a persistent torsional and vertical modulation of visually guided saccades as a function of head orientation relative to gravity is consistent with our hypothesis regarding a vestibular-driven orientation mechanism that helps to maintain and update visual spatial orientation during fast-head disturbances. Accordingly, the torsional and vertical modulation of eye orientation has been shown to be larger the larger the speed in head orientation change.[5,8,9] Moreover, slow-phase modulation that saturates at about 10°/s/g is replaced by quick phases or saccades as the speed of reorientation of the head relative to gravity increases.[5]

Dynamic Modulation of Ocular Orientation during Smooth-Pursuit Eye Movements

To study ocular orientation during a visual-motor behavior other than saccades, we trained monkeys to perform horizontal or vertical smooth-pursuit eye movements by projecting a slowly oscillating laser spot on the inner wall of the optokinetic sphere surrounding the animal. In the first series of experiments, the animal was placed inside the sphere in upright orientation. While the animal tracked the horizontally or vertically moving laser spot (0.1 Hz ± 15°), both the animal and the optokinetic sphere started to simultaneously rotate in a phase-locked fashion about the earth-vertical axis up to a constant velocity of 180°/s. The rotation induced a vigor-

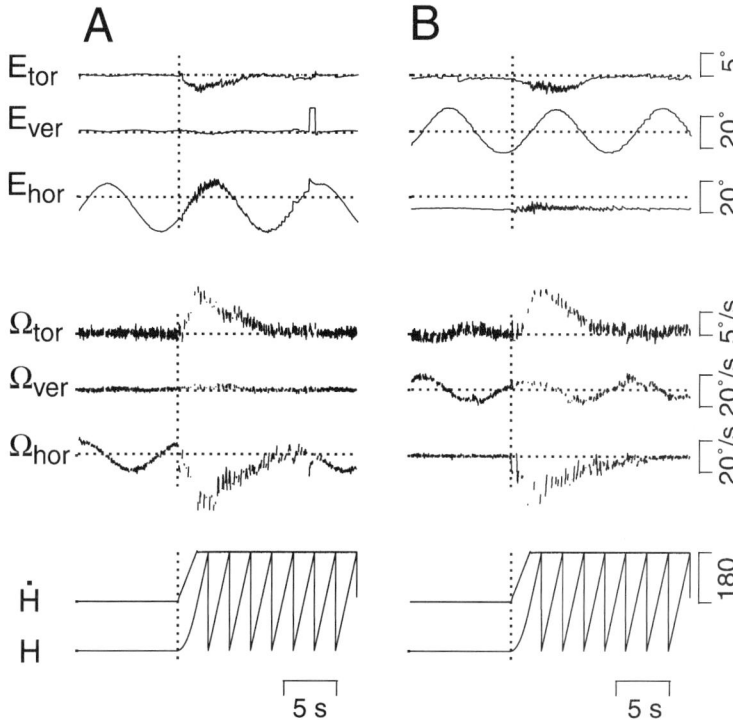

FIGURE 3. Three-dimensional organization of smooth-pursuit eye movements during earth-vertical axis rotation. Horizontal (**A**) and vertical (**B**) smooth-pursuit eye movements during in-phase rotation of the animal and the visual surround about an earth-vertical axis. At rotation onset, a strong horizontal VOR is induced that interacts with the smooth-pursuit eye movements. Note the concomitant resulting torsional shift in eye position and torsional nystagmus component. However, these effects on torsion do not correlate with the rotation cycle. H: head position (0°: nose down; +90°: right ear down; +180°: nose up; –90°: left ear down; –90°: right ear down); H-dot: head velocity (in °/s).

ous horizontal VOR that interacted with the horizontal or vertical tracking, which the animal continued during rotation, as illustrated in FIGURE 3A and B. The induced VOR was not purely horizontal, as indicated by the relatively large torsional velocity component. This torsional component was not correlated with the rotation cycle but rather with the duration of the horizontal response component. Because it was found to strongly correlate with gaze direction (data not shown), we assume that it arises from pursuit/VOR interactions[17] In the context of the ocular orientation hypothesis addressed here, the important observation is that during smooth pursuit while rotating about an earth-vertical axis, there was no change in torsional eye orientation that correlated with the head rotation cycle (FIG. 3, bottom traces). The small change in torsional eye position and velocity correlated in time with the rotation-induced horizontal VOR.

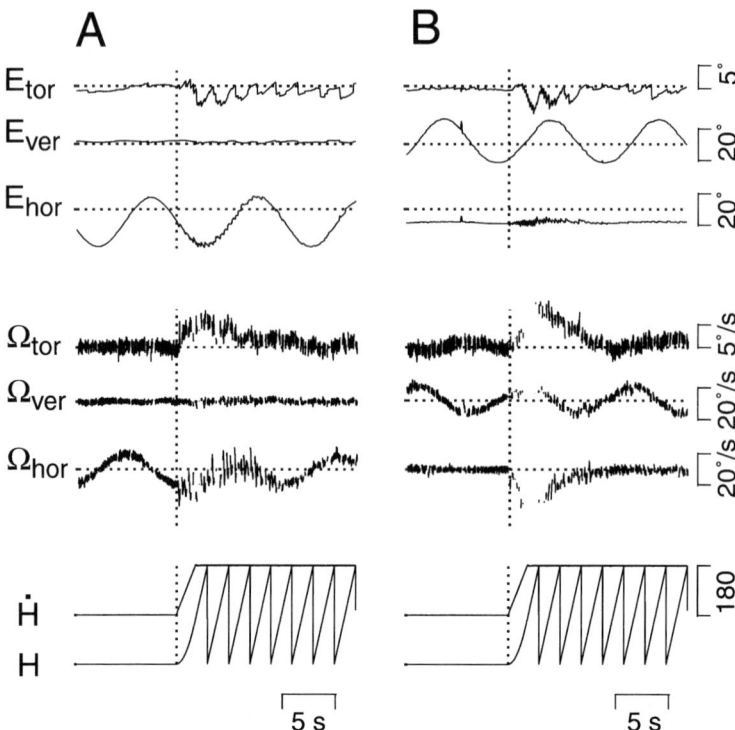

FIGURE 4. Three-dimensional organization of smooth-pursuit eye movements during off-vertical axis rotation. Responses during horizontal (**A**) and vertical (**B**) smooth pursuit while both the animal and the visual surround are rotating phase-locked about a 30° off-vertically tilted axis at a constant velocity (180°/s). Similar as with saccades, dynamic reorientation relative to gravity modulates torsional eye orientation that is phase-locked to instantaneous head orientation relative to gravity. Note that vertical eye position remains stable in **A**, as required by the smooth-pursuit task. Similar to earth-vertical axis rotations, the rotation-induced horizontal VOR exhibits a concomitant shift in torsional eye position and a torsional nystagmus component that are not correlated to the rotation cycle. H: head position (0°: nose down, +90°: right ear down; +180°: nose up, –90°: left ear down; –90°: right ear down); H-dot: head velocity (in °/s).

In the second series of experiments, we oriented the animal in a 30° nose-up position. While the animal tracked the horizontally or vertically moving laser spot, both the animal and its visual surround started to simultaneously rotate about the 30°-tilted yaw axis at 180°/s. This rotation induced a horizontal VOR that interacted with the smooth-pursuit eye movements (FIG. 4). Similar to earth-vertical axis rotation, the horizontal VOR was also accompanied by gaze-dependent torsional eye movements that were limited to the duration of the horizontal nystagmus. However, in contrast to the rotation about an earth-vertical axis, the torsional eye orientation during off-vertical axis rotation also consisted of saccadic modulations of torsional eye position. These torsional eye position modulations were mediated by fast phases and were correlated with head position relative to gravity. This saccadic-induced modulation in torsional eye orientation was strongest early during the motion and qualitatively similar to (although smaller than) those during visually guided saccades (compare FIGS. 2 & 4).

DISCUSSION

We report that dynamic reorientation relative to gravity modulates ocular orientation for both visually guided saccades and smooth-pursuit eye movements in a similar way as earlier shown for quick phases of the VOR in complete darkness.[5,8–13] During rapid off-vertical rotation about the yaw axis in the dark, quick phases of the VOR modulate torsional and vertical eye position, tightly locked with instantaneous head orientation relative to gravity. In nose-down positions, vertical quick-phase components shift the visual field upward; in right-ear-down positions, torsional quick-phase components rotate the visual field toward the left ear. In nose-up and left-ear-down positions, the reverse is true. Here we show that a similar modulation of torsional and vertical eye position occurs also during visually guided saccades in the light as well as during smooth pursuit when the animal rotates about an off-vertical axis.

Before further discussing the effects of off-vertical axis rotation on ocular orientation during smooth pursuit, we have to briefly address what requirements the brain has to meet if it is to track a target under these conflicting conditions in terms of visual and vestibular signals. Specifically, in-phase rotation of the animal and the visual surround strongly suppresses the VOR (FIG. 2A). On top of this visual-vestibular suppression due to a head-stationary visual field, the animal tries to keep tracking of the laser target. As a result of this effort, we find that the VOR shifts from a pure head horizontal to a horizontal-torsional response (FIG. 3A, B), irrespective of whether smooth pursuit occurs in a horizontal (FIG. 3A) or vertical direction (FIG. 3B). Because this shift is eye-position dependent (data not shown), our data suggest that parametric down-regulation of the gain[18–20] can explain only part of the observed suppression in our experimental paradigm. Cancellation due to superposition of vestibular and pursuit commands[17,19,21] may explain the remaining part, provided that one assumes that Listing's velocity plane shifts because of the present particular experimental context. Without such a shift, the pursuit command (peak 9.4°/s) could never overcome the vestibular drive (180°/s) by superposition because both are parallel to each other at onset of rotation (FIG. 3A). Note also that because smooth pursuit follows Listing's law,[22] the parallel vestibular velocity signal does comply entirely with Listing's law. In support of such parametric modulation of Listing's law is the slow shift in torsional eye position that parallels the VOR in duration (FIG. 3). Further experiments are required, however, to determine the nature of this postulated context-dependent modification of Listing's law.

Independently of such eye position dependence of the torsional eye orientation and slow-phase velocity, there are additional head-orientation-specific effects on visually guided saccades and smooth-pursuit eye movements that are observed only during rotations about off-vertical axes. Peak negative and positive excursions correlate with right-ear-down and left-ear-down head orientations as expected for an otolith-driven response. The same pattern of modulation of ocular torsion is found during visually guided saccades (FIG. 2B). In both the saccadic and smooth-pursuit paradigm, closer inspection reveals that this modulation is mediated by quick phases. In addition, there is a habituation of the magnitude of modulation that is particularly apparent at tilt angles of less than 90°, as earlier described.[10] We have previously shown that the otolith-driven quick-phase modulation during yaw rotation about a tilted axis can be described by a dynamic otolith-driven parametric modulation of Listing's law.[8–10] We propose that the same mechanism underlies the dynamic modulation of ocular orientation of pursuit and saccades described here. Our recent finding, that visually guided saccades and smooth-pursuit eye movements depend in the same way on gravity during static changes in head orientation relative to gravity, supports this hypothesis.[23] These orientation effects are, as already noted above, separate from the slow torsional shift that correlates with the suppression-related mechanisms described in the previous paragraph rather than with head orientation in space. This shift is much less conspicuous in the saccadic task (FIG. 2A), presumably because the fixation durations were too short for a clear expression of the suppression effects. Interestingly, there was no conspicuous head-orientation-dependent saccadic modulation in vertical direction (peak in nose-up and nose-down position) during the smooth-pursuit tasks (FIG. 3A, B) in contrast to the saccadic task (FIG. 2B). Apparently the magnitude of the ocular orientation response can be downregulated depending upon the behavioral requirements.

In conclusion, while taking account of the requirement of visual spatial constancy during motion, we have hypothesized that during off-vertical axis rotation, ocular orientation should reflect instantaneous head orientation, independent of the particular visual task, although at a reduced gain scale. We show that this appears indeed to be the case for visually guided saccades and smooth-pursuit eye movements.

ACKNOWLEDGMENTS

We thank Elena Buffone and Bernadette Disler for help with the experiments, and Urs Scheifele for developing the control software (Spike2 scripts). This study was supported by grants from the Swiss National Science Foundation (31-47287.96), the National Institutes of Health (EY-12814 and DC-04260), and the National Aeronautics and Space Administration (NAG2-1493).

REFERENCES

1. HARRIS, L.R. 1987. Vestibular and optokinetic eye movements evoked in the cat by rotation about a tilted axis. Exp. Brain Res. **66:** 522–532.
2. DARLOT, C. & P. DENISE. 1988. Nystagmus induced by off-vertical rotation axis in the cat. Exp. Brain Res. **73:** 78–90.
3. DARLOT, C., P. DENISE, J. DROULEZ, B. COHEN & A. BERTHOZ. 1988. Eye movements induced by off-vertical axis rotation (OVAR) at small angles of tilt. Exp. Brain Res. **73:** 91–105.
4. HESS, B.J.M. & N. DIERINGER. 1990. Spatial organization of the maculo-ocular reflex of the rat: responses during off-vertical axis rotation. Eur. J. Neurosci. **2:** 909–919.
5. ANGELAKI, D.E. & B.J.M. HESS. 1996. Linear acceleration responses during off-vertical axis rotation. J. Neurophys. **75:** 2405–2424.

6. HASLWANTER, T., R. JAEGER, S. MAYR & M. FETTER. 2000. Three-dimensional eye-movement responses to off-vertical axis rotations in humans. Exp. Brain Res. **134:** 96–106.
7. TWEED, D. & T. VILIS. 1987. Implications of rotational kinematics for the oculomotor system in three dimensions. J. Neurophys. **58:** 832–849.
8. HESS, B.J.M. & D.E. ANGELAKI. 1997. Kinematic principles of primate rotational vestibulo-ocular reflex. I. Spatial organization of fast phase velocity axes. J. Neurophysiol. **78:** 2193–2202.
9. HESS, B.J.M. & D.E. ANGELAKI. 1997. Kinematic principles of primate rotational vestibulo-ocular reflex. II. Gravity-dependent modulation of primary eye position. J. Neurophysiol. **78:** 2203–2216.
10. HESS, B.J.M. & D.E. ANGELAKI. 1999. Oculomotor control of primary eye position discriminates between translation and tilt. J. Neurophys. **81:** 394–398.
11. PETTOROSSI, V.E., P. ERRICO & A. FERRARESI. 1997. Difference in quick phases induced by horizontal and vertical vestibular stimulations. J. Vestib. Res. **7:** 89–99.
12. PETTOROSSI, V.E., E. MANNI, P. ERRICO, et al. 1997. Otolithic and extraocular muscle proprioceptive influences on the spatial organization of the vestibulo- and cervico-ocular quick phases. Acta Otolaryngol. **117:** 139–142.
13. PETTOROSSI, V.E., P. ERRICO, A. FERRARESI & N.H. BARMACK. 1999. Optokinetic and vestibular stimulation determines the spatial orientation of negative optokinetic afternystagmus in the rabbit. J. Neurosci. **19:** 1524–1531.
14. HESS, B.J.M. 1990. Dual search coil for measuring 3-dimensional eye movements in experimental animals. Vision Res. **30:** 597–602.
15. HESS, B.J.M., A.J. VAN OPSTAL, D. STRAUMANN & K. HEPP. 1992. Calibration of three-dimensional eye position using search coil signals in the rhesus monkey. Vision Res. **9:** 1647–1654.
16. HAUSTEIN, W. 1989. Considerations on Listing's law and the primary position by means of a matrix description of eye position control. Biol. Cybern. **60:** 411–420.
17. MISSLISCH, H., D. TWEED, M. FETTER, J. DICHGANS & T. VILIS. 1996. Interaction of smooth pursuit and the vestibulo-ocular reflex in three dimensions. J. Neurophys. **75:** 2520–2532.
18. ROBINSON, D.A. 1982. A model of cancellation of the vestibulo-ocular reflex. *In* Functional Basis of Oculomotor Motility Disorders. G. Lennerstrand, D.S. Zee & E.L. Keller, Eds.: 5–13. Pergamon. Oxford.
19. LISBERGER, S.G. 1990. Visual tracking in monkeys: evidence for short-latency suppression of the vestibulo-ocular reflex. J. Neurophys. **63:** 676–688.
20. CULLEN, K.E., T. BELTON & R.A. MCCREA. 1991. A non-visual mechanism for voluntary cancellation of the vestibulo-ocular reflex. Exp. Brain Res. **83:** 237–252.
21. BARNES, G.R., A. BENSON & A.R. PRIOR. 1978. Visual-vestibular interaction in the control of eye movements. Aviat. Space Environ. Med. **49:** 557–564.
22. HASLWANTER, T., D. STRAUMANN, K. HEPP, et al. 1991. Smooth pursuit eye movements obey Listing's law in the monkey. Exp. Brain Res. **87:** 470–472.
23. HESS, B.J.M. & D.E. ANGELAKI. 2003. Gravity modulates Listing's plane orientation during both pursuit and saccades. J. Neurophys. **90:** 1340–1345.

Mathematical Model Predicts Clinical Ocular Motor Syndromes

MARIANNE DIETERICH,[a,b] STEFAN GLASAUER,[a] AND THOMAS BRANDT[a]

[a]*Department of Neurology and Center of Sensorimotor Research, Klinikum Grosshadern, Ludwig-Maximilians University, Munich, Germany*

[b]*Department of Neurology, Johannes Gutenberg-University, Mainz, Germany*

> ABSTRACT: Clinical ocular motor syndromes were compared with ocular motor syndromes simulated by a mathematical model of the vestibuloocular reflex. The mathematical sensorimotor feedforward model of otolith control of three-dimensional binocular eye position is based on relevant anatomical connections of the vestibuloocular reflex from the utricles to extraocular eye muscles. This is the first attempt to simulate static ocular motor syndromes for unilateral utricular or vestibular nerve failure, lesions of the vestibular nucleus, and lesions of the ascending vestibuloocular reflex pathways. Comparison of the predicted syndromes with those found in patients with unilateral disorders of the vestibular nerve (herpes zoster neuritis), the vestibular nucleus (medullary infarction), and the medial longitudinal fasciculus (pontine infarction) showed good agreement as regards the direction of horizontal, vertical, and torsional eye deviations. The ability of the model to simulate complete or incomplete failures of single elements or entire pathways allows us to pose direct clinical questions about as yet unknown ocular motor syndromes or about the localization of the damage as well as the mechanism involved in syndromes already known.
>
> KEYWORDS: mathematical model; vestibuloocular reflex; otolith; ocular motor syndrome; skew deviation; ocular torsion; patients

INTRODUCTION

System analysis and the construction of algorithmic models are necessary prerequisites for the quantitative study of biological sensorimotor processes. The mathematical modeling of vestibular brainstem control of eye movements and eye position in three dimensions is based on relevant anatomical connections of the vestibuloocular reflex (VOR), which are known from electrophysiological and tracer studies in animals. Direct vestibular pathways run from the endorgan via the vestibular nuclei (VN) and ascending brainstem connections (medial longitudinal fascicle, MLF; ascending tract of Deiters, ATD; brachium conjunctivum, BC) to the ocular motor nuclei to contact their respective extraocular eye muscles.[1,2] Modeling of the VOR has so far concentrated on dynamic aspects,[3–6] especially nystagmus. We chose the tonic vestibuloocular reflexes, which are based mainly on otolith function, for modeling.

Address for correspondence: Prof. Dr. Marianne Dieterich, Department of Neurology, Johannes Gutenberg-University, Langenbeckstrasse 1, D-55131 Mainz, Germany. Voice: + 49-6131-17-2510; fax: + 49-6131-17-5697.

dieterich@neurologie.klinik.uni-mainz.de

The utricular otoliths mainly control static eye positions (in three dimensions), ocular counterroll, and conjugated vertical deviations. A pathological ocular torsion (OT) or vertical divergence of the visual axes (skew deviation) indicates a lesional tone imbalance of otolithic "graviceptive" function. Various patterns of ocular motor syndromes with monocular and binocular torsion and skew deviation have been described clinically and were attributed to separate and distinct lesions of the graviceptive vestibuloocular brainstem system.[7,8]

We developed a mathematical sensorimotor, feedforward model of otolithic control of binocular static eye position in three dimensions.[9] Model input is defined as gravitational acceleration relative to the head. The utricles represent coordinate transformations from head to utricular coordinates. The VN are assumed to transform utricular to eye muscle coordinates and to scale the afferent information.

This study determined the reliability and limitations of the current model for predicting static deviations of the eyes in three dimensions—horizontal, vertical, and torsional—due to distinct unilateral peripheral or central vestibular pathway lesions. We compared the tonic ocular deviations predicted by the model with the ocular motor findings in neurological patients in whom circumscribed lesions were identified to involve these structures. The study focuses on the differential effects of unilateral vestibular lesions of the vestibular nerve, the vestibular nucleus, and the pontomesencephalic pathways. The purpose of such modeling is to simulate not only ocular motor syndromes known to be vestibular but also to simulate the effects of single and combined pathway lesions to elucidate hitherto unexplained interrelationships between vestibular pathways and ocular motor function.

PATIENTS AND METHODS

We selected patients with a distinct clinical diagnosis of a unilateral lesion involving one of the following three structures (TABLE 1): (a) vestibular nerve, (b) vestibular nucleus, or (c) pontomesencephalic MLF. Such lesions have been shown to induce a vestibular tone imbalance with a measurable tonic deviation predominantly in the torsional (roll) direction, which is associated with a tilt of the perceived visual vertical.[7,8] Consequently, all patients showed either acute skew deviation with ocular torsion or a complete ocular tilt reaction (OTR), that is, the triad of head tilt, vertical divergence of the eyes (skew deviation), and tonic ocular torsion of both eyes. These ocular motor syndromes are known to be induced either by a unilateral peripheral or a central lesion of vestibular graviceptive pathways.[8] Exclusion criteria were ocular motor deficits from earlier peripheral or central vestibular disorders, or diplopia prior to the onset of disease. The possibility of confusing such acute clinical syndromes with strabism or decompensated childhood hyperphoria was reduced by a precise patient history and orthoptic analysis. Patients with congenital ocular motor syndromes do not show binocular tilts of the visual vertical. We selected three patients for each subgroup (a–c) and restricted the subsequent patient data to tonic ocular motor and vestibular signs. For the peripheral lesion type, we chose patients with herpes zoster neuritis because this inflammatory disease affects the entire vestibular nerve, whereas the more frequent vestibular neuritis usually affects only the superior portion of the vestibular nerve, sparing the posterior semicircular canal function.

TABLE 1. Vertical and horizontal divergence, ocular torsion, subjective visual vertical tilts, and clinical syndrome in patients with acute unilateral lesions along the graviceptive pathways

Disorders/Patients	Vertical divergence	Horizontal divergence	Ocular torsion			Subjective visual vertical tilt (degrees)	Clinical syndrome[a]
			Ipsilateral eye	Contralateral eye			
Disorder of the vestibular nerve (herpes zoster oticus)			Excyclotropia	Incyclotropia			
1. Female, 48 years, right side, day 8	−5	−0.5–1	+8	+10		+14	VIII, VII
2. Male, 65 years, right side, day 14	−10	+4	+15	+7		+11	VIII
3. Female, 56 years, left side, day 5	+3–4	+1	−4	−10		−7	VIII, VII
N/N	3/3	3/3	3/3	3/3			
Mean	6.0	1.8	9.0	9.0			
Disorder of the vestibular nucleus (medullary infarction)			Excyclotropia	Incyclotropia			
1. Male, 45 years, left side, day 5	+4.5	0	−7	−13		−23 to −24	Small VIII m
2. Male, 64 years, right side, day 10	−4	3 esotropia right	+17	+3		+17	Large VIII m, VIII l
3. Male, 44 years, left side, day 3	+1.5	1.5 exotropia left	−3	−3		−11	Large VIII m, VIII i
N/N	3/3	2/3	3/3	3/3			
Mean	3.3	2.25	9.0	6.3			
Disorder of the medial longitudinal fasciculus (pontine infarction)			Incyclotropia	Excyclotropia			
1. Male, 68 years, left side, day 1	−15	10 exotropia	+9	+6		+8–9	INO, OT, +VD
2. Male, 71 years, left side, day 2	−8	17 exotropia	+18	+21		+24–27	INO, OT, +VD
3. Female, 57 years, left side, day 3	−8	6 exotropia	+6.5	+5		+13	INO, OT, +VD
N/N	3/3	3/3	3/3	3/3			
Mean	10.3	11.0	11.2	10.7			

[a] VIII m, l, i = medial, lateral, inferior vestibular subnucleus; INO = internuclear ophthalmoplegia; +VD = vertical divergence, right over left.

Clinical Presentation

Vestibular Nerve

In the three patients (two females and one male; 48, 56, and 64 years of age, respectively) with acute herpes zoster neuritis of the seventh and eighth cranial nerves, the diagnosis was based on the typical syndrome of acute onset of prolonged severe rotatory vertigo associated with spontaneous horizontal rotatory nystagmus, postural imbalance, and nausea with concomitant auditory dysfunction. All three had blisters in the external acoustic meatus and a pleocytosis of lymphomonocytic cells in the cerebrospinal fluid (CSF). Serological tests for herpes zoster and polymerase chain reaction for varicella-zoster virus in CSF were positive. The patients presented with a complete ipsilateral OTR (TABLE 1). Unilateral vestibular paresis was confirmed by caloric testing. None had concurrent brainstem or cerebellar signs, or deficits of other cranial nerves except the facial nerve.

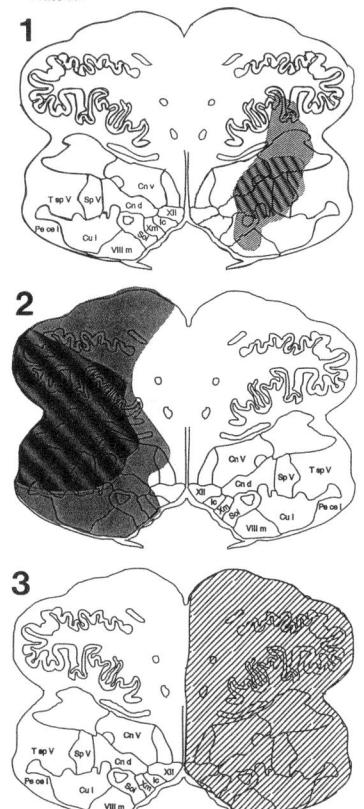

FIGURE 1. (A) Lesions of the vestibular nucleus in three patients with unilateral medullary infarctions who presented with Wallenberg's syndrome. Representative sections (plate XII) are shown indicating either involvement of the medial vestibular subnucleus (VIII m in patients 1 and 2) or the complete vestibular nucleus complex (medial, lateral, and inferior vestibular subnuclei in patient 3; only one section given).

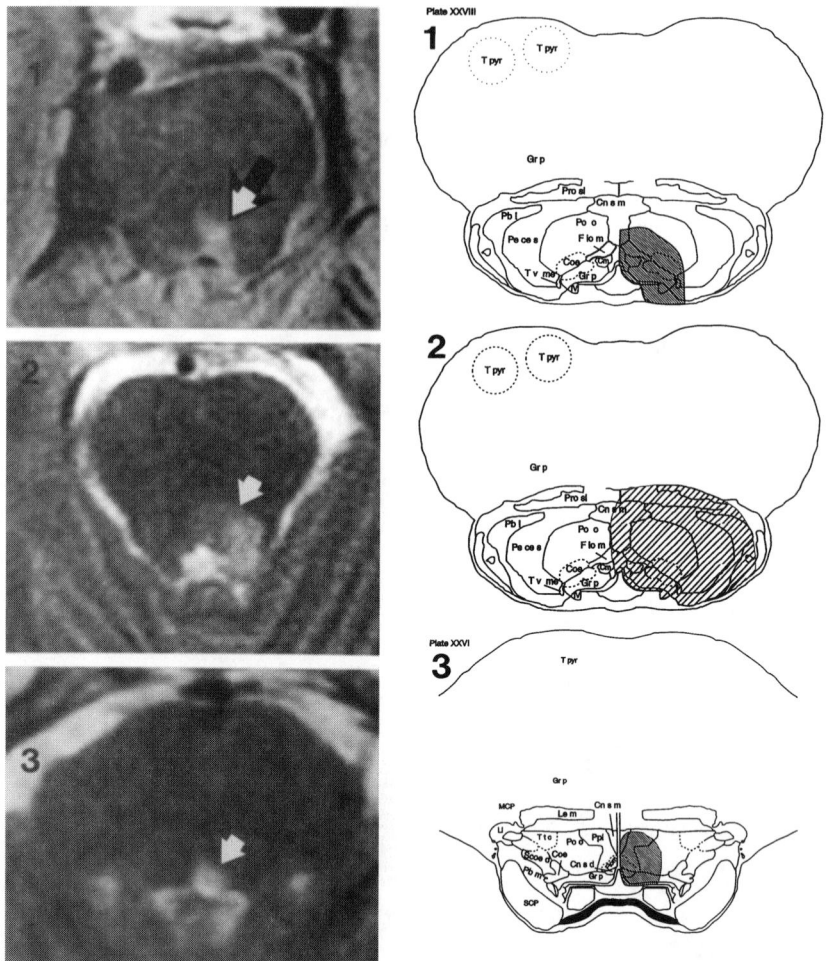

FIGURE 1. (B) Lesions of the MLF in three patients with unilateral pontine infarctions (*left*; T2-weighted sequences, TR 3464.0, TE 15.0) projected onto the appropriate transverse sections of the stereotaxic brainstem atlas (*right*; plate XXVIII in patients 1 and 2, plate XXVI in patient 3), indicate involvement of the medial longitudinal fasciculus (F lo m) at different pontomesencephalic levels.

Vestibular Nucleus

The three male patients (45, 53, and 64 years of age) with an acute right-sided infarction of the dorsolateral medulla (Wallenberg's syndrome) presented with a complete ipsilateral OTR, lateropulsion, and rightward tilts of the subjective visual vertical (TABLE 1). The extent of the infarction differed for each patient but involved smaller or larger parts of the vestibular nucleus, mainly the medial parts (for lesion site and extent see FIG. 1A).

Pontomesencephalic MLF

The three patients (one female and two males; 57, 68, and 71 years of age, respectively) presented with an acute internuclear ophthalmoplegia (INO) combined with a contralateral skew-torsion (TABLE 1). Skew-torsion means that skew deviation was associated with a tonic ocular torsion of both eyes, which represents a dysfunction of the vestibular graviceptive pathways.[7] Both INO as well as skew-torsion indicate a lesion of the MLF; a combination of the two indicates an MLF lesion at the pontomesencephalic level (FIG. 1B).

Topographic Identification of the Lesion

Magnetic resonance images (MRIs), oriented to the frontooccipital (FO) line as baseline, were used to identify the infarcted areas, which were then projected onto the appropriate transverse sections of the stereotactic atlas of the brainstem of Olszewski and Baxter.[10] Magnetic resonance imaging was performed with a Siemens Vision (1.5 T; Erlangen, Germany) with 2- or 4-mm slices (T1- and T2-weighted sequences).

Description of a Bilateral Three-Dimensional Mathematical Model

A bilateral three-dimensional mathematical model of otolith-ocular control of static eye position was used to simulate the oculomotor effects of lesions found in patients (see FIG. 2, TABLE 2). A detailed account of the model is given elsewhere[9,11] and in the Appendix (matlab/simulink model under http://www.nefo.med.uni-muenchen.de/~sglasauer/model/). In brief, the model is composed of linear (matrix operations) and nonlinear (transformations) static elements representing the known pathways from the utricles to the extraocular eye muscles, with the exception of direct utricular-abducens connections reported in the cat.[12] These latter connections are unlikely to play a major role in static otolith-ocular reflexes, but they may contribute to the linear VOR. Each brainstem nucleus (VN and ocular motor nuclei) consists of one or more model neurons. In analogy to biological neurons, each model neuron receives multiple weighted inputs, has a resting discharge, and a positive firing rate as output. The assumed operations performed on the afferent signals occur in the utricle, the VN, and ocular motor nuclei. Each utricle is composed of four neurons necessary to represent all directions of utricular sensitivity. The primary afferent output from the utricles to the VN are modeled in a nonlinear fashion according to electrophysiological studies in the squirrel monkey.[13] In the VN, each of which consists of six neurons (to contact the six extraocular eye muscles), a coordinate transformation is performed from utricular to eye muscle coordinates.[3] Commissural excitatory pathways connecting both VN are modeled to carry utricular information in the pitch plane. Pathways from the VN to the ocular motor nuclei and extraocular eye muscles are represented as excitatory, as studies of electrical stimulation of the utricular nerve in the cat suggest.[14] Afferent information ascends via several brainstem pathways (MLF, BC, and ATD) known to mediate the angular VOR. The oculomotor nuclei (III, four neurons each) weigh information from parallel pathways (MLF and BC; MLF and ATD). In the ocular motor nuclei (III, IV, and VI), an additional static input is added from other ocular motor centers such as the neural integrators (velocity to position). The ocular motor nuclei project to the extraocular eye muscles, whose innervation is related to muscle force by an approximately quadratic relationship.[15,16]

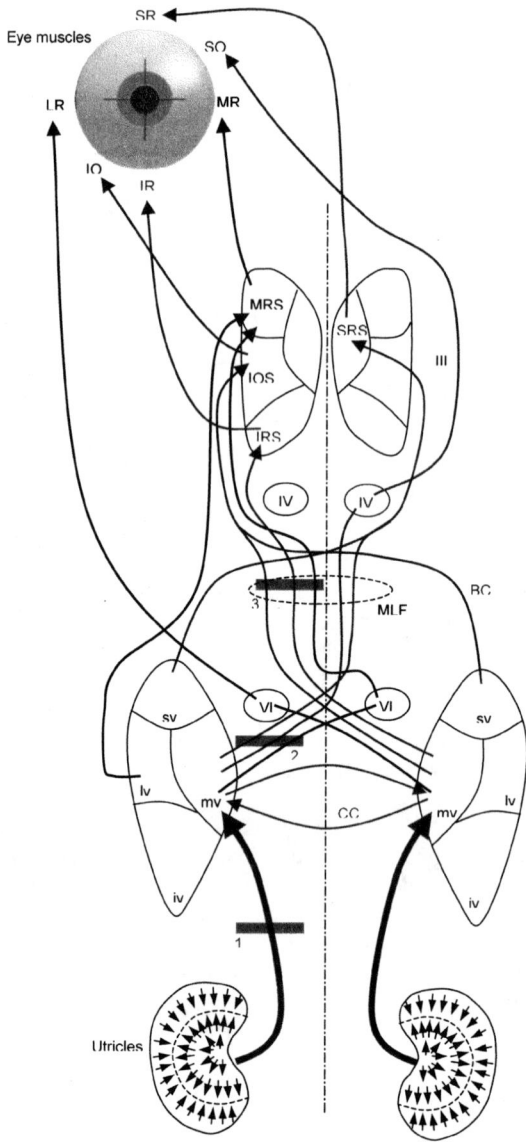

FIGURE 2. Anatomical presentation of the three-dimensional mathematical model showing the brainstem pathways from the utricles via the vestibular nuclei (sv, mv, lv, and iv = superior, medial, lateral, and inferior vestibular nucleus) and the ocular motor nuclei (MRS, SRS, IOS, and IRS = medial rectus, superior rectus, inferior oblique, and inferior rectus sections) to the extraocular eye muscles. Numbering indicates simulated lesions of the utricular/vestibular nerve (1), medial vestibular nucleus efference (2), and ascending "graviceptive" pathways in the MLF (3). The model is based on relevant anatomical connections of the vestibuloocular reflex known from electrophysiological and tracer studies in animals.

Unilateral lesions are simulated by disconnecting the respective pathways; that is, to simulate a peripheral lesion of the utricular nerve, the respective input to the VN is set to zero. Thus, the effect of a lesion on static eye position in an upright position is primarily determined by the remaining resting discharges.

TABLE 2. Model prediction

Lesion (left side)	Left eye			Right eye				
	T	V	H	T	V	H	HD	VD
No lesion	0.0	2.5	0.0	0.0	2.5	0.0	0.0	0.0
Left utricle	−3.9	2.7	0.0	−3.9	−0.3	0.0	0.0	3.0
Left vestibular nerve	−13.8	5.1	7.7	−13.6	−3.0	7.7	0.0	8.1
Left VN complete	−14.0	5.6	7.7	−14.0	−3.9	7.7	0.0	9.5
Left medial VN	−11.6	1.9	3.3	−10.3	−7.6	8.3	−5.0	9.5
Left superior VN	−2.9	8.7	−0.1	−4.2	5.7	−0.7	0.6	3.0
Left lateral VN	0.1	2.5	5.0	0.0	2.5	0.0	5.0	0.0
Left medial and superior VN	−14.0	7.2	3.2	−14.0	−4.7	7.7	−4.5	11.9
Left MLF	10.5	−7.6	5.9	11.7	2.0	1.7	4.2	−9.6
Left VN and MLF	−3.9	−3.1	8.7	−2.2	−5.0	9.4	−0.7	1.9
Left BC and MLF	7.6	−1.5	5.8	7.5	5.2	0.9	4.9	−6.7
Left MLF, only MR/IO/SO	4.3	5.7	5.7	8.8	−4.2	1.6	4.1	9.8
Left MLF, only MR/IO	4.3	5.7	5.7	0.0	2.5	0.0	5.7	3.2
Bilateral MLF	−1.2	−8.2	4.3	1.2	−8.2	−4.3	8.6	0.0
Bilateral BC	1.3	11.8	0.6	−1.3	11.8	−0.6	1.2	0.0

NOTE: The table shows the results of torsional (T), vertical (V), and horizontal (H) eye positions and horizontal and vertical divergence (HD, VD) with head upright for various vestibuloocular pathway lesions (all on the left side). Values are given in degrees. VN: vestibular nucleus; MLF: medial longitudinal fascicle; BC: brachium conjunctivum; MR: medial rectus; IO: inferior oblique; SO: superior oblique muscle; CC: commissural fibers. Parameters: c0 = 1; comgainy = 0.3; comgainx = 0; bcgain_io = 0.5; bcgain_sr = 0.5. Lesion of vestibular nerve: CC intact, no utricular input, no resting discharge. HD: − = esotopia; + = exotropia.

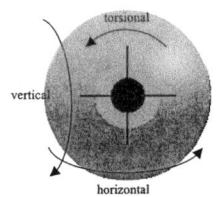

RESULTS

Comparing Model Prediction with the Patient Data

Vestibular Nerve

For a unilateral utricular lesion, the model predicts a vertical divergence of 3.0°, an ipsilateral conjugate OT of 3.9°, and no horizontal divergence (TABLE 2). For a unilateral lesion of the complete vestibular nerve, a vertical divergence of 8.1°, an ipsilateral conjugate OT of 13.6°, and no horizontal divergence are predicted. Since there is no disease affecting the utricular portion of the nerve only, we compared the ocular motor pattern of patients with herpes zoster neuritis—that affects the entire nerve—with that predicted by our static model for a unilateral utricular lesion or for a unilateral complete vestibular nerve lesion (TABLE 2). The patients with zoster neuritis presented with a mean vertical divergence of the eyes of 6.8° and a mean conjugate OT toward the ipsilateral side of 10° (TABLE 1). All three patients had a slightly horizontal divergence (mean: 1.8°). Thus, the patient data are closer to the model prediction for a complete vestibular nerve lesion than a solely utricular lesion.

Vestibular Nucleus

Lesion identification by magnetic resonance imaging did not allow an exact determination of the extent of vestibular nuclei lesions, complete or partial. Typically, the medial or superior subnuclei are involved in patients with infarctions in Wallenberg's syndrome.[17] Therefore, we contrasted our patient data not only with predictions for complete vestibular nucleus lesions, but also for separate lesions of the medial and the superior subnucleus, which differ significantly (TABLES 1 & 2). All predictions have in common an ipsilateral direction of OTR and a mainly conjugate OT, whereas the amplitudes vary between 3° and 9.5° for vertical divergence, between 3° and 14° for OT, and between 0° and 5° for horizontal divergence. Further, in complete VN lesions, a conjugate horizontal deviation of 7.7° was predicted toward the ipsilateral side. The three patients had an ipsilateral OTR with all its components (skew deviation, OT, and subjective visual vertical tilts), thus agreeing with the direction predicted (FIG. 1). However, the amounts of vertical divergence and OT differed considerably among the patients, and OT was clearly disconjugate in two of them (TABLE 1). Furthermore, two patients had a slightly horizontal divergence in opposite directions (3° esotropia in one and 2.5° exotropia in the other) and two a conjugate horizontal deviation (5° in one and 8° in the other). This heterogeneity cannot be simply explained by the different latencies between disease onset and time of investigation (days 3, 5, and 10), since the patient measured on day 3 after disease onset originally had the mildest amounts of skew deviation and OT. It can also not be attributed to the total size of infarction (FIG. 1), since the patient with the smallest lesion exhibited the largest amount of disconjugate OT (17° of the ipsilateral eye).

Pontomesencephalic MLF

For a unilateral MLF lesion, the model predicts a contralateral vertical divergence of 9.6°, a horizontal divergence of 4.2° exotropia, and a nearly conjugate OT of 10.5° for the ipsilateral eye and of 11.7° for the contralateral eye (TABLE 2). The three patients with an acute MLF lesion (TABLE 1, FIG. 1B) presented with an INO, a contralateral skew-torsion (mean vertical divergence of 10.3° and mean conjugate OT of 11°), and a mean horizontal exotropia of 11° (range: 6°–17°). Thus, the patient data corresponded well with the model prediction for direction and amplitude; however, the degree of horizontal divergence in the patients exceeded the prediction of the model.

DISCUSSION

The current three-dimensional mathematical model of the tonic vestibuloocular reflex predicts ocular motor syndromes that agree well with those found clinically in patients with acute unilateral lesions of the complete vestibular nerve and the ascending pathways in the pontomesencephalic brainstem (MLF). This supports the model approach, which is based on *utricular* ocular reflex function only. It further confirms the earlier hypothesis that skew deviation (vertical divergence), OT, OTR, and subjective visual vertical tilts are all clinical signs of *graviceptive vestibular* dysfunction.[8] Such an interpretation is not obvious, because these phenomena could also have been understood as ocular motor signs such as gaze palsies or INO independently of vestibular function.

Not only did all directions of tonic ocular deviations and subjective visual vertical tilts for the vestibular nerve and the MLF parallel those predicted by the model, but also the conjugacy and net tilt angles in degree were similar. The discrepancies, however, between prediction and clinical syndrome evident for the vestibular nucleus lesions in the three patients with Wallenberg's syndrome require further discussion.

Predictions Matching Clinical Findings

Vestibular Nerve

The ocular motor pattern of the patients with herpes zoster neuritis came close to the prediction of a complete vestibular nerve lesion. Patients with a purely utricular nerve lesion are predicted in the model to exhibit minor deviations. This agrees well with the finding that zoster neuritis involves superior and inferior parts of the vestibular nerve, which may show a contrast enhancement during magnetic resonance imaging of both parts due to viral inflammation.[18] It also confirms that postlesional static OT is caused by a lesion of not only the utricular pathway but also of the semicircular canal (SCC) pathways. This is in agreement with the finding that tonic OT induced by galvanic stimulation of the vestibular nerve is mainly due to SCC stimulation.[19] Complete OTR was also described in patients with lesions of the entire nerve due to other etiologies, that is, in the acute stage after unilateral vestibular neurectomy or labyrinthectomy.[20,21] In contrast, OTR is not a typical feature of the frequently seen "idiopathic" vestibular neuritis, which presents with horizontal rotatory nystagmus, ipsilateral conjugate OT, and subjective visual vertical tilts, but only rarely with minimal skew deviation. In our own neuroophthalmological laboratory, we saw only 4 of 60 patients (6.7%) with idiopathic vestibular neuritis who had a slight skew deviation of 1–2°. To date, idiopathic vestibular neuritis is known to be a disorder of the superior part of the vestibular nerve only.[22,23]

MLF

The model's prediction for a unilateral MLF lesion corresponded nicely with the data of acute unilateral pontomesencephalic infarctions involving the MLF (FIG. 1). The MLF conveys axons from neurons concerned with horizontal, vertical, and torsional conjugate gaze. For vertical gaze, these are axons from the vestibular nuclei, which carry signals contributing to the VOR, otolith-ocular reflexes, and gaze holding and project to the oculomotor and trochlear nuclei and the interstitial nucleus of Cajal (INC).[24] For horizontal gaze, axons from abducens internuclear neurons carrying the conjugate eye movement command project to medial rectus motoneurons in the contralateral oculomotor nucleus. In lesion studies, patients with pontine and pontomesencephalic brainstem infarctions affecting the MLF typically presented with the combination of INO and skew deviation with OT.[7,8,24,25] Here, skew deviation always occurred with a hypertropia of the eye on the side of the lesion, which was also the case in our patients. This ocular motor pattern indicates a crossing of the graviceptive pathways in the lower brainstem at the pontomedullary level.[26] Indeed, from tracer studies in animals[1,2] and lesion studies in humans,[8,25,27] it is known that the main VOR projections travel with the pathways from the (medial and superior) vestibular nuclei of one side via the contralateral MLF to the INC and ocular motor centers of the other side so that the crossing is at the rostral level of the vestibular nuclei or just above.

Predictions Deviating from Clinical Findings

Vestibular Nuclei

The only exception to this generally good agreement between the model's prediction and the patient data was seen for vestibular nuclei lesions. On the one hand, the directions for OT and vertical divergence were correct, as was the conjugate horizontal deviation of the eyes, which agrees with the "ocular lateropulsion" described earlier.[17,28,29] On the other hand, the model could not simulate the heterogeneous disconjugate patterns seen in patients with Wallenberg's syndrome. For example, the disconjugacy of OT and the amount of skew-torsion did not fit the model prediction for a common lesion of the complete vestibular nucleus or the medial or superior subnucleus. Disconjugacy of OT can probably be interpreted as a sign of SCC dysfunction; this was observed earlier in Wallenberg's syndrome.[17] The vestibular subnuclei lesions assumed in the model did not allow us to simulate single SCC pathway lesions, since the model relies on only utricular input. However, the clinical data in cases of disconjugate OT are more likely to be interpreted as a combination of VN lesions and lesions of single SCC neurons. This would nicely fit to the finding that tonic OT can also be induced by SCC stimulation only.[19]

Another interpretation for disconjugate OT is probably that of lesions of pathways to and via cerebellar structures. Animal studies have described not only pathways from the VN via the inferior olive to the cerebellar vermis (uvula-nodulus)[30,31] but also primary vestibular projections to the uvula-nodulus via mossy fibers.[32] These fibers were topographically arranged on the surface of the uvula-nodulus and distributed for vertical SCC projection, otolith input, and optokinetic projection. These fibers could be affected by the lesions. Furthermore, efferent fibers from the

VN that contact other brainstem centers and carry otolith and vertical SCC information in the SCC and/or eye muscle planes could be involved. Indeed, anatomical tracer studies and electrophysiological studies in animals have demonstrated that the otolith and SCC information converge on the same pathways from the vestibular nuclei[33] to the ocular motor nuclei[34,35] and complement each other over the whole frequency range under static and dynamic conditions.

When dealing with ischemic lesions in patients, it is to a large extent uncertain whether partial function of the vestibular nucleus survives after unilateral partial lesions. Several questions remain open, for example, the type of information resulting in the vestibular nucleus after otolith and SCC input converges; the role played by the commissural fibers between both vestibular nuclei; the importance of the downstream brainstem pathways from the integration centers (INC) to the VN; and the role of cerebellar pathways directly from the vestibular nerve to the cerebellum or from the VN to the fastigial nucleus and the vermis of the cerebellum. Thus, the next steps in refining the model will be to incorporate (1) horizontal and vertical-torsional integration centers together with their afferent and efferent connections, (2) connections from the vestibular nerve and the VN to the cerebellum, and (3) SCC function.

Role of the Integration Centers for Otolith Vestibular Ocular Motor Control

Recent evidence from human and monkey experiments indicates that the INC is essential for the control of static torsional eye position.[36] Animal experiments have shown that the INC is a vertical-torsional velocity-to-position integrator located in the rostral midbrain.[37,38] Although not a part of the direct VOR pathways, it controls the vestibular pathways from the VN via the ocular motor nuclei to the extraocular eye muscles and thus also eye-head position. Structures of the VOR have specialized functions as regards their dynamic and static velocity-to-position aspects. They are separate anatomically but cooperate during head motion and require both rapid responses with reflexive changes in position (VOR) and the maintenance of the achieved position by integration (integrator function of the INC). As Crawford and Vilis[36] have recently shown, the INC plays a crucial role in the control of static torsional eye position. They found that ocular counterroll to head tilt was completely abolished when the INC was inactivated bilaterally. Consequently, disorders of the INC and/or VOR pathways will affect both dynamic and static ocular motor aspects. Modeling of the integrators could be achieved by implementation of a bilateral neural integration network as proposed by Canon and colleagues[39] for the horizontal velocity-to-position integrator. Furthermore, direct projections from the VN to the extraocular eye muscles may be relevant, for they carry eye position information as part of a loop between the integrator and the VN.

To evaluate possible mechanisms by which otolith input may influence eye position via the INC, in a first step a dynamic mathematical model of saccade and burst generation was constructed.[40] The model simulations suggest that otolith pathways to the neural integrator that adjust Listing's plane may involve the cerebellum. According to this model, the otolith pathways dynamically determining OT via the INC operate as low-pass filters, and can thus be replaced with direct connections for static OT. Hence, the present model remains valid for the cases simulated, but has to be extended to include INC lesions, which are known to cause large amounts of OT.

ACKNOWLEDGMENTS

We wish to thank Judy Benson for critically reading the manuscript, and Claudia Frenzel and Miriam Glaser for orthoptic assistance. This work was supported by the Deutsche Forschungsgemeinschaft (DI 379/4-1, BR 639/6-1) and the Wilhelm Sander-Stiftung (2001.084.1).

REFERENCES

1. GRAF, W. & K. EZURE. 1986. Morphology of vertical canal related second order vestibular neurons in the cat. Exp. Brain Res. **63:** 35–48.
2. GRAF, W., R.A. MCCREA & R. BAKER. 1983. Morphology of posterior canal-related secondary vestibular neurons in rabbit and cat. Exp. Brain Res. **52:** 125–138.
3. ROBINSON, D.A. 1982. The use of matrices in analyzing the three-dimensional behavior of the vestibulo-ocular reflex. Biol. Cybern. **46:** 53–66.
4. VILIS, T. & D.B. TWEED. 1988. A matrix analysis for a conjugate vestibulo-ocular reflex. Biol. Cybern. **59:** 237–245.
5. TWEED, D.B., T.P. HASLWANTER, V. HAPPE & M. FETTER. 1999. Non-commutativity in the brain. Nature **399:** 281–283.
6. SMITH, M.A. & J.D. CRAWFORD. 1998. Neural control of rotational kinematics within realistic vestibuloocular coordinate systems. J. Neurophysiol. **80:** 2295–2315.
7. BRANDT, TH. & M. DIETERICH. 1993. Skew deviation with ocular torsion: a vestibular brainstem sign of topographic diagnostic value. Ann. Neurol. **33:** 528–534.
8. DIETERICH, M. & TH. BRANDT. 1993. Ocular torsion and tilt of subjective visual vertical are sensitive brainstem signs. Ann. Neurol. **33:** 292–299.
9. GLASAUER, S., M. DIETERICH & TH. BRANDT. 1998. Three-dimensional modeling of static vestibulo-ocular brain stem syndromes. Neuroreport **9:** 3841–3845.
10. OLSZEWSKI, J. & D. BAXTER. 1982. Cytoarchitecture of the Human Brain Stem. 2nd edit. Karger. Basel.
11. GLASAUER, S., M. DIETERICH & TH. BRANDT. 1999. Simulation of pathological ocular counter-roll and skew-torsion by a 3-D mathematical model. Neuroreport **10:** 1843–1848.
12. UCHINO, Y., M. SASAKI, H. SATO, et al. 1997. Utricular input to cat extraocular motoneurons. Acta Otolaryngol. Suppl. **528:** 44–48.
13. FERNANDEZ, C. & J.M. GOLDBERG. 1976. Physiology of peripheral neurons innervating otolith organs of the squirrel monkey. II. Directional selectivity and force-response relations. J. Neurophysiol. **39:** 985–995.
14. SUZUKI, J.I., K. TOKUMASU & K. GOTO. 1969. Eye movements from single utricular nerve stimulation in the cat. Acta Otolaryngol. (Stockh.) **68:** 350–362.
15. HAUSTEIN, W. 1989. Considerations on Listing's law and the primary position by means of a matrix description of eye position control. Biol. Cybern. **60:** 411–420.
16. ROBINSON, D.A. 1981. Control of eye movements. In Handbook of Physiology: The Nervous System. Vol II. Part 2. V.B. Brooks, Ed.: 1275–1320. Williams & Wilkins. Baltimore, MD.
17. DIETERICH, M. & TH. BRANDT. 1992. Wallenberg's syndrome: lateropulsion, cyclorotation, and subjective visual vertical in thirty-six patients. Ann. Neurol. **31:** 399–408.
18. ARBUSOW, V., M. DIETERICH, M. STRUPP, A. DREHER, et al. 1998. Herpes zoster neuritis involving superior and inferior parts of the vestibular nerve causes ocular tilt reaction. Neuro-ophthalmology **19:** 17–22.
19. SCHNEIDER, E., S. GLASAUER & M. DIETERICH. 2002. Comparison of human ocular torsion patterns during natural and galvanic vestibular stimulation. J. Neurophysiol. **87:** 2064–2073.
20. HALMAGYI, G.M., M.A. GRESTY & W.P.R. GIBSON. 1979. Ocular tilt reaction with peripheral vestibular lesions. Ann. Neurol. **6:** 80–83.
21. CURTHOYS, I.S., M.I. DAY & G.M. HALMAGYI. 1991. Human ocular position before and after unilateral vestibular neurectomy. Exp. Brain Res. **85:** 215–218.

22. BÜCHELE, W. & TH. BRANDT. 1988. Vestibular neuritis: a horizontal semicircular canal paresis? Adv. Oto-Rhino-Laryngol. **42:** 157–161.
23. FETTER, M. & J. DICHGANS. 1996. Vestibular neuritis spares the inferior division of the vestibular nerve. Brain **119:** 755–763.
24. LEIGH, R.J. & D.S. ZEE. 1999. The neurology of eye movements. 3rd edit. Oxford University Press. New York.
25. BRANDT, TH. & M. DIETERICH. 1994. Vestibular syndromes in the roll plane: topographic diagnosis from brainstem to cortex. Ann. Neurol. **36:** 337–347.
26. HALMAGYI, G.M., TH. BRANDT, M. DIETERICH, et al. 1990. Tonic contraversive ocular tilt reaction due to unilateral meso-diencephalic lesion. Neurology **40:** 1503–1509.
27. DIETERICH, M. & TH. BRANDT. 1993. Thalamic infarctions: differential effects on vestibular function in the roll plane (35 patients). Neurology **43:** 1732–1740.
28. HAGSTRÖM, L., G. HÖRNSTEN & B.P. SILFVERSKIÖLD. 1969. Oculostatic and visual phenomena occurring in association with Wallenberg's syndrome. Acta Neurol. Scand. **45:** 568–582.
29. BJERVER, K. & B.P. SILFVERSKIÖLD. 1968. Lateropulsion and imbalance in Wallenberg's syndrome. Acta Neurol. Scand. **44:** 91–100.
30. BARMACK, N.H., M. FAGERSON, B.J. FREDETTE, et al. 1993. Activity of neurons in the beta nucleus of the inferior olive of the rabbit evoked by natural vestibular stimulation. Exp. Brain Res. **94:** 203–215.
31. BALABAN, C.D. & R.T. HENRY. 1988. Zonal organization of olivo-nodulus projections in albino rabbits. Neurosci. Res. **5:** 409–423.
32. BARMACK, N.H., R.W. BAUGHMAN, P. ERRICO & H. SHOJAKU. 1993. Vestibular primary afferent projection to the cerebellum of the rabbit. J. Comp. Neurol. **327:** 521–534.
33. ANGELAKI, D.E., G.A. BUSH & A.A. PERACHIO. 1993. Two-dimensional spatio-temporal coding of linear acceleration in vestibular nuclei neurons. J. Neurosci. **13:** 1403–1417.
34. BAKER, R., W. PRECHT & A. BERTHOZ. 1973. Synaptic connections to trochlear motoneurons determined by individual vestibular nerve branch stimulation in the cat. Brain Res. **64:** 402–406.
35. SCHWINDT, P.C., A. RICHTER & W. PRECHT. 1973. Short latency utricular and canal input to ipsilateral abducens motoneurons. Brain Res. **60:** 259–262.
36. CRAWFORD, J.D. & T. VILIS. 1999. Role of the primate 3-D neural integrator in ocular counterroll during head tilt. Soc. Neurosci. Abstr. **25:** 6.
37. FUKUSHIMA, K. 1987. The interstitial nucleus of Cajal and its role in the control of movements of head and eyes. Prog. Neurobiol. **29:** 107–192.
38. CRAWFORD, J.D. & T. VILIS. 1993. Modularity and parallel processing in the oculomotor integrator. Exp. Brain Res. **96:** 443–456.
39. CANON, S.C., D.A. ROBINSON & S. SHIBAB. 1983. A proposed neural network for the integrator of the oculomotor system. Biol. Cybern. **49:** 127–136.
40. GLASAUER, S., M. DIETERICH & TH. BRANDT. 2001. Modeling the role of the interstitial nucleus of Cajal in otolith control of static eye position. Acta Otolaryngol. Suppl. **545:** 105–107.
41. HAUSTEIN, W. 1989. Considerations on Listing's law and the primary position by means of a matrix description of eye position control. Biol. Cybern. **60:** 411–420.

APPENDIX

Model Description

Neuronal transfer functions. For the utricle, the neuronal transfer function was as follows (Fernandez and Goldberg[13]):

$$y = F_u(x) = 2 \cdot 117.9 \cdot N(x, 1.75, 1.8) + 13)/65$$

with $N(x, \mu, \sigma)$ being the normal distribution function.

For vestibular nuclei and ocular motor nuclei, the neuronal transfer function was $y = F_n(x)$ as follows:

$$F_n(x) = x \text{ if } x > 0, F_n(x) = 0 \text{ otherwise.}$$

Utricles. The input to the utricles is gravitational acceleration $\underline{a}$ as a three-dimensional vector (in g, with $g = 9.81$ m/s^2); the output $\underline{u}$ of each utricle is a six-dimensional vector composed of two three-dimensional vectors, each being approximately proportional to gravitational acceleration in the range of 1 g (shown for the left utricle):

$$\underline{u}_l = \begin{bmatrix} u_{ll} \\ u_{lr} \end{bmatrix} = F_u \left(\frac{1}{g} \begin{bmatrix} U \\ -M \cdot U \end{bmatrix} \cdot \underline{a} \right)$$

with $g = 9.81$ m/s^2 and

$$U = \begin{bmatrix} 0 & 1 & 0 \\ \cos(30°) & 0 & \sin(30°) \\ 0 & 0 & 0 \end{bmatrix}.$$

U is a coordinate transformation reflecting the 30° pitch backward of the utricular macula and the fact that static roll causes ocular torsion, while static pitch causes vertical eye deviation. M is a 3×3 matrix that performs a mirror reflection with respect to the sagittal plane. Subscripts denote the origin and destination of the afferent information; for example, u_{ll} originates at the left utricle and mainly affects the left eye.

Vestibular nuclei. Utricular afferent information is processed by the vestibular nuclei. First, weighted utricular afferents from the ipsilateral side and excitatory commissural afferents from the contralateral side are added. Then, coordinate transformation to eye muscle coordinates (matrix T after Robinson[3]) and scaling (diagonal matrix B with gain 0.0436) are performed. The resulting two three-dimensional vectors are subsequently sent to the ocular motor nuclei. This can, for the left vestibular nuclei, be written as follows:

$$\underline{v}_l = \begin{bmatrix} v_{ll} \\ v_{lr} \end{bmatrix} = F_n \left(\begin{bmatrix} T^{-1} \cdot B \\ T^{-1} \cdot B \end{bmatrix} \cdot (V_i \cdot \underline{u}_l + V_c \cdot \underline{u}_r) + \underline{v}_0 \right)$$

with

$$T = \begin{bmatrix} -0.015 & 0.424 & 0.788 \\ 0.005 & -0.906 & 0.6 \\ -0.999 & 0.016 & 0.14 \end{bmatrix},$$

with $\underline{v}_{ll}$ and $\underline{v}_{lr}$ being the two three-dimensional output vectors of the vestibular nuclei. The weighting matrices for the commissural excitation are the diagonal matrices V_i and V_c, with $V_i = E - V_c$. In the simulations shown, the only nonzero element of V_c is $v_{c22} = 0.3$, which means that 30% of the pitch afferent information is supposed to originate in the contralateral utricle. In addition, $\underline{v}_0$ is the resting discharge of the VN; all elements are set to 0.0873.

Medial longitudinal fascicle, brachium conjunctivum, and ascending tract of Deiters. The six elements of the vestibular nuclei output vector $\underline{v}_l$ are connected to the following eye muscles: left medial rectus (lMR), left superior rectus (lSR), left superior oblique (lSO), right lateral rectus (rLR), right inferior rectus (rIR), and right inferior oblique (rIO). This afferent information is supposed to pass through different pathways that are partly parallel (TABLE A1).

Ocular motor nuclei and extraocular eye muscles. In each ocular motor nucleus (III, IV, and VI), afferent information from parallel pathways is weighted (all weights: 0.5) and a resting discharge is added: $\underline{\varrho}_0 = [0.4082, 0.3613, 0.3940]^T$. The components of $\underline{\varrho}_0$ correspond to MR, SR, and SO or LR, IR, and IO. The discharge of the ocular motor nuclei is then transformed from muscle innervation to muscle force by $y = F_m(x) = x^2 + 0.1$. The resulting muscle forces are subtracted and, after transformation back to head coordinates by T, they yield eye position expressed as rotation vector (Haustein[41]). For the left eye, this results in

$$\underline{e}_l = T \cdot (F_m(\underline{v}_{ll} + \underline{\varrho}_0) - F_m(\underline{v}_{rl} + \underline{\varrho}_0)).$$

Note that the size of $\underline{\varrho}_0$ is not arbitrary because of the nonlinear relationship between muscle innervation and muscle force. This quadratic relationship also ensures that the applied muscle force remains positive for each muscle.

Thus, for the normal case (no lesion), the relationship between left eye position and gravitational acceleration can be written in one single nonlinear vector equation. To model lesions, a MATLAB/Simulink model was used so that single or multiple connections between utricles, vestibular nuclei, and ocular motor nuclei could be disconnected.

TABLE A1. Afferents originating in the left vestibular nucleus

Elements of the VN output vector	Muscle	Destination	Pathways	Origin
1	Left medial rectus	Left oculomotor nucleus	Left ATD Right abducens, left MLF	Lateral VN Medial VN
2	Left superior rectus	Right oculomotor nucleus	Right MLF Left BC	Medial VN Superior VN
3	Left superior oblique	Right trochlearis	Right MLF	Medial VN
4	Right lateral rectus	Right abducens		Medial VN
5	Right inferior rectus	Right oculomotor nucleus	Right MLF	Medial VN
6	Right inferior oblique	Right oculomotor nucleus	Right MLF Left BC	Medial VN Superior VN

ATD: ascending tract of Deiters; BC: brachium conjunctivum; MLF: medial longitudinal fascicle; VN: vestibular nucleus.

Examining the Paradoxical Relation between Number of Spikes and Gaze Amplitude in Abducens Neurons

L. LING, J.O. PHILLIPS, AND C. SIEBOLD

Departments of Physiology and Biophysics and the Regional Primate Research Center, University of Washington, Seattle, Washington, USA

ABSTRACT: During head-unrestrained gaze shifts, the number of spikes in the burst of abducens neurons increases with gaze amplitude, even when corrected for the component of the discharge related to the change in eye position. We examine this paradoxical dissociation between the number of spikes and eye amplitude, which occurs because eye amplitude in the head saturates for larger gaze shifts. First, we show that the extra spikes are unlikely to be due to antagonist muscle loading because the abducens neurons are completely silent during large gaze shifts when the muscle acts as an antagonist. Next, we divide the firing rate profile of abducens neurons into terms that represent signals related to eye position, velocity, and acceleration; a d.c. offset term specifying the firing associated with straight-ahead gaze; and a slide term, which compensates for the zero of the oculomotor plant. Then we examine the contribution of each term to the number of spikes recorded. A comparison of the number of spikes with the integral of the fitted function, combining all of the terms, for the duration of the burst reveals that the simulation captures much of the actual data. However, even a model with a slide term cannot reproduce the nonlinear relationship of the number of spikes with amplitude that characterizes large gaze shifts.

KEYWORDS: motoneuron; burst discharge; saccades

INTRODUCTION

The first recordings of the activity in the motor nuclei of the extraocular muscles with the head restrained revealed a characteristic burst-tonic discharge pattern in association with saccades.[1-3] During fixation, the tonic firing rate is linearly related to orbital eye position. During a saccade that requires the innervated muscle to shorten, there is a burst of spikes that lasts the duration of the saccade and reaches a rate in excess of that associated with the final eye position. For saccades in the opposite (off) direction when the muscle lengthens, motoneurons exhibit a pause in activity. The number of spikes in the saccadic burst of abducens neurons show a linear increase with saccade amplitude when the spikes associated with the change in eye position due to the rate-position relationship are subtracted.[4,5]

Address for correspondence: L. Ling, Departments of Physiology and Biophysics and the Regional Primate Research Center, University of Washington, Seattle, WA.
LLING@bart.rprc.washington.edu

With the head free to rotate and contribute to the gaze shift, the number of spikes still increases, but with the amplitude of the gaze movement rather than the amplitude of the eye movement.[6] As gaze amplitudes grow larger, the eye movement contribution to gaze amplitude gradually saturates even as the number of spikes continues to increase. Therefore, for larger gaze shifts it appears that more spikes than those associated with the eye movement alone are necessary.

The paradoxical dissociation between the number of spikes and eye amplitude in abducens neurons remains unexplained. Cullen and colleagues[4] have described the net discharge profile of abducens units in terms of eye movement attributes, such as position and velocity, and have demonstrated that a model based on gaze movement trajectories does not provide a satisfactory fit. They failed, however, to explain how their fit accounts for the extra spikes during head-unrestrained gaze shifts. We also examined the neural activity and decomposed the firing pattern into signals whose contribution to the number of spikes in the burst can be evaluated separately. In particular, we investigate whether the addition of a "slide" term, which compensates for the zero of the peripheral eye movement apparatus (the plant) and is manifest late in the saccade, provides the extra spikes: this term may exhibit a nonlinear relationship with eye amplitudes because its contribution to the number of spikes in the burst is cut off during head-fixed saccades of short duration.

METHODS

We recorded neurons in the abducens nucleus of rhesus monkeys trained to follow spots of light by fixating sequentially illuminated LEDs. The abducens nucleus was identified by the characteristic discharge of its units and that of nearby cells such as inhibitory burst neurons. All units paused in the off direction, a feature that distinguishes abducens neurons from those in the nearby nucleus prepositus hypoglossi. Eye position in space was recorded by a search coil in a magnetic field.[7] Head position was measured with a precision potentiometer in line with a post that restricted the animal's head movements to the horizontal plane. Both signals were digitized at 1 kHz. The associated unit activity was recorded as interspike-intervals at a resolution of 10 μs. For details of the behavioral controls and the recording techniques, the reader is referred to our previous reports.[8,9]

We decomposed the discharge profile of abducens neurons into five separate components, consisting of terms proportional to eye position, velocity, and acceleration; a d.c. offset term and a slide term (FIG. 1A). The slide term was produced by passing eye velocity through a first-order filter.[10] The time constant of this filter is estimated for each unit by fitting a single exponential through the sagging discharge following the end of head-restrained saccades (see single arrow, FIG. 1A). The d.c. offset term represents the firing rate associated with straight-ahead gaze. The movement trajectories are sampled at the time of each action potential, then delayed to optimize the fit (that is, to produce the largest variance accounted for). This delay is larger than the average latency of the neural response by 2 to 3 ms and tends to align the time of peak velocity with the occurrence of the peak burst rate. The five coefficients of the three eye movement terms, the d.c. offset, and the slide term are then determined using a least-squares minimization procedure.

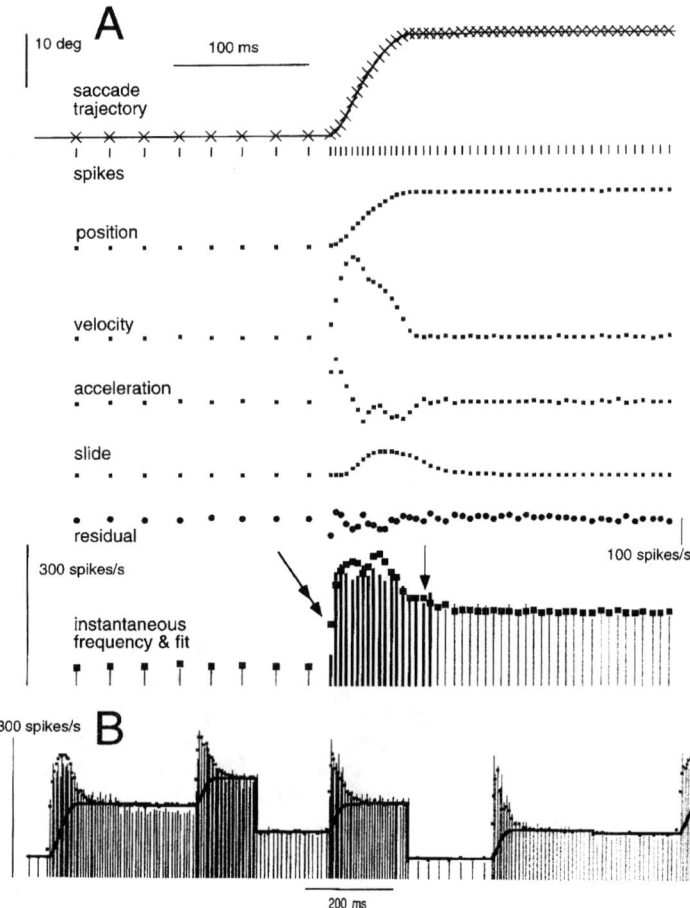

FIGURE 1. Analysis of the discharge profile of an abducens neuron during gaze shifts. (**A**) The top two traces show the time course of a saccade with the accompanying discharge of an abducens neuron. Each action potential is marked by a tic. Crosses in the eye movement trace indicate when samples are taken for the analysis. Samples of the position, velocity, acceleration, and slide terms are then displayed. Linear combinations of these terms are summed to fit the neural discharge. The results are superimposed (*filled squares*) on the instantaneous discharge frequency, which is indicated by the height of the vertical bars aligned on the occurrence of each spike. The difference between the neural data and the fit (residual) is shown at the time of each spike. (**B**) Data from several saccade trials is concatenated. The discharge profile (*vertical bars*) for a number of trials, providing an excerpt of the full dataset for one unit, is displayed with the saccadic eye movement (*black line*) and the resulting fits (*dots*).

An example of the fitting procedure is shown in FIGURE 1B. We anchor the fit by including the steady discharge preceding (about 200 ms, starting from the target step time) and following the saccade (about 180 ms unless a correction saccade occurs earlier). Nearly all trials exhibit preburst tonic activity. Data from several trials were concatenated and fit simultaneously (between 40 and 100 gaze shifts per unit). We attempt to describe the neural discharge strictly in terms of a linear system; therefore, the model does not include hysteresis, which probably is the reason for the offset of the fit during the steady firing preceding the second saccade shown in FIGURE 1B.

RESULTS

Typically, our fitting procedure utilizing functions proportional to eye position, velocity, acceleration and a slide term and a d.c. term (FIG. 1A) accounts for more than 85% of the variance of the neural data (six neurons). The variation of residuals (difference between fit and actual data) during the time course of the burst-tonic discharge indicates where the problematic parts of the fit occur. The mean absolute residual error during a period of fixation is approximately 2–5 spikes/s. The residual error increases during a burst, reaching values of 15–20 spikes/s. In particular, the fitting procedure cannot simulate the rapid rising edge of the bursts. Thus, the fit rises earlier (FIG. 1A, double arrow), causing a large negative error. However, the actual burst rates quickly surpass the fitted values, resulting in positive errors. This pattern of swing from positive to negative errors is often observed at the beginning of the burst (FIG. 1B).

When the head is unrestrained, the magnitude of the eye excursions in the orbit remains roughly constant as the size of the gaze shift increases and the head makes a growing contribution to gaze amplitude. For example, for the monkey illustrated in FIGURE 2, eye movements have a nearly constant amplitude of 30° to 35° although gaze amplitude varies between 40° and 70°. The discharge patterns associated with three gaze shifts of increasing gaze movement amplitudes but with rather similar eye movement amplitudes are shown in FIGURE 2A. As the gaze shift increases in amplitude, the number of spikes in the burst (the number of dark bars) increases. To quantify the magnitude of this transient response, we count the number of spikes occurring in the burst after subtracting the number of spikes associated with the tonic eye position sensitivity. The eye position contribution to the burst is estimated as the number of spikes represented by the gray shaded area of the burst shown in the discharge profiles in FIGURE 2A.

FIGURE 2B (inset) shows that the uncorrected number of spikes in the burst is linearly related to gaze (plus signs), not eye (open circles) amplitude. In addition, FIGURE 2B (main) shows that this pattern remains for the corrected number of spikes, which is also linearly related to the amplitudes of head-restrained saccades (open circles) and continues to increase for gaze shifts of larger amplitude during head-unrestrained movements (open squares). In contrast, the relation between the eye movement amplitude of head-unrestrained gaze shifts and the corrected number of spikes in the burst veers off from the relation obtained for head-restrained saccades as the eye amplitude saturates (filled squares).

These data seem to show that the number of spikes in the burst of large gaze shifts exceeds that needed to achieve the observed eye amplitude. Such an increase in mo-

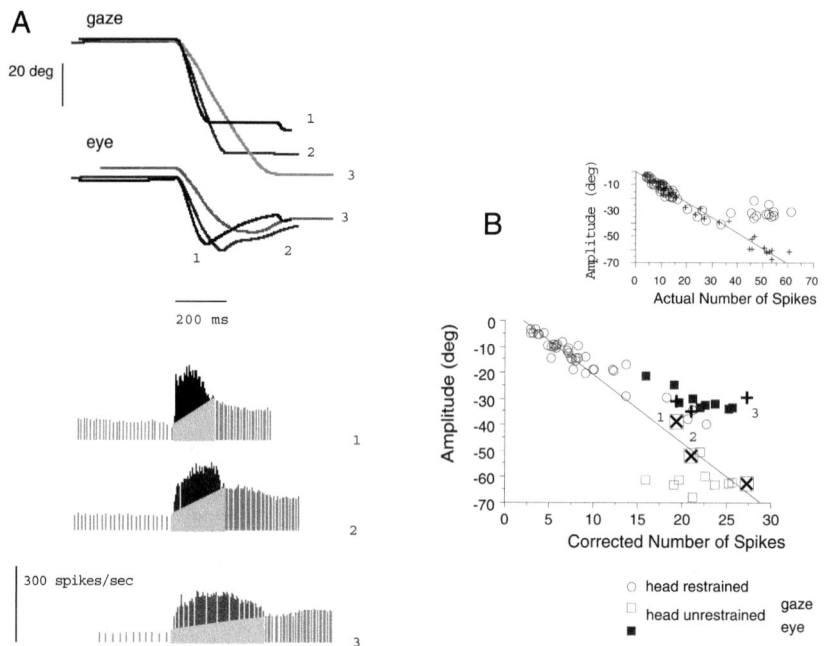

FIGURE 2. Number of spikes in burst of an abducens neuron during head-unrestrained gaze shift. (**A**) Three gaze shifts of increasing amplitude (gaze) and the accompanying eye saccades (eye) are shown together with the corresponding discharge of an abducens motoneuron. The height of the spikes in the unit raster corresponds to instantaneous frequency. The corresponding traces are labeled with numbers (1–3). The *gray portion* of the burst discharge denotes the discharge removed through the correction procedure. (**B**) The inset shows original uncorrected number of spikes re amplitude relationships for eye (*open circles*) and gaze (*plus signs*) movements. The main image displays the number of spikes corrected for the position term (that is, following removal of the gray portion of the burst discharge in **A**) plotted against amplitude for a variety of movement amplitudes. Data is displayed for head-restrained saccades (*open circles* with corresponding regression line), for gaze amplitudes during head-unrestrained gaze shifts (*open squares*), and for the amplitude of eye saccades during the same large gaze shifts (*filled squares*). The three example trials in **A** are identified (*crosses*: gaze; *plus signs*: eye) and labeled with numbers (1–3).

toneuron drive might be expected if the antagonist created an additional load during large gaze shifts. Unfortunately, no direct recordings are available from the motoneurons that innervate the antagonist medial rectus muscle during head-unrestrained gaze shifts. When the lateral rectus acts as an antagonist during head-unrestrained gaze shifts, however, abducens neurons exhibit a prominent pause, which lasts for the entire duration of the gaze movement. In fact, the pause typically continues beyond the end of the eye saccade. In FIGURE 3, two sets of gaze shifts are displayed with different mean amplitudes (36.0° vs. 56.3°) but similar eye components (27.8° vs. 33.2°). These data, which are similar for all abducens neurons we have studied, indicate that extra spikes are not needed to overcome an additional load imposed by antagonist contraction, because the antagonist is silent.

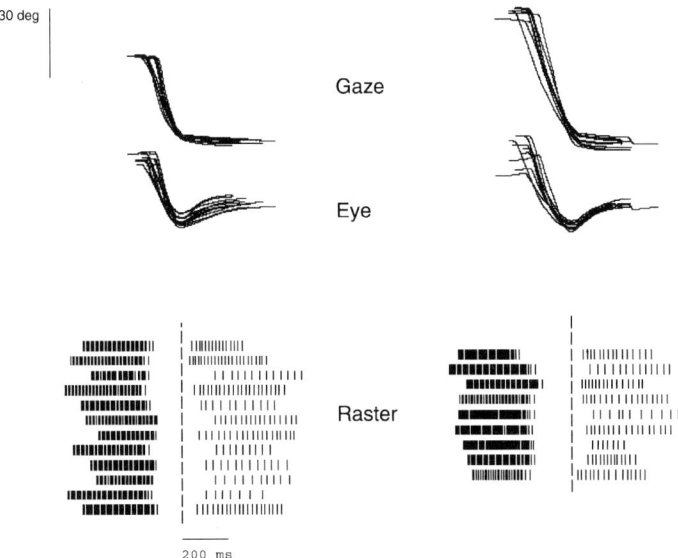

FIGURE 3. Off-direction responses of an abducens neuron during head-unrestrained gaze shifts. Gaze and eye in head are displayed for two amplitudes of gaze shift with comparable eye movement amplitudes. The accompanying neural activity is presented in the form of a raster display (raster). All traces are aligned on eye end. Each trial demonstrates a pause in tonic activity, which clearly extends beyond the end of the movement.

If not the antagonist activity, what is the explanation for the extra spikes? To address this issue we decomposed the discharge in abducens neurons during head-restrained and head-unrestrained gaze shifts in terms of components related to a d.c. offset, eye position, velocity, acceleration, and a slide term by fitting the discharge profile to a linear sum of these signals. From the fit, we can predict the actual number of spikes and ascertain the contribution of each term. This procedure allows us to locate the source of the extra spikes during head-unrestrained gaze shifts.

Our results show that the fit to the instantaneous firing rate nicely captures much of the discharge pattern associated with head restrained (FIG. 4A) and unrestrained (FIG. 4B) saccades. The position term (solid black line) follows the steady firing while the animal fixates before and after the saccade. When the velocity term is added during the head-restrained saccade in FIGURE 4A, the sum of eye position and velocity (dotted black line) describes much of the burst itself, especially when helped at the start by the acceleration term (dashed line at bottom) to produce the rapid onset of the burst. However, the sum of the position and velocity terms returns to the post-saccadic firing rate well before the actual firing rate does. To keep the firing somewhat elevated after the contributions related to parameters of the movement have dissipated, a slide term must be added.

The results of the fit provide a d.c. term, which is equal to the intercept of the relationship between steady firing rate and eye position during fixation, and a position

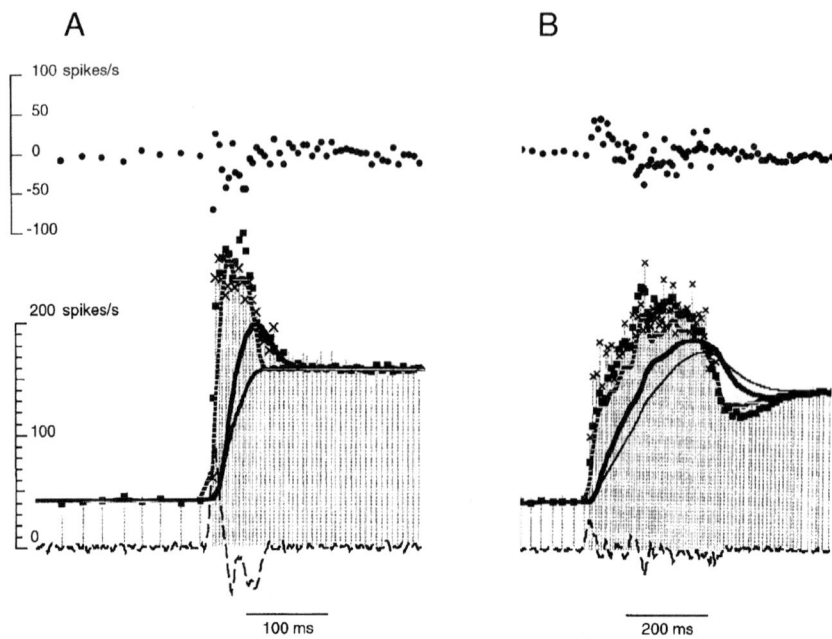

FIGURE 4. Decomposing the discharge profile of abducens neurons. (**A**) Resulting components for a head-restrained saccade exemplified in a single trial (same trial as in FIG. 1). *Top trace* displays the residual between fit and neural data. *Bottom traces* display a raster of the neural activity with the instantaneous discharge frequency represented by the height of the corresponding vertical bars. Also shown are the linear sums of the offset plus position terms (*solid black line*); the velocity plus position plus offset terms (*dotted black line*); the offset plus position plus slide terms (*solid gray line*), and the acceleration term (*dashed line* at bottom). *Filled squares* correspond to the sum of all terms in the fit. The instantaneous firing rates for spikes during the burst are denoted with *crosses*. (**B**) Resulting components for an eye movement during a head-unrestrained gaze shift. The trace definitions follow the description in **A** above.

coefficient, which corresponds to the slope of that relationship. The values are within the range of identified motoneurons[11] and confirm the numbers determined experimentally during steady fixation. Furthermore, when such data were available, the magnitude of the velocity coefficient is equal to the velocity sensitivity of the unit at 1 or 1.4 Hz, as estimated during sinusoidal pursuit or sinusoidal passive vestibular stimulation while fixating a target stationary in space.

The fit to the discharge during head-restrained saccades accounts for the total number of spikes in the burst. The integral of the actual spike density function over the burst obtained during such saccades yields the number of spikes in that burst. Because the profile of instantaneous firing rates provides a good estimate of the spike density function, a good fit to the discharge profile should also approximate the spike density function. Therefore, integrating the fitted function over the burst should re-

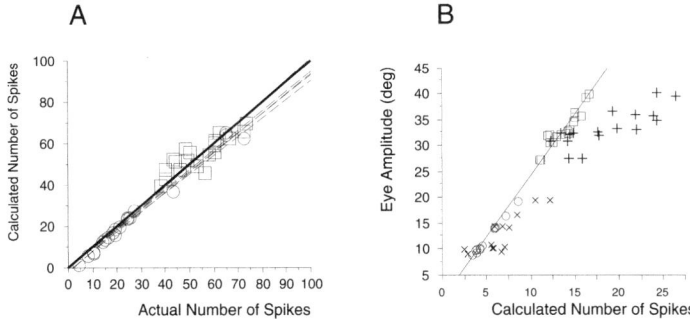

FIGURE 5. (A) Plot of the integral of the fit function over the duration of the burst against recorded number of spikes. Data from fits to head-restrained saccades (*open circles*) are combined with that to head-unrestrained gaze shifts (*open squares*) in a single regression (*solid line*). Regression lines from other units are also shown (*dotted lines*). (**B**) The calculated number of spikes remaining after the position component and d.c. offset have been removed, that is, the sum of the velocity, acceleration, and slide components is plotted against eye amplitude for head-restrained saccades (*open circles*) and head-unrestrained gaze shifts (*open squares*). The slide term does not make the relationship nonlinear. The number of spikes corrected by the position component and d.c. term (*crosses* for head-restrained data; *plus signs* for head-unrestrained data), however, retain a nonlinear relationship with eye amplitude.

sult in values close to the actual number of spikes. FIGURE 5A (open symbols) shows that this is indeed the case for a representative abducens unit. Each point represents the result from a single gaze shift with data for head-restrained saccades in open circles and those for head-unrestrained gaze shifts in open squares. The data is nicely fit by a straight line with a slope of nearly one and an intercept close to the origin, indicating that the observed and the calculated number of spikes are in close agreement. Similar linear fits (dashed lines) pertain to five other units (mean slope: 0.96 ± 0.05 (SD); intercept: –0.40 ± 1.03; r^2: 0.977 ± 0.014). The mean absolute error for the unit selected in FIGURE 5A is 3.2 spikes; however, a larger error may occasionally arise. The error tends to be less pronounced for the fit to head-restrained saccades than for that to the larger head-unrestrained gaze shifts (for example, the mean absolute errors were as follows: 1.5 vs. 4.4 spikes).

We divided the number of spikes calculated from the fit into two groups. First, we combined the velocity, acceleration, and slide components and plotted the spikes of a fit with the position term removed against the eye amplitude of head-restrained saccades (open circles) and head-unrestrained gaze shifts (open squares). The resulting data points fall on a straight line indicating that the neither of these terms gives rise to the nonlinearity of the number of spikes re the amplitude relationship. Second, we subtract the part of the fit that derives from the position component plus the d.c. term from the actual number of spikes to establish a corrected number of spikes. In FIGURE 5B, we plot the corrected number of spikes against eye amplitude. For large gaze shifts, when the eye amplitudes are saturated, the corrected number of spikes still increases. The model has in fact failed to account for the spikes that cause the nonlinearity. Similar patterns were obtained for four other units.

DISCUSSION

This study shows that during head-unrestrained gaze shifts the relationship between the number of spikes and amplitude does not have much predictive value in discerning what variables the discharge encodes (FIG. 1), in agreement with previous studies.[4,6] For the data set in FIGURE 2, we observe a dissociation between the number of spikes and eye amplitude. The subsequent analysis of fitting the entire discharge profile does provide a more complete description of the unit's behavior. However, our more comprehensive model still fails to account for the excess spikes. A full explanation may require a nonlinear model.

For head-restrained saccades, abducens neurons consistently exhibit a robust linear relationship between the number of spikes in the saccadic burst and the amplitude of the movement. The integral of the spike density function over the duration of the burst furnishes the number of spikes accumulated during the burst. Several factors conspire to result in a linear relationship. To a first approximation, the spike density function consists of the sum of a d.c. offset plus terms that are proportional to eye position and velocity. The integral of the d.c. term is equal to a constant times the duration of the burst, which is proportional to the amplitude of the saccade for main sequence movements. The integral of the position component is linearly related to amplitude as long as the rate-position curve of the unit is linear and, critically, the movement durations do not vary over a wide range. Finally, the velocity component obviously integrates to be proportional to eye amplitude. The sum total of the individual integrals is thus linearly related to eye amplitude as each component in turn is proportional to eye amplitude. With the removal of the position term, the sum of the d.c. and the position components, the linearity of the relationship is even more robustly determined.

The function of a saccade, the realignment of the line of sight, would be optimally served by a trajectory that approximates a step function as closely as possible. A step change in firing rate in the motoneuron will be distorted by the ocular plant. The discharge of abducens units reflects a control strategy that attempts to compensate for the plant dynamics. From this point of view, the signal decomposition of the discharge profile into terms related to parameters of the movement trajectory describe how the activity accounts for different components of the plant. For instance, the position, velocity, and acceleration terms deal with the poles of the system. Should the plant actually be more complex, containing also zeros, additional signals such as the slide term would be required.

If the discharge of abducens neurons is related to the eye movement, as one would expect, why then does a parametric description of the such units fail during head-unrestrained gaze shifts? A simple first-order system would require only signals proportional to eye position and velocity. As the duration of gaze shifts increases, the contribution of the position component will be nonlinear and will grow with gaze amplitude. But, after the position term has been removed, the relationships between number of burst spikes and eye amplitude can only be linear.

However, the dynamics of head-unrestrained gaze shifts may reveal the complexities of the oculomotor plant and require signals in the neural activity that compensate for such complexities. In particular, a slide term needs to be added to deal with the zero of the system. After removing the position term, the integral of all the other terms cannot add spikes beyond those proportional to the eye amplitude. During head-restrained saccades, the slide term can be neglected during the burst as it affects the discharge predominantly after the end of the movement. However, as head-unrestrained gaze shifts have much longer durations, the slide term could theoretically make a substantial contribution during the burst, providing the surplus spikes that are observed during such movements. However, the slide term is also linearly related to eye amplitude for large gaze shifts. Furthermore, the nonlinear effect brought about by the truncation of the slide term during head-restrained saccades is not large enough to create the nonlinearity observed in the number of spikes re amplitude relationship.

In the vicinity of the abducens nucleus in the brainstem, one encounters several units that display a robust burst in association with saccades. Some of these project directly to abducens neurons. Such prenuclear elements provide one of the sources of the burst observed in motoneurons during saccades. They also provide the pause in the antagonist motoneurons. These burst units exhibit a linear relationship between the number of spikes in the burst and the amplitude of head-restrained saccades in their on-direction.[12,13] FIGURE 6 plots the response of one such burst neuron, an excitatory burst neuron, during gaze shifts of varying magnitude when the head is restrained and when the head is allowed to contribute. The relationship between number of spikes and the amplitude of head-unrestrained gaze shifts follows the head-restrained data and extends it to larger amplitudes. On the other hand, the relationship for the accompanying eye amplitude deviates from the progression of head-restrained data as the eye amplitudes saturate with increasing gaze shift ampli-

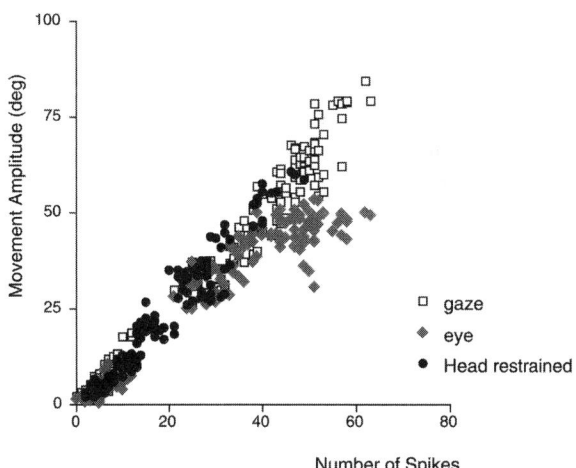

FIGURE 6. Response of an excitatory burst neuron (EBN) in the paramedian pontine reticular formation during head-restrained saccades and head-unrestrained gaze shifts. The number of spikes in the burst recorded during gaze shifts is plotted against the amplitude of the head-restrained saccade (*filled circles*), the gaze amplitude of head-unrestrained gaze shifts (*open squares*), and the amplitude of the associated eye movement (*filled diamonds*). The relationship for head-unrestrained gaze amplitudes is linear and superimposes on the head-restrained data points, whereas head-unrestrained eye amplitudes show a nonlinear relationship.

tude. This pattern is reminiscent of the behavior of abducens cells (cf. FIG. 2). The fact that the signals in excitatory burst neurons and abducens neurons are separated by only a single synapse suggests that a common rationale should be applied to both phenomena. We propose that to compensate for the complexities of the oculomotor plant, the pre-nuclear burst neurons and the abducens motoneurons carry more than just a simple velocity command. The additional component becomes apparent only during head-unrestrained gaze shifts when the longer durations require more spikes to produce the same change in eye amplitude.

REFERENCES

1. FUCHS, A.F. & E.S. LUSCHEI. 1970. Firing patterns of abducens neurons of alert monkeys in relationship to horizontal eye movement. J. Neurophysiol. **33**: 382–392.
2. ROBINSON, D.A. 1970. Oculomotor unit behavior in the monkey. J. Neurophysiol. **33**: 393–403.
3. SCHILLER, P.H. 1970. The discharge characteristics of single units in the oculomotor and abducens nuclei of the unanesthetized monkey. Exp. Brain Res. **10**: 347–362.
4. CULLEN, K.E., H.L. GALIANA & P.A. SYLVESTRE. 2000. Comparing extraocular motoneuron discharge during head-restrained and head-unrestrained gaze shifts. J. Neurophysiol. **83**: 630–637.
5. LING, L., J.O. PHILLIPS & A.F. FUCHS. 1999. Abducens neuron activity during head-unrestrained gaze shifts: unexpected associations between firing and gaze, not eye. Arch. Ital. Biol. **137**: 23.
6. LING, L., A.F. FUCHS, J.O. PHILLIPS & E.G. FREEDMAN. 1999. Apparent dissociation between saccadic eye movements and firing patterns of premotor neurons and motoneurons. J. Neurophysiol. **82**: 2808–2811.
7. ROBINSON, D.A. 1963. A method of measuring eye movement using a scleral search coil in a magnetic field. IEEE Trans. Biomed. Electron. **10**: 137–145.
8. PHILLIPS, J.O., L. LING, A.F. FUCHS, *et al.* 1995. Rapid horizontal gaze movement in the monkey. J. Neurophysiol. **73**: 1632–1652.
9. PHILLIPS, J.O., L. LING & A.F. FUCHS. 1999 Action of the brain stem saccade generator during horizontal gaze shifts. I. Discharge patterns of omnidirectional pause neurons. J. Neurophysiol. **81**: 1284–1295.
10. OPTICAN, L.M. & F.A. MILES. 1985. Visually induced adaptive changes in primate saccadic oculomotor control signals. J. Neurophysiol. **54**: 940–958.
11. FUCHS, A.F., C.A. SCUDDER & C.R. KANEKO. 1988. Discharge patterns and recruitment order of identified motoneurons and internuclear neurons in the monkey abducens nucleus. J. Neurophysiol. **60**: 1874–1895.
12. STRASSMAN, A., S.M. HIGHSTEIN & R.A. McCREA. 1986. Anatomy and physiology of saccadic burst neurons in the alert squirrel monkey. I. Excitatory burst neurons. J. Comp. Neurol. **249**: 337–357.
13. STRASSMAN, A., S.M. HIGHSTEIN & R.A. McCREA. 1986. Anatomy and physiology of saccadic burst neurons in the alert squirrel monkey. II. Inhibitory burst neurons. J. Comp. Neurol. **249**: 358–380.

Signal Processing of Semicircular Canal and Otolith Signals in the Vestibular Nuclei during Passive and Active Head Movements

ROBERT A. McCREA AND HONGGE LUAN

Department of Neurobiology, Pharmacology, and Physiology, University of Chicago, Chicago, Illinois, USA

> ABSTRACT: The vestibular nerve sends signals to the brain that code the movement and position of the head in space. These signals are used by the brain for a variety of functions, including the control of reflex and voluntary movements and the construction of a sense of self-motion. If many of these functions are to be carried out, a distinction must be made between sensory vestibular signals related to active head movements and those related to passive head movements. Current evidence is that the distinction occurs at an early stage of sensory processing in the brain, and the results are evident in the firing behavior of neurons in the vestibular nuclei that receive direct inputs from the vestibular nerve. Several specific examples of how sensory information related to passive and active head movements is transformed in the vestibular nuclei are discussed.
>
> KEYWORDS: vestibular nuclei; otolith; vestibulo-ocular reflex; head movements

INTRODUCTION

The vestibular sensory receptors are located within the bony labyrinths embedded in the petrous temporal bone of the head. Their function is to detect the position and motion of the head in space. The signals produced by the vestibular nerve are important for spatial perception and for producing a variety of reflexes that help maintain balance and equilibrium. An essential feature of the central processing required of this head movement sensory system, like all sensory systems, is the ability to distinguish between sensory experiences that are due to self-stimulation and those that are produced by passive, external forces.

The distinction between passive and active head movements is important for constructing an internal estimate of self-motion as well as producing coordinated responses to head perturbations. When the head is moved by passive, external forces, the vestibular system, together with other sensory systems, such as visual and proprioceptive systems, construct an internal estimate of head motion.[1–3] The estimate is

---

Address for correspondence: Robert A. McCrea, Department of Neurobiology, Pharmacology, and Physiology, University of Chicago, 947 East 58th Street, MC0926, Chicago, IL 60637. Voice: 773-702-6374; fax: 773-702-3736.
  ramccrea@uchicago.edu

Ann. N.Y. Acad. Sci. 1004: 169–182 (2003). © 2003 New York Academy of Sciences.
doi: 10.1196/annals.1303.015

used to produce a variety of postural reflex movements of the trunk, limbs, neck, and eyes, movements that help stabilize gaze and the orientation of the body and limbs. The estimate of passive head movement allows subsequent estimates of the motion of the body and limbs, and by comparison the relative motion of objects in the external world.[4]

The process of distinguishing between vestibular signals related to self-generated head movements and passive head movements in space could begin as early as the vestibular sensory epithelium by way of efferent vestibular pathways.[5,6] However, it is more likely that the distinction between passive and active head movements is carried out centrally by structures that receive these sensory signals. The main recipient of vestibular afferent information, the vestibular nucleus, receives inputs from the cerebellum, cerebral cortex, reticulospinal collaterals, and spinal cord that could modify sensory processing during passive or self-generated head on trunk movements.[7] The latter inputs usually reduce the vestibular nucleus unit responses to head-on-trunk rotation.[8]

The results of our recent studies suggest that the signals carried by secondary vestibular neurons in the vestibular nuclei are different during passive and active head movements[9,10] and during the vestibulocollic reflex (VCR).[11,12] The vestibular nuclei are not homogeneous. The region gives rise to several important descending and ascending pathways.[13] In this paper, we summarize how sensory signals related to active, self-generated head movements vary in different classes of vestibular nucleus neurons that have been examined to date.

METHODS

Recording Techniques

Single-unit recordings were done in alert squirrel monkeys that were free to move their head in the yaw plane while seated on a vestibular rotator. The monkeys wore a tightly fitting jacket and were perched on a Plexiglas foot rest on a vestibular turntable. They were allowed to grasp a handrail that surrounded them at chest height. The head was attached to a rod that permitted angular head movements in the plane of the horizontal semicircular canals. The axis of head motion was placed either in line with the interaural plane ("on-axis" rotation) or 5–8 cm forward of the interaural plane. The latter "off-axis" head movements stimulated both otolith and semicircular canal afferents. Head and body movements were restrained by attaching the monkey's jacket to the turntable and the monkey's head to a rod that allowed free head movements in the yaw plane.

Eye and head movements were recorded with the magnetic search-coil technique. Stimulating electrodes were implanted bilaterally in the middle ear to allow orthodromic identification of neurons that receive synaptic inputs from the vestibular nerve and to allow verification of the location of recording sites in the vestibular nuclei using evoked field potential analysis. In some animals, stimulating electrodes were implanted in the ventromedial funiculi of the spinal cord at C1 or the thalamus to allow antidromic identification of neurons that project to the thalamus or the spinal cord.

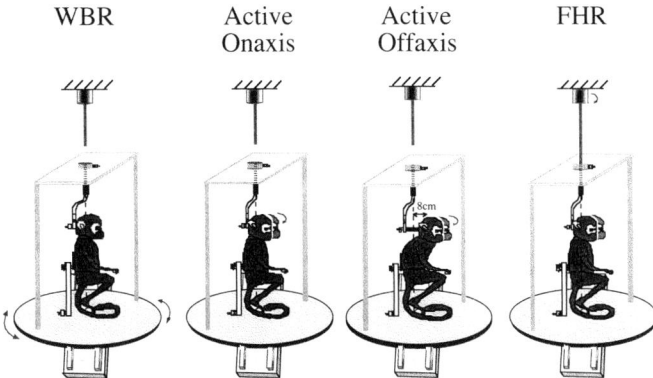

FIGURE 1. Experimental setups used for comparing passive and active head movement signals in squirrel monkeys: passive whole-body rotation or translation with head fixed to vestibular turntable; active on-axis (self-generated saccadic, VCR, or pursuit head movements allowed in the plane of the horizontal semicircular canal); axis of head rotation intersects interaural axis; active off-axis (self-generated head movements allowed in the plane of the horizontal semicircular canal). Axis of head rotation passes 5–8 cm behind the interaural plane. FHR: Forced, passive head-on-trunk rotation by attaching head to ceiling motor.

Experimental Protocols: Passive and Active Head, Neck, and Body Rotation

FIGURE 1 illustrates the methods used to compare single-unit responses to passive and active head movements. Single-unit responses were studied during passive whole-body rotation (WBR) at two stimulus frequencies (0.5 Hz, 40°/s; 2.3 Hz, 20°/s) either with the head fixed with respect to the vestibular turntable or with the head free to move in the yaw plane. The axis of head-on-trunk rotation was positioned so that it either intersected the interaural axis (on-axis position), allowing head-on-trunk movements that minimized stimulation of otolith receptors, or in an off-axis position that allowed head-on-trunk movements that stimulated both the semicircular canals and otoliths. The responses of some units were also studied during passive sinusoidal translation produced by a linear sled mounted on top of the turntable. Forced, passive head-on-trunk rotations (FHRs) were produced by rotating the rod attached to the animal's head either manually or with a ceiling-mounted motor. In some cases, a recording of active head movements was made that was then used to produce similar passive head-on-trunk rotations (HTRs) with the ceiling motor. Neck proprioceptive inputs to vestibular neurons were studied by holding the head stationary in space while passively rotating the turntable.

Three types of active, self-generated head movements were studied: (1) vestibulocollic reflex head movements evoked by passive WBR, (2) spontaneous gaze saccades, and (3) smooth tracking head movements of sinusoidal moving visual targets.

Data Analysis

Neural sensitivity to passive and active head movements was estimated using multiple linear regression analysis. The factors contributing to fitting functions included variables related to eye movement, neck rotation, as well as movement of the head in space. Estimates of neuronal sensitivity to neck rotation alone were based on parametric analysis of responses evoked when the head was kept stationary in space while the body was passively rotated by the turntable. Responses related to quick phases of nystagmus, and periods when the monkey was not alert, were not included in the averages. The records obtained during paradigms that used visual targets were also excluded from averages if the behavioral performance was poor. During head-fixed paradigms, the amount of data excluded during quick phases of nystagmus was based on the response during ocular saccades. During head-unrestrained paradigms, responses during quick phases of head-nystagmus were also excluded from the rotational analysis.

Unit responses during gaze saccades were evaluated by averaging the response to groups of saccades that had similar direction and peak head velocities. Head velocities typically ranged between 50° and 150°/s. The vestibular sensitivity during active head movements was compared to an estimate of the unit's head velocity and acceleration sensitivities during high-frequency WBR with the head restrained.

RESULTS

Vestibular nerve fibers generate similar responses to head movements during passive and active head movements. FIGURE 2 shows the response of a primary vestibular afferent fiber during simultaneous passive and active head movements. The monkey generated a series of active head movements while its body was passively

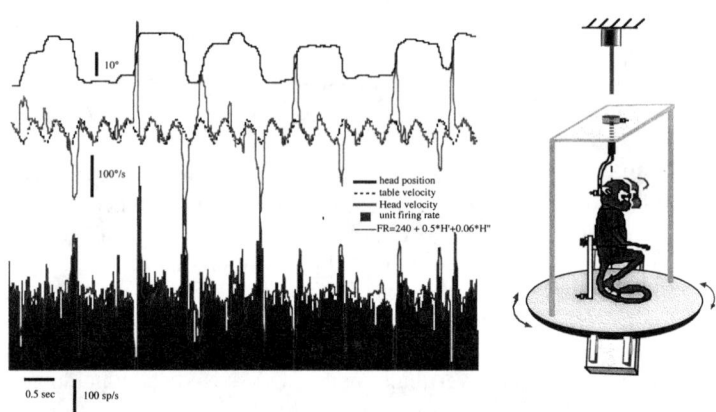

FIGURE 2. Primary vestibular nerve afferent generates similar responses during passive and active head movements. Vestibular turntable was rotated sinusoidally at 2.3 Hz while the head was free to move. Consequently, movement of the head in space was a combination of passive and active head movements. *Top trace* is head position with respect to the turntable. *Middle traces* are angular head velocity in space (*solid trace*) and passive angular head velocity in space (*dashed trace*). The solid trace superimposed on the firing-rate histogram on the bottom is a model of the unit's firing rate based on its response to passive rotation alone.

rotated by the vestibular turntable. The top trace is a record of the monkey's head movement with respect to the turntable. The middle traces show the passive head velocity in space generated by turntable rotation (dotted middle trace) and the velocity of combined passive and active head movements (solid middle trace). The bottom histogram is the firing rate of the vestibular nerve afferent. The trace superimposed on the firing rate histogram is the response expected if the afferent were equally sensitive to passive and active head movements.

Vestibular Nucleus Neurons Sensitive to Both Passive and Active Head Movements

The firing behavior of over 160 vestibular nucleus neurons that were sensitive to rotation of the head in the plane of the horizontal semicircular canal and/or to inter-

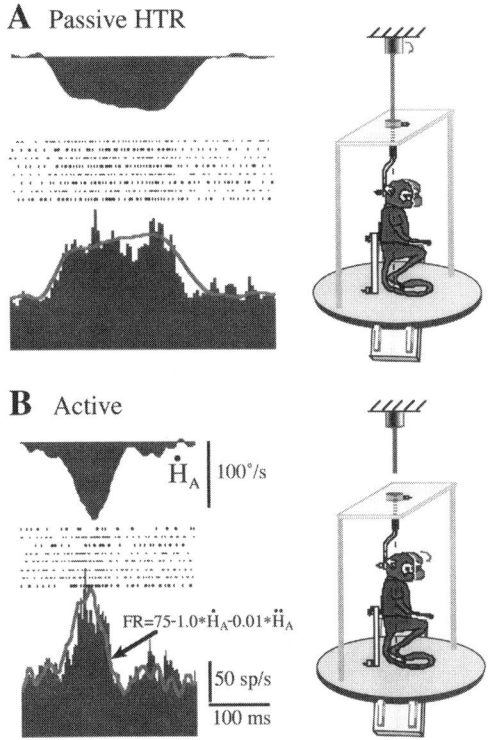

FIGURE 3. Horizontal-canal-related vestibular nucleus neuron sensitive to both passive and active head rotation. (**A**) Passive head-on-trunk rotation (average of eight steps in head velocity in the cell's excitatory on-direction). The *filled trace* at the top shows the average angular head velocity. The *middle traces* show spike rasters from individual trials. The *bottom trace* shows unit firing rate. (**B**) Responses during active head movements generated during gaze saccades. The traces superimposed on the firing-rate histograms are the responses expected on the basis of the cell's response to sinusoidal WBR at 2.3 Hz. The neuron's firing rate was not related to eye movements.

aural translation have been studied during passive and active head movements. Some vestibular nucleus neurons also generated responses to passive and active head movements that were similar. Many neurons in the vestibular nuclei are sensitive to eye movements, and most cells of this type are presumed to be related to producing or controlling the vestibulo-ocular reflex (VOR). These neurons are located primarily in the rostral parts of the vestibular nuclei. Vestibular nucleus non-eye-movement-related (NEM) neurons are located throughout the vestibular nuclei. NEM neurons project to many regions of the thalamus, brainstem, cerebellum, and spinal cord, and thus are related to a wide variety of functions. FIGURE 3 shows the firing behavior of a horizontal-canal-related NEM vestibular nucleus neuron that was sensitive to both passive and active head movements. The records in FIGURE 3A are averages of eight rapid step changes in angular head velocity produced by attaching the monkey's head to a ceiling motor. The head rotation was in the plane of the semicircular canal, and the axis of rotation was centered on the monkey's head intersecting the interaural plane. The step in head velocity produced an increase in firing rate that was proportional to head velocity (1.0 spikes/s/°/s). The comparable averaged response recorded during self-generated active angular head rotations produced during gaze saccades is shown in FIGURE 3B. The step changes in head velocity were more transient during active head movements, but the values for peak acceleration and velocity of the movements were comparable. The solid traces superimposed on the firing-rate histograms are the responses predicted on the basis of the cell's response to passive WBR (equation in FIGURE 3B). For active head movements in this cell's "on" direction (ipsilateral), the sensitivity to head rotation during active head movements was similar.

The responses of central vestibular neurons to active head translation were studied by allowing the monkey to generate head movements in the horizontal plane with the axis of head rotation moved 5–8 cm behind the center of the head. In this posture, head rotations produced a combination of linear translation and angular rotation. FIGURE 4 illustrates the response of a central otolith neuron to both passive and active head translation during off-axis head rotation. The neuron was not sensitive to angular head rotation with the head centered on the axis of rotation of the turntable. Its firing rate was modulated in phase with linear head velocity (18.7 spikes/s/cm/s) during sinusoidal linear translation at 2.0 Hz. In FIGURE 4A, the neuron's averaged response during head saccades generated with the head restrained in an off-axis position (diagram on the right) is illustrated. The spike rasters for individual saccades are illustrated. The cell was inhibited when the head was actively translated in the ipsilateral direction (left traces) and excited during contralateral head translations (right traces). The solid traces superimposed on the firing-rate histograms are the responses predicted from the cell's sensitivity to whole-body linear translation. These active head movements were stored on a computer and used to program a similar sequence of passive forced head movements using the ceiling motor (FIG. 4B). The passive head movements evoked in this manner were similar, but not identical, to the active head movements due to flexibility in the coupling of the motor to the head and to changes in resistance to movement produced by the monkey. The profiles of inhibition by ipsilateral translation, and excitation by contralateral translation, were similar to those generated during active head movements, and roughly predictable from the cell's response to passive whole-body linear translation (solid traces superimposed on firing-rate histograms in FIG. 4B).

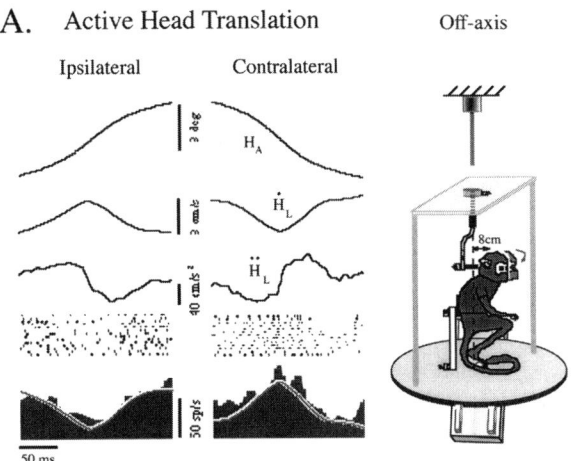

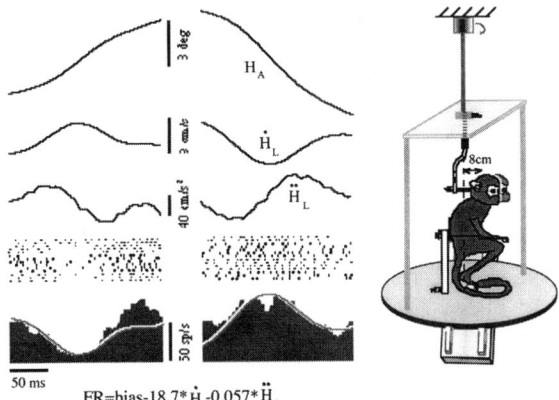

FIGURE 4. Otolith-related vestibular nucleus neuron sensitive to both passive and active head translation. (**A**) Active head-on-trunk off-axis rotations (average of 14 ipsilateral and contralateral head movements). The *top traces* show the average change in angular head position, linear head velocity, and linear head acceleration. The *middle traces* show spike rasters from individual trials. The *bottom trace* shows unit firing rate. (**B**) Responses during passive, forced head movements similar to active head movements. The traces superimposed on the firing rate histograms show the responses expected on the basis of the cell's response to sinusoidal whole body translation at 2.0 Hz. The neuron's firing rate was not related to eye movements.

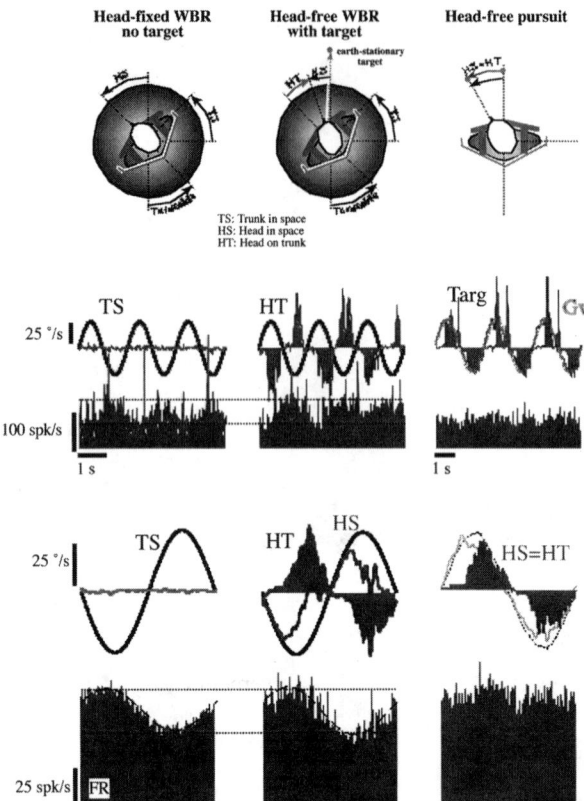

FIGURE 5. Non-eye-movement-related vestibular nucleus neuron that was differentially sensitive to passive head movements. Top pictures illustrate three different paradigms used during recording. Records in the *left column* show the cell's response to passive WBR. The *center column* illustrates the lack of a change in the neuron's response (*dashed lines* between left and center columns) when active head-on-trunk movements (HT) reduced head velocity in space (HS). The *righthand column* shows the cell's lack of a response during active head-on-trunk movements generated while tracking a visual target that was moving in space. A combination of saccades and smooth tracking head movements was produced.

Vestibular Nucleus Neurons Preferentially Sensitive to Passive Head Movements

Most vestibular nucleus neurons were unlike the cells illustrated in FIGURES 2–4, and generated dramatically different responses during passive and active head movements. The most dramatic changes were an insensitivity to active head movements. FIGURE 5 illustrates recordings obtained from a secondary horizontal-canal-related NEM neuron in the vestibular nuclei that was insensitive to active head movements. Records from three different conditions are illustrated. The records on the left were obtained during passive WBR at 0.5 Hz while the monkey's head was restrained from moving. In this condition, the movement of the trunk in space (TS) was the same as the movement of the head in space (HS). Records obtained during three representative cycles of WBR are shown as well as the average response over many cycles (bottom traces).

The center column of records was also recorded during passive WBR at 0.5 Hz, but the monkey's head was free to move, and it was encouraged to maintain its head stable in space by fixating on an earth-stationary target. In this condition, active movements of the head on the trunk (filled traces) were generated that were opposite in direction to movements of the body in space (solid sinusoidal traces). The effect was to dramatically reduce the movement of the head in space (HS trace in bottom averaged records). In spite of a reduction of head velocity in space in this condition, the modulation in the neuron's firing rate by turntable rotation was nearly the same as when the head was fixed to the turntable (dashed lines superimposed on the spike histograms).

The records in the righthand column of FIGURE 5 show responses of the same neuron when the monkey pursued a moving visual target with a combination of eye and head movements. Only a fraction of the pursuit was generated by saccadic or smooth-following head-on-trunk movements (filled traces), but the average peak head velocity in space (HS) was similar to that generated during WBR. In this condition, active head movements generated all of the head movement in space, and movement of the head in space did not modulate the neuron's firing rate. In sum, this secondary vestibular neuron was differentially sensitive to passive, non-self-generated head movements. In these contexts, its firing rate was better related to movement of the trunk in space than to movement of the head in space. The latter observation obtained for the majority of non-eye-movement-related neurons in the vestibular nuclei.[11]

Firing Behavior of Eye-Movement-Related Neurons during Active Head Movements

The majority of NEM neurons in the vestibular nuclei were differentially sensitive to passive head movements.[10] Most eye-movement-related neurons also were differentially sensitive to passive head movements, although their responses were more complex. FIGURE 6 illustrates the firing behavior of four different types of eye-movement-related vestibular nucleus neurons during gaze saccades that included a significant active head movement component. The records are averages of many gaze saccades, with spike rasters shown for individual saccades. The traces superimposed on firing-rate histograms are the responses that would be expected if the neuron's generated head-movement-related signals during both passive and active head movements. The eye-movement signals generated by eye-movement-related cells also affected their firing behavior during gaze saccades. The firing behavior of the position-vestibular-pause (PVP) and position-vestibular I and II (PVI and PVII) neurons was related to eye position. PVP and eye-head-vestibular (EHV) vestibular neurons were sensitive to eye velocity during smooth pursuit eye movements. PVP neurons characteristically paused during gaze saccades. There is considerable evidence that PVP, PVI, and EHV neurons contribute to the VOR. PVII neurons responded to contralateral head rotations, and receive direct inputs from the vestibular nerve. Many neurons, including the neuron illustrated in FIGURE 6, receive inputs from the otolith afferents and may contribute to otolith ocular reflexes.

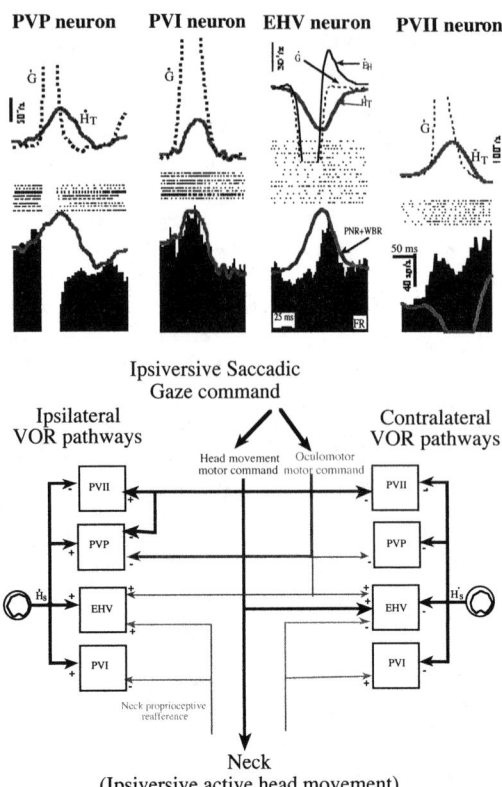

FIGURE 6. Firing behavior of four types of eye-movement-related vestibular neurons during active head movements. The *top traces* in each of the upper panels show averaged head-on-trunk velocity (*solid traces*) and average gaze velocity for several ipsiversive gaze saccades. The middle traces show spike rasters from individual saccades. The traces superimposed on firing-rate histograms are the responses expected on the basis of the cell's sensitivity to passive WBR and passive neck rotation. The diagram at the bottom of the figure summarizes oculomotor efference copy, head movement efference copy, and neck sensory reafferent inputs to different classes of VOR interneurons in the vestibular nuclei. The thickness of the lines indicates strength of inputs.

In squirrel monkeys, the head movements associated with saccadic gaze shifts typically begin at the same time as, or slightly before the initiation of saccadic eye movements and last 100 ms or more after the gaze shift is completed. Consequently, head-movement-related signals generated by these VOR-related neurons could be divided into two components: firing behavior during the combined active eye-head gaze shift, and firing behavior during the VOR eye movements that occurred immediately after the gaze shift was completed. Different types of eye-movement-related neurons generated different responses during gaze saccades and gaze-saccade-related VOR eye movements. PVP, EHV, and PVII neurons were insensitive to active head movements during active gaze shifts. PVP neurons stopped firing altogether.

EHV neurons either generated bursts of spikes related to ocular saccades or were insensitive to the active gaze shift like the cell illustrated in FIGURE 6, but they were not sensitive to active head movements until just before the end of the gaze shift when the VOR began to stabilize gaze. PVII neurons were similar to the cell illustrated in FIGURE 5, and were insensitive to active head movements related to gaze saccades. PVI neurons were exceptional, in that they were sensitive to active head movements during saccadic gaze shifts and to head movements related to VOR eye movements immediately after gaze shifts.

Contribution of Neck Proprioceptive and Efference Copy Signals to Differential Sensitivity of Vestibular Nucleus Neurons to Active Head Movements

The complex signal processing that occurs in different constituents of central VOR pathways during gaze saccades is summarized in the diagram at the bottom of FIGURE 6, which summarizes the results of several recent studies.[10,12,14] A variety of signals contributes to shaping the responses of different classes of secondary VOR neurons. Saccade-related oculomotor efference copy signals modify signal processing in PVP and, to a lesser extent, EHV neurons during active head movements. Head movement efference copy signals modify signal processing in

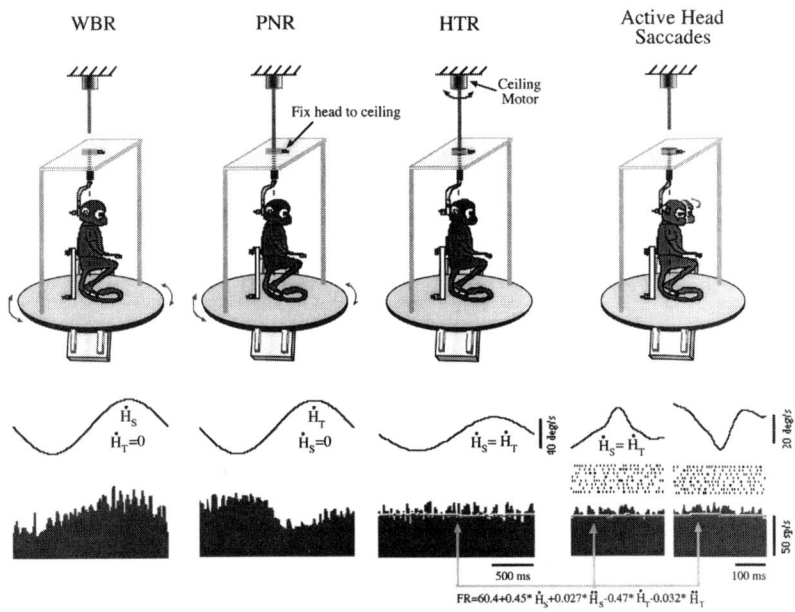

FIGURE 7. Neck sensory reafferent inputs cancel vestibular signals on a non-eye-movement-related vestibular nucleus neuron. The neuron's responses during passive WBR and passive neck rotation (PNR) were roughly equivalent and canceled each other during passive and active head-on-trunk rotation (HTR). Traces superimposed on firing-rate histograms are the responses expected on the basis of the cell's sensitivity to passive WBR and PNR.

PVII, PVP, and EHV neurons. Finally, neck proprioceptive reafferent signals modestly affect signal processing in PVI and EHV neurons.

Neck proprioceptive inputs dramatically affect signal processing in some non-eye-movement-related vestibular neurons, and effectively cause them to generate signals that are better related to movement of the trunk in space than to movement of the head in space, regardless of whether head-on-trunk movements are active or passive. The firing behavior of one such neuron is illustrated in FIGURE 7. During passive WBR, this cell's firing rate was primarily related to ipsilateral angular head velocity. Its response did not change during off-axis rotation, which suggests that it received little input from otolith vestibular receptors. On the other hand, it received a strong input from neck proprioceptors. During passive neck rotation (PNR experiment), the cell's firing rate was related to contralateral angular head-on-trunk velocity. When the head was passively rotated on the trunk with the ceiling motor (HTR condition), the neck and vestibular inputs to the neuron canceled each other. Head velocity in space was equal to head-on-trunk velocity, and the neuron's firing rate was essentially unmodulated. A similar lack of modulation was observed during active, self-generated head movements in both the ipsilateral and contralateral directions. The traces superimposed on the firing-rate histograms are the responses predicted from its responses during passive WBR and passive neck rotation (equation at the bottom of the figure).

Many vestibular neurons that were insensitive to active head movements were also insensitive to passive neck rotation and remained sensitive to passive head-on-trunk rotation. The insensitivity of these cells to active head movements was thus probably due to the addition of a head movement efference copy signal. An example of such a neuron is shown in FIGURE 8. This particular cell received direct inputs

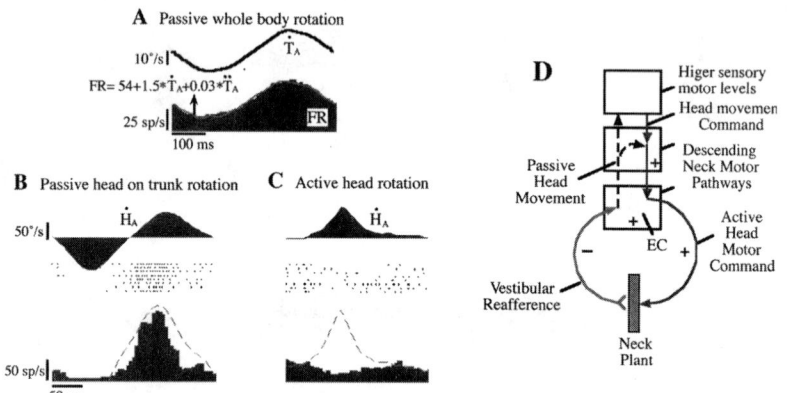

FIGURE 8. Head movement efference copy signals canceling vestibular signals on a vestibulo-spinal tract neuron. (**A**) Response to sinusoidal passive WBR at 2.3 Hz. (**B**) Response during HTR oscillations that were similar in peak velocity and acceleration to active head rotations in **C**. Traces superimposed on firing rate histograms are the responses expected on the basis of the cell's sensitivity to passive WBR. (**D**) Schematic adapted from von Holst and Mittelstaedt.[15] See text for further discussion.

from the vestibular nerve and was antidromically activated following electrical stimulation of the spinal cord. Its firing rate was strongly modulated in phase with head velocity during passive WBR (FIG. 8A) and during passive head-on-trunk rotation (FIG. 8B). The cell was not excited during comparable active head movements, which suggests that a central efference copy of head-on-trunk movements was responsible for cancellation of vestibular signals on this neuron rather than neck proprioceptive inputs. The diagram in FIGURE 8D is modified from the classic paper by von Holst and Mittelstaedt[15] on the reafference principle. Their thesis was that efference copy signals often cancel sensory reafferent signals produced by active motor commands. They argued that this cancellation probably occurred at segmental levels of central processing rather than higher centers. The scheme allowed segmental reflex motor programs to be executed without taking into account sensory reafferent consequences of ongoing intended movements. In the case of the vestibulo-collic-reflex-related neuron illustrated in this figure, the sensory reafferent signal produced by active head movement commands is a vestibular signal. Neurons of this type may project directly to neck motor neurons and produce head-on-trunk stabilizing reflex head movements when the head is passively perturbed or loaded. This reflex would work against the motor programs that produce active head movements were it not canceled. The evidence from our studies suggests that the addition of a head movement efference copy signal to vestibular signals in the vestibular nuclei may perform this function.

DISCUSSION

The vestibular nerve sends sensory signals to the brain that code the position and movement of the head in gravitoinertial space. The sensory information is used not only to construct an internal estimate of self-motion, but also to provide a reference frame for calculating the relative coordinates of motor control systems. The vestibular nuclei constitute the first place in the central nervous system that these sensory signals can be modified. What we have learned over the last 30 years is that sensory vestibular signals are profoundly modified and transformed in the vestibular nuclei. The dynamic characteristics of vestibular signals are modified. The spatial tuning of vestibular signals is transformed by convergence of information from different vestibular end organs from both labyrinths. Visual and proprioceptive estimates of self-motion are added to vestibular estimates. Finally, motor signals related to eye, head, and limb movements profoundly modify the responses of vestibular neurons. The modifications produced by these various influences produce a remarkable variety in the signals produced by individual vestibular nucleus neurons.

We have only begun to understand how and where these different signals are constructed and distributed to other sensory-motor integrative centers in the spinal cord, brainstem, cerebellum, and cerebral cortex. The approach to understanding how the vestibular system in general and the vestibular nuclei in particular contribute to the maintenance of visual stability, postural control, and sensory estimates of self-motion will have to include the use of appropriate behavioral techniques in combination with neurophysiological studies of anatomically identified central pathways in animals demonstrating alert behavior.

ACKNOWLEDGMENTS

This work was supported by the National Institutes of Health (grants DC05056 and EY08041). We would like to acknowledge the contributions of Greg Gdowski, Timothy Belton, and Stephanie Moore, who were involved in producing much of the experimental data presented in this article.

REFERENCES

1. ZACHARIAS, G.L. & L.R. YOUNG. 1981. Influence of combined visual and vestibular cues on human perception and control of horizontal rotation. Exp. Brain Res. **41:** 159–171.
2. MERGNER, T. & W. BECKER. 1990. Perception of horizontal self-rotation: multisensory and cognitive aspects. *In* Perception and Control of Self-Motion. R. Warren & A.H. Wertheim, Eds.: 219–263. Lawrence Erbaum. Hillsdale, NJ.
3. MERGNER, T. 2002. The matryoshka dolls principle in human dynamic behavior in space: a theory of linked references for multisensory perception and control of action. Curr. Psychol. Cogn. **21:** 129–212.
4. MERGNER, T., C. MAURER & R.J. PETERKA. 2003. A multisensory posture control model of human upright stance. Prog. Brain Res. **142:** 189–201.
5. GOLDBERG, J.M., A.M BRICHTA & P.A. WACKYM. 2000. Efferent vestibular system: anatomy, physiology, and neurochemistry. *In* Neurochemistry of the Vestibular System. A.J. Beitz & J.H. Anderson, Eds.: Chapt. 4: 61–84. CRC Press. Boca Raton, FL.
6. PURCELL, I.M. & A.A. PERACHIO. 1997. Three-dimensional analysis of vestibular efferent neurons innervating semicircular canals of the gerbil. J. Neurophysiol. **78:** 3234–3248.
7. BÜTTNER-ENNEVER, J.A. 1988. Anatomy of the oculomotor system. *In* Reviews of Oculomotor Research. J.A. Büttner-Ennever, Ed.: 119–176. Elsevier. Amsterdam.
8. WILSON, V.J. 1991. Vestibulospinal and neck reflexes: interaction in the vestibular nuclei. Arch. Ital. Biol. **129:** 43–52.
9. MCCREA, R.A., G.T. GDOWSKI, R. BOYLE & T. BELTON. 1999. Firing behavior of vestibular neurons during active and passive head movements: vestibulo-spinal and other non-eye-movement related neurons. J. Neurophysiol. **82:** 416–428.
10. MCCREA, R.A. & G.T. GDOWSKI. 2003. Firing behaviour of squirrel monkey eye movement-related vestibular nucleus neurons during gaze saccades. J. Physiol. **546:** 207–224.
11. GDOWSKI, G.T. & R.A. MCCREA. 1999. Integration of vestibular and head movement signals in the vestibular nuclei during whole-body rotation. J. Neurophysiol. **82:** 436–449.
12. GDOWSKI, G.T. & R.A. MCCREA. 2000. Neck proprioceptive inputs to primate vestibular nucleus neurons. Exp Brain Res. **135:** 511–526.
13. HIGHSTEIN, S.M. & R.A. MCCREA. 1988. The anatomy of the vestibular nuclei. *In* Reviews of Oculomotor Research. J.A. Büttner-Ennever, Ed.: 177–202. Elsevier. Amsterdam.
14. GDOWSKI, G.T., T. BELTON & R.A. MCCREA. 2001. The neurophysiological substrate for the cervico-ocular reflex in the squirrel monkey. Exp Brain Res. **140:** 253–264.
15. VON HOLST, E. & H. MITTELSTAEDT. 1950. Das Reafferenzprincip (Wechselwirkungen zwischen Zentralnedrvensystem und Peripherie). Naturwissenschaften. **37:** 464–476.

Morphological Properties of Vestibulospinal Neurons in Primates

RICHARD BOYLE AND CURT JOHANSON

Life Sciences Division, Ames Research Center, National Aeronautics and Space Administration, Moffett Field, California 94035, USA

ABSTRACT: The lateral and medial vestibulospinal tracts constitute the major descending pathways controlling extensor musculature of the body. We examined the axon morphology and synaptic input patterns and targets in the cervical spinal segments from these tract cells using intracellular recording and biocytin labeling in the squirrel monkey. Lumbosacral projecting cells represent a private, and mostly rapid, communication pathway between the dorsal Deiters' nucleus and the motor circuits controlling the lower limbs and tail. The cervical projecting cells provide both redundant and variable synaptic input to spinal cell groups, suggesting both general and specific control of the head and neck reflexes.

KEYWORDS: axon; eighth nerve; ventral horn; posture; synaptic boutons; intracellular labeling

INTRODUCTION

The lateral vestibulospinal tract (LVST) and medial vestibulospinal tract (MVST) communicate directly between the inner ear vestibular hair cell structures and postural musculature.[1] Specifically, the dorsal Deiters' nucleus comprises one part of the LVST and is the principal conduit through which gravito-inertial accelerations regulate the lower body's extensor musculature. The other LVST neurons are located more ventrally in the lateral nucleus, and their axons project ipsilaterally and give off collaterals to cervical levels of the spinal cord.[2] The MVST descends bilaterally through the medial longitudinal fasciculus (MLF) as far as the upper thoracic enlargements. These parallel vestibular pathways serve to regulate vestibular reflexes, such as the neck-related vestibulocollic reflex (VCR) and the limb- and ankle-related vestibulospinal reflexes.

Angular, inertial, and gravitational accelerations sensed in the semicircular canals and otolith organs are the principal inputs into the LVST and MVST.[3-6] These signals modulate the firing rate of individual spinal tract neurons in the vestibular nuclei, particularly the lateral and medial nuclei.[7] A second afferent input arises from the vestibulocerebellum and deep cerebellar nuclei, such as the fastigial

Address for correspondence: Richard Boyle, Life Sciences Division, Ames Research Center, National Aeronautics and Space Administration, Moffett Field, CA 94035. Voice: 650-604-1099; fax: 650-604-3954.

richard.boyle@nasa.gov

nucleus,[8] and may play an important modulatory role on both cervical and lumbosacral vestibulospinal reflexes or directly onto cervical neurons, as suggested by Büttner and colleagues.[9] A third input to the spinal tracts involves an efferent return pathway from muscle stretch receptors that are activated by the stabilizing movements.[10] These proprioceptive signals generated during axial and limb movements traverse spinovestibular pathways to vestibular nuclei,[11] and can modulate the firing rate of identified LVST and MVST neurons.[12,13] Like other vestibular nuclei neurons,[14,15] the vestibulospinal neurons are likely modulated during optokinetic nystagmus.[16]

In an earlier study, we mapped the location of intracellularly recorded neurons in the vestibular nuclei activated at a monosynaptic latency following electrical shocks applied to the vestibular nerve.[17] The major finding to emerge is that with the exception of lumbar LVST (L-LVST), the remaining vestibulospinal neurons and vestibuloocular reflex (VOR) cells projecting rostrally to the oculomotor nucleus (IIIrd) are intermingled, often recorded side by side in the same region of the vestibular nuclei.

This report focuses on the anatomical organization of the spinal component of LVST and MVST neurons of the squirrel monkey. We used intracellular recording, biocytin labeling, and orthodromic and antidromic stimulation protocols to map and compare descending pathways in the LVST and MVST.

METHODS

Adult male squirrel monkeys, *Saimiri sciureus*, provided the morphological data in the present study. Surgical and experimental procedures, which can be found in greater detail in Boyle,[18] were conducted in compliance with the National Institutes of Health Guide for the Care and Use of Laboratory Animals. The animal was anesthetized throughout all phases of the experiment with a continuous intravenous infusion of barbiturate anesthetic, and the systemic arterial pressure, rectal temperature, and end-tidal P_{CO2} were closely monitored. Teflon-coated Ag/AgCl silver electrodes were implanted bilaterally in the middle ear to electrically excite both the inferior and superior branches of the eighth nerve for orthodromic identification of secondary neurons. A pair of insulated tungsten wires, separated from one another by ~3 mm, were placed about the midline in the rostral MLF between the IIIrd and IVth cranial nuclei to identify possible ascending projection from bifurcating vestibuloooculocollic (VOC) neurons. The monkeys underwent dorsal laminectomies to expose the spinal segments of C_1 to C_6 for recordings from single neurons and at T_{12} for placement of 200-µm Ag/AgCl silver wires to identify lumbar projecting LVST cells.

FIGURE 1 shows a schematic representation of the recording and stimulation techniques. Intracellular recordings were made from axons with glass micropipettes filled with 3% biocytin (Sigma) in a buffered salt solution. Positive current pulses (5–20 nA, 1/s, 70% duty cycle) passed through the microelectrode were used to inject biocytin into the cell. Antidromic activation was confirmed by a constant latency of the antidromic spike for near-threshold shocks and by collision of the antidromic spike with an orthodromic action potential evoked by vestibular nerve stimulation or by applying depolarizing currents. We selected all vestibulospinal neurons based on the cell's latent period of orthodromic response to electrical stimulation of the eighth

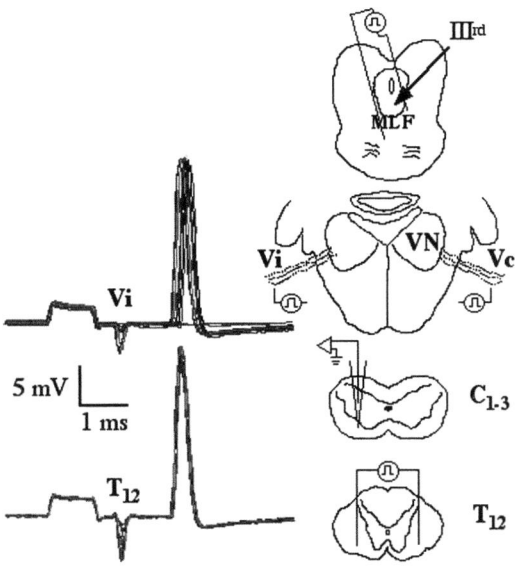

FIGURE 1. Methods to identify vestibulospinal neurons in the squirrel monkey. *Right:* Placement of stimulating electrodes in the rostral MLF, on the ipsilateral vestibular (Vi) and contralateral vestibular (Vc) nerves, and ventrolateral funiculi of both sides at T_{12}. Intraaxonal recordings and biocytin labeling were made at C_1 to C_3. *Left:* Individual responses of a secondary, L-LVST: short-latency evoked action potentials from single shocks applied to Vi (*top trace*) and antidromic responses from single shocks applied at T_{12}.

nerve at < 1.6–2.0 ms from C_1 to C_3, respectively, indicating a monosynaptic connection to the vestibular nerve afferents. L-LVST neurons were antidromically activated from the T_{12} stimulation site, and VOC neurons were antidromically activated from the rostral MLF electrode site. MVST cells were sought in the ventromedial funiculus, and we relied on the cell's orthodromic response to stimulation of the eighth nerve. We later determined the laterality of the vestibular nerves with respect to the recorded axon as ipsilateral (Vi) or contralateral (Vc) by the identification of the labeled axon from stained sections.

To prevent finding false results, we made no attempt to first extracellularly record spontaneous or induced discharges before penetrating the axon. Some vestibular neurons recorded at C_1, such as the VOC neuron, receive both Vi and Vc inputs, and are antidromically activated from the rostral MLF and can also be driven from electrodes placed in some experiments at C_6. On the basis of the cell's responses to applied stimuli from multiple sites, we repeatedly observed that fibers extracellularly recorded first were not the same as that immediately penetrated, even though several responses could have comparable latencies. To avoid confusion, we identified and labeled only those fibers recorded directly inside the nerve.

After a brief survival period under anesthesia, the animal was transcardially perfused with saline and formaldehyde solutions, and the brain and spinal cord were removed for histological processing. We derived our principal histological data from our work with three blocks of processed tissue: precollicular midbrain to obex, obex to T_1, and T_2 to T_6. Labeled processes were visualized from 60-μm serial sections collected in the sagittal (brain) and horizontal (spinal cord) planes using a modified Vectastain/diaminobenzidine method (Elite ABC kit, Vector Laboratories). We examined and reconstructed the individually labeled axons using a drawing tube (camera lucida) at a magnification of ×16 to ×40. After reconstruction, we captured the images on 35-mm film, imported them through a Nikon slide scanner, and loaded them into Adobe Photoshop for examination.

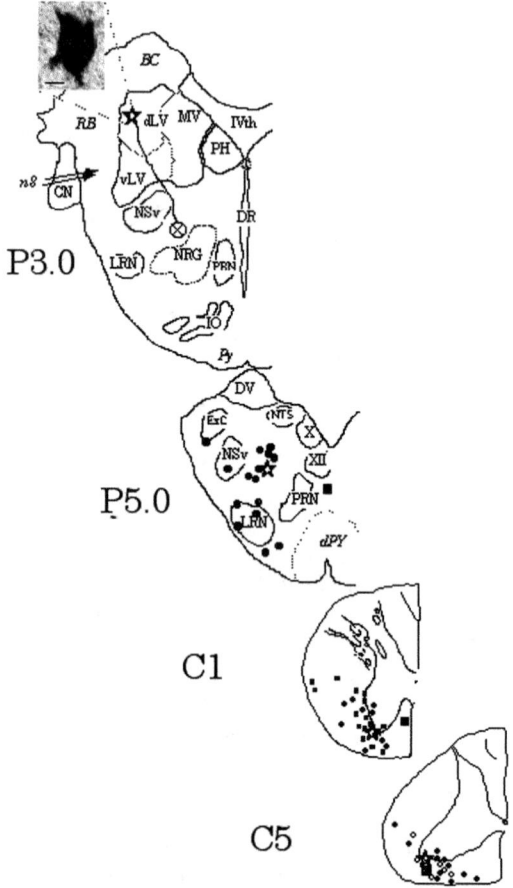

FIGURE 2. Axon location of 37 L-LVST neurons. Four drawings (rostral to caudal) show the recovered location of the individual axons in the brainstem at P3.0 and P5.0 (*upper two*) and in the cervical spinal cord at C_1 and C_5 (*lower two*). Insert shows a photomicrograph of the soma of a labeled L-LVST neuron in dorsal Deiters' nucleus (calibration bar: 20 μm); this neuron is represented by a *star* in the drawings. A *filled circle* symbolizes 35 L-LVST neurons. The last L-LVST neuron is marked by the *filled square*: the axon of this L-LVST neuron traveled in the descending MLF through the caudal brainstem and beyond the first cervical segment, but left the ventromedial funiculus between C_1 and C_2 to assume a projection course more typical of the other L-LVST neurons.

RESULTS

Using biocytin as a neural marking agent, we examined individual cervical and lumbar LVST, MVST, and VOC fibers to describe their morphological features in the caudal brainstem, where possible, and their connections to cervical spinal segments. The intraspinal conduction velocities of the L-LVST axons ranged from 55 to 95 m/s (76 ± 10 m/s, mean $\pm$ SD; $n = 37$).

L-LVST Axon Location and Extent in Brainstem and Spinal Cord

FIGURE 2 shows four transverse drawings (at P3 and P5 and at C_1 and C_5) and illustrates the axon location and its path through the brainstem and into the cervical spinal segments of L-LVST cells. The L-LVST axon maintains pathway laterality along its trajectory. We located the soma in dorsal Deiters' nucleus of one labeled neuron (insert). The cell's axon (star) followed a ventrocaudal course medial to the nucleus of the spinal tract of V (NSv), ventral to the cuneate nucleus, and entered the spinal cord in the ventrolateral funiculus. The axon maintained course near the ventral horn until it faded at C_6. The other L-LVST axons took either a similar course or traversed varied trajectories. For example, we found axons by the external cuneate nucleus and inferior olive, running through the NSv and the lateral reticular nucleus, and even one in the MLF (filled square). This axon followed an unpredictable weaving path (marked as L_4 in FIG. 4). It entered the upper cervical segment in the MLF; but then the L_4 axon snaked ventrolaterally, passing through lamina VIII of the ventral horn and finally back into the ventrolateral funiculus when the biocytin faded at C_6. At C_1, most L-LVST axons ran in the lateral funiculus near the ventral horn; by C_5, they assumed a position more in the ventral funiculus.

We measured the extent of recovered axons in the caudal brainstem to the obex, and in the cervical spinal segments C_1 to C_8. Although no axon was fully recovered over its length from soma to termination in the lumbosacral segments (a distance exceeding 150 mm), the extent of biocytin labeling adequately revealed axon morphology in the cervical segments. The average distance of recovered axons was 17.3 mm ($\pm$ 8.6 mm, SD; range: 4.5–31.7 mm).

L-LVST Innervation of the Cervical Ventral Horn

One L-LVST neuron provided innervation of the ventral horn of the cervical spinal cord. FIGURE 3 details this sole collateral input to the cervical cord. The axon entered the spinal cord in the lateral funiculus about 700 µm from the lateral border (see arrow, FIG. 3A) and issued the solitary collateral input (FIG. 3B). The collateral input projected medially and produced 42 *en passant* and terminal boutons in the ventral horn of rostral C_1 (FIG. 3C). FIGURE 3D shows the horizontal plane reconstruction of the process, and its representation in the transverse plane is shown in FIGURE 3E. The collateral input bifurcated before entering the ventral horn, with one branch innervating spinal accessory motoneuron regions within lamina VIII and the other branch extending to terminate in the region of the splenius motoneuron pool of the dorsomedial nucleus, and in lamina VII.

188   ANNALS NEW YORK ACADEMY OF SCIENCES

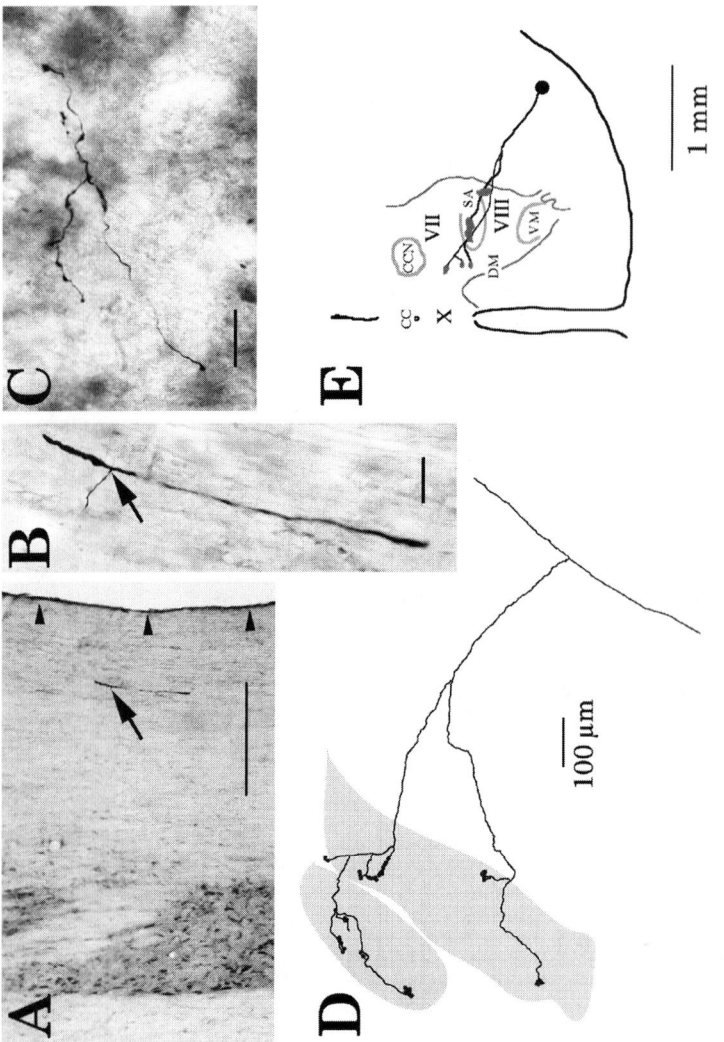

FIGURE 3. *See following page for legend.*

Comparison with Cervical-Projecting LVST Neurons

Analysis of collateral branching and specificity in terminal endings in L-LVST neurons in comparison to cervical projecting LVST (C-LVST) neurons illustrated the complete separation of these cell groups in the control of reflex movement of the head and neck. FIGURE 4 demonstrates the rudimentary nature of secondary L-LVST neurons in comparison to their C-LVST counterparts. Cells labeled L1, L2, and L3 are L-LVST neurons recorded during the same experiment as the reconstructed C-LVST neuron (label C, FIG. 4). Axon L4 shows the unique ambling trajectory of many L-LVST neurons in comparison to C-LVST fibers. The four L-LVST neurons entered the spinal cord in the ventrolateral to ventral funiculi below the ventral horn by 100–150 μm. They then merged back on course in the ventral funiculus near the base of the spinal cord. The C-LVST neuron issued its first collateral at C_1. Twelve collaterals (filled arrows) branched from the parent axon as it coursed in the ventral funiculus to its terminus at mid-C_4 (open arrow). We found a mean intercollateral spacing of 1.29 ± 0.46 mm with an average of 131 ± 136 boutons per collateral. The axon's primary target was the cell groups of C_2 to C_3, where we found 1,530 of the 1,705 (90%) specialized terminations, *en passant,* and terminal boutons. The lower panel of the figure is a schematic of the spinal cord at C_2; the axon position of the four L-LVST neurons is indicated with circles, and the terminal field of the C-LVST neuron is shaded. Innervation of the C-LVST neuron was densest in the spinal motor pools, ventromedial IX, and lamina VIII, illustrating the sophistication and broad targeting of these LVST fibers compared to the L-LVST family.

Comparison with Cervical-Projecting MVST and VOC Neurons

The structure of MVST and VOC cells indicated preferential targeting of specific cell groups in the spinal cervical region. FIGURE 5 shows horizontal reconstructions of an ipsilateral and contralateral MVST and a VOC neuron innervating cervical segments. The three cells received biocytin injections in the same experiment. The VOC neuron issued 10 collaterals between C_1 and C_4 before the labeling diminished. The pattern of innervation was similar to other MVST cells, except the VOC axon projected more dorsally within lamina VII, targeting the central cervical nucleus. The ipsilateral MVST cell bypassed the upper cervical segments of C_1 and C_2 and issued its first collateral at C_3. The branch provided five separate terminal areas within C_3 to C_4, skipping a segment before fading at C_5. The contralateral MVST cell bypassed the entire upper cervical segments from C_1 to C_5 and began collateral formation at

---

FIGURE 3. Innervation of the cervical ventral horn of a L-LVST neuron. (**A–C**) Photomicrographs in horizontal plane. (**A**) Axon location in the lateral funiculus (lateral wall of spinal cord is marked by arrowheads) and the single collateral (indicated by the *arrow*) (calibration bar: 500 μm). (**B**) Enlarged view of the branch point (*arrow*) (calibration bar: 50 μm). (**C**) View of *en passant* and terminal boutons in the ventral horn (calibration bar: 20 μm). The collateral input's innervation of the ventral horn is shown in the reconstructions of **D** (horizontal view) and **E** (transverse view). The primary target of this collateral input was the region of the sternocleidomastoid and trapezius motoneurons. *Abbreviations*: CC, central canal; CCN, central cervical nucleus; DM, dorsomedial motor nucleus; VM, ventromedial motor nucleus; SA, spinal accessory nucleus of eleventh nerve; VII, VIII, X, Rexed laminae.

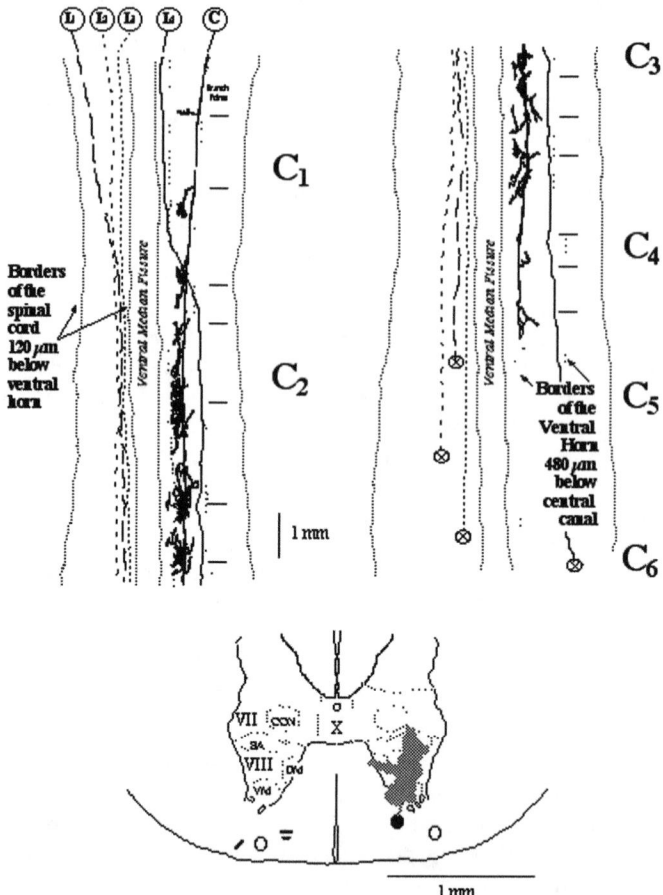

FIGURE 4. Comparison of L-LVST neurons with a LVST neuron terminating in the cervical cord. The axon course of four L-LVST neurons (labeled L1 through L4) is given together with the reconstruction of the collateral innervation pattern of a LVST neuron terminating below C_4 (terminus is marked by the *open arrow*; *solid arrows* give the individual branch points in the upper two sections). *Upper panel:* Two sections of the cervical cord from the obex to C_6 in the horizontal plane. The ventral median fissure separates the cord into left and right sides, which are represented at different depths relative to the dorsal surface of the cord: on the left side of each section the borders (*dashed lines*) mark the medial and lateral walls of the white matter 120 μm below the ventral horn; and on the right side of each section the medial and lateral walls of the spinal cord (*dashed lines*) and ventral horn (*shaded lines*) are given at 480 μm below the central canal. The caudal extent of the recovered L-LVST axon is symbolized by an X within a circle. Note the trajectory of L-LVST axon labeled L4 as it courses out of the MLF and into the ventrolateral funiculus. *Lower panel:* A drawing of the spinal cord at C_2 in the transverse plane. The location of the four L-LVST axons is given by separate symbols and the terminal field of the cervical-only LVST neuron is represented by the shaded area. Note this cell's dense input to the ventral horn below lamina VII: ventromedial motoneurons of lamina IX, motoneurons of spinal accessory nucleus, dorsomedial motor region (including splenius motoneurons), and lamina VIII.

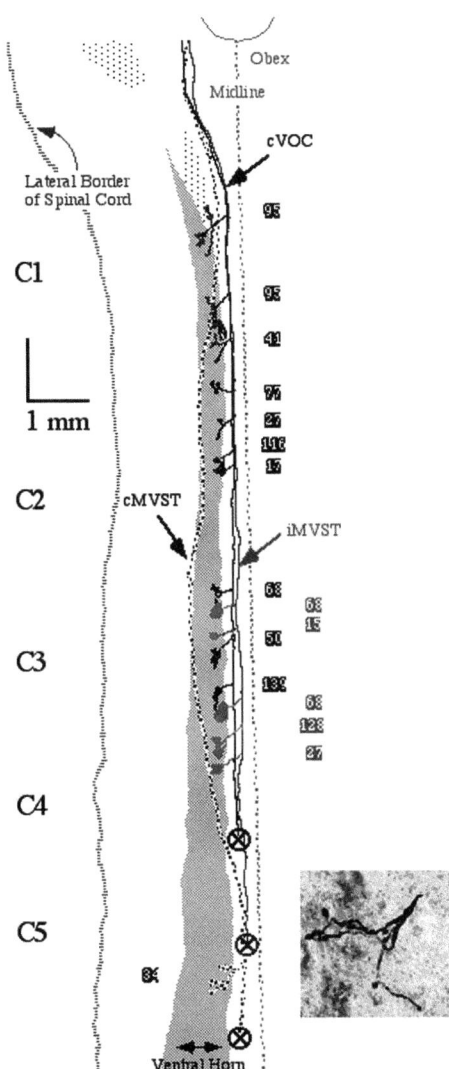

FIGURE 5. Reconstructions in the horizontal plane of an ipsilateral and contralateral MVST and a VOC neuron, and their innervation of the cervical segments; the three cells were individually labeled in the same experiment. The VOC neuron issued 10 collaterals between C_1 and C_4, at which point the label faded. The pattern of innervation was similar to that of the MVST cell shown in FIGURE 4, except the VOC cell projected more dorsally within lamina VII to target the central cervical nucleus. The ipsilateral MVST cell bypassed the upper cervical segments of C_1 and C_2, and issued its first collateral at C_3, provided five separate terminal areas within C_3 to C_4, skipped the next segment, and the label faded at C_5. The contralateral MVST cell bypassed the entire upper cervical segments from C_1 to C_5, and issued its first collateral at mid-C_5. The three axons preferentially targeted the medial wall of lamina VIII. Unlike MVST neurons that target the entire cervical spinal cord (example shown in FIG. 4), neurons like those of FIGURE 5 preferentially innervate more selected regions, such as C_1 to C_2 and C_3 to C_4, or bypass the upper segments entirely.

mid-C_5. Unlike MVST neurons that projected onto the entire cervical spinal cord, the three axons specifically targeted the medial wall of lamina VIII. MVST and VOC neurons preferentially innervated selected regions such as C_1 to C_2 or C_3 to C_4, frequently bypassing the upper segments entirely.

FIGURE 6 gives a schematic of the generalized secondary vestibulospinal morphology in the primate. FIGURE 6A shows the soma location of three idealized vestibulospinal neurons, an L-LVST (star), a C-LVST (filled circle), and an MVST (open circle) neuron. The L-LVST neuron is located in dorsal Deiters', and the cell bodies of C-LVST and MVST neurons are intermingled in the ventromedial portions of the vestibular nuclei at the entry zone of the eighth nerve. The averaged course

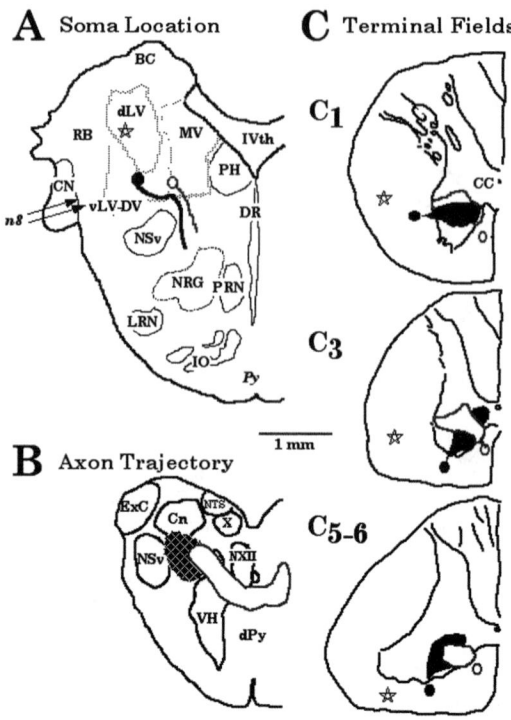

FIGURE 6. Schematic of secondary vestibulospinal morphology in squirrel monkey. (**A**) Soma location. Three idealized neurons are shown, a cervical projecting LVST neuron (*filled circle*), an MVST neuron (*open circle*), and an L-LVST neuron (*star*). The cell bodies of cervical projecting neurons are intermingled in the ventromedial portions of the vestibular nuclei at the entry zone of the eighth nerve. (**B**) Axon trajectory. The averaged course through the caudal brainstem of axons of the cervical projecting neurons depicted in **A** is shown (see FIG. 2 for L-LVST cells). MVST fibers project both ipsilaterally and contralaterally to the spinal cord. (**C**) Terminal fields. The averaged terminal field of each neuron is shown at three segments in the cervical cord.

through the caudal brainstem of axons of the C-LVST and MVST neurons depicted in FIGURE 6A is shown in panel B; see FIGURE 2 for L-LVST cells.

The C-LVST axon projects caudally through the brainstem, often coursing in fascicles below the cuneate nucleus (FIG. 6B, filled area), and enters the spinal cord from the lateral to the ventral funiculi. Most C-LVST axons enter the ventral-ventrolateral funiculus by the cervical enlargement. MVST axons follow a more varied trajectory through the caudal brainstem to reach the ventromedial funiculus of the cervical cord, with considerable variation in the location at which the contralaterally projecting MVST neuron crosses the midline before the first cervical dorsal root (FIG. 6B, open area). FIGURE 6C shows an idealized representation of the averaged terminal field of MVST neurons (open fields) and C-LVST neurons (filled fields) at three cervical segments. Both neurons target the spinal accessory nucleus and wide areas of laminae VIII and VIII. On the whole, MVST cells innervate the more dorsomedial motoneuronal cell groups, and the C-LVST cells supply the more ventromedial motoneuronal cell groups.

DISCUSSION

The present review explored the morphology of secondary lumbosacral projecting LVST (L-LVST) neurons in relation to their counterparts in the cervical LVST and MVST neurons. L-LVST neurons do not target cell groups in the caudal brainstem or in the ventral horn of the cervical spinal cord as do other vestibulospinal projections. L-LVST axons course to lower segments of the spinal cord with greater simplicity than their cervical-projecting counterparts. In addition, the L-LVST neuron appears to be the only central vestibular neuron that does not issue collaterals within the brainstem. Squirrel monkey vestibulocollic neurons project through the LVST to the ipsilateral cervical cord and through the MVST in the medial longitudinal fasciculus to bilaterally innervate the cervical cord.[2] Similar generalizations also appear to be a feature of the vestibular neurons studied in the cat.[19]

For the squirrel monkey, the caudal projection of the LVST is a simple and rapid communication pathway between the dorsal Deiters' nucleus and the lumbosacral cord. Bilateral innervation and specific targeting of small regions of the cervical cell groups by MVST and VOC projections are perhaps the closest in structure and specificity to the C-LVST fibers. Although the C-LVST axons were the most collateralized of any we studied, the MVST and VOC tended to slightly lower numbers of collaterals and targeted fewer cervical segments. The relationship between the three types of vestibulospinal neurons is not completely clear, but the morphological data indicates that variance in fiber conductance, branch points, and synaptic ending allow for redundancy and variation in function.

The morphological characteristics of L-LVST neurons at a higher latency with polysynaptic connections could be of interest; however, we excluded those cells because verifying soma location to unequivocally identify them as L-LVST neurons would be impossible using distance delay calculations. Therefore, we can only firmly conclude that the secondary L-LVST neurons do not target the ventral horn of the cervical spinal cord. Higher-order L-LVST neurons might distribute collateral inputs to the cervical cord; this might account for the high percentage of synaptic action in the cervical ventral horn from stimulating L-LVST axons as described by Abzug and colleagues.[20]

In conclusion, L-LVST neurons do not collateralize in the brainstem, and with the rare exception entirely bypass the cervical ventral horn as they project to their caudal target sites. Interestingly, one L-LVST axon was found to travel in the descending MLF in the brainstem and through the C_1 segment before coursing out of this track and into the ventrolateral fasciculus. The vestibular-related signals carried along the reflex pathways to the head, neck, and forelimbs thus can be segregated from those affecting the lower trunk and limbs. In the alert squirrel monkey, orthodromically and antidromically identified secondary LVST neurons recorded in dorsal Deiters' nucleus show tightly tuned responses dependent on head angle along the earth-horizontal plane; secondary LVST neurons recorded more ventrally show a more processed signal, reflecting semicircular canal, utricular, and eye-in-orbit signals.[5]

This redundant and often reverse processing of parallel information allows for greater refinement in postural control and coordinated motion, especially for multi-limbed animals. The somatotopic organization of Deiters' nucleus[1] provides the structural basis upon which to distribute the requisite control signals to the body. Comparative research illustrates the structural basis for physiology in that cats rely more on coordinated lower limb movement than squirrel monkeys or humans. Therefore, research observing species-specific reliance on varying distributions of vestibulospinal cell types can be correlated through species behavior, morphology, and physiologic function.

REFERENCES

1. BRODAL, A. 1984. The vestibular nuclei in the macaque monkey. J. Comp. Neurol. **227:** 252–266.
2. WILSON, V.J., R. BOYLE, K. FUKUSHIMA, P.K. ROSE, et al. 1995. The vestibulocollic reflex. J. Vestib. Res. **5:** 147–170.
3. BOYLE, R. 1993. Activity of medial vestibulospinal tract cells during rotation and ocular movement in the alert squirrel monkey. J. Neurophysiol. **70:** 2176–2180.
4. BOYLE, R., T. BELTON & R.A. MCCREA. 1996. Responses of identified vestibulospinal neurons to voluntary and reflex eye and head movements in the alert squirrel monkey. Ann. N.Y. Acad. Sci. **781:** 244–263.
5. BOYLE, R. 1997. Activity of lateral vestibulospinal neurons during applied linear and angular head acceleration in the alert squirrel monkey. Soc. Neurosci. Abstr. **23:** 753.
6. MCCREA, R.A., G. GDOWSKI, R. BOYLE & T. BELTON. 1999. Firing behavior of vestibular nucleus neurons during active and passive head movements. II. Vestibulo-spinal and other non-eye-movement related neurons. J. Neurophysiol. **82:** 416–428.
7. UCHINO, Y. 2001. Otolith and semicircular canal inputs to single vestibular neurons in cat. Jpn. Biol. Sci. Space **15:** 375–381.
8. WALBERG, F. 1975. The vestibular nuclei and their connections with the eighth nerve and the cerebellum. In The Vestibular System. R.F. Naunton, Ed.: 31–53. Academic Press. New York.
9. BÜTTNER, U., A.F. FUCHS, G. MARKERT-SCHWAB & P. BUCKMASTER. 1991. Fastigial nucleus activity in the alert monkey during slow eye and head movements. J. Neurophysiol. **65:** 1360–1371.
10. LINDSAY, K.W., T.D. ROBERTS & J.R. ROSENBERG. 1976. Asymmetric tonic labyrinth reflexes and their interaction with neck reflexes in the decerebrate cat. J. Physiol. **261:** 583–601.
11. POMPEIANO, O. & A. BRODAL. 1957. Spino-vestibular fibers in the cat: an experimental study. J. Comp. Neurol. **108:** 353–380.
12. BOYLE, R. & O. POMPEIANO. 1981. Relation between cell size and response characteristics of vestibulospinal neurons to labyrinth and neck inputs. J. Neurosci. **1:** 1052–1066.
13. KASPER, J., R.H. SCHOR & V.J. WILSON. 1988. Response of vestibular neurons to head rotations in vertical planes. I. Responses to neck stimulation and vestibular-neck interaction. J. Neurophysiol. **60:** 1765–1778.
14. WAESPE, W. & V. HENN. 1977. Neuronal activity in the vestibular nuclei of the alert monkey during vestibular and optokinetic stimulation. Exp. Brain Res. **27:** 523–538.
15. BUETTNER, U.W. & U. BÜTTNER. 1979. Vestibular nuclei activity in the alert monkey during suppression of vestibular and optokinetic nystagmus. Exp. Brain Res. **37:** 581–593.
16. BOYLE, R., U. BÜTTNER & G. MARKERT. 1985. Vestibular nuclei activity and eye movements in the alert monkey during sinusoidal optokinetic stimulation. Exp. Brain Res. **57:** 362–369.
17. BOYLE, R., J.M. GOLDBERG & S.M. HIGHSTEIN. 1992. Inputs from regularly and irregularly discharging vestibular nerve afferents to secondary neurons in the vestibular

nuclei of the squirrel monkey. III. Correlation with vestibulospinal and vestibuloocular output pathways. J. Neurophysiol. **68:** 471–484.
18. BOYLE, R. 2000. Morphology of lumbar-projecting lateral vestibulospinal neurons in the brainstem and cervical spinal cord in the squirrel monkey. Arch. Ital. Biol. **138:** 107–122.
19. MCCREA, R.A., K. YOSHIDA, C. EVINGER & A. BERTHOZ. 1981. The location, axonal arborization, and termination sites of eye-movement related secondary vestibular neurons demonstrated by intra-axonal HRP injection in the alert cat. *In* Progress in Oculomotor Research. A. Fuchs & W. Becker, Eds.: 379–386. Elsevier/North Holland. New York.
20. ABZUG, C., M. MAEDA, B.W. PETERSON & V.J. WILSON. 1974. Cervical branching of lumbar vestibulospinal axons. J. Physiol.(Lond.) **243:** 499–522.

Role of the Dorsolateral Pontine Nucleus in Visual-Vestibular Behavior

MICHAEL J. MUSTARI,[a,b] SEIJI ONO,[a] VALLABH E. DAS,[a,b] AND RONALD J. TUSA[a,b]

[a]*Division of Visual Science, Yerkes National Primate Research Center and*
[b]*Department of Neurology, Emory University, Atlanta, Georgia 30022, USA*

ABSTRACT: Visual-vestibular behavior depends on signals traveling in climbing and mossy fiber pathways. Our study examined the role of the dorsolateral pontine nucleus (DLPN), a major component of the cortico-ponto-cerebellar mossy fiber pathway. DLPN neurons discharge in relation to smooth pursuit and during visual stimulation, indicating a potential role in visually guided motor learning in the vestibulo-ocular reflex (VOR). We used unilateral muscimol injections to determine the potential role of the DLPN in short-term VOR gain adaptation. Preinjection adaptation of VOR gain was achieved by sinusoidal rotation (0.2 Hz, 30°/s) for 2 h while the monkey viewed a stationary visual surround through either magnifying (×2) or minifying (×0.5) lenses. VOR gain increases (23–32%) or decreases (22–48%) as measured in complete darkness (VORd) were achieved. Following DLPN inactivation, initial acceleration of ipsilateral smooth-pursuit was reduced by 35–68%, and steady state gain was reduced by 32–61%. Furthermore, the monkey's ability to cancel the VOR was impaired. In contrast to these significant deficits in ipsilesional smooth pursuit, the VOR during lens viewing was similar to that measured in preinjection control experiments. Similarly, following 2 h of adaptation, VORd gain adaptation was indistinguishable from control adaptation values for either ipsilesional or contralesional directions of head rotation. Our results suggest that visual error signals for short-term adaptation of the VOR are derived from sources other than the DLPN, such as those from the accessory optic system.

KEYWORDS: vestibular ocular; smooth pursuit; eye movement; pontine

INTRODUCTION

During locomotion, the vestibulo-ocular reflex (VOR) generates eye movements that compensate for head movements to preserve high-acuity vision.[1] If VOR gain is less then unity, residual visual slip signals can activate optokinetic mechanisms, including those involving the accessory optic system, to produce further compensation.[2] VOR gain and phase in light (VORl) and dark (VORd) have been characterized for a wide range of head perturbation frequencies in humans and nonhuman pri-

Address for correspondence: Michael J. Mustari, Ph.D., Division of Visual Science, Yerkes National Primate Research Center and Department of Neurology, Emory University, 954 Gatewood Road N.E., Atlanta, GA 30022. Voice: 404-727-9194; fax: 404-727-7729.
  mjmustar@rmy.emory.edu

mates.[1] VOR gain is typically higher when viewing a stationary target in the light than when imagining a target in complete darkness, indicating interaction between the VOR and visually mediated eye movements. This interaction is essential for normal visual-vestibular behavior, including adjusting the gain of the VOR when residual retinal slip signals remain during head rotations.[3–5] The source of visual signals necessary for modifying the gain of the VOR has long been a subject of interest.[6] Numerous studies have identified the accessory optic system and pretectal nucleus of the optic tract as crucial visual afferent sources driving the inferior olivary neurons, the source of complex spikes.[2,7] Recent studies have indicated that complex spike activity of horizontal gaze-velocity Purkinje (HGVP) cells in the flocculus/ventral paraflocculus was appropriately modulated to support visual modification of the VOR at high frequency (>5 Hz).[8] In contrast, simple spike activity of HGVP cells was not found to modulate appropriately during high-frequency stimulation to support VOR gain adaptation. At low frequencies of head rotation (<2 Hz), both the complex spike and the simple spike activity were modulated, and therefore either could support VOR gain adaptation. The source of the simple spike modulation could have involved both vestibular and visual-mossy fibers.

Our studies were directed at considering the potential role of dorsolateral pontine nucleus (DLPN)-derived visual mossy fibers in short-term modification of VOR gain at low frequency. The DLPN receives inputs from extrastriate visual cortex, including middle temporal (MT) and medial superior temporal (MST) areas,[9] which play a significant role in processing visual motion. The DLPN projects to the contralateral ventral paraflocculus and dorsal paraflocculus and vermal lobule VI and VII.[10] Both single-unit recording[11–15] and lesion studies[16] demonstrate that DLPN neurons carry appropriate signals for initiation and maintenance of smooth pursuit, optokinetic, and ocular following eye movements. We wanted to determine whether DLPN-derived signals could also play a role in visual-vestibular behavior.

METHODS

Three normal juvenile rhesus monkeys (*Macaca mulatta*) weighing 3–7 kg were used in our behavioral studies. A detailed description of our surgical procedures can be found in previous publications.[17] Briefly, surgical procedures were carried out under aseptic conditions using isoflurane anesthesia (1.25–2.5%) to stereotaxically implant a head-stabilization post, DLPN recording chamber, and scleral search coils. All procedures were performed in strict compliance with guidelines promulgated by the National Institutes of Health, and the protocols were reviewed and approved by the Institutional Animal Care and Use Committee at Emory University.

During all experiments, monkeys were comfortably seated in a primate chair with the head stabilized in the horizontal stereotaxic plane. Eye movements were detected and calibrated using standard electromagnetic methods and appropriate hardware (CNC Electronics, Seattle, WA). Monkeys were trained to perform a fixation task and track a small diameter (0.2°) target spot moved with a two-axis mirror galvanometer (General Scanning, Watertown, MA) in sinusoidal or step-ramp trajectories. Stimulus generation was computer controlled with custom Labview software and hardware (National Instruments, Austin, TX). Eye, head, and target position feedback signals were processed with anti-aliasing filters at 200 Hz using six-pole Bessel filters prior to digitization at 1 kHz with 16-bit precision. Velocity arrays were generated by digital differentiation the position arrays using a central difference algorithm in Matlab (Mathworks, Natick, MA).

We used functional criteria to localize the DLPN, which contains neurons that are modulated for motion of either a large-field (75° × 75°) stimulus or during smooth pursuit of a small diameter (0.2°) target spot moving (± 10°; 0.1–0.75 Hz) over a dark background.[12,16] Once we determined the location of DLPN, muscimol injections (0.5 µL; 2%) were delivered using a picoliter pump (WPI-PV830) and a small diameter (<50 µm) micropipette.[17] The efficacy of muscimol injections was confirmed by measuring the gain of smooth pursuit during step-ramp tracking.[16] Smooth-pursuit measurements were taken 15 min after the injection and in some experiments also at the conclusion of gain modification experiments (>2 h post injection). We estimate that our injections blocked most of the DLPN, based on the volume and concentration of our muscimol injections compared to those of other investigators.[18] DLPN injection sites were confirmed histologically using standard methods as described in our earlier studies.[12]

We produced adaptive changes in VOR gain by delivering sinusoidal whole-body rotation (0.2 Hz, 30°/s) for 2 h while the monkey viewed a earth-stationary visual surround with magnifying (×2) or minifying (×0.5) lenses (Designs for Vision, Ronkonkoma, NY), conditions that produced either increases or decreases of VOR gain. We characterized the gain of the VOR by measuring VORd and VOR1. We measured VORd before and after adaptation, at the adapting frequency.

To quantify smooth-pursuit performance, we used the initial acceleration and steady-state smooth-pursuit velocity during step-ramp tracking at 20°/s. Pursuit initiation was taken as the time that average eye speed reached at least three standard deviations above the pretrial value during fixation. Initial acceleration was calculated as the average eye acceleration in the first 100-ms period of pursuit to the step-ramp stimulus. Average steady-state velocity was defined as the region where eye velocity reached a plateau, typically taken between 200 and 300 ms after pursuit initiation. At least 10 trials of rightward or leftward step-ramp tracking were averaged to quantify initial acceleration and steady-state velocity. VORd gain was calculated as the ratio of peak eye velocity to peak head velocity, measured in darkness. The peak eye and head velocities over the oscillation period were determined by fitting sinusoids to each half-cycle. Average gains and their standard deviations were calculated separately for rightward and leftward head rotations from at least 10 cycles.

RESULTS

Smooth Pursuit following Muscimol Injections in the DLPN

We always observed deficits in the monkey's ability to initiate and maintain smooth pursuit toward the side of muscimol injection (ipsilesional). FIGURE 1 illustrates representative smooth-pursuit deficits for one of our monkeys. We measured the initial acceleration (first 100 ms) and average steady-state smooth-pursuit speed to characterize the quality of smooth pursuit in all of our monkeys (TABLE 1). Control values taken prior to muscimol injection (FIG. 1, solid lines) show that steady-state eye speed was close to target speed (20°/s) during leftward and rightward track-

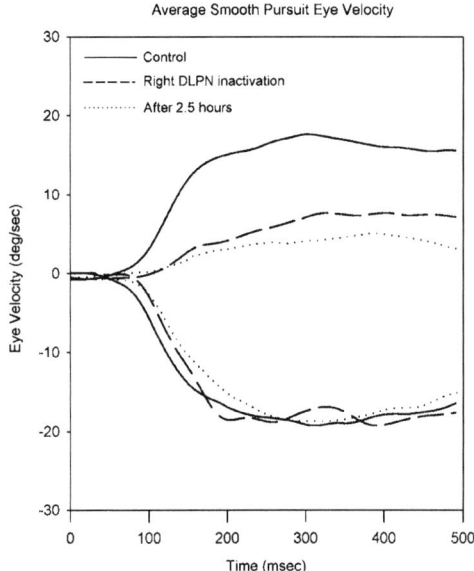

FIGURE 1. Effects of right DLPN inactivation by muscimol on smooth pursuit for monkey C. Ipsiversive and contraversive tracking in control and DLPN inactivation experiments. Averages from 10 trials of smooth eye velocity as a function of time for target motion at 20°/s are shown. Upward deflections show rightward eye velocity. Solid and dashed lines indicate average velocity for control and inactivation data. Dotted line indicates eye velocity 2.5 h after muscimol injection.

ing. After muscimol injection in the right DLPN, eye speed for ipsilesional pursuit (rightward) was reduced to only 32–61% of preinjection values (FIG. 1, dashed lines). The impairments observed during ipsilesional smooth pursuit were statistically significant ($P < 0.01$) with initial acceleration reduced by 35–68%. There were no significant deficits in pursuit in the contralesional direction. We also observed deficits in the monkey's ability to generate and maintain vertical smooth pursuit (TABLE 1). The pursuit deficit was stable for at least 2.5 h following muscimol injection (FIG. 1, dotted lines) with ipsilesional steady-state velocity reaching only 4.8°/s.

Cancellation of the VOR

We moved the target spot in phase with the rotary chair to produce a condition that allowed our monkeys to cancel their VOR. Ideally, cancellation would be complete, but most monkeys are unable to achieve this condition. FIGURE 2 shows that prior to muscimol injection, cancellation of the VOR was *symmetric* (control). After muscimol injection in the right DLPN, cancellation was *asymmetric,* such that right head rotation (positive values) was associated with a significant amount of residual VOR. In contrast, cancellation during leftward head rotation was similar to preinjection values (FIG. 2, bar graph). The directional deficit in cancellation of the VOR is consistent with the rightward smooth-pursuit deficit seen after right DLPN inactiva-

TABLE 1. Smooth pursuit performance pre- and post-DLPN inactivation

Animal, experiment number	Direction	Initial Acceleration (°/s²)		Steady State Velocity (°/s)		Performance Change (%)
		Pre	Post	Pre	Post	
E, 1	Ipsi	127.7 ± 17.1	74.9 ± 8.4	19.8 ± 1.7	12.7 ± 1.3	59[a]
	Contra	129.4 ± 6.1	126.5 ± 11.4	18.3 ± 1.6	15.5 ± 0.8	98
	Up	106.8 ± 32.3	40.9 ± 7.2	19.8 ± 1.7	14.8 ± 1.6	38[a]
	Down	119.7 ± 16.4	69.6 ± 9.6	12.3 ± 1.8	5.9 ± 1.3	58[a]
E, 2	Ipsi	123.4 ± 79.1	59.9 ± 7.7	20.5 ± 3.4	13.9 ± 3.3	49[a]
	Contra	125.1 ± 12.9	120.4 ± 8.0	18.4 ± 1.4	18.8 ± 2.4	96
C, 1	Ipsi	131.8 ± 43.1	41.6 ± 12.5	17.8 ± 1.6	6.9 ± 0.4	32[a]
	Contra	135.8 ± 18.5	138.1 ± 39.7	18.1 ± 2.4	17.9 ± 1.3	101
	Up	102.3 ± 17.4	60.3 ± 12.4	17.0 ± 0.4	14.1 ± 1.9	59[a]
	Down	104.8 ± 10.5	100.2 ± 13.4	17.1 ± 1.8	15.4 ± 2.9	96
C, 2	Ipsi	132.3 ± 27.5	48.0 ± 14.9	17.9 ± 0.5	8.4 ± 2.9	36[a]
	Contra	133.2 ± 14.7	142.0 ± 19.1	18.3 ± 2.7	18.2 ± 2.5	107
R, 1	Ipsi	103.9 ± 8.0	67.5 ± 12.9	18.6 ± 1.9	9.9 ± 0.6	65[a]
	Contra	67.3 ± 9.4	70.9 ± 17.5	18.7 ± 2.6	16.1 ± 0.5	105
	Up	85.1 ± 7.7	80.5 ± 5.3	15.5 ± 1.3	13.0 ± 1.4	95
	Down	74.7 ± 9.8	70.3 ± 5.4	13.5 ± 1.1	13.1 ± 1.7	94
R, 2	Ipsi	111.9 ± 17.8	67.7 ± 8.4	18.7 ± 0.7	11.8 ± 0.2	61[a]
	Contra	101.8 ± 17.9	75.8 ± 18.8	17.6 ± 1.3	16.4 ± 0.3	74[a]

Each value is a mean ± SD of 10 step-ramp tracking results. The performance change (%) was calculated from the ratio of eye accelerations (post/pre × 100).
[a]Significant difference between pre- and post-inactivation ($P < 0.01$; t-test).

tion because rightward head rotation produces a leftward VOR that could be cancelled by rightward smooth pursuit.

Visual Modification of the VOR

Before adaptation experiments, VORd gain was less then unity (range: 0.89 to 0.96), and VORl gain was significantly increased (range: 0.98 to 1.06) when the animals viewed a stationary target. When monkeys viewed through ×2 or ×0.5 lenses, during 0.2 Hz, 30°/s head rotations, VORl showed significant and immediate *symmetric* increases (41–43%) or decreases (39–63%; FIG. 3C, D). After 2 h of lens viewing, the VORd gain was tested to measure the degree of adaptation and showed appropriate changes in both adaptive conditions (FIG. 3E, F). The VORd gain following ×2 adaptation was increased by 23–32% and 24–32% for ipsiversive and con-

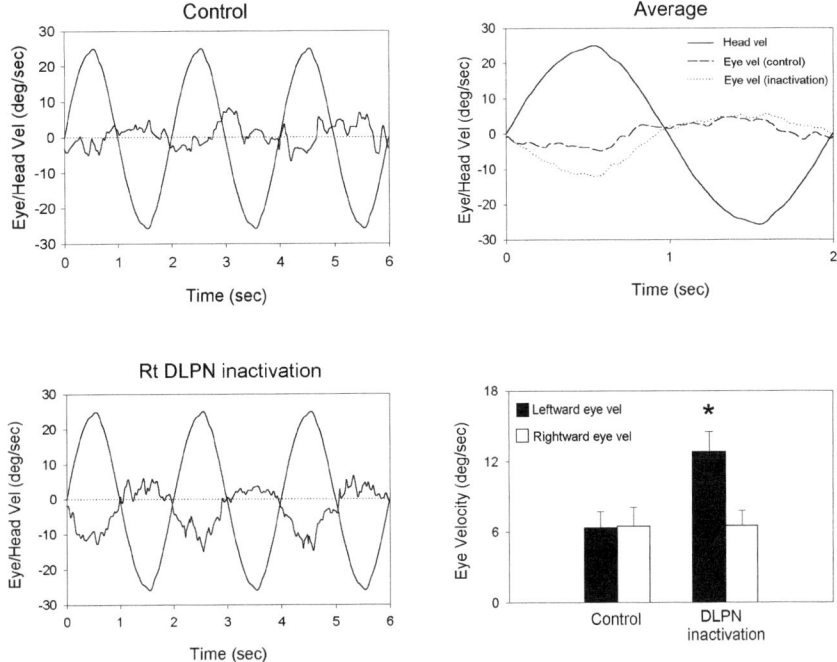

FIGURE 2. Cancellation of the VOR (VOR × 0). Cancellation of the VOR before (control) and after right DLPN inactivation (*lower left*). Average traces are shown in *upper right panel*. Average eye velocity in all conditions is shown in the bar graph (*lower right panel*). Asterisk indicates statistically significant ($P > 0.01$) effects.

traversive eye velocities, respectively. Likewise, following ×0.5 adaptation, the gain was reduced by 22–48% and 23–43% for ipsiversive and contraversive eye velocities, respectively. These values served as controls for our muscimol experiments.

During muscimol injection experiments, we first verified the efficacy of DLPN inactivation using smooth-pursuit tracking criteria. Before adaptation experiments commenced, we found that postinjection VORd gain (FIG. 3A) was not significantly different than preinjection gain values (t-test; $P > 0.93$). Similarly, the VORl gain was not significantly different (t-test; $P > 0.86$) between preinjection and postinjection conditions when viewing a stationary target (FIG. 2B). In the ×2 and ×0.5 viewing conditions immediately after muscimol injection, the VORl gain increased (40–43%) and decreased (32–68%) symmetrically in spite of strictly unilateral DLPN inactivation. These values were not significantly different from preinjection values (t-test; $P > 0.43$; FIG. 2C, D). Following 2 h of lens viewing, the VORd gain associated with ×2 adaptation conditions was increased by 25–31% and 26–32% for ipsilesional and contralesional eye velocities after muscimol injection, respectively. These values were not significantly different from preinjection adaptation values (t-test; $P > 0.75$; FIG. 3B). Likewise, following 2 h of ×0.5 viewing, the VORd gain was reduced by 24–48% and 23–48% for ipsilesional and contralesional eye velocities, re-

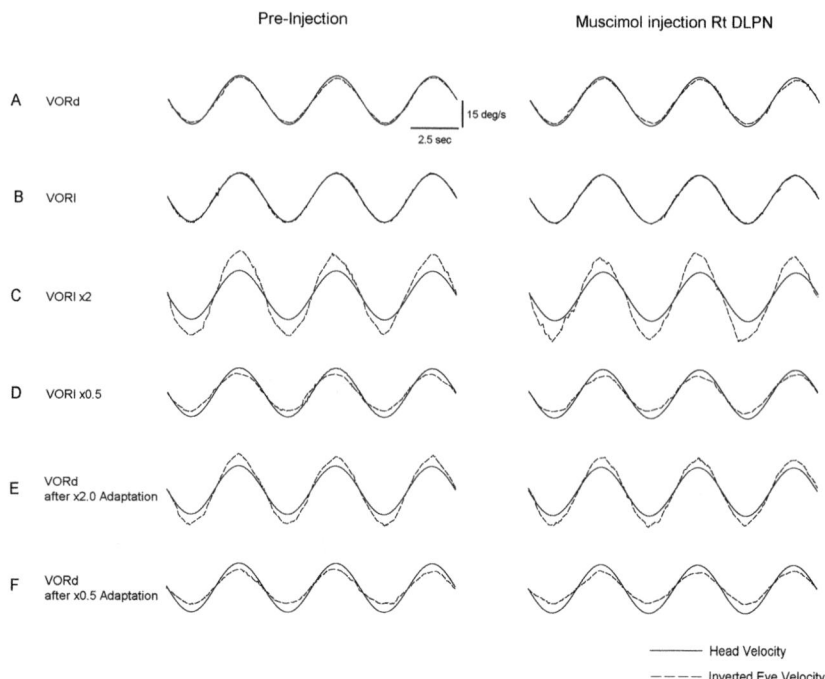

FIGURE 3. Effects of right DLPN inactivation on the VOR for monkey C. From *top to bottom* (**A** to **F**), the traces indicate eye and head velocity during sinusoidal head rotation in darkness (**A**), viewing a stationary surround in the light (**B**), viewing a stationary surround through ×2 lenses before adaptation (**C**), viewing a stationary surround through ×0.5 lenses before adaptation (**D**), in darkness after ×2 adaptation in darkness (**E**), and after ×0.5 adaptation (**F**). *Solid and dashed traces* show head and eye velocities, respectively. Eye velocities are inverted, and saccades have been removed.

spectively. These were similar to preinjection adaptation values (t-test; $P > 0.61$; FIG. 3C). Importantly, even after 2 h of adaptation, there was still a clear deficit in ipsilesional smooth pursuit, indicating that our DLPN block was stable throughout the adaptation period (FIG. 1C, dotted line). Our results demonstrate that after unilateral DLPN inactivation, there was a strong ipsilesional smooth-pursuit deficit but no effect on short-term VOR adaptation.

DISCUSSION

Our studies were designed to consider whether visual signals derived from DLPN mossy fibers could play a role in visual-vestibular behavior, including short-term plasticity in the VOR. We found that VOR adaptation proceeds *symmetrically* in the presence of a unilateral DLPN inactivation that produces an *asymmetric* deficit in smooth pursuit or cancellation of the VOR. The fact that visual enhancement of the VOR was unaffected following DLPN inactivation suggests another source of visual slip signals to support this role. The most likely source of these signals is the pretectal nucleus of the optic tract (NOT) and related terminal nuclei of the accessory optic system (AOS).

Our muscimol injections in the DLPN produce ipsilesional smooth-pursuit deficits that persist for the full 2-h duration of our adaptation paradigm. These deficits are similar those reported in earlier studies.[16] We suggest that if the DLPN played a significant role in short-term adaptation of the VOR, then some *asymmetry* in the adapted VOR would be present. Current modeling studies suggest that the cortical projections from areas MT and MST to the DLPN play a role in smooth pursuit but not necessarily in the VOR.[19] Anatomical studies show that the DLPN projects most heavily to the ventral paraflocculus,[10] which contributes to both smooth pursuit and VOR adaptation.[20] The apparent lack of DLPN contribution to short-term adaptation of the VOR argues for other structures supporting this role.

Raymond and Lisberger[8] analyzed the phase relationship of simple spike and complex spike firing in HGVP cells recorded during conditions that would result in a VOR gain increase or decrease, and found that only complex spikes carry appropriate information to drive visually guided motor learning at high frequencies (>5 Hz). However, at lower frequencies, either mossy-fiber-driven simple spikes or climbing-fiber-driven complex spikes could play a role in VOR adaptation. Correlated but not necessarily coincident signals arriving over visual climbing fibers and vestibular mossy fibers could be essential for visually guided motor learning in the VOR.[6,21] It is possible climbing fiber inputs mediate their effect by evoking long-term depression in Purkinje cells.[3] Simple spike modulation produced by correlated activity of vestibular and visual inputs carried over mossy fiber pathways could potentially induce low-frequency adaptation through different mechanisms. Our studies do not address the site of motor learning in the VOR,[5,6] but they could further constrain possible sources of visual information necessary for visual modification of the VOR.

There is strong direct evidence that visual climbing fibers are essential for adaptation of the VOR, produced in a visual-vestibular mismatch paradigm like ours. For example, Yakushin and colleagues[7] found that VOR gain could not be adaptively reduced during short-term adaptation experiments following unilateral muscimol inactivation of NOT. Lesions of the NOT remove much of the visual afferent drive for the inferior olive, which is the sole source of visual climbing fibers.[2,22] The NOT contains visual direction and velocity-sensitive neurons suited to supporting visual-vestibular interactions. It is important to point out that the visual sensitivity of NOT and DLPN neurons have many similarities, including overlapping visual latencies and speed sensitivity during ocular following, smooth pursuit, and passive visual stimulation.[11–14] Therefore, the differential effect of NOT and DLPN lesions on short-term adaptation of the VOR probably reflects their different functional-anatomical pathways. The NOT and AOS are responsible for producing modulation of visual climbing fibers, but the DLPN provides only mossy fibers. These results taken together with the constraining findings indicate that the visual climbing fiber pathways play an essential role in VOR adaptation at both high and low frequencies of head rotation.

ACKNOWLEDGMENTS

We thank Ms. Tracey Brozyna for expert technical assistance. This work was supported by National Institutes of Health grants EY06069, EY13308, RR00165, and NS007480.

REFERENCES

1. LEIGH, R.J. & D.S. ZEE. 1999. The Neurology of Eye Movements. Oxford University Press. New York.
2. FUCHS, A.F. & M.J. MUSTARI. 1993. The optokinetic response in primates and its possible neuronal substrate. Rev. Oculomotor Res. **5:** 343–369.
3. ITO, M. 1972. Neural design of the cerebellar motor control system. Brain Res. **40:** 81–84.
4. LISBERGER, S.G., T.A. PAVELKO & D.M. BROUSSARD. 1994. Neural basis for motor learning in the vestibuloocular reflex of primates. I. Changes in the responses of brain stem neurons. J. Neurophysiol. **72:** 928–953.
5. HIRATA, Y. & S.M. HIGHSTEIN. 2001. Acute adaptation of the vestibular ocular reflex: signal processing by floccular and ventral parafloccular Purkinje cells. J. Neurophysiol. **85:** 2267–2288.
6. DU LAC, S., J.L. RAYMOND, T.J. SEJNOWSKI & S.G. LISBERGER. 1995. Learning and memory in the vestibulo-ocular reflex. Annu. Rev. Neurosci. **18:** 409–441.
7. YAKUSHIN, S.B., H. REISINE, J. BÜTTNER-ENNEVER, et al. 2000. Functions of the nucleus of the optic tract (NOT). I. Adaptation of the gain of the horizontal vestibulo-ocular reflex. Exp. Brain Res. **131:** 416–432.
8. RAYMOND, J.L. & S.G. LISBERGER. 1998. Neural learning rules for the vestibulo-ocular reflex. J. Neurosci. **18:** 9112–9129.
9. DISTLER, C., M.J. MUSTARI & K.P. HOFFMANN. 2002. Cortical projections to the nucleus of the optic tract and dorsal terminal nucleus and to the dorsolateral pontine nucleus in macaques: a dual retrograde tracing study. J. Comp. Neurol. **444:** 144–158.
10. GLICKSTEIN, M., N. GERRITS, I. KRALJ-HANS, et al. 1994. Visual pontocerebellar projections in the macaque. J. Comp. Neurol. **349:** 51–72.
11. SUZUKI, D.A. & E.L. KELLER. 1984. Visual signals in the dorsolateral pontine nucleus of the alert monkey: their relationship to smooth-pursuit eye movements. Exp. Brain Res. **53:** 473–478.
12. MUSTARI, M.J., A.F. FUCHS & J. WALLMAN. 1988. Response properties of dorsolateral pontine units during smooth pursuit in the rhesus macaque. J. Neurophysiol. **60:** 664–686.
13. THIER, P., W. KOEHLER & U.W. BUETTNER. 1988. Neuronal activity in the dorsolateral pontine nucleus of the alert monkey modulated by visual stimuli and eye movements. Exp. Brain Res. **70:** 496–512.
14. SUZUKI, D.A., J.G. MAY, E.L. KELLER & R.D. YEE. 1990. Visual motion response properties of neurons in dorsolateral pontine nucleus of alert monkey. J. Neurophysiol. **63:** 37–59.
15. KAWANO, K., M. SHIDARA & S. YAMANE. 1992. Neural activity in dorsolateral pontine nucleus of alert monkey during ocular following responses. J. Neurophysiol. **67:** 680–703.
16. MAY, J.G., E.L. KELLER & D.A. SUZUKI. 1988. Smooth-pursuit eye movement deficits with chemical lesions in the dorsolateral pontine nucleus of the monkey. J. Neurophysiol. **59:** 952–977.
17. MUSTARI, M.J., R.J. TUSA, A.F. BURROWS, et al. 2001. Gaze-stabilizing deficits and latent nystagmus in monkeys with early onset visual deprivation: role of the pretectal NOT. J. Neurophysiol. **86:** 662–675.
18. ARIKAN, R., N.M.J. BLAKE, J.P. ERINJERI, et al. 2002. A method to measure the effective spread of focally injected muscimol into the central nervous system with electrophysiology and light microscopy. J. Neurosci. Methods **118:** 51–57.

19. TABATA, H., K. YAMAMOTO & M. KAWATO. 2002. Computational study on monkey VOR adaptation and smooth pursuit based on the parallel control-pathway theory. J. Neurophysiol. **87:** 2176–2189.
20. RAMBOLD, H., A. CHURCHLAND, Y. SELIG, et al. 2002. Partial ablations of the flocculus and ventral paraflocculus in monkeys cause linked deficits in smooth pursuit eye movements and adaptive modification of the VOR. J. Neurophysiol. **87:** 912–924.
21. QUINN, K.J., A.J. DIDIER, J.F. BAKER & B.W. PETERSON. 1998. Modeling motor learning in the brainstem and cerebellar sites responsible for VOR plasticity. Brain Res. Bull. **46:** 333–346.
22. MUSTARI, M.J., A.F. FUCHS, C.R. KANEKO & F.R. ROBINSON. 1994. Anatomical connections of the primate pretectal nucleus of the optic tract. J. Comp. Neurol. **349:** 111–128.

Cerebellar Contribution to Saccades and Gaze Holding

A Modeling Approach

STEFAN GLASAUER

Center for Sensorimotor Research, Department of Neurology, Klinikum Grosshadern, Ludwig-Maximilians-University, Munich, Germany

ABSTRACT: The possible role of the cerebellum for the control of saccades and gaze holding is reconsidered using a computational modeling approach. As suggested by previous research, control of gaze holding is assumed to be enhanced by the floccular lobe, whereas control of the saccadic pulse is governed by the oculomotor vermis and fastigial nucleus. In the present work, a negative feedback loop via the paramedian tract neurons and the floccular lobe that contains a forward model of the oculomotor plant is supposed to enhance the time constant of the brainstem integrator. Control of saccadic amplitude is hypothesized to be achieved by a more complex network: feedforward projections from the superior colliculus via the nucleus reticularis tegmenti pontis to the oculomotor vermis and fastigial nucleus cooperate with feedback connections from excitatory burst neurons to overcome the sluggishness of the assumed local feedback loop formed via the superior colliculus and to implement inverse dynamics of downstream neural and motor processing.

KEYWORDS: eye movements; cerebellum; fastigial nucleus; flocculus; mathematical modeling

INTRODUCTION

Current theories of cerebellar function for motor control[1–4] propose that the cerebellum enhances motor and/or sensory function to overcome slow motor dynamics and sensory feedback delays. To achieve this goal, the cerebellum is supposed to implement internal inverse and/or forward models of sensors and actuators to predict the consequences of motor commands,[4] to compare the prediction with the desired action, and to use the error between both to enhance the motor command.

If a desired action (for example, a step-like gaze shift) is directly fed to a motor system such as the eye plant (described by a low-pass filter), the resulting action is slowed by the dynamics of the motor system. An inverse model transforms the desired action into an appropriate motor command, thereby effectively cancelling the dynamics of the motor system. It yields the best results but is difficult to learn and cannot always be realized. One example of an inverse model is the oculomotor sys-

Address for correspondence: Stefan Glasauer, Department of Neurology, Klinikum Grosshadern, LMU München, 81377 München, Germany. Voice: +49 89 7095 4839; fax: +49 89 7095 4801.
sglasauer@nefo.med.uni-muenchen.de

tem. The input to the system is desired gaze velocity. For example, gaze stabilization by the vestibuloocular reflex (VOR) is driven by negative head velocity conveyed by the semicircular canals. The subsequent combination of appropriately weighted direct and integrator pathways acts as an inverse model of the eye plant dynamics.[5] For the saccadic system, the change in position of a visual target, which is equal to the desired gaze step, is converted to a velocity command by the burst generator that is then sent through the direct and integrator pathways.

An internal forward model has the advantage of providing an internal prediction of the action to be performed (cf. reafference principle[6]). Its basic principle is to predict the motor action, compute the error between predicted and desired action, and use this error in a feedback loop to enhance the motor command. However, forward models in feedback loops can only enhance motor output, but not completely cancel motor dynamics.

Evidently, inverse and feedback models may both be used in the same premotor circuit. FIGURE 1 shows a possible implementation applied to the VOR and the oculomotor system: the inverse model is realized by direct and indirect integrator pathways, and a forward model predicting eye velocity together with the comparator between predicted and desired eye velocity resides in a side loop that is hypothesized to be located in the cerebellar flocculus and ventral paraflocculus. This structure closely resembles that of the current models of cerebellar function for adaptation of the VOR.[7–10]

Lesions of the cerebellum are known to cause severe eye movement deficits (for review, see Robinson and Fuchs[11]). Specifically, lesion of the cerebellar flocculus causes defective gaze holding, and lesion of the oculomotor vermis or the oculomotor region of the fastigial nuclei (FN) causes deficits in saccadic eye movements. This observation prompted Optican and Robinson[12] to hypothesize that gaze holding

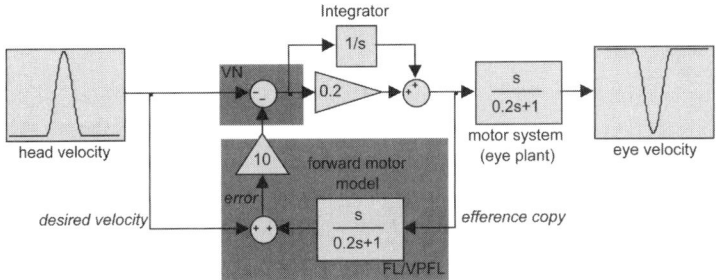

FIGURE 1. Structure of VOR pathways containing an inverse and a forward model of the eye plant, which, in its basic constituents, closely resembles models for vestibuloocular reflex adaptation.[7–10] Model input is head velocity; model output, eye velocity. The inverse model is composed of the direct and integrator pathways. The cerebellar flocculus and ventral paraflocculus (FL/VPFL) receive afferent connections from the vestibular system and an efference copy of eye velocity (possibly via the paramedian tract neurons). The Purkinje cells in the FL/VPFL inhibit floccular target neurons in the vestibular nuclei. Transfer functions are given in Laplace notation, with s denoting the Laplace operator. The motor system is modeled as a low-pass filter with a dominant time constant of 0.2 s. The motor output is differentiated to yield eye velocity as model output.

and saccades are enhanced by separate cerebellar mechanisms. In the following, I shall propose computational models based on this hypothesis to elucidate the contribution of the cerebellum to oculomotor control based on current theories of cerebellar motor control.

GAZE HOLDING

Gaze holding is an important aspect of oculomotor control. After a shift in gaze direction by saccadic or VOR-driven eye movements, the gaze-holding mechanism ensures that the eyes hold their final position even without visual input. In the following, a model for cerebellar contribution to gaze holding is developed.

Background

Robinson[5] proposed on theoretical grounds that a common final integrator is necessary to achieve gaze holding following gaze shifts, since motor commands originating in the semicircular canals or the saccadic burst generator only provide a velocity command. It turned out that this final integrator is distributed over several anatomical structures. For horizontal eye movements, the medial vestibular nuclei and the adjacent nucleus prepositus hypoglossi (NPH) are crucial (for review, see Moschovakis[13] and Fukushima and Kaneko[14]), as shown by lesion studies.[15,16] Further structures that cause impairment of gaze holding include the cerebellar flocculus and ventral paraflocculus[17–20] and cell groups in the brainstem that project to the flocculus, the paramedian tract (PMT) neurons.[21,22] From these studies, it becomes evident that the final oculomotor integrator is composed of several subsystems: the direct pathway together with the eye plant form an integration with a leakage time constant of approximately 200 ms; the brainstem integrator enhances this time constant to about 2 s; and the PMT-flocculus loop further increases the time constant to the known 25 s.

Model

Given that the time constant of the brainstem circuit is only around 2 s, the basic circuit of the VOR can be modeled as shown in FIGURE 2A. Adding the floccular loop to this structure is straightforward and similar to that shown in FIGURE 1: floccular Purkinje cells (PCs) project onto floccular target neurons (FTNs) in the vestibular nuclei, which in turn project directly onto motor neurons.[23] Additionally, FTNs send collaterals to the NPH, which is assumed to perform basic brainstem integrator function, and to the PMT neurons. The flocculus receives mossy fibers from PMT neurons, floccular projection neurons in the vestibular nuclei, and directly from the semicircular canals. Finally, the flocculus computes predicted eye velocity from the PMT signal, compares it to desired eye velocity (equal to negative head velocity) and projects the error signal back to the vestibular nuclei.

During fixation, floccular PCs carry eye position information.[24] In the present model, if there is no input from the canals, the floccular loop effectively computes a signal proportional to residual eye velocity. During attempted gaze holding in darkness, this slow ocular drift is proportional to eye position. Hence, the discharge of

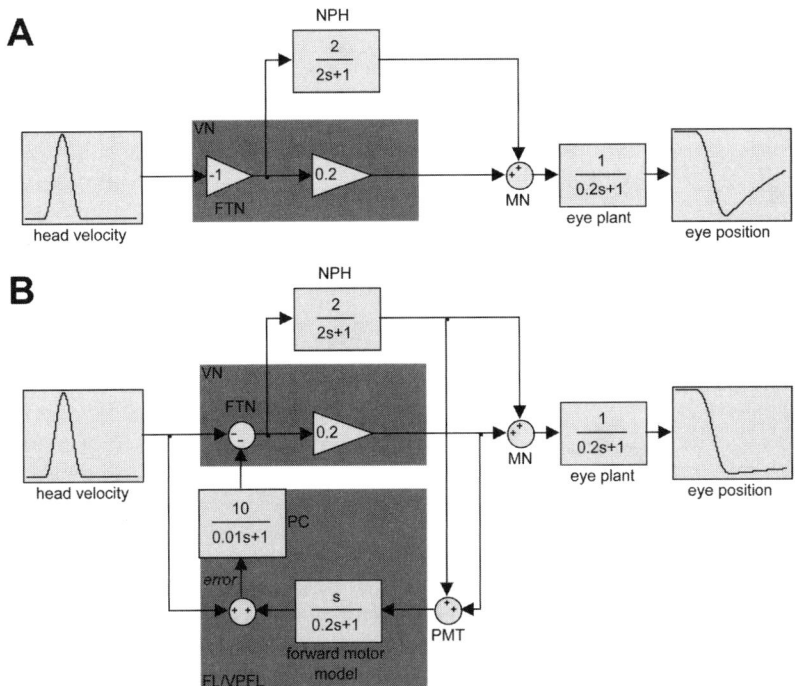

FIGURE 2. Gaze holding and integration. (**A**) Direct and indirect pathways from the semicircular canals to the vestibular nuclei and via the nucleus prepositus hypoglossi (NPH) to the motor neurons (MN). After a smooth change in head position, eye position drifts back with a time constant of the NPH of about 2 s (leaky integration). As in FIGURE 1, the eye plant is modeled as low-pass filter with a time constant of 0.2 s. (**B**) The flocculus (FL/VPFL) contributes to brainstem integration by implementing an internal model of the eye plant, thereby predicting eye velocity on the basis of an efferent copy of the motor command mediated via the paramedian tract (PMT). The predicted eye velocity is compared to the desired velocity as in FIGURE 1; the error is fed back via the Purkinje cells (PCs) to the floccular target neurons (FTNs). For a feedback gain of 10, the integration time constant is enhanced to about 25 s. PCs are modeled as low-pass filters with a time constant of 10 ms to avoid algebraic loops in the model.

the model floccular PCs is indeed proportional to eye position, and thus compatible with the experimental data.[24]

How are saccadic eye movements included in this scheme? One possible solution is that saccadic burst neurons project onto the same targets as vestibular afferents. However, this is not the case. For example, FTNs do not burst for saccadic eye movements.[25] Even more relevant: most floccular PCs pause during saccades[25] but carry eye position information.[24]

Therefore, I suggest that the floccular feedback loop is shut off during the saccadic burst (FIG. 3) via inhibitory burst input to the PCs. Hence, during a saccadic eye movement, the overall time constant of the integrator is reduced to that of the brainstem (2 s). This, however, is sufficient because the duration of a saccade usually

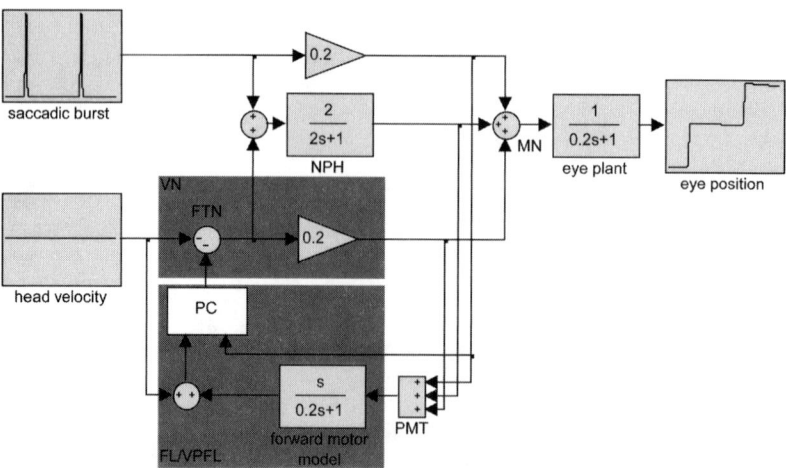

FIGURE 3. Complete structure of floccular contribution for brainstem integration. Simulation of two consecutive saccades is shown in inserts. Compared to FIGURE 2B, the saccadic burst generator that has been added projects to the extraocular motor neurons (MNs) and the nucleus prepositus hypoglossi (NPH), via the PMT neurons to the flocculus (FL/VPFL). In the model, the saccadic burst, conveyed via mossy fiber input, completely inhibits floccular Purkinje cells (PCs), thereby effectively interrupting the floccular loop.

is much shorter (around 0.1 s). The saccadic burst charges the NPH integrator, and after the saccade, the floccular loop resumes working to enhance the integrator time constant.

Discussion

While most models of the oculomotor system assume that the brainstem integrator operates perfectly and do not care about how this is accomplished, there are some models specifically concerned with the neural mechanisms of gaze holding, that is, with the oculomotor velocity-to-position integrator (for review, see Sklavos and Moschovakis[26]). Most of these models assume that the brainstem integrator operates via positive feedback loops (recent models are more realistic[26]) and performs gaze holding independently of the cerebellum. Theories about how the improvement of the time constant of the brainstem integrator may be achieved by the cerebellum are rare. Zee and colleagues[27] proposed that a positive feedback loop via the cerebellum improves the time constant. This theoretical approach has two major drawbacks: (1) positive feedback is very sensitive to minor variations in feedback gain, and (2) cerebellar PCs exert inhibitory projections on the deep cerebellar nuclei and the vestibular nuclei. Another approach to model floccular contribution to gaze holding, given by Darlot and colleagues,[28] exhibits some similarities to the present approach, specifically concerning the proposed forward model predicting eye velocity in the cerebellar cortex. However, in contrast to the present approach, their model fails to replicate experimental evidence such as floccular PCs pausing during saccades, or unaffected saccades after lesion of the flocculus.

The present model is, of course, not complete. For example, position-vestibular-pause neurons, which contribute directly to the VOR, are currently not included in the model. However, their firing properties[23] (pause during saccades, eye position sensitivity), which are, in this respect, similar to those of floccular PCs, make them likely candidates to participate in a brainstem feedback loop[29] that achieves the basic 2-s integrator time constant, similar to the floccular loop proposed here. Also, it is not clear whether FTNs project back to the flocculus via the PMT, as assumed in FIGURE 3, or whether their projection is only indirect via the NPH and the PMT. If the latter were the case, the floccular feedback loop would be less sensitive to time delays and the simulated response of floccular PCs would be closer to experimental data,[30] but the internal model would then no longer be an exact replica of the eye plant dynamics.

An important aspect of oculomotor control related to floccular function that has not been touched upon in the present model are slow, visually driven eye movements such as smooth pursuit or optokinetic nystagmus. However, the model is easily extendable to include these important features as shown by its similarity to current VOR adaptation models.[10]

SACCADIC EYE MOVEMENTS

Saccadic eye movements shift the direction of gaze rapidly in response to visual stimuli or to explore a visual scene. The neuronal substrate for the generation of a motor command has been the focus of extensive research (for review, see Moschovakis and colleagues,[31] Scudder and colleagues,[32] and Sparks[33]). In the following, a model for cerebellar contribution to saccadic eye movements is proposed. Retinal target position is used as input to the model, and the output is the saccadic burst arising at the level of the brainstem burst neurons. Thus, the model output may serve as input to the gaze-holding model presented above.

Background

Retinal input arrives at the superior colliculus (SC) directly and via different cortical pathways. Target positions are coded retinotopically in the SC.[34,35] Before a saccadic eye movement, neurons in the deeper layers of the SC discharge a burst that arrives at long-lead burst neurons in the brainstem. These neurons contact excitatory and inhibitory burst neurons that project to extraocular motor neurons. A saccade is initiated when omnipause neurons (OPNs) release inhibition onto excitatory burst neurons. Several experimental observations suggest that the saccadic burst is subject to feedback control; for example, saccades disrupted by stimulation of the omnipause region in the brainstem still reach their target.[36] However, it is not clear which anatomic structures participate in the internal feedback loop.[32] On the basis of the finding that inactivation of the oculomotor vermis[37,38] or the caudal FN of the cerebellum[38–41] causes marked deficits of saccadic eye movements, it has been suggested that the cerebellum is part of the feedback loop.[32,42] However, evidence from a lesion study of the FN suggests that the cerebellum is not the only feedback pathway.[43]

Anatomical studies have elucidated possible pathways subserving this function. The SC projects to the nucleus reticularis tegmenti pontis (NRTP), which in turn projects to the caudal FN and vermal lobules VI and VII (for review, see Moschovakis and colleagues[31]). The discharge of precerebellar burst neurons in the NRTP is not correlated with saccade metrics; it is independent of saccadic size and duration.[44] FN neurons receive input from vermal PCs that discharge with saccades[45–47] and from mossy fiber collaterals to these PCs. FN neurons project to regions containing excitatory burst neurons and, notably, back to the SC (for review, see Moschovakis and colleagues[31]). Additionally, there is a feedback pathway from the brainstem burst generator to the FN and oculomotor vermis.[48,49] Lesions of the FN cause slow, hypermetric saccades and disrupt the ability for adaptive changes of saccadic amplitude.[50,51]

Model

In the following, it is assumed that the basic internal feedback loop for control of saccades includes the SC.[32,52,53] Recent experimental evidence supports this assumption.[54] In such a case, the postulated "resettable integrator"[55] could implicitly be implemented in the burst layer of the SC[52] that receives feedback about eye velocity (see FIG. 4).

However, there are several observations showing that the SC burst neurons do not determine saccadic amplitude. For example, during multiple gaze shifts, the SC encodes distance to target rather than saccade amplitude.[35] Furthermore, SC activity does not change during short-term saccadic adaptation.[56] Since saccadic adaptation depends on an intact oculomotor vermis and FN,[50,51] these structures must participate in determining saccade amplitude.

In the following, slow hypermetric saccades after bilateral FN deactivation are supposed to be due to the slow and ineffective local feedback loop involving the SC, as suggested previously.[57] Additionally, the proposed cerebellar pathway may also account for inaccuracy of the downstream inverse motor model composed of direct and integrator pathways.

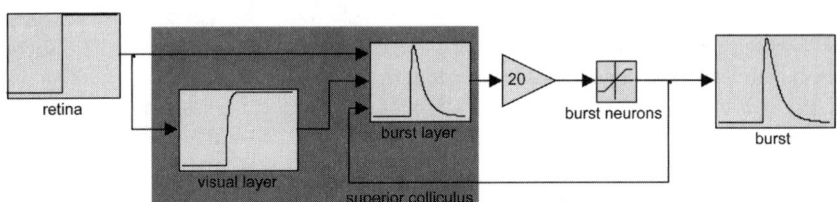

FIGURE 4. Basic model structure for burst generation in the superior colliculus (SC) and brainstem. A target jump on the retina (*left*) is converted into a burst by processing in the visual and motor layers of the SC. A negative feedback loop projecting back from the brainstem ensures that the saccade is terminated. The gain of the feedback loop was chosen to produce slow saccades, as seen following cerebellar lesions. A nonlinear saturation limits the discharge rate of brainstem burst neurons. The simulation time is 0.5 s with a target step at 0.2 s. The burst layer is a leaky integrator (time constant: 1 s) with excitatory input from the retina and inhibitory input from visual layer and burst neurons. The model output is the discharge of brainstem burst neurons and may thus be used as model input to the gaze-holding model presented in FIGURE 3.

To increase the speed of a feedback loop, a feedforward command can be added to the loop.[1,4] However, the application of this principle of control theory directly to the SC feedback loop does not help to explain the neural discharge observed in the FN, because it would result in adding an eye velocity signal rather than a signal that is similar to eye acceleration as observed in the FN.[58] Therefore, I propose that the direct forward projection from the NRTP to the FN codes the desired saccadic burst. The necessary spatial-to-temporal transformation from the spatially coded SC signal to a temporally coded burst signal may be achieved by NRTP and appropriate weighting of NRTP output reaching the FN. The same signal is sent to the vermis,[59] where a predicted burst is computed and relayed, via PCs, to the FN. Thus, with respect to the feedforward pathways, the FN acts as a comparator computing the error between desired and predicted burst (FIG. 5, feedforward pathways). This error signal is fed to the excitatory burst neurons and back to the SC, resulting in an accelerated eye movement.

Although this feedforward hypothesis captures some of the main anatomical and physiological properties of the FN, there are reasons to believe that the FN is also part of a cerebellar feedback loop, as previously suggested.[32] Feedback connections from the brainstem burst areas to the FN[48] and oculomotor vermis[49] have been dem-

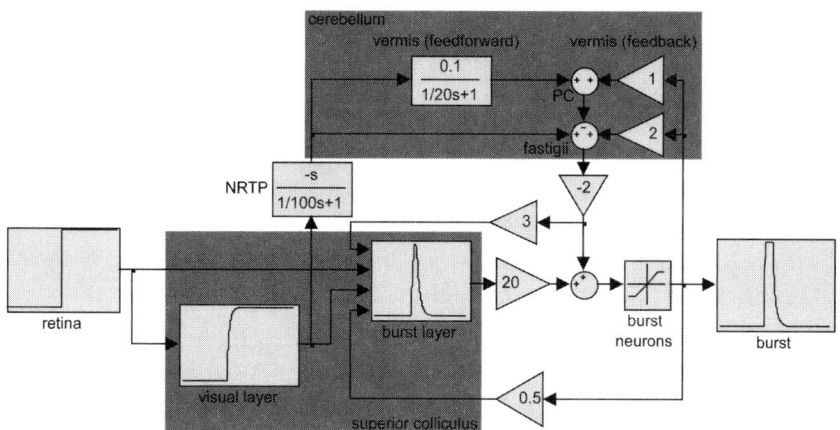

FIGURE 5. Combined feedforward-feedback hypothesis of cerebellar contribution to saccadic eye movements. To increase the speed of the local feedback loop involving the SC, the FN computes an error signal between a desired fast burst relayed via the NRTP, a predicted slow SC burst computed by the oculomotor vermis, and a feedback signal supplied by the burst neurons. This error signal between desired, predicted, and actual bursts is added to the loop at the level of the burst neurons and the SC. Note that the final burst is clipped because of the excitatory burst neuron nonlinearity. The negative gains of NRTP and FN account for the fact that excitatory input connections from SC to NRTP and excitatory output connections from FN to burst neurons cross the midline. Because the feedback loop from the burst neurons via FN and SC is negative (because of to the crossed output connections of the FN), it substitutes for the primary feedback loop shown in FIGURE 4. The gain factors involved have been adjusted to yield fast normometric saccades in the intact model, hypermetric saccades for complete lesion of the FN, and hypometric saccades for complete lesion of the oculomotor vermis.

onstrated anatomically. The proposed role of the FN concerning the feedback signal is to enhance its error signal by accounting for differences not only between desired and predicted, but also desired and actual burst profiles. The feedback pathway from the burst neurons to the FN is anatomically divided into two parts: (1) a direct pathway via mossy fiber collaterals to the FN, forming a negative feedback loop due to the crossed output connections of the FN,[48] and (2) an indirect pathway via the oculomotor vermis to the FN (FIG. 5, feedback pathways), forming a positive feedback loop due to the combination of inhibitory PC function and crossed FN output. In the model, both pathways are weighted appropriately to yield, in combination, a negative feedback loop. The vermal part of the feedback pathway can be shaped further by a forward model of downstream dynamics to adaptively account for downstream inaccuracies, for example, a weak direct projection to the oculomotor neurons.

The crossed output connections of the FN to the brainstem burst neurons[48] and SC[60] are represented by a negative FN output gain, and those of the SC to the NRTP[61] by a negative gain of the NRTP transfer function. To account for the fact that lesions of the FN cause not only slower, but also hypermetric saccades,[39] it is assumed that the feedback loop via the SC has a gain value lower than unity. Proper adjustment of the input gains to the FN as well as the dynamics of the vermal PCs is supposed to compensate for this low feedback gain and allows for adaptive control of saccadic amplitude.

A valuable test to verify the present model is to simulate lesions of the structures involved. Clearly, simulated complete lesions of the FN successfully replicate the finding of slow hypermetric saccades due to the slow feedback loop with a feedback gain smaller than unity (FIG. 6, column 2). Simulated lesion of the oculomotor vermis leads to the experimentally observed saccadic hypometria[37,38] (FIG. 6, column 3) due to the missing PC inhibition enhancing the gain of the negative feedback loop via burst neurons and FN. Also, simulated unilateral lesions of the FN show the experimentally found side-specific hypermetric or hypometric responses[39–41] (FIG. 6, columns 4 and 5). Interestingly, the proposed cerebellar feedback loop can now al-

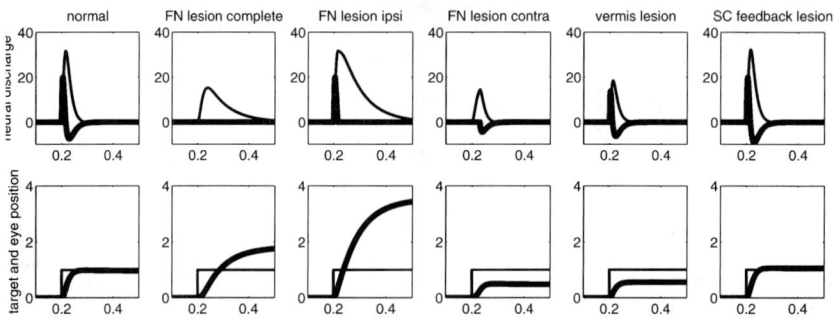

FIGURE 6. Simulations of the saccade generation model shown in FIGURE 5. Upper row shows burst (*thin line*, equal to eye velocity) and population discharge of the FN (*thick line*); lower row shows target step (*thin line*) and eye position (*thick line*). Columns show various simulations, as indicated in the titles. The first column shows a normal saccade; subsequent columns depict simulated lesions.

most completely take over the function of the previously important direct feedback loop. Simulated complete lesion of the direct feedback loop only leads to a very small increase in saccadic gain (see FIG. 6, column 6). This may explain why lesions of the NPH, which is supposed to supply velocity feedback to the SC, do not significantly affect saccadic amplitude except for a minor gain increase.[16]

Discussion

Only a few models have attempted to explain how the FN is involved in the control of saccadic eye movements. The present approach shows similarities to some aspects of each of these models. Although Dean's model[57] did not explain how the signal issued by the FN is generated, another more complex model[42] tried to overcome this disadvantage by proposing that the FN implements a spatial resetable integrator similar to that originally proposed for the SC. However, this approach is not compatible with the known anatomy and physiology of the FN (for further discussion, see Scudder and colleagues[32]). In contrast, the present approach proposes how FN discharge may be generated on the basis of current motor control theories without the need for spatially distributed processing in the cerebellum. This approach can successfully simulate various lesions (FIG. 6), including the experimentally found difference for ipsilateral and contralateral saccades following unilateral FN lesions.[38–41] Note that the simulated larger saccade gain for ipsilateral compared to complete FN lesion, which is not supported by experimental data,[39] critically depends on the exact shape of the desired burst signal. If the desired burst increases less rapidly than in the present model, the simulated contribution of the FN to saccade acceleration decreases, and the gains following unilateral or bilateral lesions become more similar. Similarly, the combination of gain factors shown in FIGURE 6 is not the only possible solution. Changing the gain factors or transfer dynamics of the vermal feedforward and feedback pathways causes changes in saccade amplitude and dynamics. The latter may aid in overcoming inaccuracy of the downstream inverse model of plant dynamics.

Some important aspects of saccade generation (for example, involvement of cortical structures such as the frontal eye fields) have been left out of the present model to keep it as simple as possible. The most important feature, however, concerns the OPNs, which are responsible for starting and shutting off the saccadic burst. Nonetheless, simulations show that OPNs can easily be implemented without changing the main aspects of the model. In the model, OPNs are inhibited by the initially increasing SC burst layer activity, thereby activating the feedback loops leading to the burst, and resume firing as soon as the burst is finished. Moreover, after short OPN stimulation braking the ongoing saccade, the present model successfully simulates that the saccade restarts and finally reaches the target, as found experimentally.[36] The (over)simplification of the SC, another aspect of the model, is likely to be less critical, because it is not the main goal of the model to explain SC function. However, it should be noted that the spatial-to-temporal transformation is thought to be achieved by appropriate spatial weighting of the SC afferents, as previously suggested.[53,62,63] The feedback from the FN to the SC may either contribute to a shift in the SC activity,[64,65] or may even simply inhibit the whole SC burst layer to terminate the burst. The latter might explain contradictory reports (for discussion, see

Sparks[63]) of whether there is a "moving hill" or not, because it would suppress the moving SC burst before it could reach the midline.

CONCLUSION

The present modeling approach attempts to explain cerebellar contribution to saccade generation and gaze holding by relatively simple structures. It is, as much as possible without compromising simplicity, compatible with known anatomy and physiology of the modeled brainstem and cerebellar regions. Model simulations capture the main features of lesion studies as well as single-cell recordings. Both models, following earlier suggestions about functional decoupling of cerebellar contribution to saccades and gaze holding,[12] can be combined to yield a complete model from retinal input to eye movement as output. In the present approach, which is based on current hypotheses about cerebellar function for motor control,[1–4] the cerebellum evaluates differences between desired and predicted motor commands, and uses this error to enhance the function of the underlying basic premotor brainstem mechanisms.

ACKNOWLEDGMENTS

I wish to thank U. Büttner and Th. Brandt for their support; J. Kleine and E. Schneider for their participation in discussion; R. McCrea, S. Highstein, and M. Goldberg for their encouraging comments; and U. Büttner, T. Eggert, and A. Koene for their critical remarks on the manuscript and models. This work was supported by the Fritz Thyssen Stiftung.

REFERENCES

1. KAWATO, M. & H. GOMI. 1992. The cerebellum and VOR/OKR learning models. Trends Neurosci. **15:** 445–453.
2. DARLOT, C. 1993. The cerebellum as a predictor of neural messages. I. The stable estimator hypothesis. Neuroscience **56:** 617–646.
3. MIALL, R.C., D.J. WEIR, D.M. WOLPERT & J.F. STEIN. 1993. Is the cerebellum a Smith predictor? J. Mot. Behav. **25:** 203–216.
4. WOLPERT, D.M., R.C. MIALL & M. KAWATO. 1998. Internal models in the cerebellum. Trends Cogn. Sci. **2:** 338–347.
5. ROBINSON, D.A. 1981. The use of control systems analysis in the neurophysiology of eye movements. Annu. Rev. Neurosci. **4:** 463–503.
6. VON HOLST, E. & H. MITTELSTAEDT. 1950. Das Reafferenzprinzip. Naturwissenschaften **37:** 464–476.
7. LISBERGER, S.G. 1994. Neural basis for motor learning in the vestibulo-ocular reflex of primates. III. Computational and behavioral analysis of the sites of learning. J. Neurophysiol. **72:** 974–998.
8. QUINN, K.J., A.J. DIDIER, J.F. BAKER & B.W. PETERSON. 1998. Modeling learning in brain stem and cerebellar sites responsible for VOR plasticity. Brain Res. Bull. **46:** 333–346.
9. HIRATA, Y. & S.M. HIGHSTEIN. 2001. Acute adaptation of the vestibuloocular reflex: signal processing by floccular and ventral parafloccular Purkinje cells. J. Neurophysiol. **85:** 2267–2288.

10. TABATA, H., K. YAMAMOTO & M. KAWATO. 2002. Computational study on monkey VOR adaptation and smooth pursuit based on the parallel control-pathway theory. J. Neurophysiol. **87:** 2176–2189.
11. ROBINSON, F.R. & A.F. FUCHS. 2001. The role of the cerebellum in voluntary eye movements. Annu. Rev. Neurosci. **24:** 981–1004.
12. OPTICAN, L.M. & D.A. ROBINSON. 1980. Cerebellar-dependent adaptive control of primate saccadic system. J. Neurophysiol. **44:** 1058–1076.
13. MOSCHOVAKIS, A.K. 1997. The neural integrators of the mammalian saccadic system. Front. Biosci. **2:** 552–577.
14. FUKUSHIMA, K. & C.R. KANEKO. 1995. Vestibular integrators in the oculomotor system. Neurosci. Res. **22:** 249–258.
15. CANNON, S.C. & D.A. ROBINSON. 1987. Loss of the neural integrator of the oculomotor system from brain stem lesions in the monkey. J. Neurophysiol. **57:** 1383–1409.
16. KANEKO, C.R.S. 1997. Eye movement deficits after ibotenic acid lesions of the nucleus prepositus hypoglossi in monkeys. I. Saccades and fixations. J. Neurophysiol. **78:** 1753–1768.
17. ZEE, D., A. YAMAZAKI, P.H. BUTLER & G. GÜCER. 1981. Effects of ablation of flocculus and paraflocculus on eye movements in primate. J. Neurophysiol. **46:** 878–899.
18. LUEBKE, A.E. & D.A. ROBINSON. 1994. Gain changes of the cat's vestibulo-ocular reflex after flocculus deactivation. Exp. Brain Res. **98:** 379–390.
19. CHIN, S., K. FUKUSHIMA, J. FUKUSHIMA, M. KASE & S. OHNO. 2002. Ocular torsion produced by unilateral chemical inactivation of the cerebellar flocculus in alert cats. Curr. Eye Res. **25:** 133–138.
20. CHELAZZI, L., M. GHIRARDI, F. ROSSI, P. STRATA & F. TEMPIA. 1990. Spontaneous saccades and gaze-holding ability in the pigmented rat. II. Effects of localized cerebellar lesions. Eur. J. Neurosci. **2:** 1085–1094.
21. BÜTTNER-ENNEVER, J.A., A.K. HORN & K. SCHMIDTKE. 1989. Cell groups of the medial longitudinal fasciculus and paramedian tracts. Rev. Neurol. (Paris) **145:** 533–539
22. NAKAMAGOE, K., Y. IWAMOTO & K. YOSHIDA. 2000. Evidence for brainstem structures participating in oculomotor integration. Science **288:** 857–859.
23. MCCREA, R.A. & G.T. GDOWSKI. 2003. Firing behaviour of squirrel monkey eye movement-related vestibular nucleus neurons during gaze saccades. J. Physiol. **546:** 207–224.
24. NODA, H. & D.A. SUZUKI. 1979. The role of the flocculus of the monkey in fixation and smooth pursuit eye movements. J. Physiol. **294:** 335–348.
25. LISBERGER, S.G., T.A. PAVELKO & D.M. BROUSSARD. 1994. Responses during eye movements of brain stem neurons that receive monosynaptic inhibition from the flocculus and ventral paraflocculus in monkeys. J. Neurophysiol. **72:** 909–927.
26. SKLAVOS, S.G. & A.K. MOSCHOVAKIS. 2002. Neural network simulations of the primate oculomotor system. IV. A distributed bilateral stochastic model of the neural integrator of the vertical saccadic system. Biol. Cybern. **86:** 97–109.
27. ZEE, D.S., R.J. LEIGH & F. MATHIEU-MILLAIRE. 1980. Cerebellar control of ocular gaze stability. Ann. Neurol. **7:** 37–40.
28. DARLOT, C., L. ZUPAN, O. ETARD, et al. 1996. Computation of inverse dynamics for the control of movements. Biol. Cybern. **75:** 173–186.
29. YAMAMOTO, K., Y. KOBAYASHI, A. TAKEMURA, et al. 2000. A mathematical analysis of the characteristics of the system connecting the cerebellar ventral paraflocculus and extraoculomotor nucleus of alert monkeys during upward ocular following responses. Neurosci. Res. **38:** 425–435.
30. NODA, H. & D.A. SUZUKI. 1979. The role of the flocculus of the monkey in saccadic eye movements. J. Physiol. **294:** 317–334.
31. MOSCHOVAKIS, A.K., C.A. SCUDDER & S.M. HIGHSTEIN. 1996. The microscopic anatomy and physiology of the mammalian saccadic system. Prog. Neurobiol. **50:** 133–254.
32. SCUDDER, C.A., C.R. KANEKO & A.F. FUCHS. 2002. The brainstem generator for saccadic eye movements: a modern synthesis. Exp. Brain Res. **142:** 439–462.
33. SPARKS, D.L. 2002. The brainstem control of saccadic eye movements. Nat. Rev. Neurosci. **3:** 952–964.

34. KLIER, E.M., H. WANG & J.D. CRAWFORD. 2001. The superior colliculus encodes gaze commands in retinal coordinates. Nat. Neurosci. **4:** 627–632.
35. BERGERON, A., S. MATSUO & D. GUITTON. 2003. Superior colliculus encodes distance to target, not saccade amplitude, in multi-step gaze shifts. Nat. Neurosci. **6:** 404–413.
36. KELLER, E.L., N.J. GANDHI & J. M. SHIEH. 1996. Endpoint accuracy in saccades interrupted by stimulation of the omnipause region in the monkey. Vis. Neurosci. **13:** 1059–1067.
37. TAKAGI, M., D.S. ZEE & R.J. TAMARGO. 1998. Effects of lesions of the oculomotor vermis on eye movements in primate: saccades. J. Neurophysiol. **80:** 1911–1931.
38. BÜTTNER, U. & A. STRAUBE. 1995. The effect of cerebellar midline lesions on eyemovements. Neuro-Ophthalmol. **15:** 75–82.
39. ROBINSON, F.R., A. STRAUBE & A.F. FUCHS. 1993. Role of the caudal fastigial nucleus in saccade generation. II. Effects of muscimol inactivation. J. Neurophysiol. **70:** 1741–1758.
40. GOFFART, L. & D. PÉLISSON. 1998. Orienting gaze shifts during muscimol inactivation of caudal fastigial nucleus in the cat. I. Gaze dysmetria. J. Neurophysiol. **79:** 1942–1958.
41. IWAMOTO, Y. & K. YOSHIDA. 2002. Saccadic dysmetria following inactivation of the primate fastigial oculomotor region. Neurosci. Lett. **325:** 211–215.
42. QUAIA, C., P. LEFEVRE & L.M. OPTICAN. 1999. Model of the control of saccades by superior colliculus and cerebellum. J. Neurophysiol. **82:** 999–1018.
43. GOFFART, L., A. GUILLAUME & D. PÉLISSON. 1998. Compensation for gaze perturbation during inactivation of the caudal fastigial nucleus in the head-unrestrained cat. J. Neurophysiol. **80:** 1552–1557.
44. CRANDALL, W.F. & E.L. KELLER. 1985. Visual and oculomotor signals in nucleus reticularis tegmenti pontis in alert monkey. J. Neurophysiol. **54:** 1326–1345.
45. HELMCHEN, C. & U. BÜTTNER. 1995. Saccade-related Purkinje cell activity in the oculomotor vermis during spontaneous eye movements in light and darkness. Exp. Brain Res. **103:** 198–208.
46. OHTSUKA, K. & H. NODA. 1995. Discharge properties of Purkinje cells in the oculomotor vermis during visually guided saccades in the macaque monkey. J. Neurophysiol. **74:** 1828–1840.
47. THIER, P., P.W. DICKE, R. HAAS & S. BARASH. 2000. Encoding of movement time by populations of cerebellar Purkinje cells. Nature **405:** 72–76.
48. NODA, H., S. SUGITA & Y. IKEDA. 1990. Afferent and efferent connections of the oculomotor region of the fastigial nucleus in the macaque monkey. J. Comp. Neurol. **302:** 330–348.
49. YAMADA, J. & H. NODA. 1987. Afferent and efferent connections of the oculomotor vermis in the macaque monkey. J. Comp. Neurol. **265:** 224–241.
50. SCUDDER, C.A. 2002. Role of the fastigial nucleus in controlling horizontal saccades during adaptation. Ann. N.Y. Acad. Sci. **978:** 63–78.
51. ROBINSON, F.R., A.F. FUCHS & C.T. NOTO. 2002. Cerebellar influences on saccade plasticity. Ann. N.Y. Acad. Sci. **956:** 155–163.
52. GALIANA, H.L. & D. GUITTON. 1992. Central organization and modeling of eye-head coordination during orienting gaze shifts. Ann. N.Y. Acad. Sci. **656:** 452–471.
53. ARAI, K., S. DAS, E.L. KELLER & E. AIYOSHI. 1999. A distributed model of the saccade system: simulations of temporally perturbed saccades using position and velocity feedback. Neural Netw. **12:** 1359–1375.
54. SOETEDJO. R., C.R. KANEKO & A.F. FUCHS. 2002. Evidence that the superior colliculus participates in the feedback control of saccadic eye movements. J. Neurophysiol. **87:** 679–695.
55. JÜRGENS, R., W. BECKER & H.H. KORNHUBER. 1981. Natural and drug-induced variations of velocity and duration of human saccadic eye movements: evidence for a control of the neural pulse generator by local feedback. Biol. Cybern. **39:** 87–96.
56. FRENS, M.A. & A.J. VAN OPSTAL. 1997. Monkey superior colliculus activity during short-term saccadic adaptation. Brain Res. Bull. **43:** 473–483.

57. DEAN, P. 1995. Modelling the role of the cerebellar fastigial nuclei in producing accurate saccades: the importance of burst timing. Neuroscience **68:** 1059–1077.
58. KLEINE J., Y.F. GUAN, S. LANGER, H. STRAKA, T. TCHELIDZE & U. BÜTTNER. 2002. Discharge properties of saccade-related neurons in the oculomotor region of the primate fastigial nucleus. Ann. N.Y. Acad. Sci. **987:** 526–528.
59. OHTSUKA, K. & H. NODA. 1992. Burst discharges of mossy fibers in the oculomotor vermis of macaque monkeys during saccadic eye movements. Neurosci. Res. **15:** 102–114.
60. SUGITA, S. & H. NODA. 1991. Pathways and terminations of axons arising in the fastigial oculomotor region of macaque monkeys. Neurosci. Res. **10:** 118–136.
61. SATO, A. & K. OHTSUKA. 1996. Projection from the accommodation-related area in the superior colliculus of the cat. J. Comp. Neurol. **367:** 465–476.
62. MOSCHOVAKIS, A.K. 1996. The superior colliculus and eye movement control. Curr. Opin. Neurobiol. **6:** 811–816.
63. SPARKS, D.L. 1999. Conceptual issues related to the role of the superior colliculus in the control of gaze. Curr. Opin. Neurobiol. **9:** 698–707.
64. MUNOZ, D.P., D. PELISSON & D. GUITTON. 1991. Movement of neural activity on the superior colliculus motor map during gaze shifts. Science **251:** 1358–1360.
65. DROULEZ, J. & A. BERTHOZ. 1991. A neural network model of sensoritopic maps with predictive short-term memory properties. Proc. Natl. Acad. Sci. USA **88:** 9653–9657.

Saccade Dysmetria during Functional Perturbation of the Caudal Fastigial Nucleus in the Monkey

LAURENT GOFFART,[a] LONGTANG L. CHEN,[b] AND DAVID L. SPARKS[b]

[a]INSERM U534, Bron, France

[b]Division of Neuroscience, Baylor College of Medicine, Houston, Texas 77030, USA

ABSTRACT: The caudal fastigial nucleus (cFN) is the output nucleus by which the medioposterior cerebellum influences the brainstem saccade generator. In the monkey, inactivation of one cFN by local injection of muscimol impairs all saccades: ipsiversive saccades become hypermetric, contraversive saccades become hypometric, and saccades aimed at a target located in the upper or lower visual fields are biased horizontally toward the injected side. The pharmacological action of muscimol does not allow deficits that are presaccadic to be distinguished from those occurring during saccade execution. To determine the interval during which altered cFN activity affects saccade accuracy, we applied low-frequency electrical microstimulation (100 Hz for 100–300 ms) to the cFN of three monkeys while they were making saccades toward a flashed target. Similar to the effect of muscimol injection in cFN, low-frequency microstimulation biased all saccades toward the ipsilateral side. When the microstimulation was applied after target flash and before saccade onset, the ipsilateral bias was absent. However, when the stimulation was applied during the ongoing movement, the saccade trajectory was biased toward the stimulated side. The muscimol-like effect of the microstimulation suggests that the stimulation inhibits cFN activity, possibly by recruiting the inhibitory afferents from the cerebellar vermis (axons of Purkinje cells). Low-frequency microstimulation had to be applied during the saccade to bias its trajectory. These data suggest that the ipsilateral horizontal bias observed during muscimol inactivation results from an imbalance in the intrasaccadic activity between the two caudal fastigial nuclei.

KEYWORDS: saccades; cerebellum; fastigial; reversible inactivation; microstimulation; monkey

INTRODUCTION

The medioposterior cerebellum is one of the most important brain regions involved in the transformation of target-related visual signals into motor commands that move the line of sight accurately toward the target location. Indeed, damage of this cerebellar region severely impairs the accuracy of goal-directed gaze shifts (for

Address for correspondence: Laurent Goffart, Ph.D., INSERM U534, 16 avenue Doyen Lépine, 69500 Bron, France. Voice: 33 472 91 34 01; fax: 33 472 91 34 03.
goffart@lyon.inserm.fr

review, see Robinson and Fuchs[1] and Pélisson and colleagues[2]). The medioposterior cerebellum consists of the lobules VIc–VII in the vermis and of their two output nuclei: the caudal fastigial nuclei.

In the head-restrained monkey, the unilateral disinhibition of neuronal activity in the caudal fastigial nucleus (cFN) by local injection of bicuculline[3] or by lesion of the vermal lobules VI–VII[4] impairs the accuracy of visually triggered saccades. Saccades toward the disinhibited side (ipsiversive saccades) become hypometric, and saccades toward the opposite side (contraversive saccades) become hypermetric. Conversely, the inactivation of the cFN by local injection of muscimol leads to hypermetric ipsiversive saccades and hypometric contraversive saccades.[5–7] In the head-unrestrained cat, after unilateral injection of muscimol in the cFN, ipsiversive combined eye-head gaze shifts become hypermetric, and contraversive ones become hypometric,[8,9] without change in the contribution of the head to the overall gaze displacement.[10]

Although most cFN neurons show a steady firing rate during intersaccadic intervals, the dysmetria observed during muscimol injection in the cFN has been proposed to result from the suppression of saccade-related bursts of activity in cFN.[11–13] According to this hypothesis, the hypermetria of ipsiversive saccades would be due to the suppression of the burst generated during the late period of the saccades, whereas the hypometria of contraversive saccades would be due to the suppression of the burst that precedes the onset of saccades.

An alternative hypothesis, based on several observations made in the head-unrestrained cat, has been proposed to account for the dysmetria resulting from unilateral muscimol injections into cFN. According to this hypothesis, the dysmetria results from an impaired specification of the movement metrics *prior to* movement onset, rather than an intrasaccadic deficit. Indeed, the observation of misdirected and inappropriately initiated ipsiversive gaze shifts suggests more than a deficit in the control of movement deceleration.[8,9] All these ipsiversive gaze shifts overshoot the target, producing a constant horizontal error: the endpoints are horizontally shifted with respect to the target position, irrespective of the starting gaze position. Moreover, no consistent modifications in the dynamics of the eye, head, and gaze displacements or in the eye-head coupling are observed. Occasional muscimol-induced modifications in dynamics are unrelated to the magnitude of the dysmetria.[10] Finally, changes in the latency of the gaze and head displacements during cFN inactivation[14] or after ablation in the oculomotor vermis[4] support the idea of a deficit unfolding prior to movement onset.

Some observations in the head-restrained monkey suggest that muscimol injection in the cFN can lead to deficits in the primate that are similar to those observed in the cat. In particular, saccades initiated from various eccentric eye positions and aimed at a visual target located straight ahead all end at approximately the same final position, one that is horizontally shifted relative to the target. This is very reminiscent of the constant horizontal error observed in the cat (see Figure 2H in the article by Ohtsuka and colleagues[6]).

PERTURBING THE CAUDAL FASTIGIAL NUCLEUS BY LOCAL INJECTION OF MUSCIMOL

The effects of inactivating the saccade-related area in the cFN was studied in three head-restrained monkeys to determine if saccades initiated from various start-

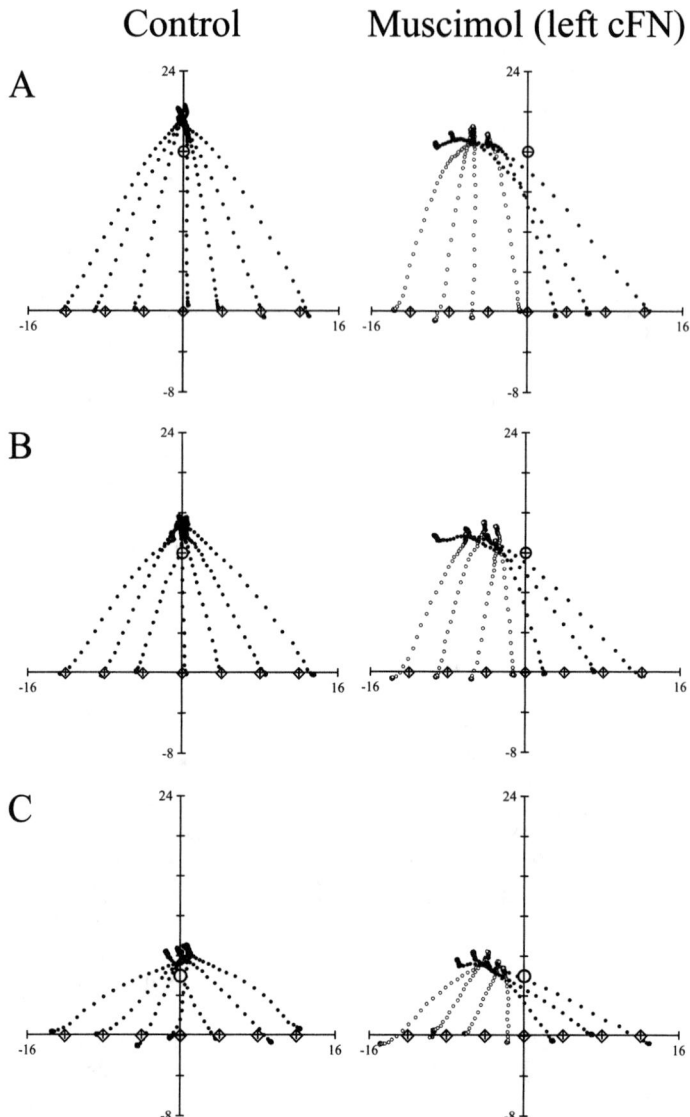

FIGURE 1. Effects on saccade direction and amplitude of perturbation of the cFN by local injection of muscimol. The saccades were aimed at flashed (duration = 100 ms) target LEDs (circles) located (**A**) 16°, (**B**) 12°, or (**C**) 6° on the vertical meridian. Variation in the starting position of the eyes was obtained by using seven different fixation LEDs (diamonds): ±12°, ±8°, ±4°, and 0° along the horizontal meridian. For clarity, saccades starting from fixation LEDs located to the left are plotted with a different symbol (open) from those starting from fixation LEDs located to the right (filled). Volume injected: 0.8 µL (1 µg/µL).

ing positions and aimed at the same visual target missed the target with a similar constant horizontal error. FIGURE 1 shows the effect of injecting a small volume of muscimol in the cFN on the trajectories of representative saccades initiated from various starting positions along the horizontal meridian and aimed at a brief target light-emitting diode (LED) (duration = 100 ms). Target LEDs (circles) were located 16° (A), 12° (B), or 6° (C) on the vertical meridian (FIG. 1A–C, respectively). The left panel shows the fixation and the saccade performance before the injection (control). After muscimol injection in the left cFN (right panel), a leftward offset in starting eye position was observed when the animal was viewing the fixation LEDs. This fixation offset was to the right following the injection in the right cFN (results not shown, but see Robinson and colleagues[5] and Goffart and Pélisson[9]). With respect to saccades toward the 16° upward target (FIG. 1A), the horizontal component of leftward (ipsiversive) saccades was too large, whereas the horizontal component of rightward (contraversive) saccades was too short to acquire the target. Moreover, after the muscimol injection, the initial direction of saccades starting from the straight-ahead fixation LED was to the left, and saccades in this direction increased, rather than decreased, the horizontal distance between gaze and target positions. Saccades initiated from the 4° leftward fixation LED had no rightward component even though the target for these trials was located more than 4° to the right. Saccades starting from fixation LEDs located further to the left had *less* of a rightward initial direction than would be required for target acquisition. The amplitude of their horizontal component was hypometric. The initial direction of saccades starting from fixation LEDs located to the right had *more* of a leftward component than that required to look to the target. The amplitude of the horizontal component was hypermetric with an overshoot that increased with more eccentric starting position (or with larger horizontal target eccentricity). Similar effects upon the initial direction were apparent for saccades directed to the 12° and 6° targets (FIG. 1B, C, respectively). However, when the vertical eccentricity of the target was reduced, the horizontal error at the end of the saccades was also significantly reduced (-3.9 ± 0.7, -2.9 ± 0.7, and $-1.9 \pm 0.5°$ for targets 16°, 12°, and 6° upward, respectively; Mann–Whitney U test, $P < 0.01$ for each comparison). The endpoints of saccades starting from the straight-ahead fixation LED were offset relative to the target with a magnitude that increased with the vertical target eccentricity (see also Iwamoto[7]). Moreover, when the saccades initiated from the most eccentric fixation LEDs to the left ($-8°$ or $-12°$) were examined, the amplitudes of their horizontal components were larger when the vertical target position decreased from 16° to 6° upward.

In summary, saccades initiated from various starting positions did not end at the same final eye position that was shifted relative to the target location by a constant horizontal error. Rather, ipsiversive saccades missed the target with a horizontal error that increased as the eccentric starting deviation of the eyes in the orbit increased and, concomitantly, as horizontal target eccentricity and saccade duration increased. Statistical analysis indicates that the horizontal error of oblique ipsiversive saccades aimed at target with similar eccentricity (for example, 12° leftward and upward) was not statistically different between saccades initiated from the 12° eccentric fixation LED and saccades initiated from the central fixation LED (Mann–Whitney U test, P level >0.10). Contraversive saccades toward one given target seemed to reach the same final eye position, but the location of saccade endpoints was different for different targets.

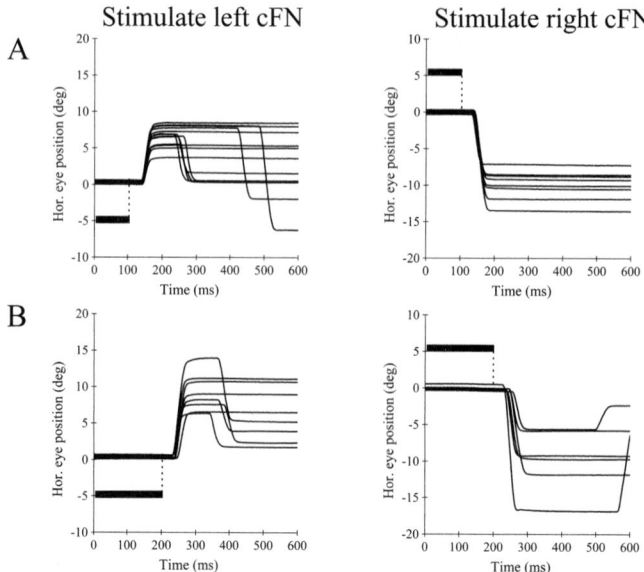

FIGURE 2. Electrical microstimulation of the dorsocaudal portion of the fastigial nucleus. The stimulation train (*black horizontal bar*; 100-Hz, 0.2-ms pulse; duration = 100 ms in **A**, 200 ms in **B**) was applied while the animal was waiting for the appearance of a visual target. Current intensity was 35 µA and 20 µA for the left cFN and right cFN of the same animal, respectively.

PERTURBING THE CAUDAL FASTIGIAL NUCLEUS BY LOW-FREQUENCY ELECTRICAL MICROSTIMULATION

From the inactivation data, it is impossible to determine whether the dysmetria is due to presaccadic or intrasaccadic imbalances in the activity of the two cFNs. Thus, we developed a technique that allowed more transient inhibition of the activity of one cFN. This technique relies on the assumption that electrical microstimulation of the dorsocaudal portion of the fastigial nucleus inhibits cFN neurons by activating the inhibitory axons of Purkinje cells from the vermis.[15] By manipulating the duration of the microstimulation and its delay with respect to the target presentation, we were able to determine the critical period during which cFN activity influences saccade accuracy within the time interval between the onset of the target and the end of the saccade.

FIGURE 2 illustrates the effect of microstimulating the dorsocaudal portion of the left and right fastigial nucleus with a 100-Hz train during a gap interval (500 ms) when the animal was waiting for the appearance of a visual target. Eye position was stable during the entire period of microstimulation (black horizontal bar; duration = 100 ms in FIG. 2A, 200 ms in FIG. 2B), but a "rebound" saccade was generated 40 to 60 ms after the offset of the microstimulation train. This rebound saccade was always directed toward the side contralateral to the stimulated side, that is, rightward

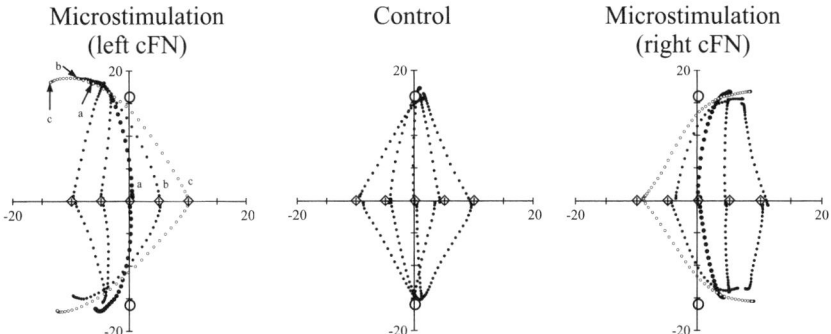

FIGURE 3. Effects on saccade direction and amplitude produced by microstimulation of the cFN. Saccades were directed toward a brief target (circles; duration = 100 ms) presented 16° above or below the central fixation LED. The stimulation train was synchronized with respect to the target offset. It overlapped the interval during which the line of sight was moving toward the target. Variations in the horizontal starting position of the eyes were obtained by using five different fixation LEDs (diamonds): ±10°; ±5°, and 0° along the horizontal meridian. Stimulation parameters for left cFN (same site as in FIG. 2, *left panels*): 100 Hz, 100 or 200 ms, 20 µA; stimulation parameters for right cFN: 100 Hz, 300 ms, 100 µA.

when the left cFN was stimulated (left panels in FIG. 2), and leftward when the right cFN was stimulated (right panels in FIG. 2). Previous work has shown that contralateral saccades are also evoked by microstimulating the axons of cFN neurons.[15] The contralateral saccades illustrated in FIGURE 2 could thus result from the rebound depolarization and spike bursting by cFN neurons following a prolonged microstimulation-induced hyperpolarization.[16] When applied while the monkey was preparing a goal-directed saccade, the microstimulation train had an effect on saccade trajectory that did indeed suggest that the microstimulation inhibits the activity in the cFN.

FIGURE 3 shows the effect of a microstimulation train at 100 Hz on the trajectory of saccades initiated from different horizontal starting positions and aimed at a brief target (duration = 100 ms) presented either 16° upward or downward. The stimulation was synchronized with target offset. The rebound saccades were generated after the saccades shown (and elicited after stimulation offset) and removed for clarity. Like the muscimol injection in the cFN (see FIG. 1), the trajectory of saccades was biased toward the perturbed side; the horizontal component of all saccades was impaired without change in the vertical component. The horizontal component of ipsiversive saccades was hypermetric, whereas for contraversive saccades it was hypometric. The greater the target eccentricity relative to the starting eye position, the larger the hypermetria of ipsiversive saccades. The muscimol-like effect of the microstimulation on visually triggered saccades strongly suggests that the stimulation inhibits the activity of cFN neurons by recruiting the inhibitory influence of Purkinje cells axons innervating the nucleus, a conclusion that is in accordance with conclusions reached by Noda's group.[15]

FIGURE 4 shows the effect of varying the interval during which the microstimulation was applied upon the trajectory and the accuracy of saccades. In the trials

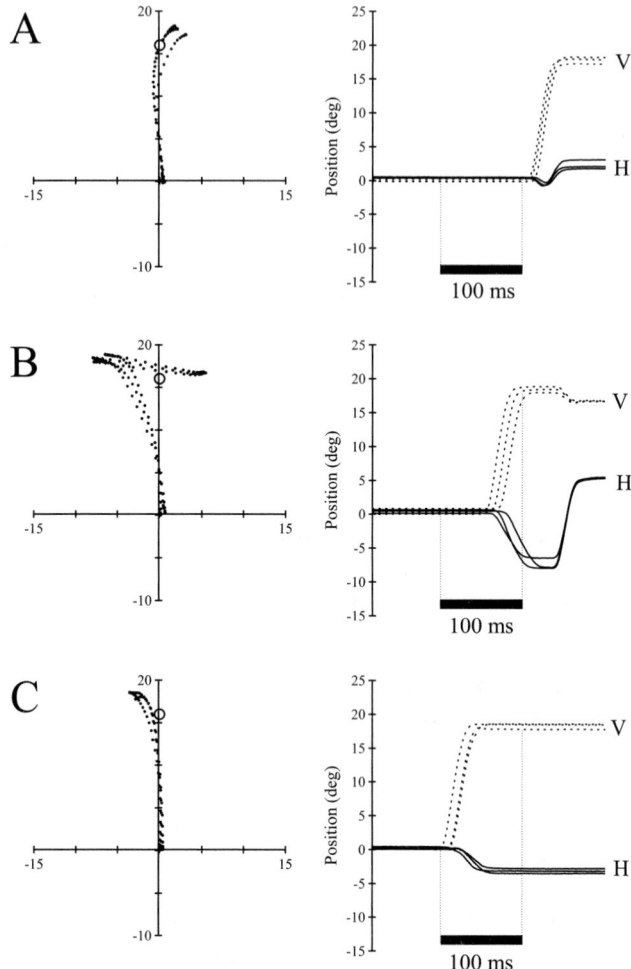

FIGURE 4. Effects of varying the period of stimulation within the target-offset/saccade-end interval. The fixation LED was located straight ahead, and the target LED was flashed 16° above the fixation stimulus. The microstimulation (*black horizontal bar*; 100-Hz, 0.2-ms pulse; 100-ms duration; 45 µA) was applied (**A**) immediately, (**B**) 50 ms, or (**C**) 100 ms after the target LED was extinguished. The *x–y* plots of eye position are shown on the left, and plots of horizontal (H) and vertical (V) eye positions as a function of time are shown on the right. The *black horizontal bar* represents the period when microstimulation was delivered. The traces are aligned on the onset of the microstimulation train.

shown as examples, the fixation LED was located straight ahead, and the target LED was flashed 16° above the fixation LED. The microstimulation was applied immediately, 50 ms, or 100 ms (FIG. 4A–C, respectively) after the target LED was extinguished. The stimulation duration was set to 100 ms so that on some trials it could be restricted to the period prior to saccade initiation. In that particular case (FIG. 4A), only small effects on vertical saccades were observed: a slight final deviation away from the stimulation side occurred. When the microstimulation was applied during the overall saccade period (FIG. 4B), a much larger leftward bias was observed in the trajectory. A rightward rebound saccade immediately followed the stimulation offset. The ipsilateral bias in saccade trajectory was less important when the microstimulation was applied slightly before saccade onset (FIG. 4C). The figure also shows that the amount of microstimulation (duration) applied before (up to 10 ms before) the saccade was launched toward the visual target is not critical in determining the amount of deviation in saccade trajectory.

CONCLUSION

Low-frequency microstimulation of the dorsocaudal portion of the fastigial nucleus biases the trajectory of saccades toward the stimulated side. This effect is similar to the effect of muscimol injection in the cFN. The microstimulation must be applied during the saccade to bias its trajectory (see also Keller and colleagues[17]). More experiments using a larger range of intervals between stimulation onset and saccade onset are needed. But when an efferent delay of approximately 10 ms is taken into account, our data suggest that it is only the microstimulation immediately before saccade onset and during the execution period that is effective in modifying the trajectory of a saccade.

Further experiments are required to verify that these conclusions also hold in the head-unrestrained monkey. If so, the particular dysmetria observed in the head-unrestrained cat[9] may be due to the nature of the behavioral responses evoked by the target. Indeed, in the cat experiments, the food target was triggering an orienting gaze shift but also an orienting movement of the mouth (and thus of the head). In the monkey experiments, target acquisition required only a shift of the line of sight.

ACKNOWLEDGMENTS

We thank Kathy Pearson for invaluable programming assistance. This work was supported by the National Institutes of Health (EY02520, EY01189 to D.L.S. and EY13444 to L.L.C.); the Human Frontier Science Program (LT 59/96); and the Centre National de la Recherche Scientifique (to L.G.).

REFERENCES

1. ROBINSON, F.R. & A.F. FUCHS. 2001. The role of the cerebellum in voluntary eye movements. Annu. Rev. Neurosci. **24:** 981–1004.
2. PÉLISSON, D., L. GOFFART & A. GUILLAUME. 2003. Control of saccadic eye movements and combined eye/head gaze shifts by the medio-posterior cerebellum. Prog. Brain Res. **142:** 69–89.

3. SATO, H. & H. NODA. 1992. Saccadic dysmetria induced by transient functional decortication of the cerebellar vermis. Exp. Brain Res. **88:** 455–458.
4. TAKAGI, M., D.S. ZEE & R.J. TAMARGO. 1998. Effects of lesions of the oculomotor vermis on eye movements in primate: saccades. J. Neurophysiol. **80:** 1911–1931.
5. ROBINSON, F.R., A. STRAUBE & A.F. FUCHS. 1993. Role of the caudal fastigial nucleus in saccade generation. II. Effects of muscimol inactivation. J. Neurophysiol. **70:** 1741–1758.
6. OHTSUKA, K., H. SATO & H. NODA. 1994. Saccadic burst neurons in the fastigial nucleus are not involved in compensating for orbital nonlinearities. J. Neurophysiol. **71:** 1976–1980.
7. IWAMOTO, Y. 2002. Saccadic dysmetria following inactivation of the primate fastigial oculomotor region. Neurosci. Lett. **325:** 211–215.
8. GOFFART, L. & D. PÉLISSON. 1994. Cerebellar contribution to the spatial encoding of orienting gaze shifts in the head-free cat. J. Neurophysiol. **72:** 2547–2550.
9. GOFFART, L. & D. PÉLISSON. 1998. Orienting gaze shifts during muscimol inactivation of caudal fastigial nucleus in the cat. I. Gaze dysmetria. J. Neurophysiol. **79:** 1942–1958.
10. GOFFART, L., D. PÉLISSON & A. GUILLAUME. 1998. Orienting gaze shifts during muscimol inactivation of caudal fastigial nucleus in the cat. II. Dynamics and eye-head coupling. J. Neurophysiol. **79:** 1959–1976.
11. OHTSUKA, K. & H. NODA. 1991. Saccadic burst neurons in the oculomotor region of the fastigial nucleus of macaque monkeys. J. Neurophysiol. **65:** 1422–1434.
12. FUCHS, A.F., F.R. ROBINSON & A. STRAUBE. 1993. Role of the caudal fastigial nucleus in saccade generation. I. Neuronal discharge patterns. J. Neurophysiol. **70:** 1712–1740.
13. HELMCHEN, C., A. STRAUBE & U. BÜTTNER. 1994. Saccade-related activity in the fastigial oculomotor region of the macaque monkey during spontaneous eye movements in light and darkness. Exp. Brain Res. **98:** 474–482.
14. GOFFART, L. & D. PÉLISSON. 1997. Changes in initiation of orienting gaze shifts after muscimol inactivation of the caudal fastigial nucleus in the cat. J. Physiol. (Lond.) **503:** 657–671.
15. NODA, H., S. MURAKAMI, J. YAMADA, *et al.* 1988. Saccadic eye movements evoked by microstimulation of the fastigial nucleus of macaque monkeys. J. Neurophysiol. **60:** 1036–1052.
16. AIZENMAN, C.D. & D.J. LINDEN. 1999. Regulation of rebound depolarization and spontaneous firing patterns of deep nuclear neurons in slices of rat cerebellum. J. Neurophysiol. **82:** 1697–1709.
17. KELLER, E.L., D.P. SLAKEY & W.F. CRANDALL. 1983. Microstimulation of the primate cerebellar vermis during saccadic eye movements. Brain Res. **288:** 131–143.

The Role of the Fastigial Nucleus in Saccadic Eye Oscillations

CHRISTOPH HELMCHEN, HOLGER RAMBOLD, CHRISTIAN ERDMANN, CHRISTIAN MOHR, ANDREAS SPRENGER, AND FERDINAND BINKOFSKI

Department of Neurology, University of Lübeck, Lübeck, Germany

ABSTRACT: For the first time, we provide functional magnetic resonance imaging evidence for a recent hypothesis that saccadic oscillations in opsoclonus may result from a disinhibition of the cerebellar fastigial nuclei. Two patients with severe opsoclonus were examined during fixation in the light and during eye closure and in darkness where opsoclonus disappeared. Their activation during opsoclonus was compared with 10 healthy subjects performing visually guided and self-paced saccades in the light and darkness. In contrast to the control subjects, the patients showed a strong bilateral midline cerebellar activation that involved the deep cerebellar nuclei. This is probably not just a secondary finding in the fastigial nuclei due to the high frequent saccadic activity because there was, concomitantly, no oculomotor vermal activation, which is normally seen in healthy subjects. We propose that cerebellar activation of the fastigial nuclei may cause opsoclonus via their projections to the brainstem saccadic generator.

KEYWORDS: opsoclonus; cerebellum; saccades; fastigial nucleus; functional magnetic resonance imaging (fMRI)

INTRODUCTION

Saccadic oscillations without intersaccadic interval are known as ocular flutter, in case of horizontal oscillations, or opsoclonus (OC), if it is multidirectional, that is, if it consists of combined horizontal, vertical, and torsional components. Both disorders extremely impair patients' visual acuity and visual orientation. Little is known about their lesion sites, because conventional imaging studies (MRT and CCT) have largely failed to detect structural brainstem or cerebellar lesions. Moreover, controversy surrounds the pathophysiological causes as to whether ocular flutter and OC are cerebellar or brainstem disorders. According to one hypothesis, the oscillations are caused by a brainstem lesion in the region of the saccade generator,[1,2] whereas other hypotheses attribute them to a form of cerebellar dysmetria.

Address for correspondence: Prof. Dr. Christoph Helmchen, Department of Neurology, University of Lübeck, Ratzeburger Allee 160, D-23538 Lübeck, Germany. Voice: +49-451-500-2927; fax: +49-451-500-2489.

helmchen_ch@neuro.mu-luebeck.de

However, neither focal brainstem[3] nor cerebellar lesions[4–6] have been shown to elicit OC. Recently, new concepts have been suggested to explain OC. These new concepts imply functional rather than structural (lesion) abnormalities.[7,8] Specifically, theoretical considerations as derived from modeling simulations proposed that an activation of the deep cerebellar nuclei, that is, the fastigial oculomotor region (FOR), causes OC.[7]

To elucidate this hypothesis we performed—for the first time—functional magnetic resonance imaging (fMRI) in two patients with OC. Because both patients showed a decrease of or no OC with the eyes closed, there were two conditions of task-related activations in fMRI (open eyes with OC vs. closed eyes without OC), and these were compared with a control group of 10 healthy subjects who performed frequent, self-paced (internally guided), and visually guided saccades of a large amplitude in the light and darkness. Preliminary data have been reported elsewhere.[9]

PATIENTS

A 65-year-old man (patient 1) presented with rapidly progressive dizziness, blurred vision, oscillopsia, and gait unsteadiness. The symptoms deteriorated over 4 weeks. On initial clinical examination 3 days after onset of symptoms, the patient showed intermittent bursts of large conjugate horizontal eye oscillations. They could not be observed when the eyes were closed, but the reoccurred immediately when the patient opened his eyes. At that time, the rest of the patient's oculomotor performance was normal. In addition, he showed severe postural trunk ataxia with only mild bilateral limb ataxia and some mild dysarthria but no myoclonus. Otherwise, the neurological examination was normal. The trunk ataxia deteriorated severely over the next week, preventing walking. Concomitantly, the eye oscillations changed, becoming very large combined vertical, horizontal and torsional oscillations resembling opsoclonus. The patient got relief only by closing his eyes; this stopped the eye oscillations on clinical examination. This opsoclonus was suspected to be of paraneoplastic origin because of a concomitant malignant bladder tumor. Cranial computed tomography (CT) and high-resolution magnetic resonance imaging (MRI) of the brainstem, particularly the pons and cerebellum, did not show any structural lesion.

A 38-year-old woman (patient 2) presented with a 3-day history of rapidly progressive dizziness, fatigue, blurred vision, oscillopsia, and gait unsteadiness. On clinical examination, she initially showed intermittent bursts of only horizontal eye oscillations. Within a few days, she also had large conjugate multidirectional eye oscillations, indicating opsoclonus that decreased but did not completely disappear on eye closure. In particular, the fixation of a target in the light or attempted shifts of fixation vigorously enhanced the opsoclonus. There was severe truncal and limb ataxia (intention tremor) and postural tremor that prevented her from walking and standing upright. There was no evidence of a malignant tumor. Cranial CT and high-resolution MRI of the brainstem and cerebellum did not reveal any structural lesion.

In both patients, routine blood samples and cerebrospinal fluid were normal. Tests included screening for infectious agents, tumor markers, and antineuronal antibodies (Anti-HuD/Ri/Yo, glutamic acid decarboxylase, and Purkinje cells). All tests were negative.

METHODS

Scleral Search-Coil Recordings of Eye and Lid Movements

Binocular three-dimensional eye and lid movements were recorded with the Remmel Search-Coil System (Remmel Labs, Ashland, MD), which has three orthogonal magnetic fields and a frame size of 180 cm^3. After the patients had given their informed consent, scleral search coils (combination annulus) (Skalar, Delft) were placed in each eye following topical anesthesia. Both eyes and the right eyelid were calibrated using a combined offline *in vitro* calibration based on previous studies.[10,11] Rightward, upward, and clockwise directions of eye rotation from the view of the subject were defined as positive.

The subject's head was comfortably stabilized in a natural upright position with a chin rest and a firm head support that kept the forehead stationary. Eye and lid movements were recorded unfiltered with a 16-bit AD converter (PCI 6071E, National Instruments, Munich) at a sampling rate of 600 Hz. After calibration, all position data were filtered by using a 100-Hz (3-dB value) Gaussian filter. Eye velocities were calculated as angular velocities, not derivatives of all eye positions. For visual stimulation, a red laser spot (∅: 0.25 mm) (Lisa Laser Systems, Katlenburg-Lindau. Germany) was front-projected by mirror galvanometers (GSI Lumonics, Munich) onto a flat, white tangent screen that was 145 cm from the subject's eyes. The following paradigms were examined: (1) fixation of gaze straight ahead, (2) spontaneous eye movements in light and darkness, and (3) eye movements during voluntary blinks.

IMAGING STUDIES

Structural MRI was performed on a 1.5-T unit (Siemens Magnetom Symphony, Erlangen, Germany) by using axial T2 Turbo spin echo, diffusion-weighted images of the brainstem, and high-resolution (slice thickness: 3 mm) T1 spin echo before and after contrast (gadolinium) administration. An additional anatomical high-resolution, three-dimensional, T1-weighted GE sequence (TR = 40 ms; TE = 5 ms; matrix size = 256 × 256; slice thickness = 2.5 mm) including the whole brain with cerebellum and brainstem was obtained. The slices of this sequence were aligned to the AC-PC line.

fMRI was conducted in both patients using gradient echo echo-planar (EPI) T2*-sensitive (TR/TE = 187/81 ms per slice; matrix size = 128 × 128; flip angle = 90°; voxel size = 2.0 × 2.0 × 5.0 mm) sequences as previously described.[12,13] For comparison, 10 healthy subjects were investigated (TR = 83 ms per slice, 36 slices; matrix size = 64 × 64; voxel size = 4.0 × 4.0 × 4.0 mm). A standard rf head coil was used and packed with foam pads to reduce the head movement artefacts. In a block design, six alternating periods of baseline (eyes closed, fixation target off) and six of active condition (eyes opened with fixation, opsoclonus) were used, each containing four pulses with a TR of 6 s (healthy subjects: six pulses with a TR of 3 s). This resulted in a total of 48 (114) pulses and an overall measurement time of 288 (342) s. Image analysis was performed using Matlab (Mathworks, Natick, MA) and SPM 99 (Statistical Parametric Mapping package, Wellcome Department of Cognitive Neurology, London).[14] Images of each condition was corrected for head movements. Low-frequency artifacts (aliased cardiac and other cyclical components) and other effects of global volume activity and time were removed as confounding factors using linear regression and sine/cosine functions. After spatial smoothing with a Gaussian kernel of 8 mm was accomplished, a categorical comparison between the baseline and active conditions was calculated using the t-test and the boxcar reference function. Activated voxels passing a statistical significance threshold of $T > 4.79$ ($P < 0.05$ corrected for multiple comparisons) in patients and of $T > 8$ in the healthy subjects, and belonging to a cluster of more than 20 voxels, were considered significant. In the patients, the significantly activated voxels were superimposed on high-resolution magnetic resonance scans of the individual patients. The scans of both patients were normalized into a standard stereotactic space (MNI space). The significantly activated voxels were superimposed onto an MNI template.

The MRI-compatible Eyetracker (Cambridge Research Systems, Rochester, UK) was used as previously described during the fMRI recordings[13,15] to monitor (1) the state of eye closure, (2) the fixation performance, and (3) the saccadic eye oscillations (opsoclonus).

EXPERIMENTAL TASK DURING fMRI

During the scanning procedure, patients were instructed to keep their eyes closed (baseline condition: minor or no opsoclonus) until they received an external signal (tap on the right lower leg) indicating they should open their eyes and fixate the target spots (active condition: opsoclonus). Fixation targets (diameter: 0.36°) were projected onto a transluminant screen in the scanner room by a computer visual stimulus generator. They could be recognized through a mirror that was adjusted over the patient's head. In the dark condition, the strongly dimmed projector was the only light-emitting source in the otherwise completely darkened scanner room.

Ten healthy subjects were examined with the following paradigms: (1) fixation in the light vs. fixation in darkness and (2) horizontal visually guided saccades of 30° in the light vs. in darkness (strongly dimmed room). Eyes closed were taken as resting condition. In addition, horizontal self-paced saccades were examined in two healthy subjects. Target displacements were presented pseudorandomized (fixation periods of excentric targets lasting 800–1500 ms) to prevent anticipatory effects. Using a block design analysis, each paradigm lasted for 18 s and was repeated six times.

RESULTS

Eye Movement Recordings

Binocular three-dimensional scleral search-coil recordings were obtained in both patients. These recordings revealed typical OC.

Patient 1

Three weeks after the onset of oscillopsia, the search-coil recordings showed typical OC with large (up to 50°, on average 30°) vertical, horizontal, and torsional os-

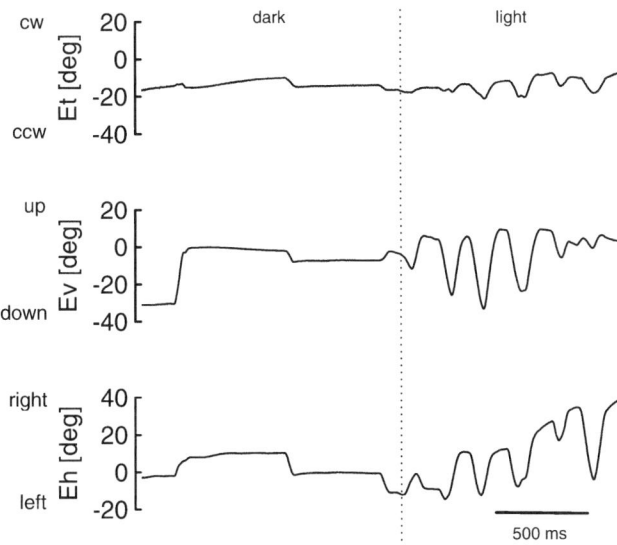

FIGURE 1. Original three-dimensional scleral search-coil recordings of the torsional, vertical, and horizontal eye positions (*from top to bottom*) of patient 1 in darkness and in the light. There is no OC in the dark. In contrast, in the light (onset: *vertical dashed line*) there is profound opsoclonus on fixation in all traces. Eh: horizontal eye position; Ev: vertical eye position; Et: torsional eye position; CW: clockwise; CCW: counterclockwise.

cillations without intersaccadic intervals and variable differences in amplitude. Binocular saccadic oscillations were conjugate, with no phase and amplitude difference between both eyes. There were saccadic oscillations not only on the horizontal and vertical, but also the torsional component (FIG. 1). However, OC only occurred on fixation in the light and disappeared in the dark (FIG. 1) or on eye closure (FIG. 2). In contrast, brief voluntary lid movements or complete blinks were sometimes but in most cases not immediately followed by OC with irregular fixation intervals. Reflexive blinks did not regularly elicit OC. This allowed us to compare two conditions of action in fMRI, that is, eyes closed without OC vs. eyes opened with OC on attempted fixation of gaze straight ahead. In darkness, saccades had normal velocities and did not show OC. Because of the severity of OC, other oculomotor tasks (smooth pursuit and visually guided saccades) could not be tested.

Patient 2

Search-coil recordings of patient 2 were obtained 1 week after the onset of oscillopsia. Opsoclonus was observed with large (up to 30°) conjugate vertical, horizontal, and torsional eye oscillations. On eye closure, OC was diminished, but as soon as the target at gaze straight ahead was fixated, OC immediately reoccurred.

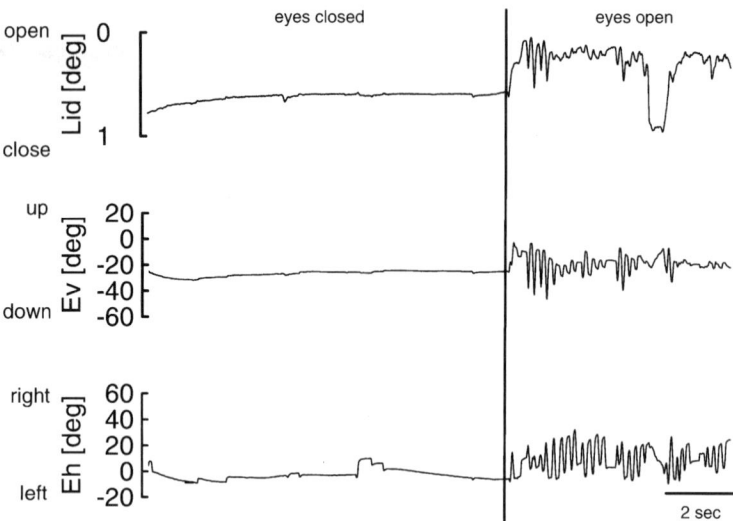

FIGURE 2. Scleral search-coil recordings of the lid position and the vertical and horizontal eye positions (*from top to bottom*) of patient 1 while the eye lids were closed (*left*) and open (*right*) (onset: *vertical line*). There is no OC when the eyes are closed. Eh: horizontal eye position; Ev: vertical eye position; Lid: normalized lid position.

fMRI Recordings

Patients

fMRI recordings in both patients were performed 3 weeks (patient 1) or 2 weeks (patient 2) after the onset of oscillopsia, that is, at a time when OC severely disabled the patients. The Eyetracker revealed reliable intervals of severe opsoclonus in the "open eyes and fixation" condition, whereas there was no OC in patient 1 and only little OC in patient 2 in the "eyes closed" condition. Brainstem activation was absent in both patients, as determined using the threshold at $P < 0.05$ (corrected). In contrast, both patients showed bilateral midline cerebellar activation that involved the deep cerebellar nuclei, including the fastigial nuclei (coordinates according to the MRI atlas of Schmahmann and colleagues[16] for patient 1 ($x = 0$, $y = -54$, $z = -28$ for patient 1; Z-value = 5.25) and for patient 2 ($x = 0$, $y = -56$, $z = -25$; Z-value = 4.85) as presented on individual data sets superimposed on the MNI template ($x = 0$, $y = -54$, $z = -27$) (FIG. 3). Additional cerebellar activation was found more posteriorly, presumably in the left hemispheric lobule VII ($x = -38$, $y = -70$, $z = -32$; Z-value = 4.05) in patient 1, and presumably at vermal lobule IX ($x = 2$, $y = -60$, $z = -40$; Z-value = 3.93) in patient 2, according to the MRI atlas of the human cerebellum.[16]

Healthy Subjects

In the healthy subjects, there was consistent posterior vermis activation (lobules VI and VII, T >10) during self-paced and visually guided (FIG. 4) horizontal saccades, in

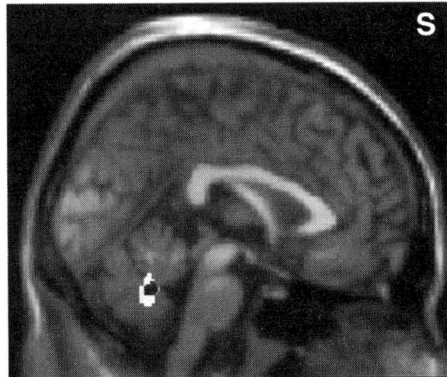
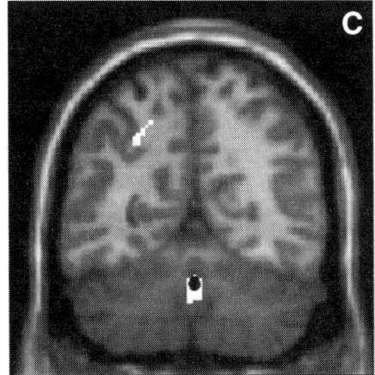
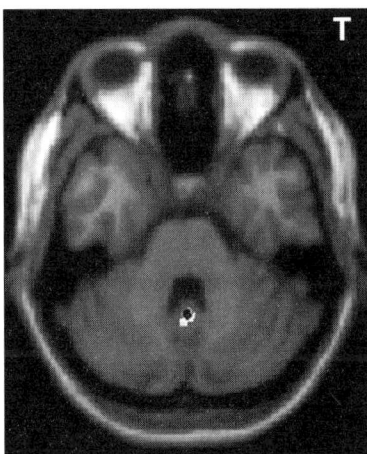

FIGURE 3. fMRI during opsoclonus. With the given thresholds ($P < 0.05$ corrected), activation is found in the cerebellum but not in the pontine brainstem in both patients. Responses in bold are shown on individual brain images for the sagittal (S), coronal (C), and transversal (T) slices at the level of highest activation in the midline cerebellum superimposed on the MNI template for both patients. For better discrimination without color gradients, activation of patient 1 is shown with *white symbols*, and that of patient 2 is shown with *black symbols*. The common midline activation in both patients aligns with the medial deep cerebellar nuclei and involves the fastigial nucleus.

the light (FIG. 4A) and darkness (FIG. 4B). However, with the given threshold (T > 10) there was no activation in the fastigial nuclei during horizontal saccades, neither in the light nor in darkness. In a contrast analysis ($P < 0.05$, random effect analysis) utilizing boxcar function, there was no cerebellar activation, indicating that there is no significant difference in vermal activation between saccades in the light and darkness. In addition, there was activation in vermal lobule IX, bilaterally in the flocculus/paraflocculus complex and bilaterally in hemispheric lobules VI (FIG. 4). There was no pontine brainstem activation (without region of interest analysis). In the fixation-only paradigm, subjects revealed no cerebellar activation when compared with the rest condition (eyes closed).

DISCUSSION

On the basis of our search-coil recordings, we classified the eye oscillations with horizontal and vertical components without intersaccadic intervals in both patients

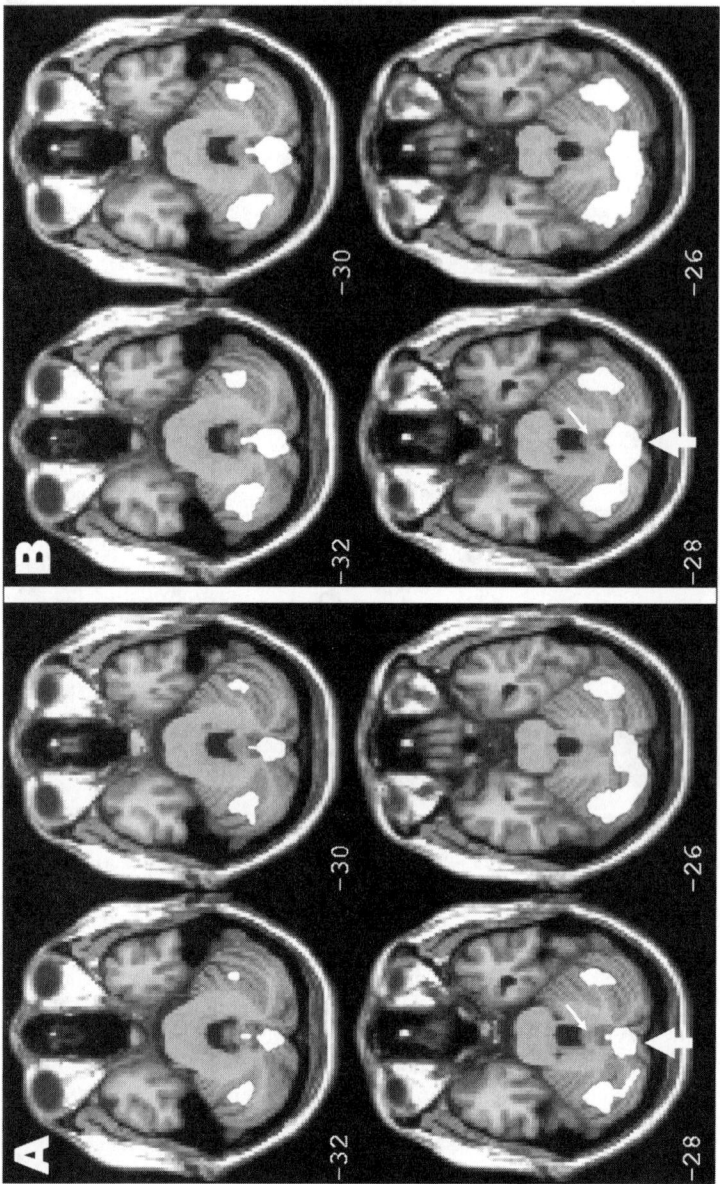

FIGURE 4. fMRI during visually guided saccades in the light (**A**) and darkness (**B**) in healthy subjects (group analysis, $N = 10$) superimposed on the MNI template. Representative transversal slices of the cerebellum are shown (from $z = -32$ to $z = -26$).[16] Activation ($T > 8$) is found in the oculomotor vermis (*thick arrow*), but not in the fastigial nuclei (*thin arrow*). For better black/white discrimination, activations are shown with *white symbols* without gradients of activation.

as OC. The three-dimensional search-coil recordings revealed that oscillations involve the torsional component, indicating that OC is a three-dimensional saccadic disorder.[7] Previous pathohistological,[17,18] imaging,[19] and physiological[20] evidence indicated that saccadic oscillations are caused by cerebellar abnormalities. For the first time, we provide fMRI evidence for a recent hypothesis that saccadic oscillations in opsoclonus may result from a disinhibition of the deep cerebellar nuclei, that is, the fastigial nuclei.[7] These results will be discussed in the light of the fastigial nuclei contribution to saccade generation.

The hallmark of cerebellar saccadic dysfunction known as saccadic step-size dysmetria,[21–23] is largely controlled by saccade-related neurons in the posterior vermis[4,24,25] and the fastigial nuclei.[26,27] The saccade-related neurons in the oculomotor vermis (lobuli VI, VII) project almost exclusively to the caudal part of the fastigial nuclei in the deep cerebellar nuclei, that is, the FOR. The FOR projects to the brainstem saccade generator, that is, the burst neurons in the paramedian pontine reticular formation and the rostral interstitial nucleus of the medial longitudinal fascicle and possibly the omnipause neurons,[28,29] and may thereby influence multidirectional saccade generation in a feedback loop.[30] The vermis-nucleus fastigii complex accelerates and decelerates saccades in a direction-specific manner[5,31] by augmenting the ongoing discharge of pontine excitatory and inhibitory burst neurons,[26] thus ensuring saccadic accuracy. Accordingly, unilateral lesions of the oculomotor vermis[4,5] and fastigial nuclei[6] cause direction-specific saccade dysmetria: unilateral lesions of the FOR elicit ipsilesional hypermetric and contralesional hypometric saccades. Bilateral FOR inactivations (muscimol) lead to bilateral saccadic hypermetria[6] but no saccadic oscillations.

The cerebellum is thought to be part of a feedback-control system. The capacity of the cerebellum to produce saccadic oscillations crucially depends on its location within the feedback loop of the saccade generation. However, controversy surrounds the question as to whether the cerebellum is embedded in a feedback or feedforward mechanism impinging on the brainstem burst generator.[32] The cerebellum can only affect saccade size in a feedback-controlled system if it is part of the feedback loop or influences the feedback gain of current eye displacement. Increasing the saccadic gain in models of the saccade generation may elicit macrosaccadic oscillations,[20] but they still have preserved intersaccadic intervals, indicating a form of saccadic pulse dysmetria. In contrast, OC is defined as eye oscillation without intersaccadic intervals. Recently, it has been proposed that a disinhibition of the FOR in combination with an increase in the gain *and* central delay of a saccade will eventually lead to saccadic oscillations.[7]

Using fMRI, we identified activation in the caudal midline cerebellum, involving the medial deep cerebellar nuclei, that is, the fastigial nuclei, and possibly the vermal lobules VIII and IX according to the atlas of Schmahmann and colleagues.[16]

Although the area of activation is larger than the size of the fastigial nuclei, which is at least in part due to the spatial filter used (methods), we suggest that it is the fastigial nuclei that are most likely to be involved in OC because the neighboring structures are not known to contain saccade-related neurons. However, the fastigial nuclei are quite small, which is probably the reason why our study with healthy subjects and the two previous fMRI studies[33,34] focusing on cerebellar activation have failed to identify activation in the deep cerebellar nuclei (fastigial nuclei) during voluntary, highly frequent, self-paced, as well as visually guided saccades and reflexive saccades during optokinetic stimulation. Both the fastigial nuclei and the brainstem generator have to be active during saccades, but the resolution capacity is yet not appropriate to demonstrate their fMRI activity under normal conditions. Thus, the fastigial nuclei activation in our patients is likely to be considerable larger than during saccades in normal subjects. It is therefore probably not just a secondary finding. Unfortunately, rapid oscillations, such as those in voluntary nystagmus, with frequencies and amplitudes haracteristic of OC, can hardly be produced voluntarily or reflexively. Therefore, they cannot reliably be studied in healthy controls. More important, oculomotor vermal activation, which was consistently found in normal subjects (our data and those of Stephan and colleagues[33]), was absent in OC patients. This is further evidence for the hypothesis that the fastigial nuclei are disinhibited. Whether this disinhibition is due to posterior oculomotor vermal dysfunction, for example, by paraneoplastic Purkinje cell lesions, remains to be shown.

Pathophysiologically, OC is thought to be caused by the inappropriate, repetitive, and alternating discharge pattern of different burst neurons in the brainstem saccadic burst generator.[35] Thus, saccadic oscillations require (1) an abnormally high discharge of burst neurons, (2) a central delay, or (3) abnormalities of the omnipause neurons (OPNs).[35] The OPNs in the caudal pons[36] control saccadic burst neurons that generate horizontal and vertical saccades. Thus, during fixation, OPNs are active and inhibit burst neurons and therefore prevent saccades. Physiological inhibition of OPNs, for example, by blinking,[37,38] and dysfunction of OPNs in disease may therefore lead to involuntary saccadic oscillations.[1,39] However, experimental lesions of OPNs elicited slowing of horizontal saccades but did not cause OC,[3] and histopathologically OPNs were not affected in patients with OC.[7,40]

FOR neurons meet these criteria in two ways: they have excitatory projections to most of the excitatory and inhibitory burst neurons and may inhibit OPNs.[29] Thus, FOR activation may be twofold: it directly drives excitatory and inhibitory burst neurons to an abnormally high but alternating discharge rate, and in addition, it may (sparse projection[28,29]) inhibit OPNs, an action that leads to a disinhibition of the saccadic burst neurons. In this way FOR, activation could elicit variable saccadic oscillation not only in the horizontal but also in the vertical and presumably torsional planes through its projections to the midbrain saccade generator for vertical and torsional saccades.

Vermal dysfunction with subsequent FOR disinhibition alone may not be sufficient to cause OC because, for example, vermal ablations do not elicit OC. Thus, an additional signal may be required either from climbing fibers or mossy fibers. This may be a visual signal because of the dependence of OC on visual mechanisms in our patients, mechanisms that could directly shut down the vermis. This is compatible with the fact that the oculomotor vermis[24] and FOR[27] saccade-related activity is strongly reduced in darkness, although we were unable to demonstrate this difference in activation between saccades in the light and in a strongly dimmed room using fMRI. The oculomotor vermis and FOR receive afferents from the pontine nuclei and the nucleus reticularis tegmenti pontis.[28,41,42] Both the lack of inhibitory signals from the oculomotor vermal Purkinje cells and also the presumably excitatory signals from the mossy fiber collaterals to the FOR[31] might lead to the excessive FOR activation.

Finally, the fastigial nuclei activation might in addition fascilitate brainstem postinhibitory rebound firing as one contributing factor in the development of saccadic oscillations.[8]

ACKNOWLEDGMENT

This work was supported by the Deutsche Forschungsgemeinschaft.

REFERENCES

1. ZEE, D.S. & D.A. ROBINSON. 1979. A hypothetical explanation of saccadic oscillations. Ann. Neurol. **5:** 405–414.
2. SCHON, F., T.L. HODGSON, D. MORT & C. KENNARD. 2001. Ocular flutter associated with a localized lesion in the paramedian pontine reticular formation. Ann. Neurol. **50:** 413–416.
3. KANEKO, C.R. 1996. Effect of ibotenic acid lesions of the omnipause neurons on saccadic eye movements in rhesus macaques. J. Neurophysiol. **75:** 2229–2242.
4. SATO, H. & H. NODA. 1992. Saccadic dysmetria induced by transient functional decortication of the cerebellar vermis. Exp. Brain Res. **88:** 455–458.
5. TAKAGI, M., D.S. ZEE & R.J. TAMARGO. 1998. Effects of lesions of the oculomotor vermis on eye movements in primate: saccades. J. Neurophysiol. **80:** 1911–1931.
6. ROBINSON, F.R., A. STRAUBE & A.F. FUCHS. 1993. Role of the caudal fastigial nucleus in saccade generation. II. Effects of muscimol inactivation. J. Neurophysiol. **70:** 1741–1758.
7. WONG, A.M., S. MUSALLAM, R.D. TOMLINSON, et al. 2001. Opsoclonus in three dimensions: oculographic, neuropathologic and modelling correlates. J. Neurol. Sci. **189:** 71–81.
8. RAMAT, S., R.J. LEIGH, D.S. ZEE & L.M. OPTICAN. 2002. Coupling and post-inhibitory rebound firing in brain stem excitatory and inhibitory burst neurons may explain high-frequency saccadic oscillations. Soc. Neurosci. Abstr. 716.7.
9. HELMCHEN, C., H. RAMBOLD, A. SPRENGER, et al. 2003. Cerebellar activation in opsoclonus: an fMRI study. Neurology **61:** 412–415.
10. TWEED, D. & T. VILIS. 1987. Implication of rotational kinematic for the oculomotor system in three dimensions J. Neurophysiol. **58:** 832–849.
11. RAMBOLD, H., W. HEIDE, A. SPRENGER, et al. 2001. Perilymph fistula associated with pulse-synchronous eye oscillations. Neurology **56:** 1769–1771.
12. BINKOFSKI, F., G. BUCCINO, S. POSSE, et al. 1999. A fronto-parietal circuit for object manipulation in man: evidence from an fMRI-study. Eur. J. Neurosci. **11:** 3276–3286.
13. HEIDE, W., F. BINKOFSKI, R.J. SEITZ, et al. 2001. Activation of fronto-parietal cortices during memorized triple-step sequences of saccadic eye movements: an fMRI study. Eur. J. Neurosci. **13:** 1177–1189.
14. FRISTON, K.J., A.P. HOLMES, J.B. POLINE, et al. 1995. Analysis of fMRI time-series revisited. Neuroimage **2:** 45–53.
15. KIMMIG, H., M.W. GREENLEE, F. HUETHE & T. MERGNER. 1999. MR-eyetracker: a new method for eye movement recording in functional magnetic resonance imaging. Exp. Brain Res. **126:** 443–449.
16. SCHMAHMANN, J.D., J. DOYON, A. TOGA, et al. 2000. MRI Atlas of the Human Cerebellum. Academic Press. San Diego.
17. ELLENBERGER, C., J.F. CAMPA & M.G. NETSKY. 1968. Opsoclonus and parenchymatous degeneration of the cerebellum: the cerebellar origin of an abnormal eye movement. Neurology **18:** 1041–1046.
18. ZITER, F.A., P.F. BRAY & P.A. CANCILLA. 1979. Neuropathologic findings in a patient with neuroblastoma and myoclonic encephalopathy. Arch. Neurol. **36:** 51.
19. OGURO, K., J. KOBAYASHI, H. AIBA & H. HOJO. 1997. Opsoclonus-myoclonus syndrome with abnormal single photon emission computed tomography imaging. Pediatr. Neurol. **16:** 334–336.
20. SELHORST, J.B., L. STARK, A.L. OCHS & W.F. HOYT. 1976. Disorders in cerebellar ocular motor control. II. Macrosaccadic oscillation: an oculographic, control system and clinico-anatomical analysis. Brain **99:** 509–522.

21. BÖTZEL, K., K. ROTTACH & U. BÜTTNER. 1993. Normal and pathological saccadic dysmetria. Brain **116:** 337–353.
22. BARASH, S., A. MELIKYAN, A. SIVAKOV, *et al.* 1999. Saccadic dysmetria and adaptation after lesions of the cerebellar cortex. J. Neurosci. **19:** 10931–10939.
23. ROBINSON, F.R. & A.F. FUCHS. 2001. The role of the cerebellum in voluntary eye movements. Annu. Rev. Neurosci. **24:** 981–1004.
24. HELMCHEN, C. & U. BÜTTNER. 1995. Saccade-related Purkinje cell activity in the oculomotor vermis during spontaneous eye movements in light and darkness. Exp. Brain Res. **103:** 198–208.
25. THIER, P., P.W. DICKE, R. HAAS, *et al.* 2002. The role of the oculomotor vermis in the control of saccadic eye movements. Ann. N.Y. Acad. Sci. **978:** 50–62.
26. FUCHS, A.F., F.R. ROBINSON & A. STRAUBE. 1993. Role of the caudal fastigial nucleus in saccade generation. I. Neuronal discharge pattern. J. Neurophysiol. **70:** 1723–1740.
27. HELMCHEN, C., A. STRAUBE & U. BÜTTNER. 1994. Saccade-related activity in the fastigial oculomotor region of the macaque monkey during spontaneous eye movements in light and darkness. Exp. Brain Res. **98:** 474–482.
28. NODA, H., S. SUGITA & Y. IKEDA. 1990. Afferent and efferent connections of the oculomotor region of the fastigial nucleus in the macaque monkey. J. Comp. Neurol. **302:** 330–348.
29. SCUDDER, C.A., D.M. MCGEE & C.D. BALABAN. 2000. Connections of monkey saccade-related fastigial nucleus neurons revealed by anatomical and physiological methods. Soc. Neurosci. Abstr. **26:** 971.
30. QUAIA, C., P. LEFEVRE & L.M. OPTICAN. 1999. Model of the control of saccades by superior colliculus and cerebellum. J. Neurophysiol. **82:** 999–1018.
31. KLEINE, J. *et al.* 2003. Saccade-related activity in the primate fastigial oculomotor region. Ann. N.Y. Acad. Sci. **1004:** this volume.
32. SCUDDER, C.A., C.S. KANEKO & A.F. FUCHS. 2002.The brainstem burst generator for saccadic eye movements: a modern synthesis. Exp. Brain Res. **142:** 439–462.
33. STEPHAN, T., A. MASCOLO, T.A. YOUSRY, *et al.* 2002. Changes in cerebellar activation pattern during two successive sequences of saccades. Hum. Brain Mapp. **16:** 63–70.
34. DIETERICH, M., S.F. BUCHER, K.C. SEELOS & T. BRANDT. 2000. Cerebellar activation during optokinetic stimulation and saccades. Neurology **54:** 148–155.
35. LEIGH, R.J. & D.S. ZEE. 1999. Diagnosis of central disorders of ocular motility. *In* The Neurology of Eye Movements. 3rd edit. F.A. Davis, Ed.: 449–456. Philadelphia.
36. BÜTTNER-ENNEVER, J.A., B. COHEN, M. PAUSE & W. FRIES. 1988. Raphe nucleus of the pons containing omnipause neurons of the oculomotor system in the monkey, and its homologue in man. J. Comp. Neurol. **267:** 307–321.
37. HAIN, T.C., D.S. ZEE & M. MORDES. 1986. Blink-induced saccadic oscillations. Ann. Neurol. **19:** 299–301.
38. RAMBOLD, H., A. SPRENGER & C. HELMCHEN. 2002. Effects of voluntary blinks on saccades, vergence eye movements, and saccade-vergence interactions in humans. J. Neurophysiol. **88:** 1220–1233.
39. AVERBUCH-HELLER, L., A.A. KORI, K.G. ROTTACH, *et al.* 1996. Dysfunction of omnipause neurons causes impaired fixation: macrosaccadic oscillations with a unilateral pontine lesion. Neuro-ophthalmology **16:** 99–106.
40. RIDLEY, A., C. KENNARD, C.L. SCHOLTZ, *et al.* 1987. Omnipause neurons in two cases of opsoclonus associated with oat cell carcinoma of the lung. Brain **110:** 1699–1709.
41. THIELERT, C.D. & P. THIER. 1993. Patterns of projections from the pontine nuclei and the nucleus reticularis tegmenti pontis to the posterior vermis in the rhesus monkey: a study using retrograde tracers. J. Comp. Neurol. **337:** 113–126.
42. GONZALO-RUIZ, A. & G.R. LEICHNETZ. 1990. Afferents of the caudal fastigial nucleus in a New World monkey (*Cebus apella*). Exp. Brain Res. **80:** 600–608.

Multimodal Signal Integration in Vestibular Neurons of the Primate Fastigial Nucleus

U. BÜTTNER, S. GLASAUER, L. GLONTI, Y. GUAN, E. KIPIANI, J. KLEINE, C. SIEBOLD, T. TCHELIDZE, AND A. WILDEN

Department of Neurology, Ludwig-Maximilians University, 81377 Munich, Germany

> ABSTRACT: The rostral fastigial nucleus contains vestibular neurons, which presumably are involved in spinal mechanisms (neck, gait, posture) and which are not modulated with individual eye movements. Single-unit recordings in the alert behaving monkey during natural stimulus conditions reveal that virtually all neurons demonstrate integration of several sensory inputs. This applies not only for canal–canal and canal–otolith interaction, but also for otolith–otolith interaction. There is also some evidence that most neurons receive not only an utriculus but also a sacculus input. Furthermore, most neurons also respond to large-field optokinetic stimulation, reflecting visual–vestibular interaction. Neurons are also affected by the head on trunk position, which would allow these neurons to operate in a body-centered rather than a head-centered reference frame. These complex, multisensory features could permit fastigial nucleus neurons to rather specifically affect spinal motor functions.
>
> KEYWORDS: fastigial nucleus; monkey; vestibular; semicircular canals; otolith

INTRODUCTION

The fastigial nucleus (FN), the most medial deep cerebellar nucleus, can be divided into a rostral and a caudal part. The caudal part also has been labeled the fastigial oculomotor region (FOR), because neurons here are modulated with saccades[1–3] or smooth pursuit eye movements.[4,5] Neurons in the rostral FN are modulated during natural vestibular stimulation,[6–8] but they are not modulated with individual eye movements.[4] Based on this, they have been labeled "vestibular-only" neurons. In this article, only these vestibular-only neurons in the rostral FN are considered.

The rostral FN receives its Purkinje cell (PC) input from the overlying anterior vermis (lobulus I to V).[9] PCs in the anterior vermis also have been shown to respond to vestibular stimulation.[10,11] Other inputs to the FN as mossy fiber collaterals derive from the vestibular nuclei on both sides.[12] The rostral FN mainly projects to the contralateral medial and superior vestibular nucleus.[12]

Address for correspondence: Prof. Dr. U. Büttner, Department of Neurology, Ludwig-Maximilians University, Marchioninistrasse 15, D-81377 Munich, Germany. Voice: 0049-89-7095-2560; fax: 0049-89-7095-5561.
  ubuettner@brain.nefo.med.uni-muenchen.de

The precise functional role of the rostral FN is not very well understood. Lesions here lead to a falling tendency to the ipsilateral side[13,14] and to disturbed eye-head coordination during gaze shifts.[15] Based on this evidence, it is generally assumed that the rostral FN is involved in vestibulospinal mechanisms (neck, posture, gait).[14] To obtain a better understanding of the neuronal mechanisms underlying the control of these motor functions, we recorded vestibular-only neurons in the rostral FN in the alert monkey during various vestibular stimulus conditions, different head on trunk positions, and large-field optokinetic stimuli. It will be shown that virtually every vestibular-only neuron reflects the integration of various sensory inputs.

METHODS

Monkeys were chronically prepared for single-unit recordings.[7] A recording chamber for single-unit recordings and a head holder was attached to the skull. Eye position was recorded with the scleral search-coil method[16] and single-unit activity with varnished tungsten microelectrodes. During the experiment, the monkey sat erect with the head fixed, in a primate chair on a vestibular turntable.

Vestibular Stimulation

Earth Vertical and Earth Horizontal Axis Rotation

For vestibular stimulation, the monkey could be rotated by a motor-driven device around an earth vertical and an earth horizontal axis. Rotation around the earth vertical axis mainly activates horizontal semicircular canals, whereas rotation around the earth horizontal axis leads mainly to stimulation of vertical semicircular canals and the utriculus. A second motor allowed the head of the monkey to be positioned in different orientations. This allowed for stimulation in pitch, roll, and vertical canal planes (LARP: left anterior–right posterior; RALP: right anterior–left posterior). Sinusoidal rotation around the earth horizontal axis ranged from 0.1 to 1.4 Hz with amplitudes of $\pm 10°$ to $\pm 15°$.

Earth Fixed Vertical Axis Rotation

For this, the monkey in the primate chair was tilted $\pm 15°$ off the vertical axis.[17] The tilt could be nose down (ND) or nose up (NU), left ear down (LED) or right ear down (RED), or in intermediate orientations. Rotation around the earth vertical axis with different tilt positions leads only to activation of semicircular canals, in contrast with the stimulation around the earth horizontal axis described above, which activates semicircular canals (mainly vertical) and otolith organs (mainly utriculus).

Different Head on Trunk Position

For this, the monkey wore an individually molded corselet, which allowed the trunk to be brought into $\pm 45°$ positions relative to the head. Vestibular stimulation consisted of rotation around the earth horizontal axis as described above.

Large-Field Optokinetic Stimuli

The monkey was completely surrounded by a large cylinder covered with vertical black and white stripes. The cylinder moved in the horizontal plane in both direction at velocities between 10° and 120° per second.

Analysis

Signals (single-unit activity, eye position, vestibular stimuli) were digitized and stored for off-line analysis. With constant head and trunk orientation, 3 to 20 sinusoidal stimulus cycles were averaged. When the head orientation altered continuously, responses of neighboring orientations were included for averaging. The averaged neuronal activity was fitted by a least squares best-sine function. Sensitivity (imp • s^{-1}/deg) and phase were determined relative to head position if not stated otherwise. Positive phase values indicate that neuronal activity leads head position. Sensitivity and phase at different head orientations were used to determine the optimal response orientations (response vector orientation [RVO])[18] (see below).

Spatiotemporal Convergence

The response of vestibular neurons can be described by phase and sensitivity in relation to the sinusoidal stimulus. The response is also determined by the plane of head stimulation. Vestibular nerve afferents from the left anterior (LA) and right posterior (RP) canal show the best modulation for stimulation in this canal plane (LARP). For different head orientations, the modulation decreases to zero at an orientation 90° apart (null response). The changes in sensitivity with head orientation can be described by a cosine function. The convergence of two such inputs with the same phase leads (by linear superposition) to a similar response pattern with an optimal response (RVO) at a different orientation. The phase relation remains the same except for a 180° phase shift around the null position.

If the phase relation of the two inputs differs, the response pattern of the output changes. There is now modulation at all orientations with an optimal response (RVO) and a minimal response (no null response). Accordingly, the phase changes gradually around the minimal response. In the extreme case, when the inputs have a phase difference of 90°, the output shows the same sensitivity at all orientations and phase changes continuously with head orientation. It could be shown that for all vestibular FN neurons responses can be explained by linear superposition of inputs with the same or different phase relations.[18]

RESULTS

Canal–Canal Interaction

During stimulation around an earth horizontal axis many "vestibular-only" neurons in FN have a RVO in a canal plane (LARP or RALP). The modulation (sensitivity) decreases monotonously, when the head orientation deviates from this plane. At a head orientation 90° apart, there is no modulation (null response). Phase is stable and close to head velocity except for a 180° phase shift around the null response.

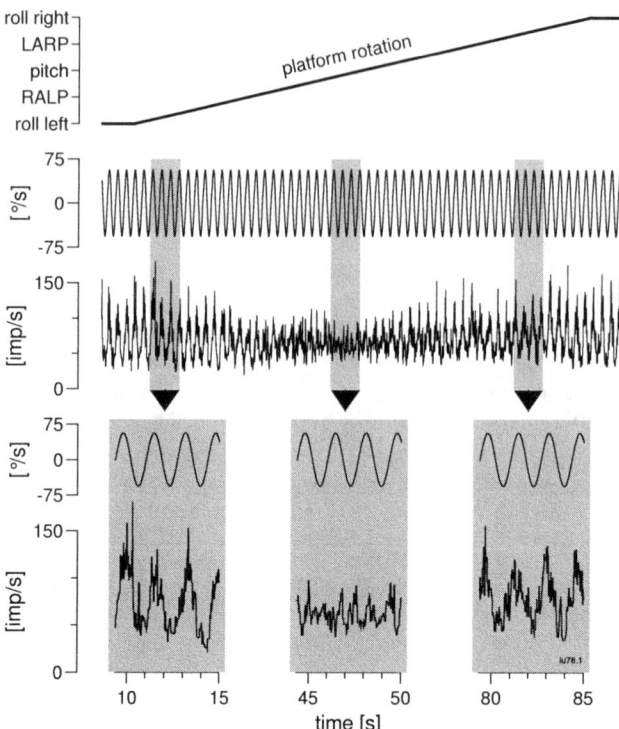

FIGURE 1. Vestibular-only neuron in the rostral fastigial nucleus during stimulation (0.6 Hz) around an earth horizontal axis at different head orientations. During the sinusoidal stimulation (*third trace from top*), the head orientation changes continuously from roll (90°) to pitch (0°) to roll (–90°). Enlargements at certain orientations (as indicated) are shown below. This neuron is not modulated close to pitch (*middle row*) and shows best modulation close to roll stimulation.

Canal–canal interaction leads to RVOs in the roll or pitch plane, which is also commonly seen for fastigial neurons[7,19] (FIG. 1).

At a stimulus frequency of 0.6 Hz, most neurons (53%) had their RVO for ipsilateral canal planes (i.e., anterior and posterior canal ipsilateral to the recording side). Convergence was found for neurons (33%) with RVOs in the roll plane more common than in the pitch plane. In general, neurons with RVOs to the ipsilateral side were found more often (66%) than those to the contralateral side (22%).

Canal–Otolith Interaction

Traditionally, otolith responses have been assumed when neurons show a phase relation close to head position during sinusoidal stimulation.[20] Based on this criteria, 23% of the neurons in the FN show at the RVO a response in phase with head position.[7] RVOs for these neurons were in all orientations except for pitch.

As outlined above, the absence of a null response and gradual phase changes at different head orientations indicate convergence, usually canal–otolith interaction but possibly also otolith–otolith interaction, as will be shown below. Such signs of convergence were seen for 35% of the neurons at 0.6 Hz.[19] If tested over a wide frequency range (0.1–1.4 Hz), this percentage is much higher, because most neurons shows signs of convergence at one frequency which is not present at other frequencies.

In recent years, there has been increasing evidence that central otolith neurons can also encode velocity.[21] Thus, a distinction between canal and otolith input can no longer be made on phase relation. To get a better estimate of the otolith contribution to FN responses, we compared two stimulus conditions: (1) rotation around an earth horizontal axis with different head orientations, which leads to semicircular canal and otolith (mainly utriculus) stimulation, and (2) tilted stimulation around an earth vertical axis, which only activates canals.[17] The second paradigm allows the canal response of a given neuron to be determined in isolation. This response then can be subtracted from the response in the first paradigm to obtain the otolith contribution. With this approach, 74% of the vestibular FN neurons revealed an otolith input. In 64% of the neurons, the otolith component was in phase with head velocity,[17] a pattern not found for otolith-afferent neurons.[22] Canal–otolith convergence occurred in 61% of the neurons.[17] Interestingly, many neurons with canal–otolith interaction did not show a minimal response as a sign of spatiotemporal convergence.

Otolith–Otolith Interaction

The previous paragraph showed that certainly more than 50% of the vestibular FN neurons reflect an otolith input. This refers to dynamic stimulation. During static tilt, the sensitivity is usually much lower compared with dynamic stimulation, or neurons do not respond at all.[7] One reason could be that the input is determined by irregular otolith afferents, which increase their sensitivity with higher frequencies.[22] Based on modeling, there is also evidence that irregular and regular otolith inputs to FN neurons might have opposing RVOs[23] (FIG. 2). With the same sensitivity during static tilt, these otolith contributions would cancel each other out.

If tested over a large frequency range (0.06–1.4 Hz), vestibular FN neurons show several features which are not compatible with convergence of a canal and one otolith input. As already mentioned above, minimal responses (as a sign of spatiotemporal convergence) can be present at one stimulus frequency but not at others. Furthermore, phase changes can exceed 90° over a frequency range of 0.1–1.0 Hz. In addition, for many neurons the RVO changed with frequency, often exceeding 90°.[19] This raises the question whether such complex responses can be achieved by the convergence of peripheral canal or regular and irregular otolith inputs or if some specific additional central processing is required. Modeling the transfer characteristics of vestibular FN neurons based on these three types of peripheral inputs showed that the response characteristic of most neurons (79%) can be simulated by assuming only convergence of peripheral inputs.[23] Additional central processing had to be assumed for only a small minority of neurons. Virtually all neurons reflected some canal–otolith convergence. The RVOs of irregular and regular otolith inputs often were opposing, that is, inhibiting each other[23] (FIG. 2). As outlined above,

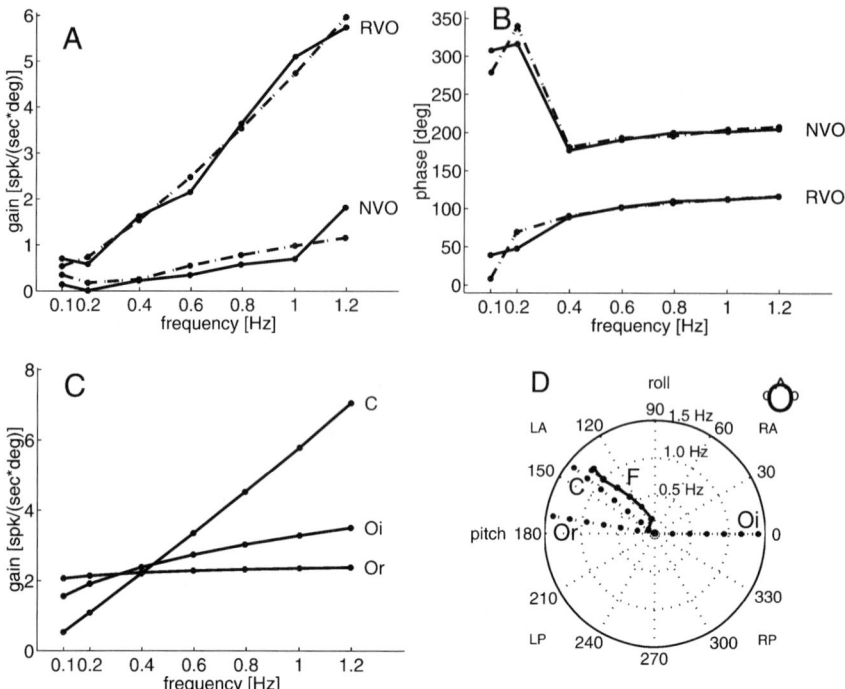

FIGURE 2. Contribution of canal neurons (C), irregular (Oi) and regular (Or) otolith neurons (C, D) to the response characteristics of a vestibular-only FN neuron (**A, B**, *solid line* in **D**). Shown are the gain (**A**) (imp·s^{-1}/deg) and the phase (**B**) for the RVO and the minimal response (NVO) for different stimulus frequencies. (*Solid line*, data; *stippled line*, fit.) The gain (sensitivities) of the input neurons in relation to stimulus frequency is shown (**C**). (**D**) Shown are the RVOs for the FN neuron and its inputs at different frequencies, increasing from the center to the outer ring. The RVO of the FN neuron mainly follows the canal input (**C**) except for low frequencies. Note that the RVO for the irregular (Oi) and regular (Or) otolith oppose each other.

such distribution of the otolith RVOs could contribute to the fact that vestibular FN neurons respond only poorly or not at all during static tilt.

There is also some preliminary evidence that afferents from the sacculus contribute to the response of vestibular FN neurons.[23] With stimulation around an earth horizontal axis and amplitudes of ±15°, it is mainly the utriculus that is activated in addition to the canals because of the stimulus component in the horizontal direction. The vertical component as a stimulus for sacculus activation is small and only 7% of the horizontal component. With sinusoidal stimulation, the sacculus-related response component should show the double stimulus frequency. This indeed can be shown despite the irregular activity pattern of FN neurons (FIG. 3). This sacculus contribution can best be demonstrated for orientations around the minimal or null response, when the horizontal response contribution of the utriculus is small or lacking. If one assumes a similar sensitivity of the neurons responding to the horizontal

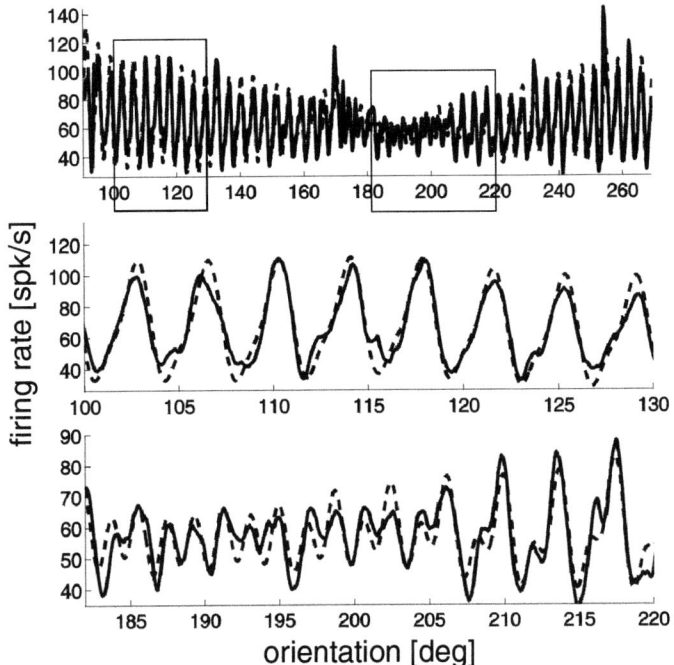

FIGURE 3. Neuronal activity (*solid line*) of a vestibular-only neuron in FN during stimulation around an earth horizontal axis and various head orientations (abscissa). This neuron had its null response (minimal modulation) around 190° (pitch) and an optimal response (RVO) at an orientation 90° apart at 110° (roll). Enlargements of the areas outlined are shown at the RVO (*middle row*) and at the null response (*bottom row*). The stippled lines indicate the fit, which includes the horizontal and the vertical stimulus component with double stimulus frequency. The fit in the *bottom row* supports a sacculus input.

(utriculus) and the vertical (sacculus) stimulus component, these preliminary data suggest a high percentage (79%) of neurons also receiving a sacculus input.[23]

Head–Neck Interaction

During locomotion, the vestibular signals are sensed by the vestibular organs in the head. However, the response (output) is mainly used to stabilize body and limbs independent of the actual head position in relation to the trunk. In the decerebrate cat, Manzoni et al.[24] could demonstrate that the RVO of vestibular Purkinje cells in the anterior vermis changes during tonic neck displacement.

This is also the case for most vestibular neurons in the rostral FN of the alert behaving monkey. The RVO changes systematically with different head on trunk positions, when vestibular stimuli around an earth horizontal axis are applied (FIG. 4). For most neurons, the RVO shift is partially compensatory (approximately 50°). Several neurons also showed full compensation (90°), and only a minority of neurons were not affected by different trunk positions (no compensation, 0°). In contrast with

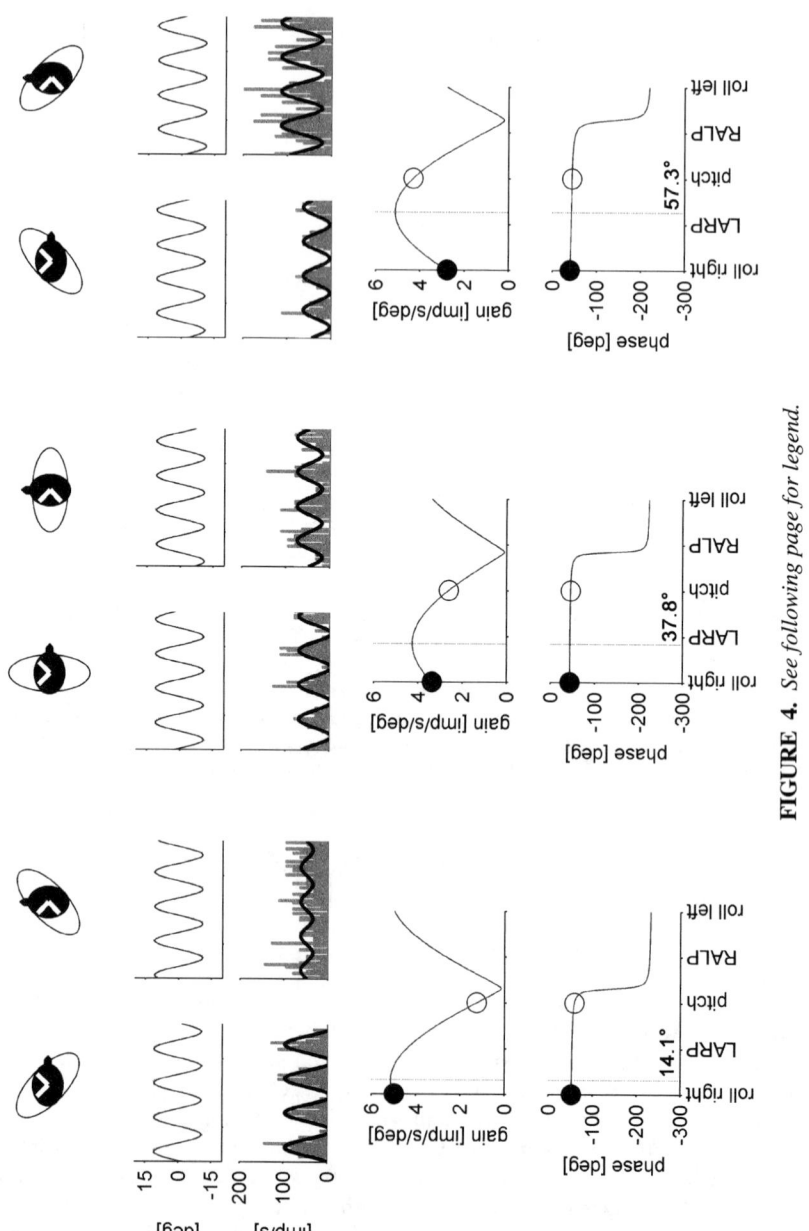

FIGURE 4. *See following page for legend.*

these RVO changes, phase and sensitivity were not affected by different head on trunk positions.

This pattern of RVO changes is also found when different stimulus frequencies (0.1–1.0 Hz) are applied. The RVO difference between the various head-on trunk positions remains the same independent of the stimulus frequency.

Visual–Vestibular Interaction

Most (89%) of the vestibular FN neurons are also modulated during full-field optokinetic stimulation in the horizontal plane at 60°/s.[4] In all instances, an activity increase occurred in the direction opposite to that which led to an activity increase during vestibular stimulation. Activity changes increased with higher optokinetic stimulus velocities. Optokinetic stimulation in the opposite direction led to a decrease in firing rate, and complete cessation of firing could occur at the highest stimulus velocities.

After prolonged (50 s) optokinetic stimulation, nystagmus continues as optokinetic after-nystagmus (OKAN) in the dark. During this period, activity of vestibular FN neurons returns gradually (>10 s) to the resting discharge level. Furthermore, the sudden onset of the optokinetic stimulus leads only to gradual activity changes. Sudden activity changes have been related to the smooth pursuit system.[25,26] It is in accordance with this that vestibular-only FN neurons are not modulated during smooth pursuit eye movements. Rather, the activity changes during optokinetic stimulation and during OKAN appear to be related to the velocity storage system.[4]

COMMENT

The results show a complex activity pattern of vestibular FN neurons reflecting multisensory integration, which would allow these neurons to specifically affect spinal motor functions. This is similar to studies performed in the vestibular nuclei. One important goal will be to better understand the contribution of the FN in relation to the anterior vermis (as a major input) and the vestibular nuclei (the major output structure). For this, a quantitative comparison of neuronal data from these structures from the same species under identical stimulus conditions is necessary. There are few studies which fulfill these criteria. It also appears to be an unsolved question which functional differences are caused by the direct transmission of anterior vermis signals to the vestibular nuclei in contrast with the indirect route via the fastigial nuclei.

FIGURE 4. Response of a vestibular FN during different head on trunk positions shown in the top trace (45° *left*, *center*, 45° *right*). Sinusoidal stimuli (0.6 Hz) around an earth horizontal axis are applied with the head oriented in roll and pitch. Stimuli and responses are shown in the *second and third traces*. Note particularly that during pitch stimulation there is no modulation with the trunk to the left but good modulation with the trunk to the right. From the gain (sensitivity) and phase values, the RVOs (*stippled lines in bottom rows*) at different head-on-trunk positions are calculated. The RVO moves in a compensatory fashion from 14.1° (close to roll) at trunk left to 57.3° (between LARP and pitch) at trunk right.

The demonstration of abundant convergence of different inputs on vestibular FN neurons is clearly caused by the application of appropriate stimuli. The studies described above show that more than 70% of vestibular FN neurons have an otolith input.[17,23] Also, otolith–otolith interaction seems to be common. This also has been demonstrated during linear acceleration with many FN neurons being broadly tuned.[8] If one takes only responses to static tilt as a sign of an otolith input, the numbers are considerably lower.[7] In the study by Gardner and Fuchs,[6] none of the neurons responded to static tilt. Ghelarducci[27] also postulated the absence of canal–otolith interaction based on his findings in the decerebrate cat that FN neurons responding to dynamic tilt did not respond to static tilt. These developments over the last 20 to 30 years suggest that probably even more complex signal interactions in FN neurons will be discovered if the appropriate stimulus paradigms are applied.

ACKNOWLEDGMENTS

This work was supported by Deutsche Forschungsgemeinschaft. The authors thank S. Langer for technical assistance, B. Pfreundner and I. Wendl for preparing the manuscript, and K. Ogston for editing the English text.

REFERENCES

1. HELMCHEN, C., A. STRAUBE & U. BÜTTNER. 1994. Saccade-related activity in the fastigial oculomotor region of the macaque monkey during spontaneous eye movements in light and darkness. Exp. Brain Res. **98:** 474–482.
2. FUCHS, A.F., F.R. ROBINSON & A. STRAUBE. 1993. Role of the caudal fastigial nucleus in saccade generation. 1. Neuronal discharge patterns. J. Neurophysiol. **70:** 1723–1740.
3. ROBINSON, F.R. & A.F. FUCHS. 2001. The role of the cerebellum in voluntary eye movements. Annu. Rev. Neurosci. **24:** 981–1004.
4. BÜTTNER, U., A.F. FUCHS, G. MARKERT-SCHWAB & P. BUCKMASTER. 1991. Fastigial nucleus activity in the alert monkey during slow eye and head movements. J. Neurophysiol. **65:** 1360–1371.
5. FUCHS, A.F., F.R. ROBINSON & A. STRAUBE. 1994. Participation of the caudal fastigial nucleus in smooth-pursuit eye movements. I. Neuronal activity. J. Neurophysiol. **72:** 2714–2728.
6. GARDNER, E.P. & A.F. FUCHS. 1975. Single-unit responses to natural vestibular stimuli and eye movements in deep cerebellar nuclei of the alert rhesus monkey. J. Neurophysiol. **38:** 627–649.
7. SIEBOLD, C., L. GLONTI, S. GLASAUER & U. BÜTTNER. 1997. Rostral fastigial nucleus activity in the alert monkey during three dimensional passive head movements. J. Neurophysiol. **77:** 1432–1446.
8. ZHOU, W., B.F. TANG & W.M. KING. 2001. Responses of rostral fastigial neurons to linear acceleration in an alert monkey. Exp. Brain Res. **139:** 111–115.
9. ARMSTRONG, D.M. & R.F. SCHILD. 1978. An investigation of the cerebellar corticonuclear projections in the rat using an autoradiographic tracing method. I. Projections from the vermis. Brain Res. **141:** 1–19.
10. PRECHT, W., R. VOLKIND & R.H. BLANKS. 1977. Functional organization of the vestibular input to the anterior and posterior cerebellar vermis of cat. Exp. Brain Res. **27:** 143–160.
11. POMPEIANO, O., P. ANDRE & D. MANZONI. 1997. Spatiotemporal response properties of cerebellar Purkinje cells to animal displacement: a population analysis. Neuroscience **81:** 609–626.

12. NODA, H., S. SUGITA & Y. IKEDA. 1990. Afferent and efferent connections of the oculomotor region of the fastigial nucleus in the macaque monkey. J. Comp. Neurol. **302:** 330–348.
13. KURZAN, R., A. STRAUBE & U. BÜTTNER. 1993. The effect of muscimol micro-injections into the fastigial nucleus on the optokinetic response and the vestibulo-ocular reflex in the alert monkey. Exp. Brain Res. **94:** 252–260.
14. THACH, W.T., H.P. GOODKIN & J.G. KEATING. 1992. The cerebellum and the adaptive coordination of movement. Annu. Rev. Neurosci. **15:** 403–442.
15. PÉLISSON, D., L. GOFFART & A. GUILLAUME. 1998. Contribution of the rostral fastigial nucleus to the control of orienting gaze shifts in the head-unrestrained cat. J. Neurophysiol. **80:** 1180–1196.
16. BARTL, K., C. SIEBOLD, S. GLASAUER, et al. 1996. A simplified calibration method for three-dimensional eye movement recordings using search-coils. Vision Res. **36:** 997–1006.
17. SIEBOLD, C., E. ANAGNOSTOU, S. GLASAUER, et al. 2001. Canal-otolith interaction in the fastigial nucleus of the alert monkey. Exp. Brain Res. **136:** 169–178.
18. KLEINE, J.F., A. WILDEN, C. SIEBOLD, et al. 1999. Linear spatio-temporal convergence in vestibular neurons of the primate nucleus fastigii. Neuroreport **10:** 3915–3921.
19. Siebold, C., J.F. KLEINE, L. GLONTI, et al. 1999. Fastigial nucleus activity during different frequencies and orientations of vertical vestibular stimulation in the monkey. J. Neurophysiol. **82:** 34–41.
20. KASPER, J., R.H. SCHOR & V.J. WILSON. 1988. Response of vestibular neurons to head rotations in vertical planes. II. Response to neck stimulation and vestibular-neck interaction. J. Neurophysiol. **60:** 1765–1778.
21. ANGELAKI, D.E. & J.D. DICKMAN. 2000. Spatiotemporal processing of linear acceleration: primary afferent and central vestibular neuron responses. J. Neurophysiol. **84:** 2113–2132.
22. FERNANDEZ, C. & J.M. GOLDBERG. 1976. Physiology of peripheral neurons innervating otolith organs of the squirrel monkey. III. Response dynamics. J. Neurophysiol. **39:** 996–1008.
23. WILDEN, A., S. GLASAUER, J.F. KLEINE & U. BÜTTNER. 2002. Modelling transfer characteristics of vestibular neurons in the fastigial nucleus of the behaving monkey on the basis of canal-otolith interaction. Neuroreport **13:** 799–804.
24. MANZONI, D., O. POMPEIANO, L. BRUSCHINI & P. ANDRE. 1999. Neck input modifies the reference frame for coding labyrinthine signals in the cerebellar vermis: a cellular analysis. Neuroscience **93:** 1095–1107.
25. BÜTTNER, U., O. MEIENBERG & B. SCHIMMELPFENNIG. 1983. The effect of central retinal lesions on optokinetic nystagmus in the monkey. Exp. Brain Res. **52:** 248–256.
26. COHEN, B., V. MATSUO & T. RAPHAN. 1977. Quantitative analysis of the velocity characteristics of optokinetic nystagmus and optokinetic after-nystagmus. J. Physiol. **270:** 321–344.
27. GHELARDUCCI, B. 1973. Responses of the cerebellar fastigial neurones to tilt. Pflügers Arch. **344:** 195–206.

Discharge Properties of Saccade-Related Neurons in the Primate Fastigial Oculomotor Region

J.F. KLEINE, Y. GUAN, AND U. BÜTTNER

Department of Neurology, Klinikum Grosshadern, LMU München, München, Germany

ABSTRACT: To clarify the mechanisms by which the cerebellar fastigial oculomotor region (FOR) contributes to the control of saccadic eye movements, we recorded saccade-related FOR units in alert monkeys that made horizontal saccades between neighboring points of a three-by-three grid of target positions (16° amplitude). As in previous studies, FOR units exhibited saccade-related bursts that occurred earlier for contralateral than for ipsilateral saccades. In addition, many FOR units reflected variations in the kinematic profiles of the saccades by exhibiting bursts with earlier onset and shorter peak latencies and higher peak discharge rates for fast as compared with slow saccades of the same amplitude. Moreover, reflecting systematic differences in saccade velocity rather than an influence of eye position itself, FOR bursts showed subtle but recurrent and, at the population level, statistically significant differences between centripetal and centrifugal saccades that closely paralleled the eye position dependency of saccadic dysmetria seen after FOR lesions. We conclude that the FOR output signal is not, as previously proposed, specifically related to the temporal properties of the saccade, but also contains information about saccade velocity. Moreover, the FOR output signal appears to change systematically depending on the actual kinematic properties of the saccade, in a way that would help to maintain saccadic accuracy.

KEYWORDS: fastigial oculomotor region; monkey; saccade; oculomotor vermis

INTRODUCTION

The cerebellar oculomotor vermis (OV) and the target zone of its Purkinje cell output, the fastigial oculomotor region (FOR), are involved in saccade control mechanisms, but their precise functional role is unknown. Early lesion studies suggested that these cerebellar midline areas might play a role in the compensation of the viscoelastic forces that arise in the orbita. In these studies, it was observed that the degree of lesion-induced saccadic dysmetria depended on the initial position of the eye: saccades from the periphery toward the center of the oculomotor range (centripetal) became distinctly more hypermetric than otherwise similar centrifugal saccades.[1–4]

Address for correspondence: Justus F. Kleine, Neurologische Klinik, Klinikum Grosshadern, Marchioninistrasse 15, 81377 München, Germany. Voice: +49 89 7095 4836; fax: +49 89 7095 4805.

jkleine@brain.nefo.med.uni-muenchen.de

Ann. N.Y. Acad. Sci. 1004: 252–261 (2003). © 2003 New York Academy of Sciences.
doi: 10.1196/annals.1303.022

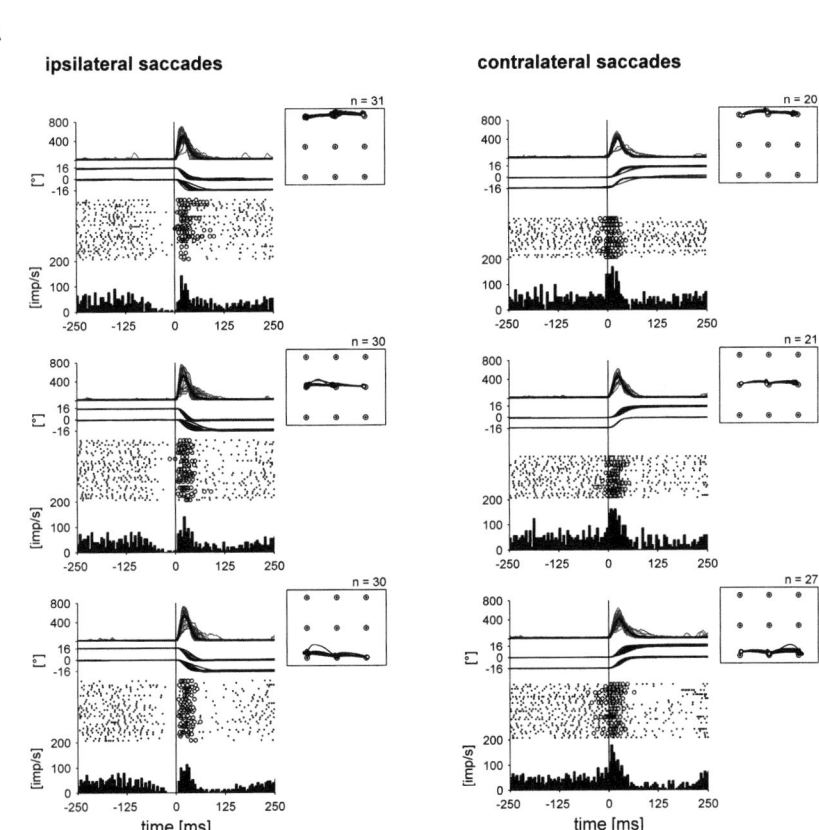

FIGURE 1. Activity of a saccade-related neuron in the fastigial oculomotor region (FOR) during 16° horizontal saccades from different starting positions, as indicated by the *dots in the insets* on the right of each panel, which show "screen views," with horizontal and vertical eye position plotted as two-dimensional traces for each saccade. Saccades were sorted according to vertical (**A**) and horizontal (**B**) starting position. Each panel shows (*from above*) horizontal eye velocity (*gray lines*: individual trials; *black line*: average), horizontal eye position, raster diagrams with spike occurrences for individual saccades (in each case restricted to a maximum of 30 randomly selected trials), and averaged neuronal activity as spike histogram. Traces are aligned with saccade onset. "Burst spikes," as identified by the computer (see METHODS), are highlighted by *circles* in the raster diagrams. There were no consistent differences between FOR bursts for saccades from different vertical starting positions (**A**). For ipsilateral, but not for contralateral saccades, however, bursts for centripetal saccades occurred and peaked slightly earlier and exhibited slightly higher peak discharge rates than bursts for centrifugal saccades (**B**). Note the variability of the velocity profiles of the saccades.

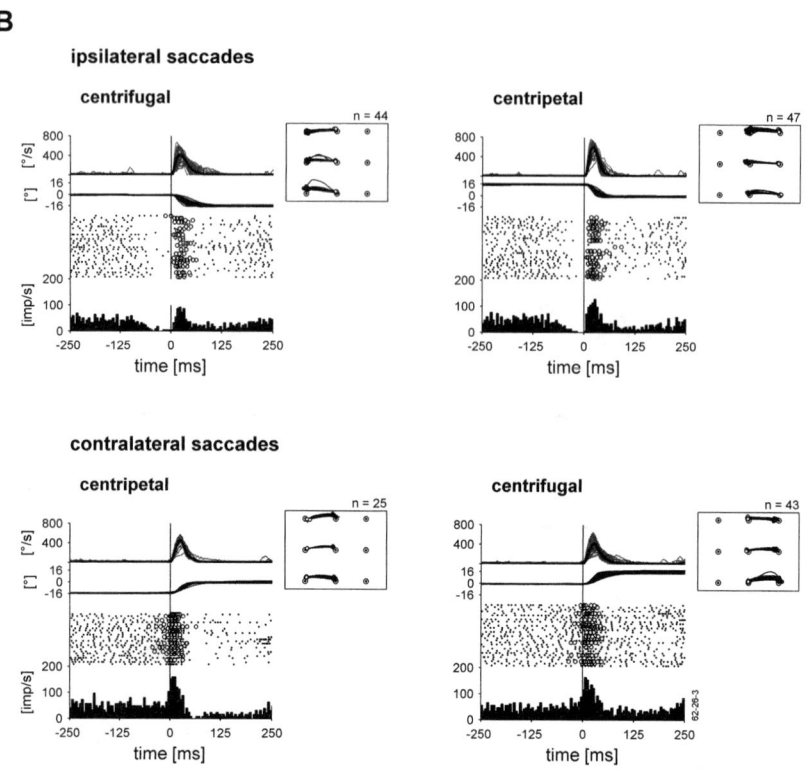

FIGURE 1. *Continued.*

However, this functional concept was not supported by single-unit recording studies, which consistently failed to demonstrate corresponding eye position dependencies in the output signals provided by FOR units.[5,6]

These single-unit studies set the focus on a seemingly unrelated aspect by revealing latency differences between FOR bursts, which occurred earlier for contralateral than for ipsilateral saccades. However, they also started another controversy. Ohtsuka and Noda,[5] who observed fairly robust correlations between burst and saccade duration in a subset of their neuronal sample, proposed that FOR signals use a *precise temporal* code that reflects saccade duration and thereby provides accurate information about desired saccade amplitude to help to control saccade metrics. This hypothesis, however, was challenged by Fuchs et al.,[6] who demonstrated that the correlations between burst and saccade properties generally were much less precise than reported by Ohtsuka and Noda.[5] They proposed the alternative view that the contralateral and ipsilateral FOR bursts constituted auxiliary accelerative and decelerative signals to supplement the burst generator, which, however, have little relation to the properties of the ongoing saccade.

To further the insight into the nature of the neuronal signals exhibited by FOR units, we recorded single units from the FOR of two monkeys that made visually guided horizontal saccades between neighboring points of a three by three grid of target positions. In contrast with previous studies, we recorded saccades of one fixed amplitude (16°). This allowed correlation of neuronal discharge patterns with the kinematic properties of the saccades without confounding influences of "main sequence" effects.

METHODS

Two monkeys (*Macaca mulatta*) were prepared for chronic single-unit recordings from the FOR by using previously described techniques and surgical procedures.[7] During the experiments, the monkeys sat, with their head fixed, in a primate chair and followed a small light spot displayed by a video monitor. Eye movements were recorded by means of a scleral search coil,[8] using previously described calibration routines.[9] The target jumped horizontally between neighbouring points of a three by three square grid centered about the straight ahead position to induce horizontal saccades (16° amplitude) ipsilaterally and contralaterally to the recording site as well as centripetally and fugally at different vertical starting positions (FIG. 1). Neuronal discharges were recorded with a temporal resolution of 20 μs using conventional recording and amplification equipment and techniques and stored on computer hard disc along with the eye position signals (500 Hz sampling frequency) for off-line analysis. Bursts of discharges related to individual saccades were detected and quantified for onset latency (re saccade onset), peak latency, burst peak amplitude, number of spikes per burst, and burst duration by computer using a modified version of the "Poisson-spike-train-analysis" originally described by Hanes and colleagues.[10] The relationships between these burst parameters and saccade velocity were assessed by linear correlation analyses. For the evaluation of eye position–related effects on neuronal responses, saccades and associated spike trains were sorted according to the vertical (FIG. 1A) and horizontal (FIG. 1B) component of the starting position, and the resultant distributions of burst parameters were compared by nonparametric ANOVA (Kruskal-Wallis). For the reconstruction of electrode tracks, tracer substances (Di I[11]) were placed at selected recording sites. At the end of all experiments, one monkey was deeply anesthetized with barbiturate and perfused transcardially with 10% formalin. Coronal sections of the brain taken every 50 μm were processed for the tract-tracing substance, confirming that the recording sites were located in the caudal part of the fastigial nucleus. Currently, the other monkey is still alive, so that a detailed histological reconstruction is not yet available for this animal. However, based on response properties and the discharge characteristics in the surrounding areas, we are confident that the recording sites also were located in the FOR in this monkey.

RESULTS

General Characteristics

Seventy-four units showing saccade-related bursts are included in the current study. Fifty-two showed a burst for both ipsilateral and contralateral saccades. Eigh-

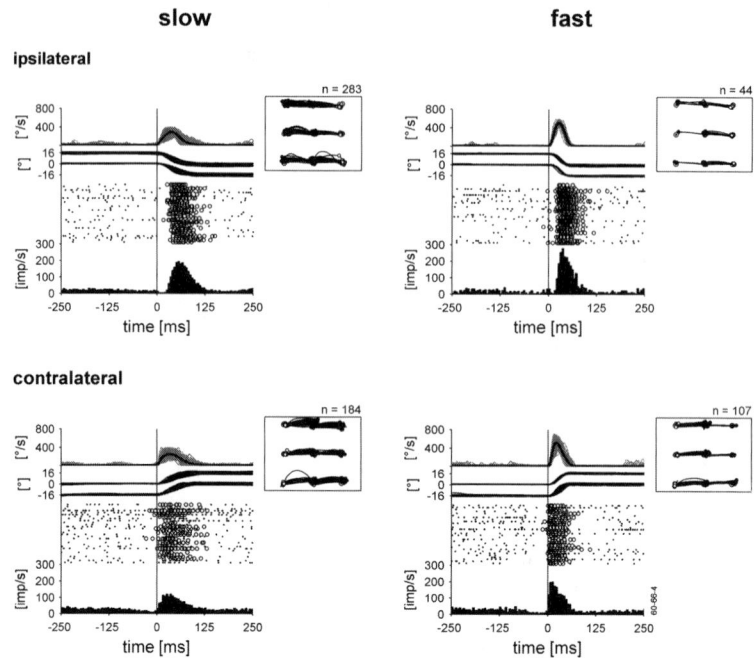

FIGURE 2. Comparison of burst activity for slow (*left*, 200–400°/s) and fast (*right*, 500–800°/s) saccades for one sample neuron. Panel layout as in FIGURE 1. For fast saccades, bursts start and peak earlier, and peak burst activity is higher than for slow saccades.

teen neurons showed a burst for ipsilateral saccades only, and four for contralateral saccades only. There were no systematic differences between the ipsilateral and contralateral bursts of these units or the corresponding bursts of the "bilaterally" bursting units. The following analyses therefore pertain to the ipsilateral bursts of 70 units and the contralateral bursts of 56 units. As in previous studies,[5,6,12] contralateral bursts occurred, on average, earlier than ipsilateral bursts (FIG. 1).

Correlations between FOR Bursts and Saccade Velocity

Although the recorded saccades were restricted to one fixed amplitude (16°), their kinematic properties varied considerably across trials even for individual units (FIG. 1), presumably because of fluctuations in the alertness level of the animals. This variability allowed to compare neuronal responses for saccades with different velocity characteristics. Saccades were included in the analysis if their peak velocity was at least 200°/s; however, actual peak velocities ranged from this lower limit up to almost 800°/s, with an average of approximately 420°/s in both monkeys. When we compared saccades from the lower end (200–400°/s) and the upper end of this velocity range (500–800°/s), distinctive differences appeared in the corresponding perisaccadic spike histograms in a considerable fraction of units. Typically, saccade-related bursts started and peaked earlier, and exhibited higher peak discharge rates for the faster than for the slower saccades (FIG. 2). Accordingly, when burst parameters, derived from computer-based analysis of single bursts (see METHODS), were correlated with the associated peak velocities of individual saccades (FIG. 3), there was clear predominance of negative correlation coefficients for burst onset and peak latency, and of positive correlation coefficients for burst peak amplitude (for onset latency in 53/70 units [ipsilateral] and 47/56 units [contralateral]; for peak latency

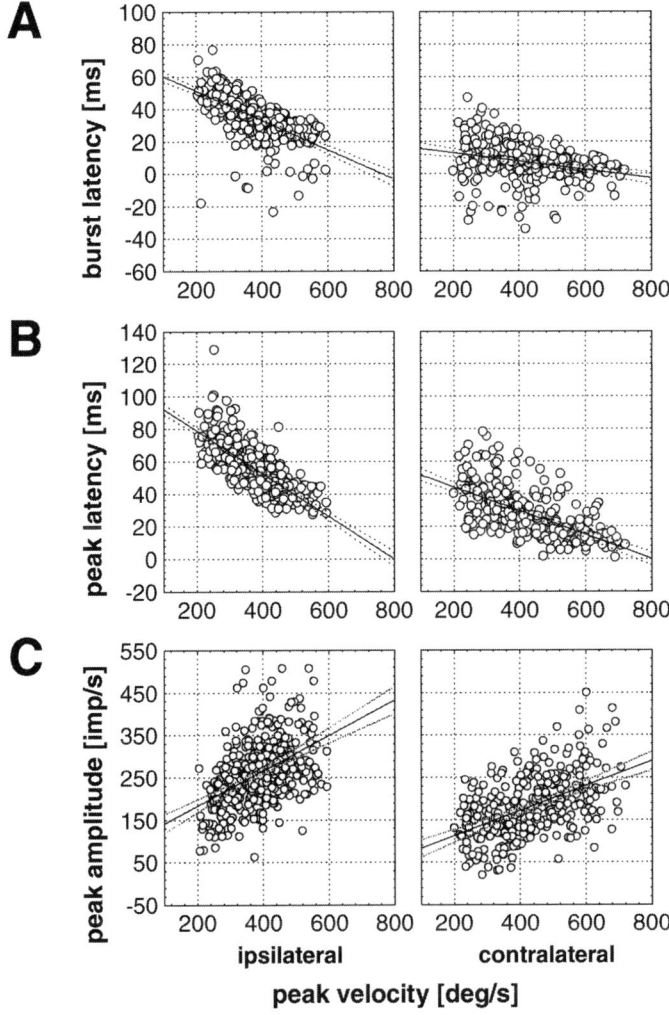

FIGURE 3. Relation of saccade peak velocity to burst latency, peak latency, and peak burst amplitude. same neuron as in FIGURE 2. Each *circle* represents data from one individual ipsilateral (*left column*) or contralateral (*right column*) saccade. Burst and peak latencies decrease and peak discharge rates increase with saccade velocity. *Solid lines*: linear regression line with 95% confidence bands.

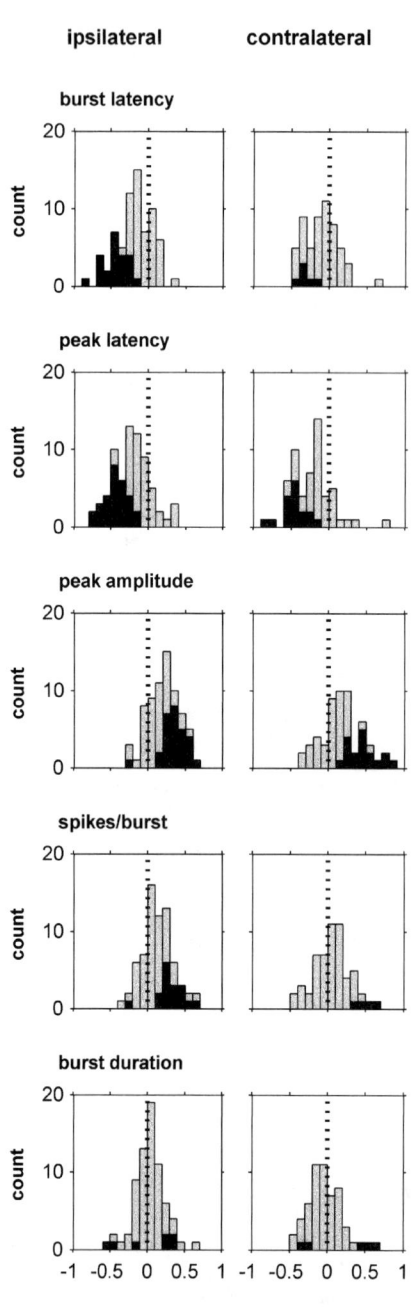

FIGURE 4. Distributions of the linear correlation coefficients of individual neurons calculated for the relations between burst parameters and saccade peak velocities (cf. FIG. 3). In the neuronal sample, negative correlations predominate for burst and peak latency; positive correlations predominate for burst peak amplitude. The *leftward* and *rightward* shifts of the distributions were, for these three parameters, statistically significant ($P < 0.05$). The *darker bars* represent data from neurons in which the correlation coefficients were statistically significant on the single-cell level.

in 59/70 and 39/56 units, and for peak burst amplitude in 58/70 and 44/56 units). These biases in the distributions of correlation coefficients, which were in each case statistically highly significant ($P < 0.01$), were even more pronounced for those neurons, in which the individual correlation coefficients were statistically significant at the single-cell level (FIG. 4).

Influence of Starting Position on Neuronal Responses

There were no systematic influences of the vertical component of the starting position (FIG. 1A) on FOR bursts. However, there were subtle, but recurrent differences in burst properties between bursts for centripetal and centrifugal saccades. Interestingly, these differences were recognizable for ipsilateral but not for contralateral eye movements. Typically (ipsilateral) centripetal saccades were accompanied by bursts that started and peaked earlier, and that showed higher peak discharge rates than bursts for otherwise similar centrifugal saccades (FIG. 1B). Although differences were statistically significant for only eight *individual* cells, there was a clear and statistically significant ($P < 0.05$) overrepresentation of units in which the difference between burst parameters for centripetal and centrifugal saccades was correspondingly negative (onset and peak latency) or positive (burst peak amplitude), over those in which these differences had the opposite signs.

Obviously, this pattern with earlier burst onset, shorter peak latencies, and higher peak discharge rates for centripetal as compared with centrifugal saccades paralleled the predominant pattern of correlations between burst parameters and saccade peak velocity described above. This correspondence raised the question of whether the subtle but systematic differences between centripetal and centrifugal saccades were related to an actual influence of eye position *per se*, or whether they rather reflected influences of saccade velocity. Indeed, the latter seems to be the case. Saccade peak velocities turned out to be on average significantly higher for centripetal than for centrifugal saccades for both monkeys (monkey #1: mean ± SD centripetal 462 ± 92°/s, centrifugal 430 ± 5°/s, $P < 10^{-5}$ (*t* test); monkey #2: centripetal 464 ± 102°/s, centrifugal 439 ± 95°/s, $P < 10^{-5}$). When these systematic differences were taken into account in the statistical analysis by considering saccade peak velocity as covariate, all differences between bursts for centripetal and centrifugal saccades were greatly attenuated or disappeared.

DISCUSSION

Our data show, for the first time, that FOR bursts correlate systematically with saccade velocity, both in their temporal properties and in their peak discharge rates. On the single-cell level, these effects are often not readily apparent in the highly variable discharge patterns of FOR neurons, and they are statistically significant for only a minority of individual units. However, they are present as a clear and, on the population level, statistically significant trend in a larger part of the neuronal population. In combination therefore, the bursts generated by individual FOR units may constitute a cerebellar output signal that reflects temporal characteristics and amplitude of the kinematic profile of the saccade. Accordingly, our data do not support the idea of Ohtsuka and Noda[5] that the cerebellar output signal would make use of a precise and specifically temporal code to determine saccade duration and, thereby, saccade amplitude. Rather, they are in line with the hypothesis that the contralateral and ipsilateral FOR bursts constitute supplementary accelerative and decelerative inputs to the burst generator.[6]

The saccade velocity sensitivity of ipsilateral and contralateral FOR bursts does not seem to be a merely passive reflection of saccade properties. If this was the case, the observed differences between bursts for centripetal and centrifugal saccades, which obviously relate to systematic direction-dependent differences in saccade velocity, should be present for both ipsilateral and contralateral saccades: these velocity differences, which are not a peculiar property of our data, but have been described previously for human primates,[13] are presumably caused by the passive mechanical forces arising in the orbital tissues that facilitate centripetal eye movements and are, of course, independent of the position of the microelectrode. Hence, they were present for contralateral saccades as well, whereas differences in centripetal and centrifugal FOR bursts were recognizable for ipsilateral saccades only. Remarkably, a parallel asymmetry was observed after unilateral FOR lesions: Robinson et al.,[4] who temporally inactivated the FOR on one side by means of muscimol injection, observed that centripetal saccades became distinctly more hypermetric than centrifugal saccades, but that this differences occurred for ipsilateral saccades only. This correspondence between response properties and lesion effects supports the notion that the observed saccade velocity sensitivity of FOR bursts has functional relevance.

CONCLUSION

Variations in the kinematic properties of saccades require dynamic changes in the muscular forces that brake the saccade to and at the targeted position and therefore require adaptive modifications of neuronal control signals. If the ipsilateral FOR bursts were involved in such function, it would make sense if they were stronger and occurred earlier or faster than for slower saccades. Our data suggest that they do indeed change in just this way. These dynamic modifications of FOR bursts not only may help to balance the mechanical forces arising in the eye plant, but may also play a relevant role in the general context of adaptive control of saccade metrics.

ACKNOWLEDGMENTS

The authors thank S. Langer for technical assistance. We are grateful thank Dr. E. Anagnostou for his participation and important contributions in the initial phase of this study. This work was supported by the Deutsche Forschungsgemeinschaft.

REFERENCES

1. RITCHIE, L. 1976. Effects of cerebellar lesions on saccadic eye movements. J. Neurophysiol. **39**: 1246–1256.
2. OPTICAN, L.M. & D.A. ROBINSON. 1980. Cerebellar-dependent adaptive control of the primate saccadic system. J. Neurophysiol. **44**: 1058–1075.

3. VILIS, T. & J. HORE. 1981. Characteristics of saccadic dysmetria in monkeys during reversible lesions of medial cerebellar nuclei. J. Neurophysiol. F**46:** 828–838.
4. ROBINSON, F.R., A. STRAUBE & A.F. FUCHS. 1993. Role of the caudal fastigial nucleus in saccade generation. 2. Effects of muscimol inactivation. J. Neurophysiol. **70:** 1741–1758.
5. OHTSUKA, K. & H. NODA. 1991. Saccadic burst neurons in the oculomotor region of the fastigial nucleus of macaque monkeys. J. Neurophysiol. **65:** 1422–1434.
6. FUCHS, A.F., F.R. ROBINSON & A. STRAUBE. 1993. Role of the caudal fastigial nucleus in saccade generation. 1. Neuronal discharge patterns. J. Neurophysiol. **70:** 1723–1740.
7. BOYLE, R., U. BÜTTNER & G. MARKERT. 1985. Vestibular nuclei activity and eye movements in the alert monkey during sinusoidal optokinetic stimulation. Exp. Brain Res. **57:** 362–369.
8. ROBINSON, D.A. 1963. A method of measuring eye movement using a scleral search coil in a magnetic field. IEEE Transactions in Bio-Medical Electronics. BME **10:** 137–145.
9. BARTL, K., C. SIEBOLD, S. GLASAUER, *et al.* 1996. A simplified calibration method for three-dimensional eye movement recordings using search-coils. Vision Res. **36:** 997–1006.
10. HANES, D.P., K.G. THOMPSON & J.D. SCHALL. 1995. Relationship of presaccadic activity in frontal eye field and supplementary eye field to saccade initiation in macaque: Poisson spike train analysis. Exp. Brain Res. **103:** 85–96.
11. SNODDERLY, D.M. & M. GUR. 1995. Organization of striate cortex of alert, trained monkeys (*Macaca fascicularis*): ongoing activity, stimulus selectivity, and widths of receptive field activating regions. J. Neurophysiol. **74:** 2100–2125.
12. HELMCHEN, C., A. STRAUBE & U. BÜTTNER. 1994. Saccade-related activity in the fastigial oculomotor region of the macaque monkey during spontaneous eye movements in light and darkness. Exp. Brain Res. **98:** 474–482.
13. PELISSON, D. & C. PRABLANC. 1988. Kinematics of centrifugal and centripetal saccadic eye movements in man. Vision Res. **28:** 87–94.

Neurons in the Caudal Frontal Eye Fields of Monkeys Signal Three-Dimensional Tracking

SERGEI KURKIN,[a] NORIHITO TAKEICHI,[a] TEPPEI AKAO,[a] FUMIE SATO,[a] JUNKO FUKUSHIMA,[b] CHRIS R.S. KANEKO,[c] AND KIKURO FUKUSHIMA[a]

[a]*Department of Physiology, School of Medicine, Hokkaido University, Sapporo 060-8638, Japan*

[b]*College of Medical Technology, Hokkaido University, Sapporo 060-8638, Japan*

[c]*Department of Physiology and Biophysics and Washington National Primate Research Center, University of Washington, Seattle, Washington 98195, USA*

ABSTRACT: To maintain optimal clarity of objects moving in three dimensions, precise coordination of binocular eye movements is required in frontal-eyed primates. Caudal parts of the frontal eye fields (FEFs) contain smooth pursuit neurons and the discharge of the majority of them is related to vergence eye movements as well. However, whether or not those pursuit neurons carry true binocular signals has not been tested critically. Using dichoptic stimuli that dissociate horizontal movements of the left and right eyes, we found that all pursuit-related, FEF neurons tested carried binocular signals.

KEYWORDS: frontal eye fields; smooth-pursuit; vergence; binocular coordination

INTRODUCTION

The evolution of binocular visual fields and high-acuity fovea conferred the advantage that three-dimensional visual information can be accurately obtained by aiming the foveae of both eyes at the objects of interest. For small objects moving slowly and smoothly, two eye movement systems are used to precisely track them and maintain their images on the foveae.[1] The smooth-pursuit system moves both eyes in the same direction (conjugately) to track movement in frontal planes (frontal pursuit), whereas the vergence system moves left and right eyes in opposite directions to track targets moving toward or away from the observer. Although the neural pathways mediating these two eye movement systems are known to be distinct,[1] recent observations have indicated that the frontal-pursuit and vergence system signals are combined in the caudal parts of the FEF.[2] Moreover, prearcuate saccade neurons also carry disparity-tuned (i.e., three-dimensional) visual responses.[3] These observations suggest that FEF neurons may carry binocular signals related to eye movements in three-dimensional space.

Address for correspondence: Kikuro Fukushima, Department of Physiology, Hokkaido University School of Medicine, West 7, North 15, Sapporo, 060-8638 Japan. Voice: 81-11-706-5038; fax: 81-11-706-5041.

kikuro@med.hokudai.ac.jp

In contrast, monocular command signals have been reported in the paramedian pontine reticular formation (PPRF).[4] Because direct projections to the PPRF are well known from the FEF,[1] it might be expected that they also contain monocular signals. However, whether FEF neurons carry true binocular signals has not been tested critically, because this question cannot be answered by monocular recording or with task conditions that induce conjugate eye movements. Apparent monocular tracking that requires asymmetric vergence eye movements in a plane aligned on one eye has been used to examine neural activity related to monocular movement,[4] but such tasks cannot exclude the possibility that apparent "monocular" discharge might be the result of cancellation of frontal pursuit by vergence tracking discharge sensitivity.[2,5] For example, FEF neurons that respond to both convergent tracking and leftward pursuit with similar sensitivity exhibit little discharge modulation during tracking in a plane aligned on the right eye[2] because the signals combine and cancel. We therefore developed a task condition that required the dissociation of left and right horizontal smooth eye movements. For this, a horizontal target trajectory was generated by combination of two different frequencies, one for each eye, and subjects tracked the fused image in a three-dimensional virtual space. We asked specifically in this study whether vergence and/or frontal-pursuit neurons in the caudal FEF carry true binocular signals.[2,6] To confirm first that subjects indeed track a single fused target, we tested this task in normal humans. We then tested identical tasks in monkeys and, by recording task-related neurons in the caudal FEF, we will show that they indeed carry true binocular signals.

METHODS

Human Studies

Three healthy subjects (aged 25–32 years) participated in this study. Informed consent was obtained from each of them. This study was approved by the Committee of Medical Ethics, Hokkaido University School of Medicine. Infrared oculography (DC-100 Hz/–24 dB/octave) was used to record horizontal and vertical movements of both eyes in each subject. The subjects were seated on a chair in a dimly lit room, facing a 22-inch computer display placed 40 cm away from their eyes. Their heads were firmly stabilized by a chin rest and a mechanical device. A virtual 0.5° red target spot was presented using a time multiplexed display acheived by using liquid crystal display shutters synchronized to independent alternating images for each eye at a 120-Hz refresh rate. Calibration of eye movements was taken before and after each session by asking the subjects to fixate a target on the display at known visual angles (±5°, ±10°) for each eye in the frontal plane.

In the control task conditions, subjects were asked to track the virtual spot either in the frontal plane (for frontal pursuit) or in depth in the midsagittal, cyclopean plane (for vergence tracking). The virtual target moved at a single frequency ranging from 0.2 to 1.9 Hz with identical anglular excursions for each eye (±5°) in these two task conditions. To dissociate horizontal components of left and right eye movements, we generated a horizontal target trajectory by combination of two different frequencies of horizontal target motion, one for each eye (e.g., FIG. 1A). In this "combined" task condition, all subjects reported that a single fused target moved in a complex trajectory in depth and frontal horizontal planes.

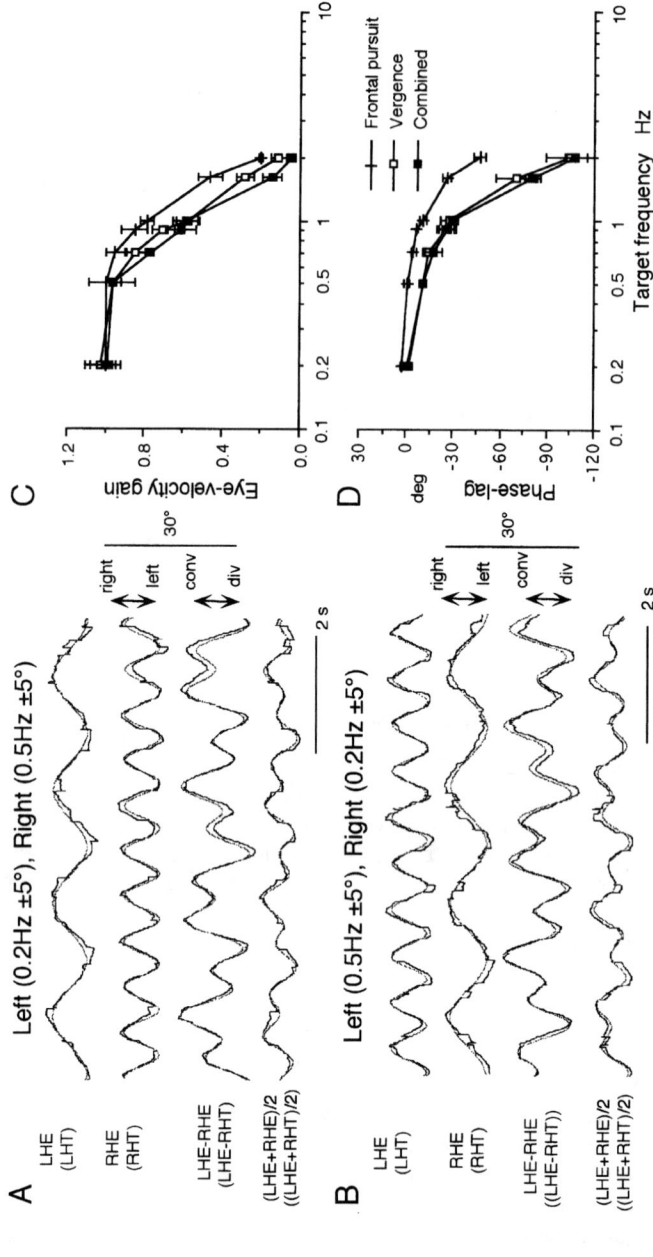

FIGURE 1. Human subject tracking. (**A, B**) The combined task. A horizontal target trajectory was generated by combination of two different frequencies of horizontal target motion for each eye as indicated. LHE and RHE indicate left horizontal eye position and right horizontal eye position, respectively. LHT and RHT indicate left horizontal target position and right horizontal target position, respectively. The third and fourth traces in **A** and **B** show vergence and version position components, respectively. In each, stimulus (*gray*) and response (*black*) traces are superimposed. (**C, D**) Eye-velocity gain and phase of a human subject during frontal-pursuit, vergence tracking, and combined task conditions as indicated.

Monkey Studies

Two male monkeys (*Macaca fuscata*, 3.8–4.5 kg) were used. All the procedures were evaluated and approved by the Animal Care and Use Committee of Hokkaido University School of Medicine. Our methods for animal preparation, training, and recording are described elsewhere in detail[2,7] and therefore are summarized here only briefly. Using apple juice reward, we trained monkeys to track the virtual target spot as in the human studies. In addition, asymmetric vergence tracking was examined by moving the target in the right or left eye–aligned plane perpendicular to the frontal plane. Extracellular recordings were made in the periarcuate cortex. Once isolated task-related neurons were located, frontal-pursuit, vergence tracking and the "combined" tasks were tested separately to examine neuronal discharge.

The data were analyzed off-line as previously described.[2,7] Position signals were differentiated to obtain velocity by analogue circuits (DC-100 Hz, −12 dB/octave). Saccades were removed using an interactive computer program. Vergence eye movements were calculated as the difference in horizontal components of the left and right eyes. A version component was calculated as the mean horizontal eye movement of the two eyes.[8,9] Eye vergence velocity, version velocity, and target velocity were averaged over 10 to 20 cycles for each eye. A least squares method was used to fit a sinusoid to eye movement responses. To quantify cell responses, we fitted a sine function to the cycle histograms of cell discharge, exclusive of the bins with zero spike rate, by means of a least squared error algorithm. Phase shift of eye version, vergence velocity, or cell response was calculated as the difference in phase between the peak stimulus velocity and the peak of the fundamental component of eye version, vergence velocity, or cell response, respectively. Gain was calculated as the peak amplitude of the fundamental component of these responses divided by target-velocity amplitude. For cell response, gain greater than or equal to 0.10 spikes/s/deg/s was taken as significant modulation. The preferred activation direction of each cell was estimated using a Gaussian function. The locations of recording sites of one monkey were histologically verified to be in the fundus of arcuate sulcus as in previous studies.[2,7,10]

RESULTS

Human Studies

All three subjects could fuse retinal images of both eyes, and they reported perceiving a single spot moving in the depth and/or frontal planes over the range of amplitudes and frequencies used in the combined task. Their eye movements were consistent with the perceived target motion. They reported that the target moved in depth when the two spots moved in opposite directions, and that it was moving in the frontal horizontal plane when the two spots moved in the same direction. Only at higher frequencies (>1 Hz) did they occasionally experience double images, suggesting that they failed to fuse those retinal images.

Representative tracking eye movements are shown in FIGURE 1A, B when two dichoptic spots moved horizontally at different frequencies in the "combined" task. Clearly, each eye followed the spot movement presented to that eye but not to the other (FIG. 1A, B). At higher frequencies (above 1 Hz), there was a tendency for cross talk between the two eyes in all subjects, that is, part of high-frequency components of one eye appeared in the other eye. However, such cross talk appeared only occasionally, was small in magnitude, and affected minimally, the calculation of phase and gain values. In the "combined" task, all subjects tracked target motion presented to each eye individually, with response characteristics similar to vergence tracking. Representative frequency response curves are illustrated in FIGURE 1C, D. Mean gain and phase (±SD) values during frontal pursuit, vergence tracking, and combined task of the right eye relative to target velocity presented to that eye for one subject are plotted against the frequencies of target motion. In the combined task, the left eye saw a target image moving at 0.5 Hz, whereas the right eye saw a target moving at different frequencies. During frontal pursuit, gain gradually dropped and phase-lags increased above 0.7 Hz and above 0.5 Hz during vergence tracking. Compared with these control responses, gain and phase curves in the combined task are quite similar to those of vergence tracking. The frequency response curves obtained from two other subjects were similar.

Monkey Studies

Tracking behavior of the virtual spot in two monkeys were similar. Frequency response curves for tracking eye movements during frontal-pursuit, vergence-tracking, and combined task conditions were like those shown in FIGURE 1. Using the combined task condition, we analyzed the activity of 38 neurons; 18 responded during vergence and frontal pursuit, 14 only during frontal pursuit with horizontal preferred directions, and the remaining 6 responded only during vergence tracking. Of the 18 vergence + frontal-pursuit neurons, preferred vergence directions were convergent ($n = 10$) or divergent ($n = 8$), and their frontal preferred directions were horizontal ($n = 11$), oblique ($n = 4$), and vertical ($n = 3$).

Discharge when two dichoptic spots moved at different frequencies is illustrated in FIGURE 2 (A1, B1) for two representative neurons. As in humans, each eye clearly followed the spot motion presented to that eye but not to the other. By comparing discharge modulation with left or right eye velocity (LHĖ or RHĖ, respectively), vergence velocity, or version velocity, we found that it is clear that discharge modulation is not closely related to velocity of a single eye (LHĖ or RHĖ). This is also shown by plotting discharge rate against velocity of one eye (FIG. 2A3, B3), and vergence (not shown), and version velocity (FIG. 2A2, B2). Higher correlation coefficients were obtained between discharge rate and version velocity (FIG. 2A2, B2) for both neurons. None of the 38 neurons tested showed a monocular preference in rate velocity plots.

To further evaluate and quantify discharge rate correlation with eye-velocity components, we approximated discharge rate by time-shifted linear combinations of the left and right eye velocities, as defined by the following equation[11]:

$$f(t - d) = gL * \text{LHĖ}(t) + gR * \text{RHĖ}(t) + C \tag{1}$$

where $f(t)$ is reconstructed firing frequency at time t; d is time lag between cell activity and eye movement; gR, gL are gains of right and left eye-velocity components; C is a bias term combining resting discharge rate and DC shift of LHĖ and RHĖ. Optimal coefficient values gR, gL, C, and time lag d were found using multiple re-

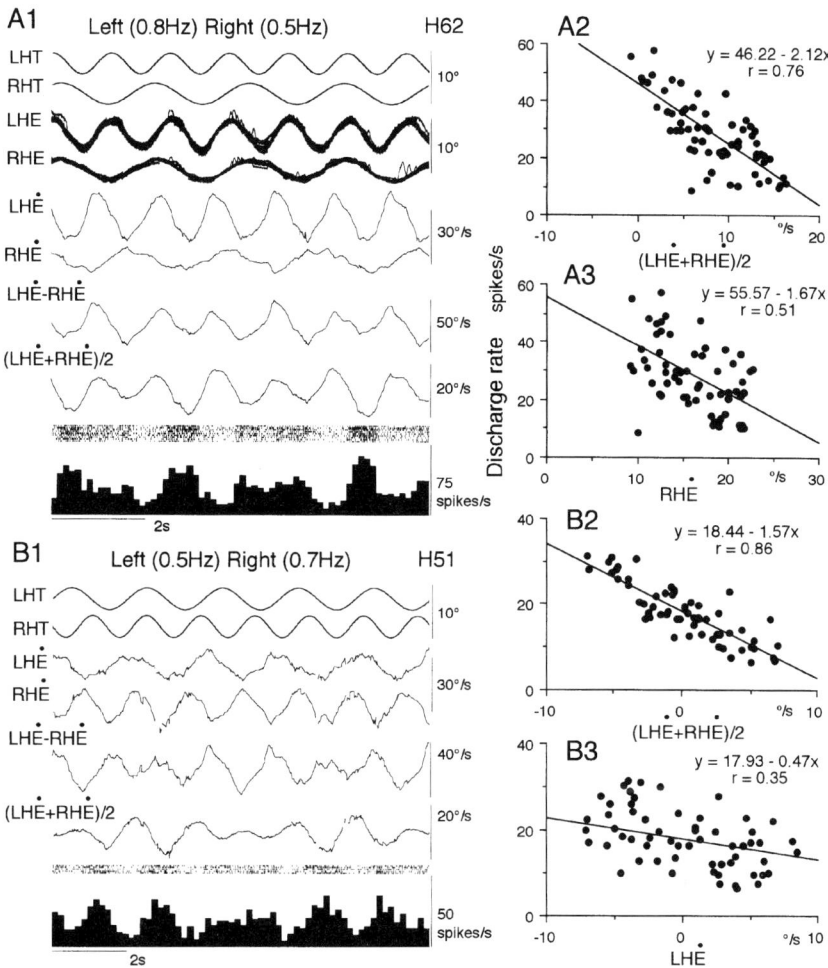

FIGURE 2. Discharge of two representative caudal FEF neurons during the combined task. (**A1–3, B1–3**) Responses of different neurons. (**A1, B1**) Discharge modulation. Traces indicated at left. (**A2, B2**) Discharge rate as a function of eye version velocity. (**A3, B3**) Discharge rate as a function of velocity of one eye. The same abbreviations are used as in FIGURE 1. Ė indicates eye velocity. Eye position traces (LHE, RHE) in **A1** were superimposed. All eye-velocity traces including version and vergence velocity in **A1** and **B1** were averaged.

gression.[11] By this method, we fit the discharge rate of the 38 neurons using either one eye or both eyes and calculated the best correlation for each neuron. Representative fitting is shown in FIGURE 3A, B for the two neurons illustrated in FIGURE 2A1, B1. In both neurons, the best correlation was obtained by fitting both left and right eyes. This result is consistent with rate-velocity correlations (FIG. 2A2 vs. A3, B2 vs. B3), where the best correlation was obtained by fitting discharge rate with the horizontal velocities of both eyes.

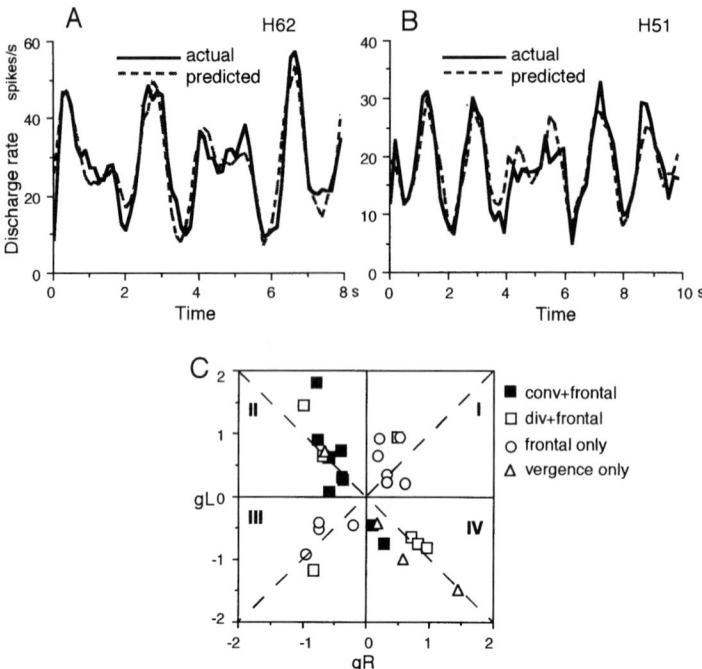

FIGURE 3. Fitting of discharge rate by left and right eye-velocity components using equation 1. **A, B**, actual (*black*), and predicted (*dashed gray*) discharge rate for the two neurons shown in FIGURE 2. gL, gR, d, and C values of equation 1 were −1.01, −2.37, +10, −7.5 for the neuron shown in **A**, and −1.07, −0.93, +20, −33.4 for the neuron shown in **B**. **C**, gR plotted against gL for four groups of neurons as indicated in the inset.

Calculation of version and vergence velocity assumes that left and right eyes contribute equally to the calculation (see METHODS).[8,9] To examine this assumption in the case of neuronal responses, we checked relative weights of gL and gR values across the different neurons by parsing the 38 neurons into four groups (convergence + frontal pursuit, divergence + frontal pursuit, frontal only, vergence only). Their *g*L and *g*R values are plotted in FIGURE 3C (see *key*). All neurons with vergence components (18 vergence + frontal pursuit, 6 vergence only) except for two (FIG. 3C, quadrants II and IV for each) were best fit by subtraction of the two components, whereas all frontal-pursuit–only neurons ($n = 14$) and the above two neurons were best fit by addition of left and right eye velocity (FIG. 3C, quadrants I and III). These two neurons had higher horizontal pursuit sensitivity than vergence-velocity sensitivity (1.92 vs. 0.77 and 1.98 vs. 0.29 spikes/s/deg/s, respectively), suggesting the best fit might have been induced by their stronger frontal-pursuit sensitivity during the combined task. Mean (± SD) gL/gR ratio for the 38 neurons was 1.33 (±1.25), close to one (*dotted lines* in FIG. 1C).

DISCUSSION

Using our "combined" task, we correlated discharge rates for all 38 neurons tested best with either vergence or version velocity and not the velocity of a single eye (FIG. 2). Moreover, discharge modulation of these neurons was best approximated by combinations of both left and right horizontal eye velocities with the mean gL/gR ratio close to one (FIG. 3). These results suggest that caudal FEF neurons carry true binocular signals for both vergence tracking and frontal pursuit. Although our inability to find monocular neurons in the caudal FEF does not completely rule out the possibility of monocular signals there, it would be reasonable to conclude that the caudal FEF codes primarily binocular signals for smooth tracking eye movements in three-dimensional space. Because true vergence and version signals are available in the caudal FEF, "monocular" commands can be easily extracted in the downstream pathways by taking a weighted sum of the activity of neurons with different combinations of binocular signals.[2] Thus, binocular signals in the caudal FEF can provide signals sufficient for individual movements of each eye.[4,5] Monocular signals would be necessary in some behavioral conditions.[1] Although it is still unknown where this extraction occurs for smooth tracking eye movements, the cerebellar floccular lobe (flocculus and ventral paraflocculus) is a potential site.[12,13] The flocculus projects to the vestibular nuclei which may provide the output signals.[1] The ventral paraflocculus projects both to the vestibular nuclei and to the deep cerebellar nuclei that could furnish ascending signals.[14] The latter projection may provide feedback signals to the caudal FEF for elaboration of binocular signals.[12]

ACKNOWLEDGMENTS

This work was supported in part by the Japanese Ministry of Education, Culture, Sports, Science, and Technology and Marna Cosmetics.

REFERENCES

1. LEIGH, R.J. & D.S. ZEE. 1999. The Neurology of Eye Movements. 3rd edit Oxford University Press. New York.
2. FUKUSHIMA, K., T. YAMANOBE, Y. SHINMEI, *et al.* 2002. Coding of smooth eye movements in three-dimensional space by frontal cortex. Nature **419:** 157–162.
3. FERRAINA, S., M. PARE & R.H. WURTZ. 2000. Disparity sensitivity of frontal eye field neurons. J. Neurophysiol. **83:** 625–629.
4. ZHOU, W. & W.M. KING. 1998. Premotor commands encode monocular eye movements. Nature **393:** 692–695.
5. KING, W.M. & W. ZHOU. 2000. New ideas about binocular coordination of eye movements: is there a chameleon in the primate family tree? New Anat. **261:** 153–161.
6. GAMLIN, P.D. & K. YOON. 2000. An area for vergence eye movement in primate frontal cortex. Nature **407:** 1003–1007.
7. FUKUSHIMA, K., T. SATO, J. FUKUSHIMA, *et al.* 2000. Activity of smooth pursuit-related neurons in the monkey periarcuate cortex during pursuit and passive whole body rotation. J. Neurophysiol. **83:** 563–587.
8. RASHBUSS, C. & G. WESTHEIMER. 1961. Independence of conjugate and disjunctive eye movements. J. Physiol. **159:** 361–364.
9. ERKELENS, C.J. & H. COLLEWIJN. 1985. Eye movements and stereopsis during dichoptic viewing of moving random-dot stereograms. Vision Res. **25:** 1689–1700.

10. FUKUSHIMA, K., T. YAMANOBE, Y. SHINME & J. FUKUSHIMA. 2002. Predictive responses of periarcuate pursuit neurons to visual target motion. Exp. Brain Res. **145:** 104–120.
11. GOMI, H., M. SHIDARA, A. TAKEMURA, *et al.* 1998. Temporal firing patterns of Purkinje cells in the cerebellar ventral paraflocculus during ocular following responses in monkeys. I. Simple spikes. J. Neurophysiol. **80:** 818–831.
12. FUKUSHIMA, K. 2003. Roles of the cerebellum in pursuit-vestibular interactions. Cerebellum **2:** 223–232.
13. CHIN, S., K. FUKUSHIMA, J. FUKUSHIMA, *et al.* 2002. Ocular torsion produced by unilateral chemical deactivation of the cerebellar flocculus in alert cats. Curr. Eye Res. **25:** 133–138.
14. NAGAO, S., T. KITAMURA, N. NAKAMURA, *et al.* 1997. Location of efferent terminals of the primate flocculus and ventral paraflocculus revealed by anterograde axonal transport methods. Neurosci. Res. **27:** 257–269.

Vestibular Signals of Posterior Parietal Cortex Neurons during Active and Passive Head Movements in Macaque Monkeys

FRANÇOIS KLAM AND WERNER GRAF

Laboratory de Physiologie de la Perception et de l'Action, CNRS/Collège de France, 11, place Marcelin Berthelot, 75231 Paris Cedex 05, France

ABSTRACT: The posterior parietal cortex may function as an interface between sensory and motor cortices and thus could be involved in the formation of motor plans as well as abstract representations of space. We have recorded from neurons in the intraparietal sulcus, namely, the ventral and medial intraparietal areas (VIP and MIP, respectively), and analyzed their head-movement–related signals in relation to passive and active movements. To generate active head movements, we made the animals track a moving fixation spot in the horizontal plane under head-free conditions. When under certain circumstances the animals were tracking the fixation spot almost exclusively via head movements, a clear correlation between neuronal firing rate and head movement could be established. Furthermore, a newly employed paradigm, the "replay method," made available direct comparison of neuronal firing behavior under active and passive movement conditions. In such case, the animals were allowed to make spontaneous head movements in darkness. Subsequently, the heads were fixed and the previously recorded active head-movement profile was reproduced by a turntable as passive stimulation. Neuronal responses ranged from total extinction of the vestibular signal during active movement to presence of activity only during active movement. Furthermore, in approximately one-third of the neurons, a change of vestibular on-direction depending on active versus passive movement mode was observed, that is, type I neurons became type II neurons, etc. We suggest that the role of parietal vestibular neurons has to be sought in sensory space representation rather than reflex behavior and motor control contexts.

KEYWORDS: parietal cortex; vestibular; monkey; head movement; active movement; efference copy; self-motion perception

INTRODUCTION

Distinction between active and passive movements is an important function in everyday life for goal directed movements without interference by reflex mechanisms, and to allow vital reflexes to happen when necessary. In this context, seminal concepts have been developed, such as the reafference principle[1] about how we move about and control and correct our own movements.

Address for correspondence: Werner Graf, CNRS-LPPA, Collège de France, 11, place Marcelin Berthelot, 75231 Paris Cedex 05, France. Voice: +33-1-44-27-16-30; fax: 33-1-44-27-13-82.
werner.graf@college-de-france.fr

Recent studies on vestibular nuclei neurons during passive and active head movements showed that vestibular signals were strongly influenced by self-generated movements as early as the first vestibular projection neurons,[2-4] and furthermore neurons in the vestibular nuclei related to head and eye movements subserving the vestibuloocular reflex are found in a similar proportion as neurons that signal only head velocity, without any eye-movement relatedness.[3] The latter are thought to be part of the vestibulocortical relay. However, some vestibuloocular neurons project to thalamic units that, in turn, then project to the vestibular cortices.[5] Vestibular thalamic and cortical units have been reported not to carry eye-movement signals.[6-8]

Several "vestibular" areas have been identified in the parietotemporal cortex of macaque monkeys, namely, the parietoinsular vestibular cortex,[9] area 2v at the anterior tip of the intraparietal sulcus,[10,11] area 3a[12] as part of somatosensory area 3, and in the posterolateral part of area PG.[13] Recent anatomical studies confirmed and extended previous findings that the ventral intraparietal area (VIP) in the fundus of the intraparietal sulcus[14] receives direct projections from vestibular areas and thus is part of a cortical vestibular network.[15-17] This work extends our previous reports on vestibular responses in VIP.[18-20] The principal aim of this study was to analyze head-movement–related signals in intraparietal vestibular neurons in relation to passive and active movements, in particular, because there exist large differences between active and passive movements as early as second-order vestibular neurons,[2-4] and also with respect of the involvement of the parietal cortex in self-motion perception and representation of extrapersonal space.

METHODS

Extracellular recordings were made in the left hemispheres of two macaque monkeys, one male rhesus *(Macaca mulatta)* and one female fascicularis monkey *(Macaca fascicularis)*. Animal care (housing, nourishment, veterinary consultations, surgical procedures, postoperative care, daily care) conformed to French government regulations (Ministries of Agriculture and Research, CNRS: approval 75-546) and European Union standards (European Communities Council Directive 86/609/EEC).

Animal Training

Head-fixed animals initially were trained to fixate a small spot of light within a narrow target window ($2 \times 2°$) for a certain time. The light spot could be kept stationary in darkness and in light to monitor a given neuron's resting activity. To determine a neuron's eye position sensitivity, we moved the spot in random order into nine different locations on the tangent screen.[21] The spot could also be moved to test smooth pursuit sensitivity (FIG. 1A). The animals' heads were fastened in a specialized head-holder system that allowed free head movements about the vertical axis (horizontal head movements) (FIG. 1B). Once the head was freed, the animals were allowed either to make spontaneous head movements or to track the light spot via head or combined eye–head movements. From the combined signals, head, eye, and gaze information could be derived.

In addition, we used a new testing paradigm to compare vestibular signals during active and passive head movements, the "replay method" (see also Robinson &

Tomko[22]). To that end, the animal was first allowed to make spontaneous head movements in the dark. Neuronal activity and the head-movement profile were recorded for various periods (up to 250 s). After that, the animal's head was fixed, and the previously recorded active head-movement trajectory was reproduced by the turntable, again recording neuronal activity. Thus, a direct comparison during active and passive neuron discharge became available.

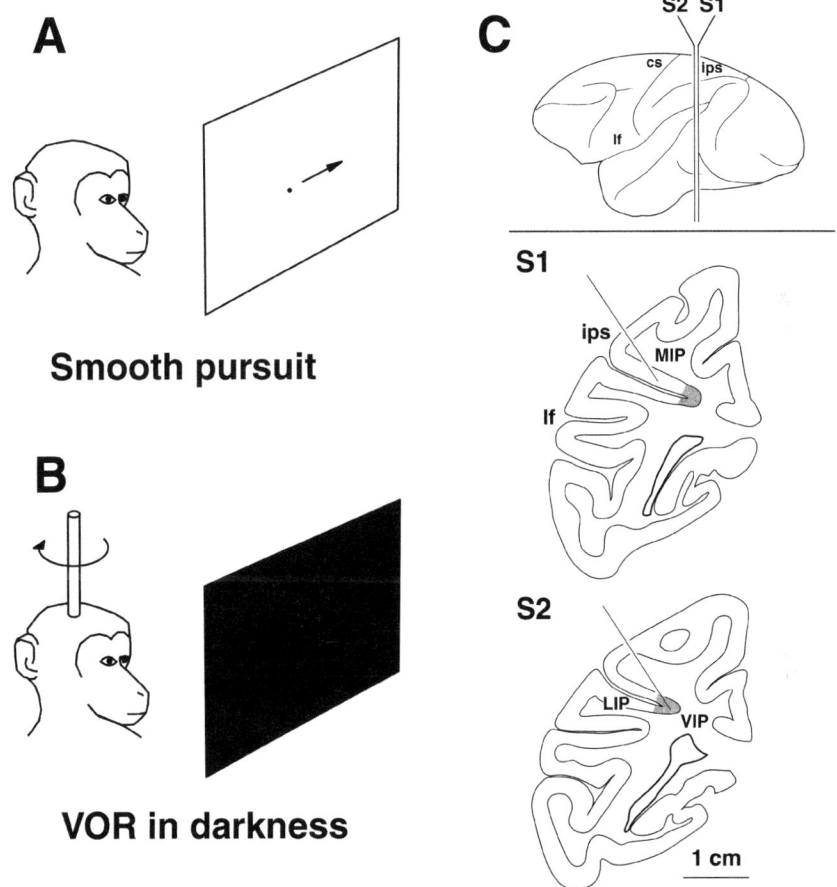

FIGURE 1. Stimulation parameters and location and reconstruction of recording sites. (**A**) Smooth pursuit: the animal was seated stationary and head-fixed in front of a tangent screen. It had to follow a light spot that was moved in eight cardinal linear directions. (**B**) Vestibular stimulation: the animal was rotated about the vertical axis in the darkened laboratory eliciting vestibular nystagmus. (**C**) Overall lateral view of the left hemisphere of a macaque monkey indicating the topographical relationship of cortical landmarks, that is, intraparietal sulcus (ips), central sulcus (cs), and the lateral fissure (lf). Vertical lines indicate the placement of two coronal sections (S1 and S2) shown below with reconstructed typical electrode tracks and recording sites (MIP, VIP) in the intraparietal sulcus. Area VIP is highlighted on the two slices in *gray*. Note that to reach VIP, electrode penetrations in some cases had to cross the intraparietal sulcus (LIP, lateral intraparietal area).

Recordings

Single cells were recorded extracellularly with glass-coated tungsten microelectrodes (F. Haer) in areas VIP and medial intraparietal area (MIP) of the two left hemispheres of the two monkeys. The animals were awake and performed several oculomotor tasks. Neurons were classified as located in area VIP on the basis of the recording sites and depth within the intraparietal sulcus, and for their response properties.[14,23–26] Neurons in MIP were characterized by absent or low visual sensitivity and strong somatosensory responses located on the fingers, hands, and forearms. In a typical recording session, the passage of the electrode from MIP into VIP was marked by a distinct change in background and resting activity of the recorded neuronal elements.

Eye movements were recorded with the magnetic search-coil method, head movements with a head-holder mounted potentiometer. Previous tests had shown that the eye-movement signal remained linear within the range of the monkey's head movements. Neuronal signals were sampled at 1000 Hz, and eye and head position at 250 Hz.

STIMULATION AND CHARACTERIZATION OF NEURONAL RESPONSIVENESS

Vestibular stimulation was delivered via a vertical axis turntable (horizontal rotation) that could be moved manually or via a servo controller. To exclude any visual influence on vestibular responses during purely vestibular testing, we covered the animals' eyes with opaque pads and darkened the laboratory. During vestibular testing, the animals, naturally, had to be left free to make compensatory eye movements (vestibuloocular reflex [VOR]) (FIG. 1B). Fixation and smooth pursuit targets were back-projected onto a translucent tangent screen. Directional selectivity was assessed as described previously.[27]

Data Analysis

Vestibular responses were evaluated according to their preferred, or on-directions[28] (type I, II, and III), for the response strength and the response latencies under the two movement conditions. Vestibular on-directions are referred according to the recording sites in the left hemisphere, that is, a neuron that reacts with excitation during leftward (ipsilateral) rotation is defined as a type I neuron, etc.

Because reflex compensatory eye movements had to be allowed in our experimental tasks (VOR), eye-movement sensitivities were evaluated separately. When judging their effect on the vestibular response by adding them in a simple multilinear regression, the R^2 never gained more than 10% of its original value, and usually less than a few percent (see also Bremmer et al.[20]). Moreover, the sensitivities to eye position usually were lower than the vestibular sensitivities by an order of magnitude. Smooth pursuit sensitivities were typically negligible as well (see FIG. 2B). We thus proceeded with our analysis without taking eye-movement effects further into account. Preferred directions of visual stimulus motion were determined using the weighted average method (for details, see Bremmer et al.[20,27]). All analyses were performed using either the SAS statistical package or programs in MATLAB and in visual C++.

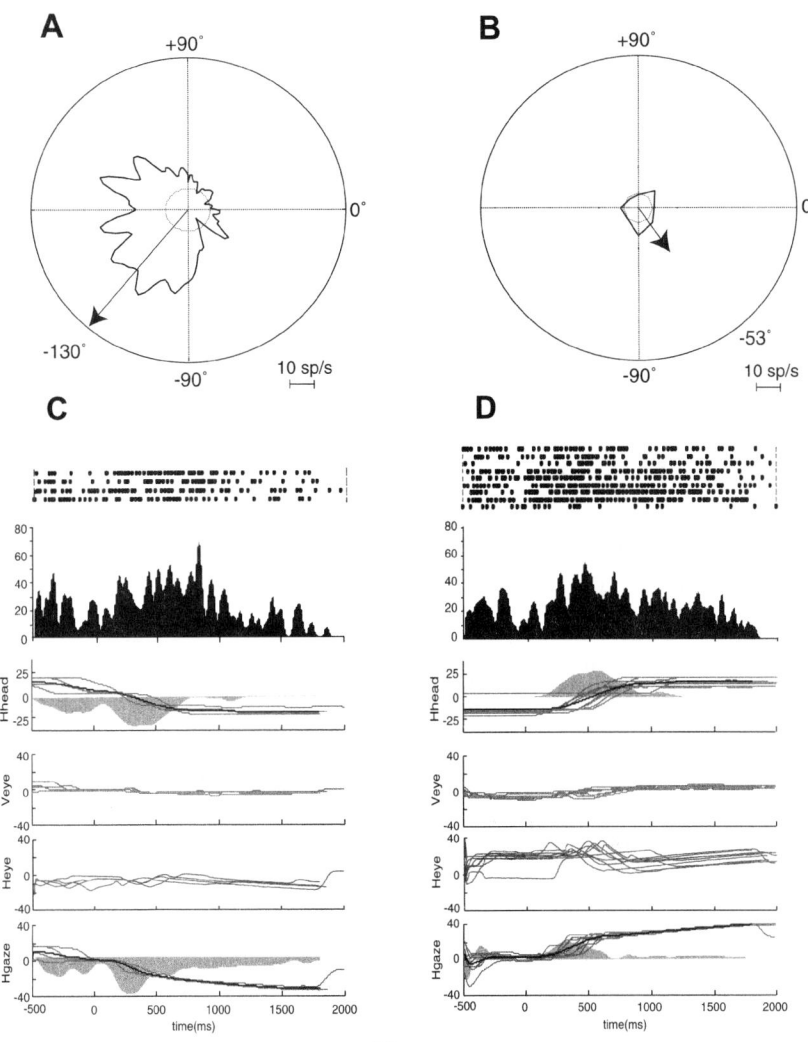

FIGURE 2. Response parameters of a posterior parietal vestibular neuron. (**A**) Polar plot of visual directional selectivity, indicating a preferred direction into the left hemifield (head-fixed condition). (*Solid black line*) Neuronal firing rate during stimulation; (*dotted circle*) resting discharge with fixation spot illuminated. (**B**) Polar plot of directional tuning during smooth pursuit (head-fixed condition). (*Outer solid line*) Firing rate during smooth pursuit; (*dotted circle*) discharge with fixation spot illuminated. (**C**) Pursuit of a horizontally moving target (head-free condition) to the left. Rows from top to bottom depict neuronal firing rate (shown as a raster plot and as a histogram); horizontal head movement (position: *line*, velocity: *gray shading*); vertical eye position; horizontal eye position; horizontal gaze (position: *line*, velocity: *gray shading*). (**D**) Pursuit of a horizontally moving target (head-free condition) to the right. Presentation sequence is as in **C**. Note that the animal, in this case almost exclusively, uses head movements to pursue the target (in particular in **C**). The neuron's firing rate (vestibular type III) seems to be related principally to head movement.

Anatomical Location of Recorded Cells and Physiological Characterization

In our experiments, neurons were recorded along microelectrode tracks determined by a grid that allowed reproducible positionings across experimental sessions with maximal precision. While descending in the intraparietal sulcus from the surface, vestibular testing was performed regularly. Besides VIP, we recorded also from MIP, a second intraparietal vestibular zone that was quite distinct from VIP for anatomical location and physiological characteristics. The recording sites have been verified in the fascicularis monkey to be located in the medial bank and in the fundus of the intraparietal sulcus (FIG. 1C). The rhesus monkey is still used in ongoing experiments.

RESULTS

A total of 106 cells were recorded in the intraparietal sulcus of two left hemispheres of two macaque monkeys in response to various visual, vestibular, and oculomotor paradigms, and active-passive head-movement comparisons.

Posterior Parietal Vestibular Neurons during Pursuit Head Movements

Posterior parietal vestibular neurons could be shown to be visually direction-selective, as reported previously (Bremmer et al.[20,27] FIG. 2A). Although all vestibular-responsive posterior parietal neurons had eye-position sensitivity (Bremmer et al.[20]), smooth pursuit activity was almost negligible at the velocities tested in our experiments (up to 20°/s; FIG. 2B). Under certain circumstances, the animals were tracking the fixation spot almost exclusively via head movements (FIG. 2C, D). In such case, a clear correlation between neuronal firing rate and head movement could be established. Surprisingly, many parietal vestibular neurons showed type III vestibular responses during active head movements, i.e., activation to ipsi- and contralateral rotation (see also FIG. 3C, D).

Comparison between Passive and Active Head Movements

Response characteristics of parietal vestibular neurons during active and passive head movements were studied by comparing the neuronal firing rate during an active head movement with that of the replay of the same head-movement profile under passive and head-fixed conditions (FIG. 3). The roster of the illustrated neuron examples shows a wide variety of responses, ranging from total extinction of the vestibular signal during active movement (FIG. 3A) to presence of activation only during active movement with absence of any neuronal reaction during passive stimulation (FIG. 3B). Neuronal signals could be diminished in the active movement condition compared with passive stimulation (FIG. 3C), or the vestibular signal could become stronger in the active movement condition (FIG. 3D). Most surprisingly, quite frequently we also found a change of directional selectivity for the vestibular on-directions of the recorded neurons (FIG. 3D). The neuron illustrated in FIGURE 3D has a type III response in the active head-movement condition but shows a type I response under passive vestibular stimulation (i.e., excitation via rotation to ipsilateral).

Quantification of change of directional selectivity was provided by plotting firing rates as a function of head velocity of selected neurons during active and passive movement conditions (FIG. 4A, B). In the illustrated examples, one neuron's firing behavior changed from type II in the active condition to type I under passive stimulation (FIG. 4A). In the other case (FIG. 4B), neuronal firing showed type I directional

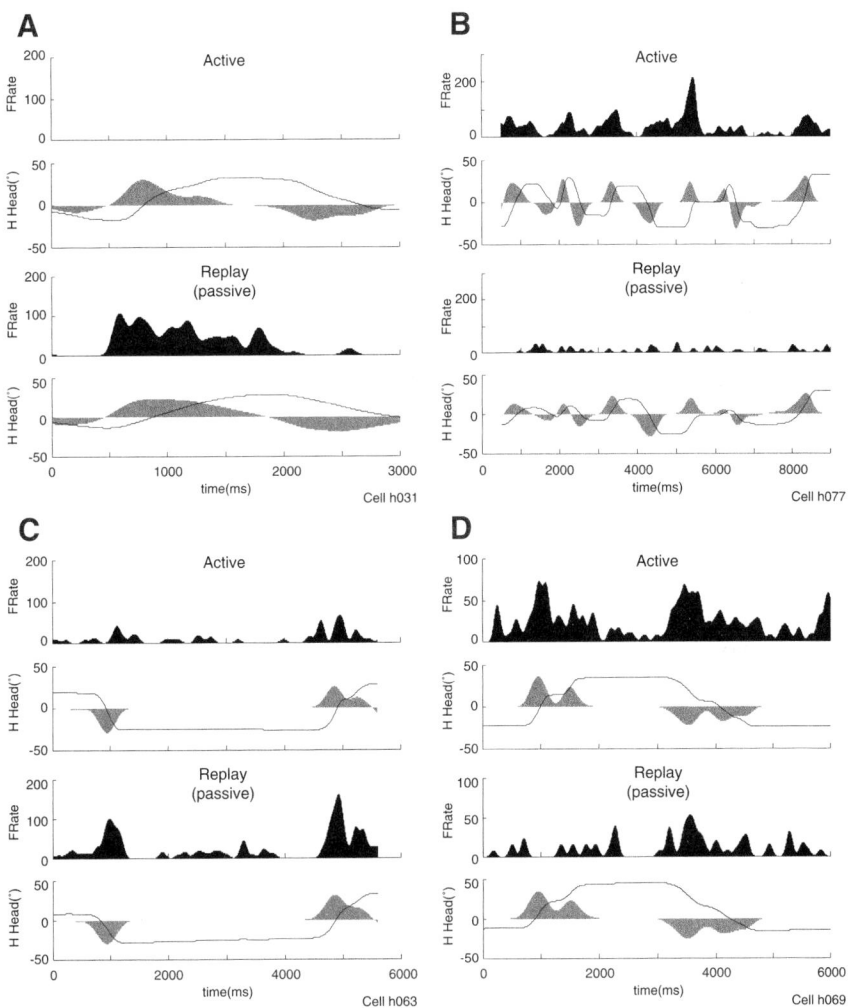

FIGURE 3. Comparison of firing behavior of parietal vestibular neurons during active and passive (replay) head movements. (**A**) Type II neuron active only during passive rotation. (**B**) Type II neuron only active during active head movement. (**C**) Type III neurons whose activity is larger during passive stimulation. (**D**) Under active movement conditions, this neuron shows type III behavior; under passive stimulation it shows type I behavior. Neuronal activity is greater during active head movements than during passive stimulation.

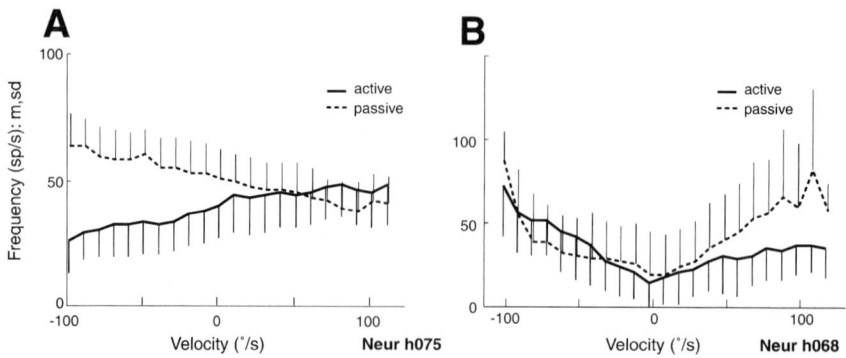

FIGURE 4. Illustration and quantification of change of on-direction of posterior parietal vestibular neurons during active and passive head movements. (**A**) Neuronal firing rate in relation to head velocity. The neuron shows type II behavior (increase of firing toward positive velocity values, i.e., rotation to the right) during active head movement and type I behavior (increase of firing toward negative velocity values; i.e., rotation to the left) during passive stimulation. (**B**) Neuronal firing rate in relation to head velocity. The neuron shows type I behavior (increase of firing toward negative velocity values) during active head movement and type III behavior (increase of firing toward negative and positive velocity values) during passive stimulation. (**C**) Quantification of neuronal responses. Approximately one-third of the tested neuron population shows a change in vestibular on-direction depending on active versus passive movement mode.

selectivity during active head movements, which then changed to type III behavior under passive stimulation conditions. The full complement of our neuron sample is illustrated in FIGURE 4C. Clearly, many neurons change directional selectivity depending on active versus passive movement mode, involving all possible combinations of the encountered vestibular response types, that is, types I, II, and III. Of a total of 86 neurons that were tested, 33 (38%), that is, more than one-third, showed the described change in vestibular on-direction.

Quantification of the strength of neuronal responses under active versus passive movement conditions (FIG. 5) also demonstrated that in most cases, neuronal responses were diminished under active movement conditions compared with passive stimulation. In approximately equal proportions, response strengths stayed the same or were even stronger in the active condition.

When determining response delays to vestibular stimulation, neurons clearly had earlier reaction times under active movement condition (FIG. 6). Naturally, under

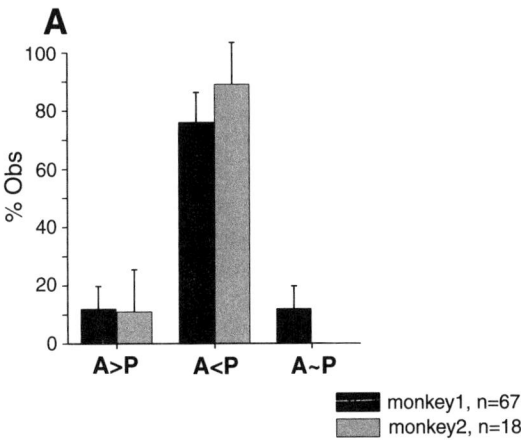

FIGURE 5. Quantification of response strengths of posterior parietal neurons for active or passive movement mode. In most neurons, responses were weaker during active movement than during passive stimulation. However, in a sizable minority, neuronal responses stayed the same or became even stronger during active movement.

passive stimulation conditions, a given neuron only reacted after the onset of turntable movement. Under active head-movement conditions, neurons could fire as early as 400 ms before the ensuing head movement, although such cases were rare exceptions. Most neurons fired up to 100 ms after movement onset. A sizable minority, however, was observed to be activated already up to 100 ms before the actual head movement.

DISCUSSION

The variety of vestibular responses in posterior parietal cortex neurons points to a complex processing pattern that is not readily accessible to traditional methods of analysis. Because our present and previous testing (Bremmer *et al.*[20]) had shown little influence of eye-movement signals on the neuronal firing of parietal vestibular neurons, we assume that these neurons are fundamentally different from brainstem vestibular neurons. Their role has to be sought in sensory space representation rather than reflex behavior and motor control contexts. Clearly, each time we perform a head movement, vestibular receptors become activated, and central processing between commands and reflexes takes place. Because vestibular receptors *per se* cannot distinguish between active and passive movements,[29] this distinction has to be furnished by central neurons. Second-order vestibular neurons, that is, two synapses away from the receptor cells already react differentially to active and passive head movements.[2–4] The question to be answered in this context now is where the actual neuronal processing of this distinction occurs. Posterior parietal cortex neurons may perform this function, or at least play an important role in it.[30]

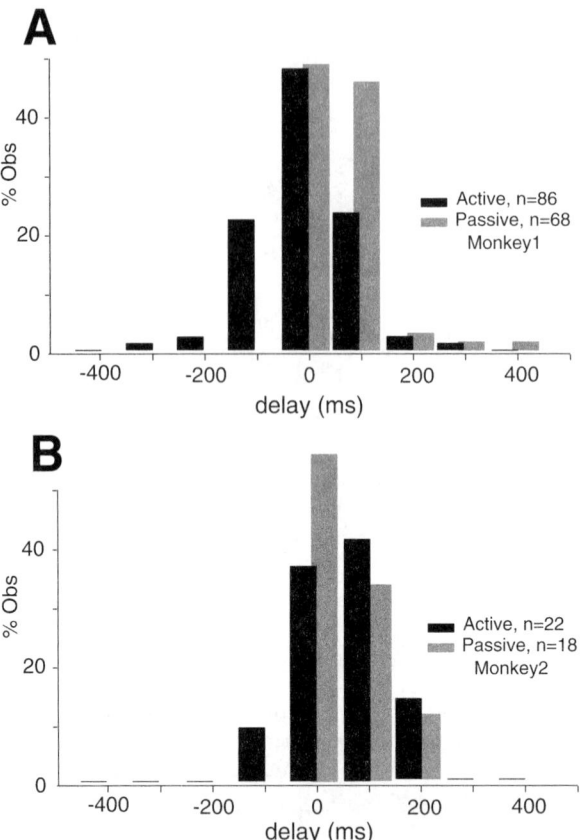

FIGURE 6. Response latencies of neuronal firing rates for onset of head movement. Bin width for analysis was set to 100 ms. Most responses to active head movement and passive stimulation occurred up to 100 ms after head movement, or stimulus onset. However, neuronal activity could precede self-initiated head movements by as much as 400 ms, although 100 ms was a value observed more often.

Although some of our posterior parietal vestibular neurons receive neck input (unpublished observation), the key to understanding active-passive movement distinction processing may be the change in vestibular on-direction of approximately one-third of these neurons (FIG. 4C). A simple combination of neurons with particular directional selectivity depending on active or passive movement mode would allow specific populations of target neurons to become active and thus provide an output signal that would be discriminating between active and passive movement. These signals, in turn, could be used to suppress reflex movements during active movement by providing the neural basis for the observed extinction of, for instance, vestibular signals during active head rotation in the vestibular nuclei.[2–4]

A change of on-direction of the vestibular signal depending on the VOR gain was reported in gaze-velocity Purkinje cells,[31] and such activity has been discussed in context of motor learning.[32] Our own data point to a much more widespread use of such change in directional selectivity. All in all, we conclude that parietal vestibular neurons may play a much more important role in the processing of self-motion detection signals than has been envisioned up to now, being part of a large network involved the perception of extrapersonal space.

ACKNOWLEDGMENTS

This work was supported by the European Union (BIO4-CT98-0546), CNRS (UMR 9950/7124), and the ATER program of the Collège de France.

REFERENCES

1. V. HOLST, E. & H. MITTELSTAEDT. 1950. Das Reafferenzprinzip. Naturwissenschaften **37:** 464–476.
2. MCCREA, R.A., G.T. GDOWSKI, R. BOYLE & T. BELTON. 1999. Firing behavior of vestibular neurons during active and passive head movements: vestibulo-spinal and other non-eye-movement related neurons. J. Neurophysiol. **82:** 416–428.
3. GDOWSKI, G.T. & R.A. MCCREA. 1999. Integration of vestibular and head movement signals in the vestibular nuclei during whole body rotation. J. Neurophysiol. **81:** 436–449.
4. ROY, J.E. & K.E. CULLEN. 2001. Selective processing of vestibular reafference during self-generated head motion. J. Neurosci. **21:** 2131–2142.
5. MATSUO, S., M. HOSOGAI, H. MATSUI & H. IKOMA. 1995. Posterior canal-activated excitatory vestibuloocular relay neurons participate in the vestibulocortical pathways in cats. Acta Otolaryngol. **520:** 97–100.
6. MAGNIN, M. & A. FUCHS. 1977. Discharge properties of neurons in the monkey thalamus tested with angular acceleration, eye movement and visual stimuli. Exp. Brain Res. **28:** 293–299.
7. BÜTTNER, U., V. HENN & H.P. OSWALD. 1977. Vestibular-related neuronal activity in the thalamus of the alert monkey during sinusoidal rotation in the dark. Exp. Brain Res. **30:** 435–444.
8. GRÜSSER, O.-J., M. PAUSE & U. SCHREITER. Vestibular neurons in the parieto-insular cortex of monkeys (*Macaca fascicularis*): visual and neck receptor responses. J. Physiol. (Lond.) **430:** 559–583.
9. GRÜSSER, O.-J., M. PAUSE & U. SCHREITER. 1990. Localization and responses of neurons in the parieto-insular vestibular cortex of awake monkeys (*Macaca fascicularis*). J. Physiol. (Lond.) **430:** 537–557.
10. SCHWARZ, D.W.F. & J.M. FREDRICKSON. 1971. Rhesus monkey vestibular cortex: a bimodal primary projection field. Science **172:** 280–281.
11. BÜTTNER, U. & U.W. BUETTNER. 1978. Parietal cortex (2v) neuronal activity in the alert monkey during natural vestibular and optokinetic stimulation. Brain Res. **153:** 392–397.
12. ÖDKVIST, L.M., D.W.F. SCHWARZ, J.M. FREDRICKSON & R. HASSLER. 1974. Projection of the vestibular nerve to the area 3a arm field in the squirrel monkey (*Saimiri sciureus*). Exp. Brain Res. **21:** 97–105.
13. SAKATA, H., H. SHIBUTANI, Y. ITO, *et al.* 1994. Functional properties of rotation-sensitive neurons in the posterior parietal association cortex of the monkey. Exp. Brain Res. **101:** 183–202.
14. COLBY, C.L. & J.-R. DUHAMEL. 1991. Heterogeneity of extrastriate visual areas and multiple parietal areas in the macaque monkey. Neuropsychologia **29:** 517–537.
15. GULDIN, W.O., S. AKBARIAN & O.-J. GRÜSSER. 1992. Cortico-cortical connections and cytoarchitectonics of the primate vestibular cortex: a study in squirrel monkeys (*Saimiri sciureus*). J. Comp. Neurol. **326:** 375–401.

16. LEWIS, J.W. & D.C. VAN ESSEN. 2000. Mapping of architectonic subdivisions in the macaque monkey, with emphasis on parieto-occipital cortex. J. Comp. Neurol. **428:** 79–111.
17. LEWIS, J.W. & D.C. VAN ESSEN. 2000. Corticocortical connections of visual, sensorimotor, and multimodal processing areas in the parietal lobe of the macaque monkey. J. Comp. Neurol. **428:** 112–137.
18. GRAF, W., F. BREMMER, S. BEN HAMED & J.-R. DUHAMEL. 1996. Visual-vestibular interaction in the ventral intraparietal area (VIP) of macaque monkeys. Soc. Neurosci. Abstr. **22:** 666.7.
19. BREMMER, F., J.-R. DUHAMEL, S. BEN HAMED & W. GRAF. 1997. The representation of movement in near extra-personal space in the macaque ventral intraparietal area (VIP). *In* Parietal Lobe Contributions to Orientation in 3D Space. P. Thier & H.O. Karnath, Eds.: 619–630. Springer Verlag. Berlin-Heidelberg–New York.
20. BREMMER, F., F. KLAM, J.-R. DUHAMEL, *et al.* 2002. Visual-vestibular interactive responses in the macaque ventral intraparietal area (VIP). Eur. J. Neurosci. **16:** 1569–1586.
21. BREMMER, F., W. GRAF, S. BEN HAMED & J.-R. DUHAMEL. 1999. Eye position encoding in the macaque ventral intraparietal area (VIP). Neuroreport **10:** 873–878.
22. ROBINSON, F.R. & D.L. TOMKO. 1987. Cat vestibular neurons that exhibit different responses to active and passive yaw head rotations. Aviat. Space Environ. Med. **58:** A247–249.
23. COLBY, C.L., J.-R. DUHAMEL & M.E. GOLDBERG. 1993. The ventral intraparietal area (VIP) of the macaque: anatomical location and visual properties. J. Neurophysiol. **69:** 902–914.
24. SCHAAFSMA, S.J. & J. DUYSENS. 1996. Neurons in the ventral intraparietal area of awake macaque monkey closely resemble neurons in the dorsal part of the medial superior temporal area in their responses to optic flow patterns. J. Neurophysiol. **76:** 4056–4068.
25. SCHAAFSMA, S.J., J. DUYSENS & C.C. GIELEN. 1997. Responses in ventral intraparietal area of awake macaque monkey to optic flow patterns corresponding to rotation of planes in depth can be explained by translation and expansion effects. Vis. Neurosci. **14:** 633–646.
26. DUHAMEL, J.-R., C.L. COLBY & M.E. GOLDBERG. 1998. Ventral intraparietal area of the macaque: congruent visual and somatic response properties. J. Neurophysiol. **79:** 126–136.
27. BREMMER, F., S. BEN HAMED, J.-R. DUHAMEL & W. GRAF. 2002. Optic flow processing in the macaque ventral intraparietal area (VIP). Eur. J. Neurosci. **16:** 1554–1568.
28. DUENSING, F. & K.-P. SCHAEFER. 1958. Die Aktivität einzelner Neurone im Bereich der Vestibulariskerne bei Horizontalbeschleunigungen unter besonderer Berücksichtigung des vestibulären Nystagmus. Arch. Psychiat. Nervenkrankh. **196:** 265–290.
29. CULLEN, K.E. & L.B. MINOR. 2002. Semicircular canal afferents similarly encode active and passive head-on-body rotations: implications for the role of vestibular efference. J. Neurosci. **22:** RC226(1–7).
30. GABEL, S.F., H. MISSLICH, C.C.A.M. GIELEN & J. DUYSENS. 2002. Responses of neurons in area VIP to self-induced and external visual motion. Exp. Brain Res. **147:** 520–528.
31. LISBERGER, S.G., T.A. PAVELKO, H.M. BRONTE-STEWART & L.S. STONE. 1994. Neural basis for motor learning in the vestibuloocular reflex of primates. II. Changes in the responses of horizontal gaze velocity Purkinje cells in the cerebellar flocculus and ventral paraflocculus. J. Neurophysiol. **72:** 954–973.
32. GREEN, A. & H.L. GALIANA. 1996. Exploring sites for short-term VOR modulation using a bilateral model. Ann. N.Y. Acad. Sci. **781:** 625–628.

Inhibitory Interhemispheric Visuovisual Interaction in Motion Perception

THOMAS BRANDT,[a] ESTHER MARX,[a] THOMAS STEPHAN,[a] SANDRA BENSE,[b] AND MARIANNE DIETERICH[b]

[a]*Department of Neurology, Ludwig-Maximilians University, Klinikum Grosshadern, 81377 Munich, Germany*

[b]*Department of Neurology, Johannes Gutenberg University, 55131 Mainz, Germany*

ABSTRACT: Findings of an earlier functional magnetic resonance imaging (fMRI) study that coherent motion stimulation of the right or left visual hemifield exhibited negative signal changes (deactivations) in the primary visual cortex and the lateral geniculate nucleus contralateral to the stimulated hemisphere were evaluated to determine the functional significance of this contralateral inhibition of the visual system. Fourteen subjects participated in a psychophysical study on the perception of single object motion (0.4°/s) in one visual hemifield with or without concurrent coherent motion stimulation of the contralateral hemifield. Mean detection times for horizontal object motion (0.5 ± 0.19 vs. 0.61 ± 0.22 s) and vertical object motion (0.53 ± 0.19 vs. 0.72 ± 0.34 s) were significantly prolonged during concurrent motion pattern stimulation in the contralateral hemifield. These data support the interpretation that the deactivation of neuronal activity in the visual system found by fMRI is associated with a functional decrement in the sensitivity needed to perceive motion and may reflect transcallosal attentional shifts between the two hemispheres.

KEYWORDS: visual hemifield; motion perception; transcallosum; visuovisual interaction; fMRI and psychophysics

INTRODUCTION

In an earlier functional magnetic resonance imaging (fMRI) study, we found that coherent motion stimulation of the right or left visual hemifield elicits a significant visuovisual interhemispheric interaction.[1] Motion stimulation of one hemisphere caused the following changes in brain activity in the nonstimulated hemisphere: first, an activation of the medial occipital gyrus including motion sensitive middle temporal/middle superior temporal areas (MT/V 5) and second, a deactivation of the primary visual cortex including the lingual and fusiform gyri, and of the lateral geniculate nucleus (FIG. 1). This interaction is most likely mediated by transcallosal pathways. Animal experiments[2,3] and brain activation studies[1,4,5] have shown that

Address for correspondence: Thomas Brandt, MD, Department of Neurology, Klinikum Grosshadern, Ludwig-Maximilians University, Marchioninistrasse 15, 81377 Munich, Germany. Voice: 49/89-7095-2570; fax: 49/89-7095-8883.
thomas.brandt@nro.med.uni-muenchen.de

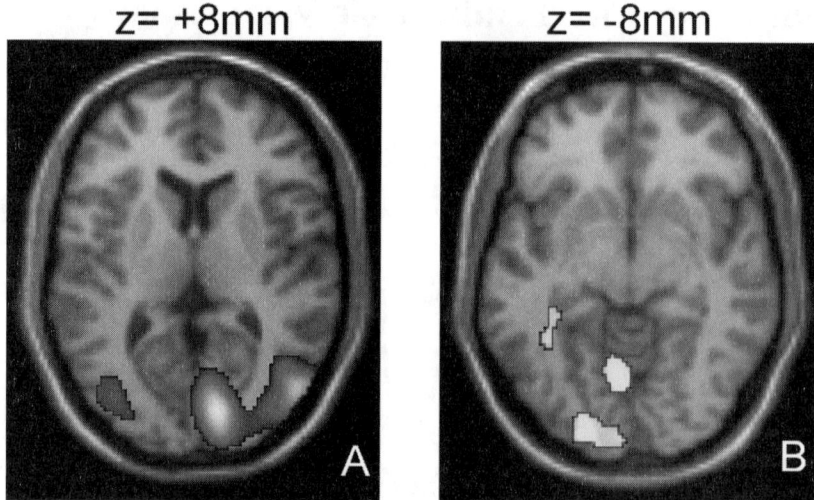

FIGURE 1. fMRI during visual hemifield motion stimulation in the roll plane while a stationary target straight ahead is fixated. Areas with signal increases (*left*) and signal decreases (*right*) during motion stimulation of the left hemifield obtained by statistical group analysis ($n = 9$; $P < 0.001$). Activation maps are superimposed onto transverse sections of a standard brain template 8 mm above or below the anterior-posterior commissure. Activations were found in the primary visual cortex contralateral to the stimulated hemifield and in the medial occipital gyrus covering MT/V 5 on both the stimulated hemisphere as well as the hemisphere without input from the ipsilateral visual cortex. Signal decreases were found in the primary visual cortex and the lateral geniculate nucleus in the hemisphere without direct visual input.

the visual cortices, especially the motion-sensitive areas MT/V5, are connected interhemispherically by commissural fibers.

The fMRI findings of contralateral activations and deactivations during visual hemifield motion stimulation raise the question of their functional significance. We argued earlier that contralateral activation of MT/V5 allows both hemispheres to interact in stimulus situations in which visual hemifields have contradictory information about motion, for example, when sitting in a train reading.[1,6] Here information about constant velocity self-motion is provided by the optic flow pattern in one hemifield, while the other hemifield is filled with stationary contrasts from inside the train. Because you cannot perceive two different states of body motion at the same time, the two hemispheres have to correspond to each other to determine an actual and unique perception of self-motion or absence of motion.

The functional significance of this contralateral inhibition of the visual cortex and the lateral geniculate nucleus may possibly be related to attentional mechanisms. It was hypothesized that the inhibitory intrasensory visuovisual interaction found in the fMRI study would allow attention to be shifted between the two hemispheres (to visual hemifields) by raising the perceptual thresholds in the hemifield with the currently less relevant input.[1] The latter hypothesis prompted us to conduct a psychophysical study on the perception of object motion in one hemifield with and without concurrent coherent motion stimulation of the opposite hemifield.

METHODS

Object motion perception was tested in 14 healthy volunteers (8 women, 6 men; 20–52 years of age; mean age 31.6 years). Volunteers sat on a chair with a headrest in darkness while fixating a stationary target straight ahead (red light-emitting diode, diameter 0.6 degrees). A second target, a projected white dot (diameter 0.9 degrees), was presented throughout the experiments in the right or left hemifield 8° horizontally beyond the vertical meridian (FIG. 2). The eccentric dot started to move haphazardly with random latencies at a constant velocity of 0.4°/s in the horizontal or vertical direction.

In a second condition, an additional motion pattern was projected onto the contralateral hemifield with the vertical edge of the pattern located 10° distant from the fixation point to avoid stimulating the vertical meridian, which is represented retin-

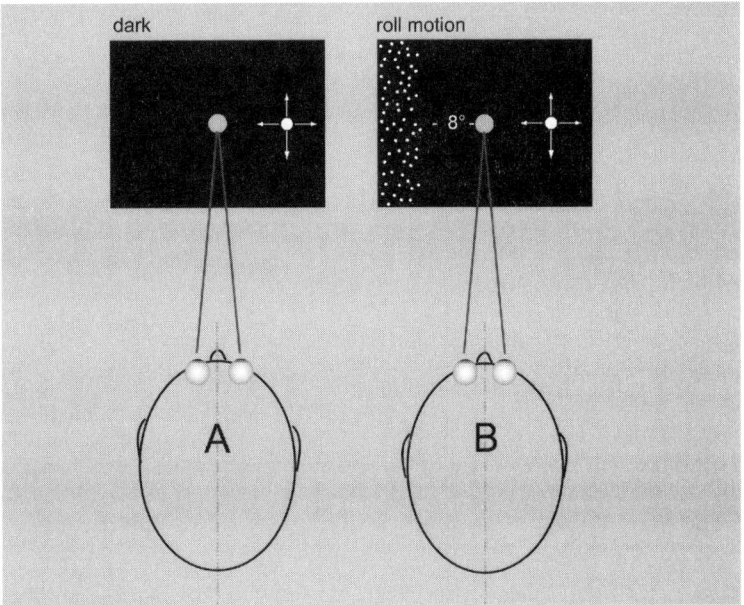

FIGURE 2. Schematic representation of the experimental conditions during the psychophysical experiments. Subjects were asked to fixate a stationary target straight ahead and to press a button when they detected horizontal or vertical motion of the eccentric white dot, which started to move with random latencies in various directions. Object motion perception was measured without (**A**) and with (**B**) concurrent coherent motion pattern stimulation in the contralateral hemifield. The vertical edge of the motion pattern and the single moving target were located 8° from the central fixation point to avoid stimulating the vertical meridian.

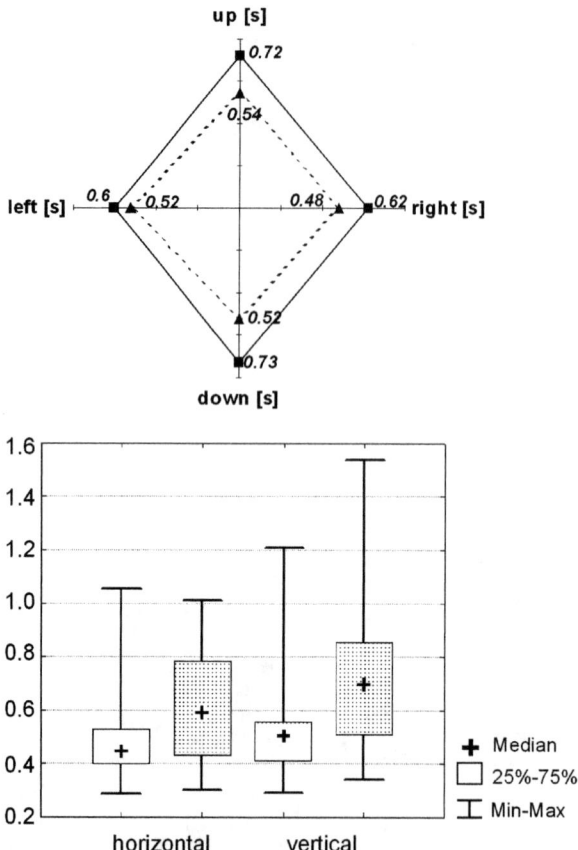

FIGURE 3. Mean detection times for vertical (*upward or downward*) and horizontal (*right or left*) target motion (0.4°/s) without (*dotted line*) and with (*solid line*) concurrent motion pattern stimulation in the contralateral visual hemifield (*left*). Box plot showing mean detection times of target motion averaged across the group ($n = 14$) with (*dotted rectangles*) and without (*plain rectangles*) concurrent motion pattern stimulation (*right*). The diagram shows the minimum, lower quartile, median, upper quartile, and maximum of the data. Mean detection times are significantly larger with concurrent motion pattern stimulation than without.

otopically in both hemispheres of macaque monkeys[7] and humans.[8] Pattern motion consisted of random white dots (diameter 1.2°) that rotated clockwise or counterclockwise at a constant velocity of 30°/s around the fixation dot. The size of the visual field was 30° in the horizontal and 20° in the vertical dimensions. Visual motion stimulation did not induce apparent self-motion (roll vection).

Horizontal eye movements were recorded by electronystagmography to monitor fixation of the stationary target.

Detection times of object motion were measured by asking the subject to press a button at each of the three conditions: (1) no pattern motion, (2) pattern motion left hemifield, and (3) pattern motion right hemifield, presented in random order 12 times for each horizontal or vertical object motion to determine mean detection times. Subjects also had to indicate the direction of dot motion; trials with incorrect directions were discarded. Detection times of object motion during unstable fixation of the stationary target straight ahead were excluded from further analysis.

RESULTS

Mean detection times for horizontal object motion were 0.61 ± 0.22 s with concurrent motion pattern stimulation and 0.5 ± 0.19 without concurrent motion pattern stimulation in the contralateral hemifield (FIG. 3). Mean detection times for vertical target motion were 0.53 ± 0.19 s without concurrent pattern motion stimulation in the contralateral hemifield and 0.72 ± 0.34 s with concurrent motion pattern stimulation. Statistical analysis of the data by ANOVA revealed a significant increase in detection times during concurrent pattern stimulation ($P = 0.015$).

DISCUSSION

The results of the psychophysical experiments showed that the sensitivity needed to perceive motion of a single target is impaired during simultaneous motion pattern stimulation in the contralateral hemifield. These findings are compatible with the earlier fMRI finding that the lateral geniculate nucleus and the visual cortex contralateral to the hemisphere stimulated by coherent pattern motion are deactivated. Thus, the deactivation of the visual neuronal assemblies appears to be associated with a functional decrement and may reflect transcallosal attentional shifts between the two hemispheres. Contrary to the fMRI study, however, attention was divided in the psychophysical study; subjects exposed to gross motion stimulation in one hemifield were asked to detect a single object moving in the opposite hemifield.

In another fMRI study using visual hemifield motion stimulation, a simple computational model of visuovisual hemispheric interaction was proposed.[9] Instead of giving a detailed account of visual processing, it illustrates a basic idea that might be helpful when interpreting fMRI data during sensory stimulation. In visuovisual interaction, the stimulation of both hemispheres may be congruent, in that visual stimuli delivered in the right and left visual hemifield indicate the same surround motion. Conversely, it may be incongruent, for example, if the left visual field is stimulated, whereas the right visual field is not. We proposed that the activation or deactivation seen in fMRI studies often does not reflect net sensory input, but rather a sensory mismatch. To compute sensory mismatch, we used the input to the left visual field to predict the input to the right visual field and vice versa. Hence, sensory mismatch occurs for incongruent visual stimuli. The basic mechanism that detects such a mismatch is a central predictor formed by a feedback loop. The prediction is compared with the actual input, and the model proposes that sensed motion of a visual hemifield which is larger than the predicted net motion causes increased activation of the respective neuropopulation. In contrast, less sensed motion causes less activation. This model is compatible with the reciprocal inhibitory visuovisual interaction described earlier.[1]

ACKNOWLEDGMENT

The authors thank J. Benson for copyediting the manuscript.

REFERENCES

1. BRANDT, TH. et al. 2000. Hemifield visual motion stimulation: an example of interhemispheric cross talk. NeuroReport **11:** 2803–2809.
2. MAUNSELL, J.H. & D.C. VAN ESSEN. 1987. Topographic organisation of the middle temporal visual area in the Macaque monkey: representational biases in the relationship to callosal connections and myeloarchitectonic boundaries. J. Comp. Neurol. **266:** 535–555.
3. WELLER, R.E., J.T. WALL & J.H. KAAS. 1984. Cortical connections of the middle temporal visual area (MT) and the superior temporal cortex in owl monkeys. J. Comp. Neurol. **228:** 81–104.
4. BRANDT, TH. et al. 1998. Bilateral functional MRI activation of the basal ganglia and middle temporal/medial superior temporal motion-sensitive areas: optokinetic stimulation in homonymous hemianopia. Arch. Neurol. **55:** 1126–1131.
5. TETTAMANTI, M. et al. 2002. Interhemispheric transmission of visuomotor information in humans: fMRI evidence. J. Neurophysiol. **88:** 1051–1058.
6. BRANDT, TH. et al. 2002. Visual-vestibular and visuovisual cortical interaction: new insights from fMRI and PET. Ann. N.Y. Acad. Sci. **956:** 230–241.
7. VAN ESSEN, D.C., W.T. NEWSOME & J.L. BIXBY. 1982. The pattern of interhemispheric connections and its relationship to extrastriate visual areas in the macaque monkeys. J. Neurosci. **2:** 265–283.
8. TRAUZETTEL-KLOSINSKI, S. & K. BRENDLER. 1998. Eye movements in reading with hemianopic field defects. The significance of clinical parameters. Graefes Arch. Clin. Exp. Ophthalmol. **236:** 91–102.
9. BRANDT, TH. et al. 2003. Expectation of sensory stimulation modulates brain activation during visual motion stimulation. Submitted.

Delayed Saccades, but Not Delayed Manual Aiming Movements, Require Visual Attention Shifts

HEINER DEUBEL AND WERNER X. SCHNEIDER

Department of Psychology, Ludwig-Maximilians-Universität, Leopoldstrasse 13, 80802 München, Germany

ABSTRACT: Several studies have shown that during the preparation of a goal-directed movement, perceptual selection (i.e., visual attention) and action selection (the selection of the movement target) are closely coupled. Here, we study attentional selection in situations in which delayed saccadic eye movements and delayed manual movements are prepared. A dual-task paradigm was used which combined the movement preparation with a perceptual discrimination task. The results demonstrate a fundamental difference between the preparation of saccades and of manual reaching. For delayed saccades, attention is pinned to the saccade target until the onset of the response. This does not hold for manual reaching, however. Although fast reaching movements require attention, reaches delayed more than 300 ms after movement cue onset can be already performed "off-line"; that is, attention can be withdrawn from the movement target.

KEYWORDS: attention; saccade; reaching; manual movements; delayed movements

INTRODUCTION

Visual attention, the ability to select a portion of the visual world for further processing, has since long been viewed to play a central role in visual perception. Attention is seen to facilitate detection,[1] to integrate features from different visual modules into "object files,"[2] to allow for object recognition,[3] and to regulate entry into visual short-term memory.[4] In contrast with this classic view of visual attention as a mechanism-supporting perception, the important role of visual attention in the control of action was emphasized only by the end of the 1980s.[5,6] Goal-directed actions such as grasping an object are normally directed to a single target and imply a mechanism that selects the target from competing distractors in the scene. Also, humans typically make many eye movements when examining a scene. Given that the visual scene often is crowded with many different stimuli, there must be a mechanism which

---

Address for correspondence: Heiner Deubel, Department Psychologie, Ludwig-Maximilians-Universität, Leopoldstrasse 13, D-80802 München, Germany. Voice: 49-(0)89-2180-5282; fax: 49-(0)89-2180-5211.

deubel@psy.uni-muenchen.de

selects one particular stimulus as the target of the saccade. The question arises how this "selection-for-action" relates to the perceptual functions of visual attention.

As to saccadic eye movements, a now well-established hypothesis is that the saccade target is chosen by allocating attention to it. A growing number of studies have supported this view.[7–10] In the study by Deubel and Schneider,[10] subjects were confronted with a dual-task situation which required a perceptual discrimination (discriminating the letter "E" from a reversed "E") while preparing a saccadic eye movement. The spatial relationship between the saccade target and the discrimination target (DT) was systematically varied. The DT disappeared before the actual eye movement started so that perceptual performance was measured during the saccade preparation phase only. If visual attention for perception and saccade target selection can be controlled independently, discrimination performance should not depend on the location of the saccade target. On the other hand, if both selection processes are coupled via a common selection mechanism, discrimination performance should be best when DT appears at the saccade target location. The results of this study indeed revealed a high degree of spatially selective coupling between saccade target position and DT position. Discrimination performance was good when both referred to the same object while performance for an object that appeared only a degree of visual angle away from the saccade target location was close to chance level. Further related experiments revealed that the coupling between perceptual processing and the selection of the saccade target is obligate; it is not possible to attend to one location in space while preparing a saccade to another.[10,11] From these studies, the question arose whether a manual reach or grasp also would bind the attentional mechanism in visual perception to the movement target. This was tested in various dual-task paradigms in which subjects had to make a fast manual pointing movement to a centrally cued item while performing a discrimination task at that or at a different location.[12–14] The results showed that perceptual performance again depended strongly on the position of the movement target, with best perceptual performance when the movement was directed to the DT. Further evidence for the relevance of a visual selection process in manual movement programming comes from several studies which analyzed the effect of task-related distractors on the preparation of manual movements. In a study by Castiello,[15] subjects had to grasp an object while counting the number of times a distractor object was illuminated by a spotlight. The results showed that the type of distractor influenced the amplitude of the peak grip aperture to the target, that is, the manipulation component of the movement. When the distractor was smaller/bigger than the target, the peak aperture was also smaller/bigger than in trials without a distractor. Craighero and colleagues[16] investigated whether a nonrelevant prime picture influenced the latency of the following grasping movement. They found a reduction of grasping latency when the prime picture depicted the object to be grasped compared with the condition when the prime depicted a different object. Hence, visual perception of an object, here the prime, influenced the programming of a movement that immediately followed the perception.

Taken together, these studies point to an important role of attentional deployment in the preparation phase, both for saccadic and manual movements: they suggest that visual attention has to be focused on the movement target and cannot be withdrawn before the onset of the movement. However, in all these previous experiments, subjects had to saccade or reach to the target immediately after the presentation of a movement cue, and they were encouraged to perform a fast response. Consequently, it remains an open question whether attention could be withdrawn from the target before movement onset, given the subject had sufficient time to completely prepare the movement. Therefore, the present study analyzed selective discrimination performance before delayed saccades and before delayed manual reaching movements, while the subject tried to attend at the movement goal or at other spatial locations.

METHODS

The first experiment investigated attentional deployment for delayed manual aiming. The experimental setup is sketched in FIGURE 1. The stimuli were presented on a 21-inch color monitor with a resolution of 1024 by 768 pixels; the frame rate was 100 Hz. Visual information was presented via a half-translucent mirror at an effective viewing distance of 60 cm. This setup made it possible to present movement targets and discrimination stimuli on the working plane in front of the subject without seeing the hand movement or having the hand obstructing the DTs during the movement. Eye fixation was controlled by an SMI-Eyelink Infrared Eye Monitoring system (SensoMotoric Instruments, Teltow, Germany). Manual movements were recorded with a Polhemus Fastrak electromagnetic position and orientation measuring system. This system provides the spatial position of a small position sensor that was mounted on the fingertip of the subject's right index finger. Attached to the sensor was a small red light-emitting diode which allowed visual feedback about the spatial position of the fingertip at the beginning of each trial.

The sequence of stimuli and the experimental task is illustrated in FIGURE 2. The subject was asked to keep fixation in the center of the screen throughout the experi-

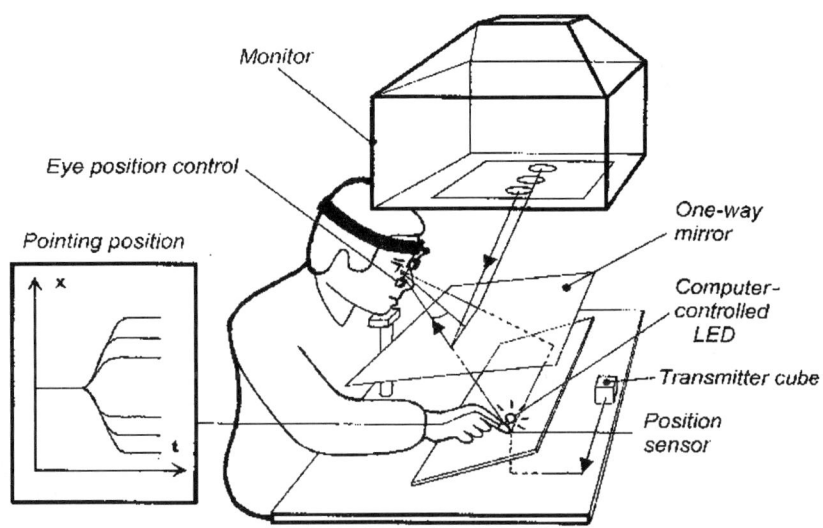

FIGURE 1. Experimental setup.

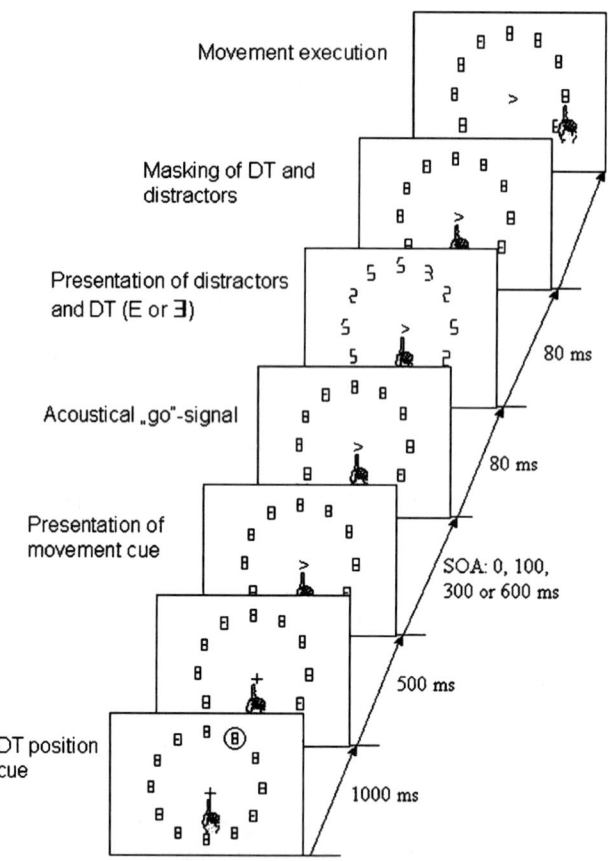

FIGURE 2. Stimulus sequence in experiment 1. See text for explanation.

ment. A circular array of 12 masking letters initially was displayed at an eccentricity of 7.2 degrees. At the beginning of each trial, the subject put her finger on the small cross in the center of the screen. At one of the letter locations, a circle was presented which served as a valid cue indicating the future location of the critical discrimination stimulus. The circle disappeared after 1000 ms. Five hundred milliseconds later, a central arrow appeared which indicated the position of the movement target. The subject was instructed to perform a pointing movement to this target, but to start the movement only after an acoustical "go" signal which was given at a delay of 0, 100, 300, or 600 ms after the presentation of the movement cue. Eighty milliseconds after this go signal, 11 of the masking letters changed into distractors (which resembled "2" or "5"). At the position cued by the circle at the beginning of the trial, however, the critical DT was presented. The DT consisted of either an "E" or a reversed "E" which was shown for 80 ms. Then, the DT and the distractors changed back to the masking letters. Because typical movement onset latencies in this experiment were in the range of 250 to 300 ms, it is obvious from the timing of stimulus sequence that the critical discrimination stimulus normally appeared and disappeared before the onset of the movement. At the end of each trial, the subject received feedback about the movement accuracy by means of a red dot displayed at the landing position of the second movements. In 50% of the trials, the position of DT coincided with the location of the movement target. Otherwise, position of DT and the location of the movement target were selected randomly from 6 of the 12 clock positions. Six paid, naïve subjects participated in the experiments. Each subject performed two experimental blocks; each block contained 120 trials.

In the second experiment, subjects were asked to produce an eye saccade, instead of a manual aiming movement, to the indicated movement target. The stimulus sequence was similar to that shown in FIGURE 2, except that three different values of Stimulus Onset Asynchrony (SOA; 100, 500, and 1200 ms) were used. Eye movements were recorded with a SRI Generation 5.5 Dual Purkinje-image eyetracker and sampled at a rate of 500 Hz. Further details of experimental setup, eyetracker calibration, and eye movement analysis are given in Deubel and Schneider.[10] Again, six subjects (different from those of experiment 1) participated.

RESULTS

FIGURE 3 provides perceptual performance (given as percentage correct) as a function of the SOA between the onset of the movement cue and the acoustical go signal. Note that a performance level of 50% would indicate chance level, whereas 100% would indicate perfect performance. The data for the manual movements (experiment 1) are displayed on the left graph; the data for the saccadic eye movements (experiment 2) are shown on the right. The data points indicate the means over the participating subjects; vertical bars indicate standard errors. Data are presented separately for those trials where DT and the movement target coincided (open squares) and for the conditions in which DT appeared at a position which was not the target for the movement (filled circles).

As expected from previous work,[9–14] perceptual performance depended on whether DT was shown at the movement target location or at a different spatial location. For the cases where movement target and DT position coincided (open squares), performance was close to perfect and independent of SOA, for both saccades and manual reaching. For the incongruent case in the reaching experiment, however, discrimination performance strongly depended on the SOA. For zero and short SOA (SOA = 0 and 100 ms), performance was significantly lower than in all congruent conditions. Note that because of the presentation of the valid DT position cue, the subjects were perfectly informed about the location of the DT. Nevertheless, subjects were not able to intentionally keep their focus of attention on the discrimination stimulus, as indicated by the inflated perceptual performance in these conditions. This implies that attention had to be focused on the movement target to prepare the manual reach. For longer SOA values, however, performance improved considerably and reached the performance level of the congruent conditions for SOA values of 300 ms and above. This indicates that for these sufficiently delayed

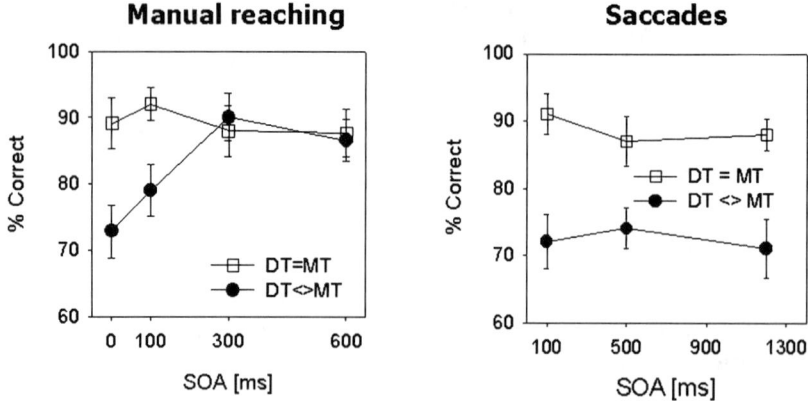

FIGURE 3. Perceptual discrimination performance in the manual reaching task (experiment 1, *left*) and in the saccade task (experiment 2, *right*). The data are shown as a function of SOA (see FIG. 2) and are plotted separately for the cases where the movement was directed to the location of the discrimination stimulus (*open squares*) and for the incongruent conditions (*filled circles*).

movements, attention can be already withdrawn from the movement target and can be deployed onto the location of the DT, allowing for DT identification.

In contrast, there is no indication of performance improvement for the case of delayed saccades, even for the longest SOA (right graph). Although discrimination was perfect at the location of the target of the planned saccade (open squares), it remained at a consistently lower performance level at the other locations (filled circles). This finding implies that even when saccades are delayed by more than a second, attention still remains bound to the saccade target in an obligatory manner. Therefore, whereas manual movements can be prepared and finally started "offline," that is, without attentional deployment, saccade preparation is always "online" in the sense that attention stays at the target location until movement onset.

DISCUSSION

The data presented here reveal an obligatory coupling of visual attention to the saccade target, even when a temporal delay should allow preparation of an internally generated, stereotyped movement. The finding that it is not possible to withdraw attention from the target before saccades adds to former findings on the relation of attention and saccade programming studied in a variety of experimental situations.[9–11] Investigations on the role of attentional in manual reaching have suggested that the same strict coupling also may hold for manual reaching and grasping.[12–14] The present findings qualify this assumption, however, demonstrating a basic difference between the control of saccades and manual movements. Whereas saccades always require attention, manual reaches can be preprogrammed, allowing to specify the movement parameters and store the motor program for use in a delayed movement. It is interesting to see that this attention-mediated parameter specification can be completed within less that 300 ms. The remarkable dissociation between mechanisms of the preparation of saccades and manual reaches is in line with another recent finding on the role of attention in the control of sequential movements.[14] In this study, subjects had to prepare a sequence of either two saccades or two sequential reaching movements to separate targets. Analysis of perceptual performance revealed that in the saccade case, only the target of the initial saccade experienced processing by attention, whereas performance at the second location was close to chance level. For the manual reaches, however, both the first and the second movement target were simultaneously selected before the onset of the initial movement.

The present findings have some implications for the ongoing discussion on the functional role of neural activity in the posterior parietal cortex. Several studies have shown that the activity of neurons in the lateral intraparietal area (LIP) is enhanced when a behaviorally relevant stimulus is presented in the neuron's receptive field, relative to when this stimulus is unimportant. This enhanced response traditionally has been interpreted as evidence that LIP is involved in the generation of attention to the stimulus. However, an alternative view has been that the activity of LIP neurons may reflect motor intention, more specifically, the intention to perform a saccade to the object on the neuron's receptive field, rather than (effector-independent) attentional focusing.[17] Because, as shown in the present and other work,[8–11] visual attention is normally pinned to the spatial location of a saccade goal until the onset of a saccade, one cannot distinguish a priori whether LIP activation before saccades is related to attention or to a motor plan. The strongest evidence for LIP activity representing motor intentions came from an electrophysiological study showing that the activity of LIP neurons is greater when the neurons are activated by the target of a saccade than when they describe the target of a simultaneously generated arm movement, directed to a different location.[18] When this finding is interpreted in the light of the current results, however, it is plausible to assume that when delayed, simultaneous hand and eye movements to different locations are required, visual attention may first move to the hand movement target to establish the spatial movement parameters of the manual move. After a short temporal interval (possibly <300 ms), attention then would be free to move on to the saccade target, which ultimately would lead to the enhanced saccade-related response until saccade onset. This hypothesis is in line with a recent study demonstrating a significant correlation of the activity of LIP neurons with a perceptual measure for the monkey's selective spatial attention.[19]

In summary, the present work demonstrates that even for delayed saccades, attention is pinned to the saccade target until the onset of the response. This does not hold for manual reaching, however; reaches delayed by more than 300 ms after movement cue onset can be already performed "off-line," that is, without attention.

ACKNOWLEDGMENT

This research was supported by the Deutsche Forschungsgemeinschaft (SFB 462/ B4 and De 336/2).

REFERENCES

1. POSNER, M.I. 1980. Orienting of attention. Q. J. Exp. Psychol. **32:** 3–25.

2. TREISMAN, A.M. & G. GELADE. 1980. A feature-integration theory of attention. Cognit. Psychol. **12:** 97–136.
3. SCHNEIDER, W.X. 1995. VAM: a neuro-cognitive model for attention control of segmentation, object recognition and space-based motor action. Vis. Cognit. **2:** 331–374.
4. DUNCAN, J. & G.W. HUMPHREYS. 1989. Visual-search and stimulus similarity. Psychol. Rev. **96:** 433-458.
5. ALLPORT, D.A. 1987. Selection for action: some behavioral and neurophysiological considerations of attention and action. *In* Perspectives on Perception and Action. H. Heuer & A.F. Sanders, Eds.: 395–419. Lawrence Erlbaum. Hillsdale, NJ.
6. NEUMANN, O. 1987. Beyond capacity: a functional view of attention. *In* Perspectives on Perception and Action. H. Heuer & A.F. Sanders, Eds.: 361–394. Lawrence Erlbaum. Hillsdale, NJ.
7. SHEPHERD, M., J.M. FINDLAY & R.J. HOCKEY. 1986. The relationship between eye movements and spatial attention. Q. J. Exp. Psychol. **38A:** 475-491.
8. HOFFMAN, J.E. & B. SUBRAMANIAM. 1995. The role of visual attention in saccadic eye movements. Percept. Psychophys. **57:** 787–795.
9. KOWLER, E., E. ANDERSON, B. DOSHER & E. BLASER. 1995. The role of attention in the programming of saccades. Vis. Res. **35:** 1897–1916.
10. DEUBEL, H. & W.X. SCHNEIDER. 1996. Saccade target selection and object recognition: evidence for a common attentional mechanism. Vision Res. **36:** 1827–1837.
11. SCHNEIDER, W.X. & H. DEUBEL. 2002. Selection-for-perception and selection-for-spatial-motor-action are coupled by visual attention: a review of recent findings and new evidence from stimulus-driven saccade control. *In* Attention and Performance XIX: Common Mechanisms in Perception and Action. W. Prinz & B. Hommel, Eds.: 609–627. Oxford University Press. Oxford, UK.
12. DEUBEL, H., W.X. SCHNEIDER & I. PAPROTTA. 1998. Selective dorsal and ventral processing: evidence for a common attentional mechanism in reaching and perception. Vis. Cognit. **5:** 81–107.
13. SCHIEGG, A., H. DEUBEL & W.X. SCHNEIDER. 2003. Attentional selection during preparation of prehension movements. Vis. Cognit. **10:** 409–431
14. DEUBEL, H. & W.X. SCHNEIDER. 2003. Attentional selection in sequential manual movements, movements around an obstacle, and in grasping. *In* Attention in Action. G.W. Humphreys & M.J. Riddoch, Eds. Psychology Press. Hove. In press.
15. CASTIELLO, U. 1996. Grasping a fruit: selection for action. J. Exp. Psychol. Hum. Percept. Perform. **22:** 582–603.
16. CRAIGHERO, L., L. FADIGA, G. RIZZOLATTI & C. UMILTÀ. 1998. Visuomotor priming. Vis. Cognit. **5:** 109–125.
17. ANDERSEN, R.A. & C.A. BUNEO. 2002. Intentional maps in posterior parietal cortex. Annu. Rev. Neurosci. **25:** 189–220.
18. SNYDER, L.H., A.P. BATISTA & R.A. ANDERSEN. 1997. Coding of intention in the posterior parietal cortex. Nature **386:** 167–170.
19. BISLEY, J.W. & M.E. GOLDBERG. 2003. Neuronal activity in the lateral intraparietal area and spatial attention. Science **299:** 81–86.

Prolonged Optokinetic Stimulation Generates Podokinetic after Rotation

CARLOS R. GORDON,[a] DROR TAL,[b] NATAN GADOTH,[a] AND AVI SHUPAK[b]

[a]*Department of Neurology, Meir General Hospital, Kfar Saba and Sackler Faculty of Medicine, Tel Aviv University, Tel Aviv, Israel*

[b]*Motion Sickness and Human Performance Laboratory, Israel Naval Medical Institute, Haifa, Israel*

> ABSTRACT: Previous studies showed that after prolonged stepping in place on the center of a rotating platform blindfolded subjects could no longer step in place on a firm floor. Instead, they invariably rotated themselves relative to space without perceiving their rotation, a phenomenon termed podokinetic after-rotation (PKAR). We speculated that prolonged optokinetic stimulation (OK) alone may generate similar PKAR. The purpose of this study was to evaluate the effects of prolonged OK on podokinetic (PK) responses. Ten healthy subjects participated in the study. After a control stepping test, they were seated in a circular closed cage and randomly (right or left) exposed to an OK (45°/s) covering the whole visual field for 30 min. After this procedure, blindfolded subjects attempted to step in place on the stationary floor for 30 min. When trying to do so, all subjects turned relative to space without any perception of rotation. The direction of this optokinetically after-rotation (oPKAR) was opposite of that of the direction of OK. Mean peak velocity of oPKAR was 7.8 ± 4.1°/s, and it was reached after approximately 6 min of stepping. After that, there was a progressive velocity decay, which exhibited a discharging time constant on the order of 42 min toward a final positive asymptote of 3.1°/s. We conclude that OK alone causes oPKAR. Long-term OK probably charges a storage element for podomotor activity with a relatively prolonged time constant. This novel form of neural interaction and adaptive plasticity may have significant implications for the treatment of vestibular and parietal lobe disorders.
>
> KEYWORDS: optokinetic; podokinetic; adaptive plasticity; vestibular; ocular motor

INTRODUCTION

In the first of a series of studies, we showed that after prolonged walk in place on the periphery of a horizontal rotating platform, blindfolded subjects could no longer walk straight ahead on firm ground. When trying to do so, all subjects generated curved walking trajectories with angular velocities well above of vestibular thresh-

---

Address for correspondence: Dr. C. R. Gordon, Department of Neurology, Meir General Hospital, Kfar Saba 44281, Israel. Voice: 972-9-7472828; fax: 972-9-7471317.
cgordon@post.tau.ac.il

old; yet all subjects perceived themselves as walking straight ahead.[1] Further studies showed that after prolonged stepping in place on the center of a rotating platform, blindfolded subjects could no longer step in place on firm floor. Instead, they invariably rotated themselves relative to space without perceiving their rotation.[2,3] Analogous to optokinetic terminology, the term "podokinetic" (PK) was introduced to describe the system responsible for this form of bottom-up sensory-motor control, and the term "podokinetic after-rotation" (PKAR) to describe the postadaptive rotation observed during walking or stepping in place without vision. PKAR exhibited exponential decay with a short-term component of discharging time constant on the order of 6–12 min and another long-term component with a time constant of 1–2 h.[3] This PKAR is not caused by sensory conflict between visual stationary signals and the somatosensory messages of feet-on-platform rotation, and it is considered a new form of adaptive motor learning.[4]

From previous observations and some data from the latter study, we speculated that prolonged optokinetic stimulation (OK) alone may generate PKAR. The aim of the present study was to evaluate the effects of prolonged OK on PK responses.

METHODS

Ten healthy subjects (nine men and one woman) whose ages ranged from 18 to 43 years (mean, 25.2 ± 9.7 years) participated in the study. All subjects gave their informed consent, and approval from the local ethics committee was obtained to perform the experiments. All subjects had a normal neurootological examination. None of the subjects had a history of otologic, neurologic, or orthopedic abnormalities or was taking medication.

Each experiment consisted on a control stepping test followed by an OK adaptation phase and a final postadaptive phase of stepping in place for 30 min. The control stepping was adapted from Fukuda (1959)[5] and consisted on five repeated attempts of blindfolded and ear-plugged stepping in place on firm ground for 1 min. During the adaptive OK phase, subjects were seated in a circular closed cage and randomly (right or left) exposed to an OK (45°/s) covering the whole visual field for 30 min using the Contraves Goerz DP-300 computerized system (Neurokinetics, Pittsburgh, PA). A close video system allowed visualizing the subject eyes and behavior during this phase, while arousal was maintained by conversation when necessary. After this procedure, and after a pause of 1–2 min to prevent after sensations, blindfolded subjects attempted stepping in place on the stationary floor for 30 min. Earphones were used to minimize auditory cues. All stepping tests were performed in a large, quiet room. The stepping frequency on both control and postadaptive conditions was fairly constant at approximately 2.0 Hz (i.e., 1 s for a complete stepping cycle). Rotational velocities were estimated from the total angle of turn during a 1-min interval using a compass rose. Occasionally during attempted stepping in place on the floor, subjects had to be passively moved away from impending obstructions because of inadvertent translational movement. Data samples spanning such events were excluded from results.

RESULTS

Control Trials

During the control stepping tests, individual average angular velocities ranged from 0.25 to 1.7°/s (mean, 0.69 ± 0.42°/s). Only one subject turned at more than 1.0°/s. The direction of rotation varied from right to left in six subjects and remained the same in four subjects.

Postadaptive OK Phase

When trying to step in place after the postadaptive OK phase, all subjects turned relative to space in the opposite direction of the OK. In other words, the five subjects exposed to right optokinetic drum rotation turned to the left and all subjects exposed to left optokinetic drum rotation turned to the right. The individual maximal angular velocities of this optokinetically after rotation (oPKAR) ranged from 2.1 to 17.7°/s, and the mean peak velocity was 7.8 ± 4.1°/s. Eight subjects exhibited maximal angular velocities above 6 degrees/s.

FIGURE 1 shows the time course of oPKAR for one subject. FIGURE 2 illustrates the averaged group response over the 30 min of postadaptive OK stepping. All subjects exhibited an initial oPKAR with an increasing velocity over the first 5–7 min. The fitted curve for the first 6 min showed an almost perfect linear rising slope (r^2 = 099). After that, the response closely followed an exponential velocity decay toward a positive asymptote. After excluding data points from the first 5 min (the rising phase), the fitted curved yielded a decay time constant of 42 min and a final estimated asymptote of 3.1°/s.

During all trials, subjects were convinced that they stepped in place with no rotation. None of the subjects experienced any sensation of unsteadiness, disequilibrium, or dizziness, whether standing still or performing the stepping test.

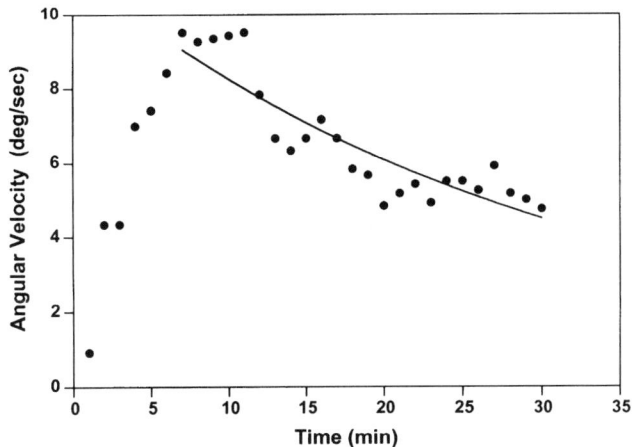

FIGURE 1. Illustration of oPKAR in one subject. Plots show angular velocity plotted versus time for the 30-min oPKAR period.

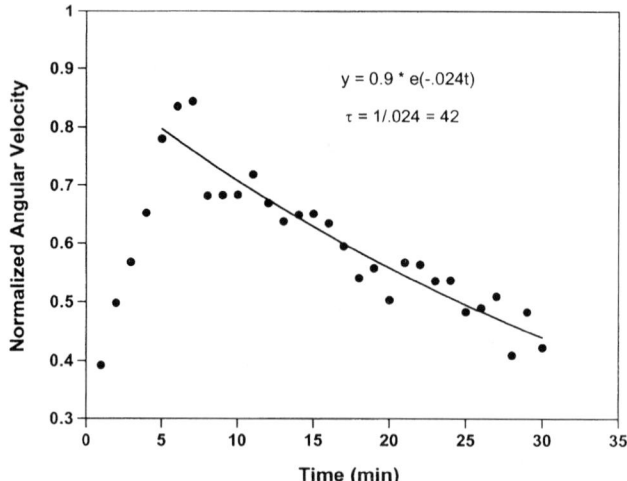

FIGURE 2. Illustration of mean angular velocity from 10 subjects plotted versus time for the 30-min oPKAR period. Individual angular velocity for every 1-min interval was normalized using the equation: actual velocity/peak velocity of oPKAR.

DISCUSSION

The results of the present study clearly show that OK alone causes a consistent oPKAR in healthy subjects. After being exposed to 30 min of OK at 45°/s, all blindfolded subjects exhibited remarkable rotation when attempting to step in place without turning, in the absence of any sensation of rotation. The direction of rotation relative to space was invariably opposite to the direction of the previous OK. Mean peak velocity of oPKAR was approximately tenfold the mean average of control stepping (7.8 ± 4.1 vs. 0.69 ± 0.42°/s). During the entire oPKAR period, the rate of individual body rotation was always above the presumed vestibular sensory threshold of 1–2°/s.[6] Nevertheless, all subjects were convinced that they stepped in place without turning. In contrast, during control stepping tests only one subject turned at more than 1.0°/s. We have reported previously that when performing the Fukuda's stepping test, healthy subjects occasionally turned at more than 1.5°/s but never at more than 2.3°/s.[2]

Our results are in agreement with those of Jürgens et al.[4] In this study, three healthy blindfolded subjects demonstrated PKAR after they stood for 10 min on a rotating platform (35°/s) and watched a grounded stationary optokinetic pattern.

All of our subjects demonstrated an oPKAR that typically accelerates over the first 5 min to reach a maximum velocity of approximately one-sixth of the velocity of the adapting optokinetic stimulus. Thereafter, the oPKAR followed a subsequent slow exponential decay of response velocity (time constant, 42 min) toward a positive asymptotic value of approximately 3.1°/s. We found a longer rising phase of oPKAR than the previously described sharp 1–2-min rising phase after PK adaptation.[3] The peak velocity of oPKAR response was slower than that obtained using PK stimulation with a rotating disc at 45°/s and exhibited a relatively long time constant decay of 42 min. The differences between oPKAR and PKAR responses could be attributed to possible different integration and modulations of the information (stimulus and response) of this bimodal (OK-PK) "learning" in comparison with a more simple and direct unimodal (PK) learning that takes place during PK adaptation.

In this context, prolonged exposure and consequently adaptation to unfamiliar vestibular, visual, and somatosensory stimuli frequently are observed during long sea voyages. When returning to land after sailing a transient sensation of swaying, swinging, unsteadiness, and disequilibrium, a phenomenon called "mal de debarquement" is experienced by approximately 80% of healthy subjects.[7] We have previously suggested that mal de debarquement represents a dynamic, multisensory motor form of central nervous system adaptive plasticity.[8]

As noted above, during the oPKAR period, the angular velocity of all our subjects was well above of the vestibular sensory threshold. The lack of perception of rotation during the oPKAR phase could be explained by a remodeled and/or remapped perception of self-rotation after OK adaptation. As we have suggested previously for PKAR responses,[1-3] this adaptive remodeling probably takes place at the level of the brainstem ocularmotor system. Similar to the well-known vestibulooptokinetic velocity storage,[9] it is probably that long-term OK also charges a storage element for podomotor activity with a relatively prolonged time constant. Our results strongly support a physiological link between the OK and PK systems in a "top-down" flow. In this context, previous studies have shown that purely arthrokinetic (the arms of a stationary subject in contact with a rotating drum)[10] or somatosensory/podokinetic (apparent walking in the dark of the periphery of a rotating treadmill)[11] stimulation can generate ocular nystagmus in a "down-top" flow. These results demonstrate that arthrokinetic and podokinetic information reach the level of the brainstem ocularmotor system.

From a clinical standpoint, the adaptive remodeling ability shown in the present study might be of practical use in rehabilitation programs for patients with vestibular and parietal lobe lesions.

A considerable number of patients with noncompensated unilateral loss of peripheral vestibular function will complain on imbalance and difficulty on walking "straight ahead." Recently, Weber et al.[12] reported PKAR asymmetry in patients with compensated unilateral vestibular ablation, suggesting a residual static vestibular imbalance. We suggest that both prolonged "bottom-up" PK and "up-down" OK activation may remodel and reinforce balance and the sense of straight ahead in patients with noncompensated vestibular loss.

Several studies in patients with parietal lobe lesions have shown that short OK or vestibular stimulation may produce a transient improvement or even remission of unilateral neglect.[13,14] However, the use of these paradigms in the process of neurological rehabilitation has not been yet systematically evaluated. We suggest that applying prolonged PK and OK to patients with neglect not only will result in the appearance of PKAR but also may improve other parietal "neglect" functions.

A very recent study showed that patients with cerebellar dysfunction had impaired PK adaptation.[15] Because of the essential role of the cerebellum in many forms of motor learning and particularly in ocular motor functions, it would be of interest to also investigate the oPKAR phenomenon in such patients.

REFERENCES

1. GORDON, C.R., W.A. FLETCHER, G. MELVILL JONES, *et al.* 1995. Adaptive plasticity in the control of locomotor trajectory. Exp. Brain Res. **102:** 540–545.
2. GORDON, C.R., W.A. FLETCHER, G. MELVILL JONES, *et al.* 1995. Is the stepping test a specific indicator of vestibulospinal function? Neurology **45:** 2035–2037.
3. WEBER, K.D., W.A. FLETCHER, C.R. GORDON, *et al.* 1998. Motor learning in the "podokinetic" system and its role in spatial orientation during locomotion. Exp. Brain Res. **120:** 377–385.
4. JÜRGENS, R., T. BOSS & W. BECKER. 1999. Podokinetic after-rotation does not depend on sensory conflict. Exp. Brain Res. **128:** 563–567.
5. FUKUDA, T. 1959. The stepping test: two phases of the labyrinthine reflex. Acta Otolaryngol. **50:** 95–108.
6. MERGENER, T., F. HLAVACKA & G. SCHWEIGART. 1993. Interaction of vestibular and proprioceptive inputs. J. Vestib. Res. **3:** 41–57.
7. GORDON, C.R., O. SPITZER, A. SHUPAK & I. DOWECK. 1992. Survey of mal de debarquement. Br. Med. J. **304:** 544.
8. GORDON, C.R., O. SPITZER, I. DOWECK, *et al.* 1995. Clinical features of mal de debarquement: adaptation and habituation to sea conditions. J. Vestib. Res. **5:** 363–369.
9. COHEN, B., V. HENN, T. RAPHAN & D. DENNET. 1981. Velocity storage, nystagmus, and visual-vestibular interactions in humans. Ann. N.Y. Acad. Sci. **374:** 421–433.
10. BRANDT, T., W. BUCHELE & F. ARNOLD. 1977. Arthrokinetic nystagmus and egomotion sensation. Exp. Brain Res. **30:** 331–338.
11. BLES, W. & S. KOTAKA. 1986. Stepping around: nystagmus, self-motion perception and coriolis effects. *In* Adaptive Processes in Visual and Oculomotor Systems. E.L. Keller & D.S. Zee, Eds: 465–473. Pergamon Press. Oxford, UK.
12. WEBER, K.D., W.A. FLETCHER, G. MELVILL JONES & E.W. BLOCK. 2002. Podokinetic after-rotation in patients with compensated unilateral vestibular ablation. Exp. Brain Res. **147:** 554–557.
13. VALLAR, G., C. GUARIGLIA, D. NICO & L. PIZZAMIGLIO. 1997. Motor deficits and optokinetic stimulation in patients with left hemineglect. Neurology **49:** 1364–1370.
14. VALLAR, G., G. BOTTINI, M.L. RUSCONI & R. STERZI. 1993. Exploring somatosensory hemineglect by vestibular stimulation. Brain **116:** 71–86.
15. EARHART, G.M., W.W. FLETCHER, F.B. HORAK, *et al.* 2002. Does the cerebellum play a role in podokinetic adaptation? Exp. Brain Res. **146:** 538–542.

A Modeling Approach to the Human Spatial Orientation System

T. MERGNER[a] AND W. BECKER[b]

[a]*Abteilung Neurologie, Neurozentrum, Universität Freiburg, 79106 Freiburg, Germany*

[b]*Sektion Neurophysiologie, Universität Ulm, 89081 Ulm, Germany*

ABSTRACT: The human spatial orientation system is highly complex and nonlinear. It is difficult, therefore, to arrive at an unequivocal model of the underlying processing by merely combining the known elementary mechanisms ("bottom-up" approach); additional "top-down" concepts are required to narrow the choice between several formally equivalent solutions. We here suggest a concept in which sensorimotor control is based on a meta-level that provides an internal representation of the physical stimuli acting upon a subject (e.g., tilt of the support surface), whereas the classic reflex concept essentially proceeds from a direct coupling between physiological stimuli, sensors and actuators. At the hypothesized meta-level, the axial body segments are represented as a stack of superimposed platforms with the lowermost platform (generally the feet) riding on a support surface that acts as the buttress for the subject's active movements. From the sensory point of view, this stack constitutes a system of nested references. This concept explains data from various experiments dealing with self- and object motion perception and body stabilization in a more exhaustive way than does the classic concept. In our view, it provides a robust, flexible, and modular framework for perception and action in space.

KEYWORDS: human; spatial orientation; sensor fusion; sensory integration; sensorimotor control; model

INTRODUCTION

During the last century, the notion that the nervous system can be viewed as a network for the transfer and processing of information became generally accepted. Accordingly, beginning in the 1940s, technical concepts derived from systems and information theory were increasingly applied to neuroscience ("cybernetics").[1] However, it soon was realized that the analytical and descriptive tools available at that time would allow only description of simple nervous mechanisms such as reflexes (which invited an interpretation as negative feedback systems), but not the more complex aspects of brain function and behavior. Bertalanffy (1969)[2] discussed the problems related to the formalization of complex and nonlinear systems in his "General System Theory." He denoted that a common problem in most if not all fields of science is that the function of a complex system cannot be understood solely

Address for correspondence: T. Mergner, Abteilung Neurologie, Neurozentrum, Universität Freiburg, 79106 Freiburg, Germany. Voice: 49-761-270-5513; fax: 49-761-270-5416.
mergner@uni-freiburg.de

by analytically investigating its elements (e.g., the laws of thermodynamics cannot be derived from the rules of molecular motion, hence the slogan "the whole is more than the sum of its elements").

Bertalanffy[2] denoted especially two problems. One problem is that an analytic mathematical treatment of complex nonlinear systems is difficult if not impossible. The second problem is that complex systems tend to have a high number of degrees of freedom. Therefore, the usual analytical approach to simple elementary mechanisms, which in a "bottom-up" way tries to establish an unequivocal solution, is no longer applicable. To cope with the many degrees of freedom of complex systems, one would have to narrow the many possible solutions by applying, in a "top-down" way, auxiliary criteria based, for example, on "biological plausibility." These problems were not solved at the time of Bertalanffy, and his considerations had little practical implications for science in general, as true also for neuroscience.

With the advent of modern computer-based simulation tools, the numerical analysis of complex nonlinear systems is no longer an insurmountable hurdle. We can combine many nonlinear subsystems, be they experimentally identified (detection thresholds, saturation characteristics, etc.) or conceptual constructs representing complex cognitive networks (decision mechanisms, memory, prediction, etc.) into models of ever-growing complexity and yet obtain a description of the resulting behavior in a short lapse of time. However, even if we find a model that produces simulation results that closely resemble the experimentally observed ones, how do we know that this is the "correct" description of the system. As mentioned above, the problem with a complex system is that there are usually a manifold of different models which can do the same job or a similar one. Thus, there is no "absolute solution," and we still face the problem of defining auxiliary criteria.

We here are interested in the human spatial orientation system, a system that certainly qualifies as complex and nonlinear. Auxiliary criteria that we can conceive of for the analysis of this system include robustness, flexibility, and modular structure.[3] Similar criteria have been suggested recently for the modeling of biological systems in a series of special articles in *Science* magazine[4-8] under the heading of "Wholistic Biology," a new term for an old problem, as acknowledged in these articles. Although the problems considered in these articles relate to molecular physiology and genetics, where it has been learned that the knowledge of a cell's elementary structures and mechanisms does not automatically lead to an understanding of its function, a similar situation is encountered in neurophysiology.

In the context of our studies into the role of intersensory interaction for human self-motion perception, and, for orientation in general, the attempt to meet auxiliary criteria of the type mentioned above led to the following basic conclusions concerning the presumptive structure of the brain's internal processing.

There exists an intermediate level of sensory processing as an interface between the low-level elementary sensory functions and the high-level behavioral functions; note that such a notion does not occur with traditional reflex concepts which assume an essentially direct sensor-actuator coupling. At this intermediate level, an internal reconstruction of the external stimuli is performed. For example (one to which we will repeatedly refer below), a head-in-space rotation may arise from rotations anywhere in the neck, along the torso (trunk), in the legs and feet, or from a rotation of the body support surface, or any combination thereof. The vestibular signal arising from this rotation is ambiguous, therefore. As a likely way to disambiguate it, we have suggested that it is canceled, to the extent that it resulted from body segment rotations, by subtraction of axial proprioceptive signals. The residual vestibular signal left over after this subtraction then must stem from a rotation of the body support. It can be viewed as an internal reconstruction of the support's kinematic state and, by the same token, as a basic reference for many purposes in the context of orientation in space and control of body posture and movement.

We hold that the control of our spatially oriented behavior, in general, strongly depends on how well our brains internally reconstruct with the help of our senses the physics (kinematics and kinetics) of our own movements and of those of the environment we interact with. Ultimately, the framework of this physics is the terrestrial "anisotropy" of space given by gravity and by the earth surface as well as by the fact that the earth surface represents the ultimate buttress for most of our movements. Therefore, when modeling human spatial behavior, a first, and actually trivial, step is to model the physical situation within this framework, considering both the kinematics and kinetics of the various elements of the body and of the environment. The second and most important step then is to conceive of an internal reconstruction of the physical situation that would draw on the information supplied by our sensory systems. In addition to the criterion of biological plausibility, we have adopted this procedure as a part of the guidelines to be followed when modeling aspects of spatial behavior and posture stabilization.[3] To illustrate this approach, we shall consider, in the following, the case of an upright human subjected to horizontal rotations.

HEAD ROTATION AS AN EXAMPLE

As pointed out above, a head movement in space can arise in various ways. One can turn the head relative to the trunk using neck muscles. Alternatively, head motion can result from a trunk motion during walking. Finally, head motion can result from a motion of the body support surface, for example, during transportation in a vehicle. Note that we can view the multisegment structure of the human body here as a stack of superimposed platforms. In this stack, a vertical hierarchy is given by the gravity-induced contact of the feet with the body support. The elements of the stack, that is, the various platforms, are linked by passive viscous-elastic elements and active intersegmental stabilization mechanism. Accordingly, any motion of the body support or lower body segments tends to take along all the respective upper segments. Kinematically, such movements entail physical coordinate transformations. For instance, whereas head motions on the stationary trunk can be described in trunk coordinates, those during walking ultimately must be specified in space coordinates.

One could argue that there may be no need for the brain to use reference frames at all when controlling spatial behavior. For example, one might propose a look-up table which for each behavioral goal and each configuration of sensory messages would have an entry determining the required motor action. However, such a solution does not meet the criterion of flexibility and modularity. The assumption of internal references reflecting the laws of physics leads to much more flexible and at the same time parsimonious solutions.

A kinetic aspect of the head-on-trunk movement is that it requires the trunk as a buttress taking up the reaction forces; in turn, the trunk will transmit these forces to the body's support (e.g., the floor of a vehicle) and ultimately to the surface of the earth. This consideration again underlines that the multisegment human body, its support, and the earth surface (as the terrestrial representation of space) can be viewed as one mechanical system composed of a chain of linked movement references in a foot-up hierarchical order.

A foot-up order of our movement control may not be intuitive on introspection. This appears to be related to our perception in two respects. (1) Our brains tend to "automatically" compensate for the forces and force fields that occur during our behavior, without representing this in conscious perception. Consider, for instance, a forward extension of the arm; the gravitational pull on the arm becomes enormous when it gets extended, without us noticing it and this independently of our momentary body orientation in space (a fact which indicates that the body kinematics are predictively taken into account). As we have argued previously,[3] the kinetics of our behavior are normally learned and then become unconsciously compensated for in a predictive way. This unburdens our conscious sensorimotor control and, in addition, makes movement imagination and planning primarily a matter of kinematics. (2) The most relevant sensors for spatial orientation, the vestibular and visual systems, are located in the head rather than in the feet. As will be described in the following section, the kinematic information carried by these signals is transferred to the internal representation of the feet and their support before being used for movement control. However, the "downward chain" of processing underlying this transfer apparently does not cause signals that are consciously perceptible. As explained previously,[3] only the signals arising in the ensuing foot-up chain are consciously perceived (provided attention is focused on them).

SCENARIO IDENTIFICATION AND REPRESENTATION

Because head rotations in space can result from a variety of scenarios (movements of either the neck, or the legs, or the support), the concomitantly arising vestibular signal has to be perceptually interpreted with the help of the proprioceptive signals of relative motion between the various body segments. Or, put the other way around, the proprioceptive motion cues require specification with the help of vestibular signals. For example, if we want to use neck proprioceptive afferents for the control of our behavior (e.g., oculomotor control or walking behavior), we have to know "what was rotated relative to what": Was the head rotated in space relative to the stationary trunk or, vice versa, the trunk relative to the stationary head, or were both rotating in space to different degrees and possibly in different directions? At first sight, there appears to be a simple solution to this problem of scenario identification. The vestibular system, as a gravitoinertial measuring device, would inform us about the head rotation in space. By combining the vestibular head-in-space signal with a proprioceptive trunk-to-head signal, we would obtain a trunk-in-space signal. Given that these sensory signals are reliable, we then would have appropriate information concerning the rotations of head-in-space, trunk-to-head (from the proprioceptive signal), and trunk-in-space.

However, our psychophysical studies of human self-motion perception during various horizontal head and trunk rotations in the absence of visual orientation cues led us to a somewhat different conclusion.[9] This conclusion was based mainly on a comparison of subjective estimates of head-in-space rotation in two different situations. (1) When head and body are (passively) rotated *en bloc*, these estimates exhibit a purely "vestibular character" in that the gain decreases at low frequencies, the detection threshold is high, and the intrasubject variability is very large (all these characteristics are typical for the vestibular signal, particularly at low frequencies[10]). (2) In contrast, when the head is rotated on the stationary trunk, the gain is similar at all frequencies and the detection threshold is low. The estimates in the latter situation closely resemble those that are obtained when subjects are asked to estimate head-on-trunk instead of head-in-space rotation, suggesting that these estimates are based on neck proprioceptive cues rather than drawing on the vestibular signal. However, neck proprioception does only signal the *relative* motion between head and trunk. Before it can be used to estimate the *absolute* motion of the head in space in the second scenario, it somehow must be established that the trunk is motionless and, hence, stationary in space. It is at this point that our conclusions start to deviate from the simplistic view sketched above.

We posit that the primordial function of the vestibular head-in-space (hs) signal is to estimate the kinematic state of the trunk. To explain our view, we refer to the signal flow diagram in FIGURE 1A, in anticipation of a more general description below (although FIG. 1A describes a kinematic control model of head and trunk movements in the sagittal plane, it can be applied to horizontal rotations as well). The vestibular hs signal is summed with a "vestibularly colored" proprioceptive trunk-to-head signal (th′) having dynamics very similar to those of the vestibular afferents. This summation yields an internal estimate of trunk in space, ts. Vestibular coloring would be achieved by passing the primary neck signal (ht) through a "vestibular *eigen*model," emulating the transfer characteristics of the vestibular channel (note that ht = –th in our terminology). To the extent that the emulation is accurate, the two signals (hs, th′) cancel each other during head rotation on a *stationary* trunk, irrespective of whether fast or slow rotations are considered. Thus, their sum can be taken as an indicator of trunk stability or, more generally, as an estimate of trunk-in-space motion ts (ts = hs + th′). However, the vestibular component (hs) of this sum is prone to considerable fluctuations (noise). Therefore, the estimate appears to be protected by a threshold element fending off these fluctuations (T in FIG. 1A; note that we assume for the moment that there is no relative movement between trunk and feet, hence ts = fs and ts′ = fs′). The threshold prevents the estimate ts′ from falsely indicating a movement when the trunk actually is stationary. Finally, the head-in-space estimate to be used for perception and postural adjustments (hs′) is obtained in a second step by combining the trunk-in-space estimate ts′ with an ideal (i.e., having unity transfer function) neck signal ht indicating head-on-trunk excursion (hs′ = ht + ts′).

As mentioned before, most passive head rotations in space during natural behaviour occur in the wake of trunk movements (during walking, turning, etc.) which may cause leg proprioceptive messages. The interpretation of these messages faces the same problem as described above for those from the neck. Did the trunk rotate with respect to the stationary feet, or vice versa, the feet relative to the trunk, or perhaps as a result of vehicle or platform motion? This consideration readily leads to a *generalization* which postulates that the vestibular signal is used in the first place to establish for each segment of the body the physical event that caused its movement. Starting with the head-trunk joint, a chain of interactions with vestibularly colored axial proprioceptive signals of increasingly "lower" origin (i.e., closer to the feet) ultimately would provide an estimate of the extent to which the observed movements

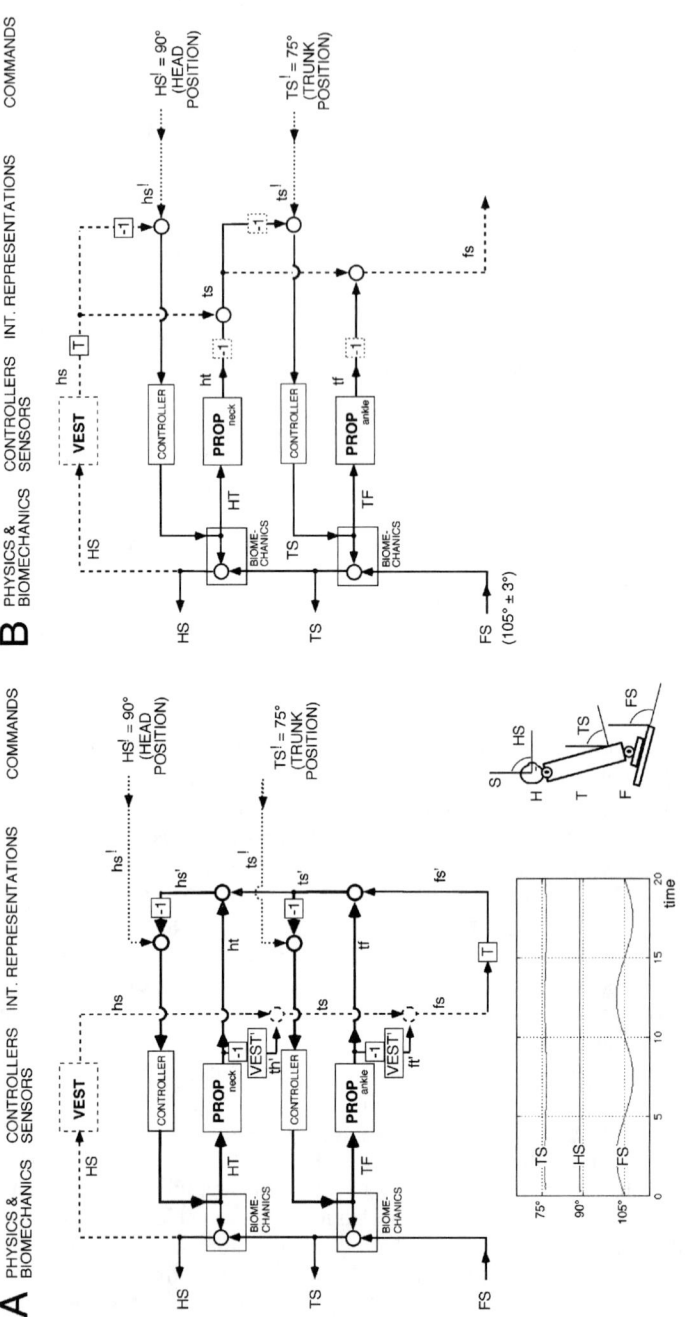

FIGURE 1. *See following page for legend.*

were caused by a motion of the body's support. Note in this context that the ecologically most relevant scenario is the one where the support (the surface of the earth in general) is stationary; the vestibular threshold mentioned above can be viewed as means to guarantee a particularly reliable representation of this case.

Experiments in which we stimulated the leg joints rather than the neck joints confirmed this generalization.[11] The observed patterns of vestibulo-proprioceptive interaction indicated that the subjects used the vestibular signal primarily to estimate the motion of the feet and the foot support. Analogous findings were also obtained with horizontal translatory movements between the body and the legs.[12] These observations led to the general conclusion that during movement on firm ground the unreliable vestibular signal (large noise at low frequency) is not used directly for our self-motion perception. Rather, its main function is to establish an internal notion of the body support kinematics. In the most frequently occurring situation of movement on firm ground, this notion is made more reliable by the intervention of a threshold and, possibly, also of cognitive mechanisms. Building then on the notion of the body support as a space reference, our self-motion perception becomes determined by proprioceptive afferents or visual signals (see below).

Although the above concept has been derived primarily from studies using rotations in the horizontal plane where the vestibular system shows no static sensitivity, we suggest that it may hold as well for the sensory control of body kinematics in the vertical planes,[13,14] where the additional intervention of otolith afferents endows the vestibular sense with static sensitivity ("broadband characteristics"). However, a re-

FIGURE 1. Two alternative models of the control of head position in space based on the three-segment kinematic body model shown in inset (HS, TS, and FS define vertical head, trunk, and foot angular positions in space, respectively). (**A**) Support reconstruction model. The physical variables and their interactions are shown on the left (trunk vs. feet, head vs. trunk: TF, HT). On top, HS induces a vestibular signal hs. Along a downward processing chain (interactions with neck and ankle proprioceptive inputs), hs is first used to obtain an estimate of foot-in-space position (fs; fs = hs + th' + ft'); the proprioceptive signals th' and ft' intervening in this process are internal sign-reversed representations of HT and TF which, for the sake of generality, are shown here to be shaped by *eigen*models of the vestibular system (VEST'). Noise (mostly of vestibular origin) affecting fs is suppressed by threshold T; stabilized in this way, signal fs' serves as a computational reference for the ensuing "upward" processing that subserves perception and motor control of head and trunk position. To control trunk in space position, we obtain an internal representation of this position (ts') by adding the proprioceptive signal tf from the trunk-to-foot joint (ankle) to the above reference signal. Signal ts' then is compared with the set point signal ts! (desired trunk position), with their difference (error) acting to readjust the trunk-to-foot position. In this way, a local control loop is established which stabilizes TS in the presence of disturbances caused by FS (internally represented by fs'). In turn, the internal trunk-in-space representation ts' is used to calculate head position in space (hs') and, thereby, to inform a local neck proprioceptive control loop about the deviations from the desired head-in-space position (hs!) resulting from movements of the trunk in space (TS). Thus, local loops acting on the *relative* positions of the various joints are put into the service of the control of *absolute* position in space. Simulated position curves for HS, TS, and FS are given in inset (instructed head and trunk positions in space: $HS^! = 90°$ and $TS^! = 75°$, respectively; FS is assumed to undergo a ± 3° sinusoidal tilt superimposed on 105° toes-down platform position). (**B**) Direct head-down control model. Here, the vestibular hs signal is used to directly control head position and, after interaction with a neck signal, also trunk position. See text for further details.

consideration of a previous simple and straightforward model of canal–otolith interaction[15] leads us to assume that in terms of its noise, the output of this mechanism cannot be better than the input from the canals. Given this is true, also the vestibular signals for the vertical planes would be unreliable because of noise. Hence, the processing scheme postulated above also would improve the perceptual reliability during *vertical* movements executed for a *stationary* body support.

The notion of an internal reconstruction of the support behavior as a basic step for orientation and posture control also in the vertical planes is, moreover, justified by the physics (kinematics and kinetics) of these movements. Indeed, also the movements in the vertical planes can be described in terms of a chain of linked movement references arranged in a foot-up hierarchical order. This point is illustrated in FIGURE 1A which shows a formal implementation of our hypotheses for a sensory control model for human upright body posture in the sagittal plane, but which also intends to illustrate our hypotheses in general. As shown in the inset, we here consider the kinematic control of a three-segment model of the human body (feet, trunk, head in space: FS, TS, HS, respectively), whose task is to maintain certain head and trunk positions during tilt of the support surface.

The angular positions of the body's segments with respect to space (FS, TS, HS) and relative to each other (trunk vs. feet, head vs. trunk: TF, HT) are represented on the left of the model in FIGURE 1A which we refer to in the following as the "support reconstruction model." On top of the chain of kinematic interactions between the physical variables is HS which induces a vestibular signal of head position in space (hs). This signal, rather than being directly used for perception and head position control, is first summed with (sign inverted) proprioceptive signals from the joints to obtain an estimate of trunk in space (ts; see above) and then of feet in space (fs = hs + th' + ft'). As mentioned before, the proprioceptive information in this "downward chain" of processing becomes vestibularly colored by *eigen*models of the vestibular system (dashed boxes VEST') such that the dynamics of the two signals become similar. To suppress fluctuations of signal fs that conceivably are caused by vestibular noise, it is passed through a threshold element which becomes effective in the ecologically most relevant case, that is, during support stationariness. Thus, the final reconstruction of foot/support position (fs') will be particularly reliable when the individual stands on firm ground. Representations of the various angular positions for space (ts', hs') then are derived by sequential summation of fs' with proprioceptive signals from increasingly higher segments; these representations are accessible to perception and serve as feedback signals for local loops that maintain or adjust the desired posture of the body segments (as shown in the inset for a simulation of the model with instructed head and trunk positions in space of $HS^! = 90°$ and $TS^! = 75°$, respectively, during a $\pm 3°$ sinusoidal tilt superimposed on a $105°$ toes-down platform position).

An obvious question with the scheme in FIGURE 1A is why proprioceptive signals of a given joint are first subtracted (during "downward processing" of the vestibular cue) and then again added ("upward processing"). Granted that, unlike with horizontal rotations, the vestibular and proprioceptive cues have similar broadband dynamics during vertical rotations, would it not be more parsimonious to use a single chain of downward processing? This (seeming) *alternative model* is depicted in FIGURE 1B. In this scheme, the vestibular signal hs is directly used to control the head, that is, without specification of what the trunk or the feet are doing and what proprioception tells about the state of the neck joint. Similarly, a trunk-in-space signal ts, derived from vestibular-neck interaction (ts = hs − ht), is used to control the trunk, again without a specification of what the foot support is doing and what the state of the ankle joint control is. The two models behave similarly as long as the vestibular signals are assumed to be free of noise (both yield the same simulation results shown as inset in FIG. 1). However, with the more realistic assumption of fairly large fluctuations of the vestibular signal in the low-frequency range, a significant difference emerges. In the support reconstruction model (FIG. 1A), the head-in-space estimate hs' profits from the stability of the reference signal fs' (which is noise protected by threshold T) and from the (presumed) precision of the proprioceptive signals tf and ht. In contrast, because in the alternative model (FIG. 1B) the head-in-space estimate depends entirely on the vestibular signal hs, either it will be as noisy as the vestibular cue or, if noise is fended off by a threshold (T in FIG. 1B), it will be insensitive to small head-on-trunk rotations.

So far, an experimental differentiation between the two models has been conducted only for the horizontal plane (this clearly favored the reconstruction model as described above[10]). Although corresponding experiments have yet to be performed to confirm our contention that the reconstruction model is also applicable to the vertical planes, we can list further theoretical reasons to prefer it. First, it would seem to be more robust than the direct head down-processing scheme in FIGURE 1B. If the vestibular sensor is damaged or completely out of function, the reconstruction model will continue to properly work during behavior on firm ground (the most relevant situation), whereas the direct model does not (see our previous discussions[16,17]). Second, the reconstruction model, but not the direct model in FIGURE 1B, faithfully reflects the physical situation starting with the body support surface as a platform for the feet, the feet in turn as the platform for the trunk, etc. Its correspondence to physics allows the model in A to be extended in a straightforward way to also include kinetic aspects in addition to the kinematic ones considered here.[18,19] Moreover, it generally is recognized that skeletal motor control is shaped to a large extent by predictive mechanisms which prepare the force compensations and postural adjustments that normally accompany movements. Conceivably, such predictions require an "internal model" of the body in its environment, similarly as it has been repeatedly envisaged to account for our ability of movement planning and imagery. We hold that the foot-up hierarchical chain of linked movement and kinetic references proposed here represents such an internal model. We assume that any solution that is detached from the kinetic aspects of physics, as the direct head-down control in FIGURE 1B, is hardly suitable for such a model because it requires auxiliary mechanisms and/or may be applicable only for specific purposes.

As often happens in biology when two theories are pondered, it ultimately may turn out that both apply, depending on the behavioral situation considered. For example, certain situations requiring fast reactions may possibly activate control loops with direct routes similar to the one outlined in FIGURE 1B. For example, the vestibuloocular reflex (VOR) directly counteracts any head-in-space movement by a compensatory eye-in-head rotation; it is not "interested" in why the head moves, because its mode of action does not require adjustments depending on whether a support or a head-versus-trunk movement occurs. One can conceive also of other case-specific "simplifications." For instance, in situations in which we have experienced the ground (or the visual scene; see below) as stationary many times before, the brain may *a priori* tend to use the ground (or the scene) as a space reference and control the action primarily with the help of proprioceptive (or visual) signals alone. Generally, in situations where we obtain optimal sensor information from many different sources, which is especially likely to happen when the body support and the visual scene are stationary, the system becomes so redundant that several functionally equivalent control strategies can be adopted, giving the brain a high degree of flexibility.

THE ROLE OF VISUAL INFORMATION

Our notion that the primordial interaction between vestibular and axial proprioceptive information is one which reconstructs the kinematic state of the body support and thereby provides the computational platform for human spatial orientation also applies to motion perception and localization of visual targets in space during self-motion. Several studies into this subject[10,20–22] concur in that the observed behavior cannot be explained by a straightforward interaction of vestibular and visuooculomotor inputs alone; to account for the dynamic and noise characteristics of the subjects' performance, the hypothesized reconstruction of body support motion must again be invoked.

More complex are situations in which, in addition to the vestibular cue, a visual scene provides visuooculomotor information on the relative motion between subjects' heads and the surroundings. In our view, the visuooculomotor system can replace the vestibular system as a space reference on the provision that a visual-vestibular interaction mechanism first establishes that the visual scene is indeed stationary in space. Experimental studies into the role of visual-vestibular interaction for human self-motion perception[23] suggest that this interaction is largely analogous to that between vestibular and proprioceptive signals. In a first step, subjects estimate the scene-in-space motion, by combining the vestibular head-in-space signal with a vestibularly colored visuooculomotor scene-to-head signal. The two signals cancel each other when the head is rotated while the scene is stationary, ecologically again the most relevant scenario as large scenes rarely move under natural conditions. In a second step, subjects then estimate the head-in-space motion by summing a visuooculomotor signal of head-to-scene position with the scene-in-space estimate.

Thus, in the presence of a stationary visual scene, the scene tends to be taken as a space reference. This then leads to the use of a visual head-in-space signal for self-motion perception, which is more stable and shows a better spatial resolution than the corresponding vestibular signal. When we use it to substitute the vestibular signal in the downward processing of FIGURE 1A, the internal estimate of foot/support motion in space (fs') becomes improved accordingly. An optimum is reached when, in addition, the support is stationary; then, both the support and the scene become representatives of space. Under these conditions, self-motion perception is determined by proprioceptive signals as outlined in FIGURE 1A and/or by congruent visual signals. Stationary visual surroundings and a stable body support (ground) are actually what we experience most often during life. Deriving our self-motion perception in this most common situation from almost ideal visual or proprioceptive motion cues rather than from the nonideal vestibular signal represents in our view a pragmatic "behavioral" optimization of the human spatial orientation system (for error and noise minimization[10]).

STILL NOT A FINAL PROOF

We would like to return to our starting point and reemphasize the problem of narrowing the many possibilities when it comes to formally describing a complex system such as the human spatial orientation system. We here have presented two models of this system, the reconstruction model and the alternative direct model. In view of the system's complexity, we doubt that there will be a direct proof for which of these models is closer to the "truth." We can only invoke circumstantial arguments. An argument that would favor the direct model is its straightforward and parsimonious structure. However, in our view, the internal reconstruction concept has a heavier argument on its side: it offers a larger explanatory and predictive power.

This applies not only to our psychophysical findings on self-motion and object motion perception, but also to postural control. The relevant aspect here is that sensorimotor control in our model is based on a meta level providing internal representations of the *physical* stimuli (e.g., support tilt or contact force such as a pull on the body), whereas most other models proceed from the idea that the *physiological* stimuli feed directly into control loops in the way envisaged by the classic reflex concept. A drawback of the latter models is the necessity of "sensory reweighting" (changes in the model's parameters) when external conditions change (cf. Peterka[24]), because the sensory cues *per se* do not sufficiently specify the external conditions. In contrast, with our concept the internal representations of all relevant kinematic and kinetic stimuli make a sensory weighting largely superfluous. Indeed, a model of postural control based on these principles allowed us to simulate the experimental responses to quite different stimuli (such as support tilt and pull on the body) with the same model parameters.[19]

Finally, another circumstantial argument in favor of our concept is the possibility of implementing increasing levels of sensory redundancy and thereby of functional robustness and flexibility. In motor control, flexibility results, among others, from the multisegment structure of the systems, which allows us to reach toward a goal in space in many different geometrical ways, for instance. We hold that our reconstruction model is able to provide the basis for the sensory control required for such a flexible motor system. Moreover, it has the flexibility that is required to deal with changes in the geometry of the body and environment; for instance, it is easily reconfigured when we change from a standing to a sitting position so that the back instead of the feet transmit the reaction forces to the body support surface. Another aspect of its flexibility is that the modular character of the concept allows us to extend its multisegment structure, for example, when we add a tool to an extremity for reaching or when we control a vehicle which constitutes an interface between the body and the earth surface.

SUMMARY

Human spatial orientation builds upon multisensory integration and upon an interplay of several motor subfunctions and thus represents a complex system with many degrees of freedom. Whereas an analytical description, for a bottom-up mathematical approach, is impossible because of the intervention of nonlinear equations, numerical solutions have become feasible with the advent of powerful computers and modeling software. Yet, these tools do not much further our understanding as long as our ignorance of the brain's internal wiring leaves room for many formally equivalent solutions. To narrow the choice, criteria for a "biological plausible" modeling must be applied in a top-down way. We here suggest, as a particular important criterion, that modeling should proceed from an internal (neural) reconstruction of the physics of the scenario under consideration, taking into account the biological constraints such as the characteristics of the available sensors and their location within the body. Following this line, we characterize the upright human body during orienting behavior as a stack of superimposed motion platforms. The common buttress of this stack is the inert earth surface which supports the body either directly or via a movable platform. A model of how the physical states of the various platforms are internally (neurally) reconstructed from sensory information leads to a concept of nested references which is well apt to deal with the high complexity of the human orientation system. Using this concept as a guide, one may explain several so far enigmatic phenomena but may also detect exceptions reflecting specific biological demands.

ACKNOWLEDGMENTS

This work was supported by DFG Me 715/5-1 and Be 783/3.

REFERENCES

1. WIENER, N. 1948. Cybernetics. MIT Press. Boston.
2. VON BERTALANFFY, L. 1969. General System Theory. George Brazillier. New York.
3. MERGNER, T. 2002. The Matryoshka Dolls principle in human dynamic behavior in space—a theory of linked references for multisensory perception and control of action. Curr. Psychol. Cogn. **21:** 129–212.
4. CHONG, L. & L.B. RAY. 2002. Wholistic biology. Science **295:** 1661.
5. KITANO, H. 2002. Systems biology: a brief overview. Science **295:** 1662–1664.
6. CSETE, M.E. & J.C. DOYLE. 2002. Reverse engineering of biological complexity. Science **295:** 1664–1669.
7. DAVIDSON, E.H. et al. 2002. A genomic regulatory network for development. Science **295:** 1669–1678.
8. NOBLE, D. 2002. Modeling the heart—from genes to cells to the whole organ. Science **295:** 1678–1682.
9. MERGNER, T., C. SIEBOLD, G. SCHWEIGART & W. BECKER. 1991. Human perception of horizontal head and trunk rotation in space during vestibular and neck stimulation. Exp. Brain Res. **85:** 389–404.
10. MERGNER, T., G. NASIOS, C. MAURER & W. BECKER. 2001. Visual object localisation in space. Interaction of retinal, eye position, vestibular and neck proprioceptive information. Exp. Brain Res. **141:** 33–51.
11. MERGNER, T., F. HLAVACKA & G. SCHWEIGART. 1993. Interaction of vestibular and proprioceptive inputs. J. Vestib. Res. **3:** 41–57.
12. HLAVACKA, F., T. MERGNER & B. BOLHA. 1996. Human self-motion perception during translatory vestibular and proprioceptive stimulation. Neurosci. Lett. **210:** 83–86.
13. MERGNER, T., W. HUBER & W. BECKER. 1997. Vestibular-neck interaction and transformations of sensory coordinates. J. Vestib. Res. **7:** 119–135.
14. MERGNER, T. & T. ROSEMEIER. 1998. Interaction of vestibular, somatosensory and visual signals for posture control and motion perception under terrestrial and microgravity conditions. Brain Res. Rev. **28:** 118–135.

15. MERGNER, T. & S. GLASAUER. 1999. A simple model of vestibular canal-otolith signal fusion. Ann. N.Y. Acad. Sci. **871:** 430–434.
16. SCHWEIGART, G., S. HEIMBRAND, T. MERGNER & W. BECKER. 1993. Role of neck input for the perception of horizontal head and trunk rotation in patients with loss of vestibular function. Exp. Brain Res. **95:** 533–546.
17. SCHWEIGART, G., R.D. CHIEN & T. MERGNER. 2002. Neck proprioception compensates for age-related deterioration of vestibular self-motion perception. Exp. Brain Res. **147:** 89–97.
18. MERGNER, T., C. MAURER & R.J. PETERKA. 2002. Sensory contributions to the control of stance: a posture control model. Adv. Exp. Med. Biol. **508:** 147–152.
19. MERGNER, T., C. MAURER & R.J. PETERKA. 2003. A multisensory posture control model of human upright stance. Prog. Brain Res. **142:** 189–201.
20. MERGNER, T., G. ROTTLER, H. KIMMIG & W. BECKER. 1992. Role of vestibular and neck inputs for the perception of object motion in space. Exp. Brain Res. **89:** 655–668.
21. MAURER, C., H. KIMMIG, A. TREFZER & T. MERGNER. 1997. Visual object localization through vestibular and neck inputs. I. Localization with respect to space and relative to the head and trunk mid-sagittal planes. J. Vestib. Res. **7:** 119–135.
22. MERGNER, T., G. NASIOS & D. ANASTASOPOULOS. 1998. Vestibular memory-contingent saccades involve somatosensory input from the body support. Neuroreport **9:** 1469–1473.
23. MERGNER, T., G. SCHWEIGART, M. MÜLLER, et al.. 2000. Visual contributions to human self-motion perception during horizontal body rotation. Arch. Ital. Biol. **138:** 139–167.
24. PETERKA, R.J. 2002. Sensorimotor integration in human postural control. J. Neurophysiol. **88:** 1097–1118.

Spatial Memory Deficits in Patients with Chronic Bilateral Vestibular Failure

FRANZ SCHAUTZER,[a,b] DEREK HAMILTON,[c] ROGER KALLA,[a]
MICHAEL STRUPP,[a] AND THOMAS BRANDT[a]

[a]*Ludwig-Maximilians University, 81377 Munich, Germany*

[b]*Department of Neurology and Psychosomatic, LKH Villach, 9500 Villach, Austria*

[c]*Canadian Centre for Behavioural Neuroscience, University of Lethbridge, Lethbridge, Alberta, Canada T1K 3M4*

ABSTRACT: The role of the vestibular system for navigation and spatial memory has been demonstrated in animals but not in humans. Vestibular signals are necessary for location-specific "place cell" activity in the hippocampus which provides a putative neural substrate for the spatial representation involved in navigation. To investigate the spatial memory in patients with bilateral vestibular failure due to NF2 with bilateral neurectomy, a virtual variant (on a PC) of the Morris water task adapted to humans was used. Significant spatial learning and memory deficits were shown in 12 patients as compared to 10 healthy controls. These data suggest that functional hippocampal deficits manifest due to a chronic lack of vestibular input in these patients. These deficits can even be demonstrated with the subjects stationary, i.e., without any actual vestibular or somatosensory stimulation.

KEYWORDS: chronic vestibular deficit; spatial memory; virtual Morris water task

INTRODUCTION

Since the early 1960s, animal studies have indicated that the vestibular system plays an important role in navigation based on self-motion cues (e.g., as in path integration; for review see Smith[1]), and more recently the effects of vestibular stimulation and lesions on navigation involving control by exteroceptive stimuli (e.g., visual) have been evaluated in tasks such as the Morris water task (MWT). In the MWT, rats are trained to navigate to an escape platform in a circular pool of water. The escape platform is made invisible by submerging it just below the surface of the water; however, normal rats are capable of directly navigating to the platform from several release points. It is generally agreed that this behavior is related to ambient visual cues in the extramaze environment which remain in a fixed spatial location to

Address for correspondence: Franz Schautzer, M.D., Department of Neurology, University of Munich, Klinikum Grosshadern, D-81377 Munich, Germany. Voice: ++49-89-7095-3678; fax: ++49-89-7095-6673.

schautzer@lkh-vil.or.at

the platform throughout training. There are no proximal (intramaze) cues that mark the goal location, and strategies based on idiothetic cues (e.g., proprioception) are not effective because several starting locations are used (i.e., a simple route cannot be learned). Furthermore, removal of most of the visual stimuli leads to deficits in spatial navigation in the Morris task.[2] Thus, based on the idea that the Morris task measures place learning for a constellation of visual stimuli and that learning in the MWT is critically dependent on hippocampal circuitry, it is not readily apparent how erroneous or lacking vestibular signals may affect this form of learning.

Semenov and Bures[3] found that stimulation of the vestibular system (via prolonged rotation) disrupts learning in the MWT. Although deficits in the ability to swim have been demonstrated in animals with vestibular lesions,[4] the deficits reported by Semenov and Bures[3] appear to be related to the lack of good correspondence between visual and vestibular signals. Because vestibular lesions lead to impaired swimming, place learning in the MWT has not been systematically evaluated in animals with vestibular lesions (D.G. Wallace, personal communication). In other comparable spatial learning tasks, vestibular lesions do not appear to cause deficits in learning to navigate to a goal based on its fixed spatial relationship to a set of visual stimuli. Thus, spatial learning of the type measured in the MWT appears to be intact in animals with vestibular lesions,[4,5] whereas other spatial behaviors that depend on idiothetic cues are clearly disrupted after vestibular lesions.[5]

Perhaps paradoxically, both vestibular stimulation and lesions disrupt physiology in circuitry that is known to be involved in place learning. For example, Stackman et al.[6] found that vestibular signals are necessary for location-specific "place cell" activity in the hippocampus, which provides a putative neural substrate for the spatial representation involved in navigation (see also Smith[1] for review). Recent animal studies also have reported long-term changes in activity of hippocampal neurons[7] and expression of N-methyl-D-aspartate receptors subunits[8] which is critical for normal synaptic plasticity. One possibility is that chronic alteration in hippocampal physiology may lead to hippocampal-dependent learning deficits in navigation tasks that do not involve salient vestibular signals.

Human patients with bilateral vestibular failure (BVF) are capable of executing goal-directed linear locomotion without impairment;[9] however, they fail to accurately negotiate corners when walking along a triangular path.[10] Thus, navigation is expected to be particularly impaired in BVF patients; however, the relative contributions of idiothetic and exteroceptive stimulus control to this type of impairment have not been investigated. In the present study, we asked whether patients with chronic BVF are impaired at learning to navigate relative to exteroceptive visual stimuli (as in the MWT). We used a computerized (virtual) version of the MWT (VMWT)[11,12] to measure spatial learning and memory in patients with BVF as a result of bilateral neurectomy for neurofibromatosis type 2 (NF2). The VMWT simulates first-person visual experiences associated with navigation and requires participants to control navigation to a hidden goal based on its relationship to a set of conspicuous visual cues. Idiothetic signals that are generated during real-world navigation are absent in the VMWT, particularly vestibular signals because the body and head are kept still. This methodology allowed us to determine whether a spatial learning and memory deficit can be demonstrated in humans with BVF independently of impairments related to the processing of self-motion cues and related behaviors. Place learning and navigation in the VMWT used here appear to require and engage hippocampal circuitry; therefore, place learning deficits in BVF would suggest a deficit related to hippocampal circuitry that may occur as a result of the chronic absence of vestibular input. In addition, we tested BVF patients in a cued navigation (visible-platform) task which is intact in animals with hippocampal damage and in humans the display place learning deficits in the VMWT.[11,12]

METHODS

Subjects

Ten patients (four women, six men; mean ± SD = 38.0 ± 6.7 years) with neurofibromatosis type 2 and 10 sex- and age-matched controls (mean ± SD = 38.7 ± 5.4 years) with no known neurological history participated in the study. All patients had undergone a bilateral labyrinthectomy between 5 and 10 years before the test and subsequently had complete BVF. Only one patient lacked a complete postoperative hearing loss.

Materials and Apparatus

The virtual environment used here has been described in detail elsewhere.[11,12] In brief, the basic features of the environment consisted of a circular pool located in the center of a room with a square floor plan. FIGURE 1A depicts the layout of the environment and FIGURE 1B shows a representative view of the environment from a participant's perspective.

Four conspicuous distal cues of equal size were placed around the distal walls (see FIG. 1A). The cues were positioned such that one cue was on each of the four distal room walls, and the platform could not be found by directly approaching a sin-

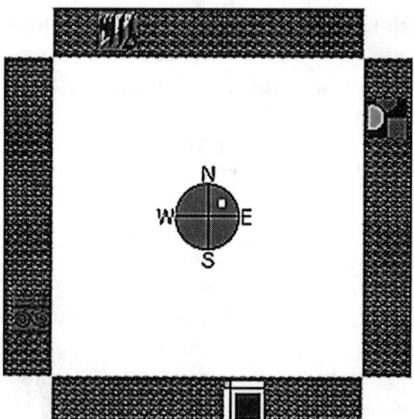

FIGURE 1. (**A**) Layout of the virtual environment. Distal walls and cues are laid flat. The circular pool was centered in the room. The platform (*white square*) was located in the N/E quadrant of the pool. The four starting locations are labeled "N," "E," "S," and "W".

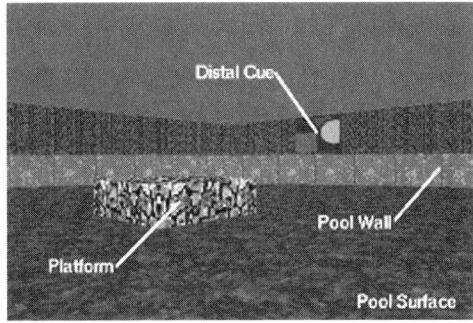

FIGURE 1. *Continued.* (**B**) A representative view of the virtual environment from the center of the circular pool. The pool surface, pool wall, distal wall, the visible platform, and a single distal cue are labeled.

gle cue from any release point. The platform was positioned in the center of one quadrant (N/E) and occupied approximately 2% of the pool area. A first-person view of the virtual environment was displayed on a 17-inch PC laptop monitor with a 45° field of view (see FIG. 1B). The observer's position was always slightly above the surface of the water, and forward movement was controlled by the UP (↑) arrow key on the keyboard. Rotation was controlled by the LEFT (←) and RIGHT (→) arrow keys. Backward navigation or up–down movement within the pool was not possible. A full, 360° rotation in the absence of forward movement required approximately 2.5 s, and a straight path from one side of the pool to the other took approximately 4 s to complete.

Design and Procedure

VMWT training and testing were done in three phases that required a total of approximately 30 min to complete. During Phase I, participants completed five hidden platform training blocks, which consisted of four trials each. Starting locations during Phase I were sampled pseudorandomly without replacement from four locations that corresponded to the cardinal compass points (see FIG. 1A). The latency and path length to navigate to the hidden platform was measured for each trial. Phase II consisted of a single 45-s probe trial during which the platform was removed from the environment. The starting location for the probe trial was selected pseudorandomly from the two starting locations furthest from the platform location (W & S). Five dependent measures were recorded for the probe trial: (1) latency to enter the platform quadrant, (2) path length to enter platform quadrant, (3) initial heading error (the angular deviation from a straight trajectory to the platform measured 1 s after movement was initiated, (4) percentage of time spent in the platform quadrant, and (5) percentage of the total probe trial path length spent in the platform quadrant (N/E quadrant in FIG. 1A). During Phase III the platform was slightly raised above the surface of the water (as illustrated in FIG. 1B) for two blocks of four trials. Starting locations were determined as in Phase I, and the latency and path length to navigate to the visible platform were measured for each trial.

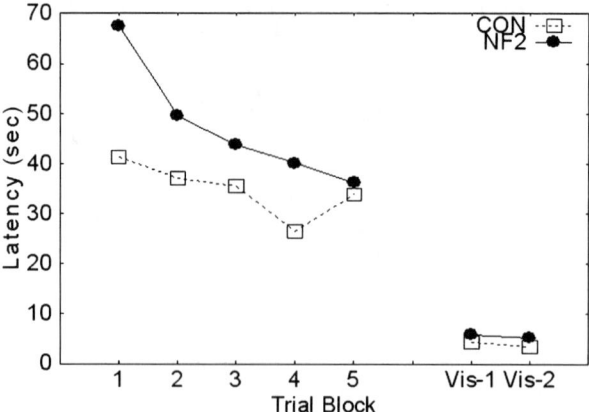

FIGURE 2. Mean path latency for each group to navigate to the platform during hidden platform (place learning).

RESULTS

Phase I

Eight of the 10 controls consistently navigated directly to the hidden platform, whereas only five of the 10 NF2 patients consistently displayed direct navigation to the platform. Note, however, that two of the NF2 patients were able to directly navigate to the platform because they consistently waited for the platform to become visible (after 60 s). Thus, their improved path length performance was at the cost of longer latencies to navigate to the platform. Given that some patients routinely adopted this strategy at various points during training, our analyses will focus on latency as a measure of place learning. Patients consistently took longer to navigate to the hidden platform during Phase I than controls; this was particularly evident during the first four trial blocks. An overview of the latency values for the groups to navigate to the platform during the Phase I hidden platform and Phase III visible trial blocks is provided in FIGURE 2A. An analysis of variance (ANOVA) on latency for the groups to navigate to the hidden platform was conducted with Group and Trial Block as independent variables. Sex was not included as a factor because there were only four women in each group. The Group main effect failed to reach statistical significance [$F(1, 18) = 3.54, P = 0.076$]. There was a significant main effect for Trial Block [$F(4, 72) = 12.91, P < 0.001$] as well as a significant interaction [$F(4, 72) = 3.54, P = 0.011$]. The interaction was caused by a significant Group difference during the first Trial Block [$F(1, 18) = 8.48, P = 0.009$] which was not detected in the remainder of the training blocks. (The Group difference approached significance during Block 4 [$P = 0.063$].) NF2 patients and controls did not differ in rate of navigation during the Phase I trials [$F(1, 18) = 2.10, P = 0.16$].

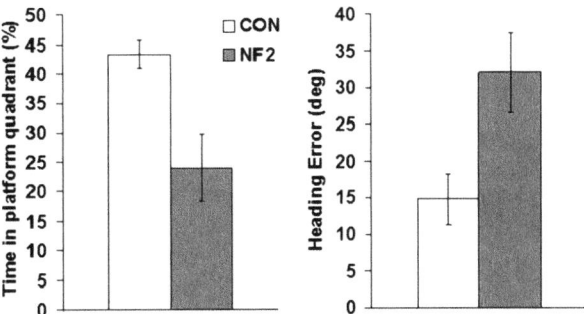

FIGURE 3. (*Left*) Mean percentage of search time each group spent in the platform quadrant during the no-platform probe trial of Phase II. (*Right*) Mean initial heading error for each group during the no-platform probe trial of Phase II. Error bars are ± 1 SEM.

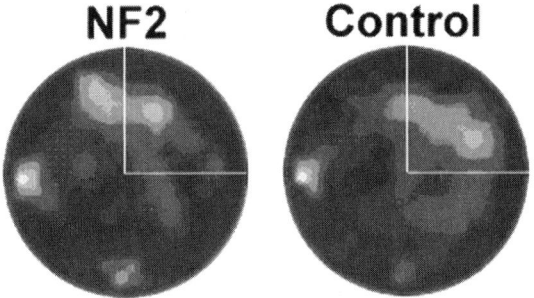

FIGURE 4. Dwell time for the 10 patients (NF2) and normal controls (CON) during the no-platform probe trial. Light areas indicate regions where a relatively large amount of time was spent; dark areas indicate regions where a relatively small amount of time was spent. The platform quadrant is demarcated by the white lines.

Phase II (Probe Trial)

During the no-platform probe trial, controls spent most of their time searching in the quadrant of the virtual pool where the platform had been during the 20 hidden platform trials of Phase I (see FIG. 3A), whereas the NF2 patients spent only approximately 25% of their search time in the platform quadrant. FIGURE 4 is a diagram portraying the composite dwell time for each group during the no-platform probe trial. Light areas depict regions occupied for a relatively large percentage of time, and dark areas indicate those occupied for a relatively small percentage of time. As shown in FIGURE 4, the NF2 group spent less time in the platform quadrant than controls and more time in other regions of the pool. An ANOVA detected a significant Group difference in the percentage of time spent in the platform quadrant [$F(1, 18) = 9.41$, $P = 0.007$]. Although controls also had lower heading errors than patients, this difference did not reach statistical significance [$F(1, 18) = 7.24$, $P = 0.015$ (see

FIG. 3B)]. The controls performed numerically better than NF2 patients on the other three dependent measures during the probe trial; however, none of these effects approached statistical significance (all Ps >0.26). The means ± 1 SEM for each dependent measure were as follows: (1) latency to enter the platform quadrant (M_{CON} = 10.30 s ± 2.63; M_{NF2} = 15.28 s ± 4.64); (2) path length to enter the platform quadrant (M_{CON} = 0.714 ± 0.082; M_{NF2} = 0.836 ± 0.101); and (3) percentage of path length spent in the platform quadrant (M_{CON} = 35.7% ± 4.02; M_{NF2} = 27.0 ± 6.48). Future research with this patient population should include more participants to increase the statistical power of these measures. NF2 patients and controls did not differ in rate of navigation during the Phase II probe trial (F < 1).

Phase III (Cued Navigation)

The NF2 and control groups were similar in latency to navigate to a visible platform in the same environment as used in Phases II and III (see FIG. 2), and all control participants and NF2 patients were consistently able to navigate directly to the visible platform. An ANOVA failed to detect a significant Group main effect or a significant Trial Block effect (both Ps >0.076). The interaction term was also nonsignificant (P >0.84). NF2 patients and controls did not differ in rate of navigation during the Phase III cued navigation trials [$F(1, 18) = 3.10, P = 0.095$].

DISCUSSION

The current study provides evidence of spatial learning and memory deficits in humans with chronic BVF in a computerized version of the MWTs (the VMWT).[11,12] The MWT is the gold standard for measuring hippocampal-dependent learning and memory in rats, and the VMWT represents a human analogue which appears to require and engage hippocampal circuitry, despite the fact that proprioceptive and vestibular signals that are present in real-world navigation are completely lacking. Thus, NF2 patients were impaired relative to controls in a hippocampal-dependent spatial learning in a task which does not require vestibular signals for accurate performance. In contrast, patients were able to navigate to a cue that marks a goal location (cued navigation). Cued navigation has been shown to be independent of hippocampal circuitry in rats; thus, the present results provide a neurobehavioral dissociation which is similar to that observed in rats with hippocampal damage. The lack of a BVF-related impairment in cued navigation suggests that deficits in visual perception, motor skills, or motivation were not the cause of the place-learning impairment observed in the NF2 patients. The present findings are novel in humans with BVF and suggest that functional deficits of hippocampal circuitry may be a consequence of chronic lack of vestibular input.

Various anatomical connections have been demonstrated between the vestibular nuclei via the thalamus to the hippocampus directly or by back projections from the vestibular cortex. Several reports have suggested spatial learning deficits in animals after vestibular lesions or stimulation and similar manipulations have been linked to physiological changes in circuitry critical for place learning and navigation. For example, vestibular stimulation was able to modulate "head direction cells" in the anterior thalamic nuclei and "place cells" in the hippocampus (for review, see Smith[1]), both of which are involved in navigation. We hypothesize that this type of chronic alteration in hippocampal physiology may lead to long-term changes in how the hippocampus processes information. It is difficult to explain these results based on the lack of vestibular input, because the VMWT does not involve interoceptive cues. It is possible, however, that virtual navigation may elicit potentially complex forms of "top-down" signals in circuitry that normally respond to the idiothetic cues related to movement in real navigation. Such signals could be altered in BVF in which case there may be a critical lack of correspondence between perceived self-motion and visual cues. Future research should (1) devise methods to address the influence of such top-down signals in virtual place learning and apply them to the BVF populations and (2) replicate and extend the present research to include assessment of whether chronic BVF patients demonstrate deficits in nonspatial forms of hippocampal-dependent learning and memory.

CONCLUSION

VMWT was used to measure spatial learning and memory in 10 patients with chronic BVT as a result of bilateral neurectomy for neurofibromatosis type 2. The patients took longer to navigate to the hidden platform, required longer path latencies, spent less time in the platform quadrant during the no-platform probe trial, and had larger heading errors than age-matched controls. No difference was found for cued navigation to a visible platform.

The VMWT requires and engages hippocampal circuitry despite the fact that the proprioceptive and vestibular signals, present in real-world navagation, are completely lacking. Thus, patients with BVF were impaired relative to the controls in hippocampal-dependent spatial learning in a task which does not require vestibular signals. These findings are novel and suggest that functional hippocampal deficits are a consequence of the chronic lack of vestibular input.

REFERENCES

1. SMITH, P.F. 1997. Vestibular-hippocampal interactions. Hippocampus 7: 465–471.
2. SUTHERLAND, R.J., I.Q. WHISHAW & B. KOLB. 1983. A behavioral-analysis of spatial localization following electrolytic, kainite-induced or colchicine-induced damage to the hippocampal formation in the rat. Behav. Brain Res. 7: 133–153.
3. SEMENOV, L.V. & J. BURES. 1989. Vestibular stimulation disrupts acquisition of place navigation in the Morris water tank task. Behav. Neural Biol. 51: 346–363.
4. CHAPUIS, N., M. KRIMM, C. DE WAELE, et al. 1992. Effect of post-training unilateral hemilabyrinthectomy in a spatial orientation task by guinea pig. Behav. Brain Res. 51: 115–126.
5. WALLACE, D.G., D.J. HINES, S.M. PELLIS & I.Q. WHISHAW. 2002. Vestibular information is required for dead reckoning in the rat. J. Neurosci. 22: 10009–10017.
6. STACKMAN, R.W., A.S. CLARK & J.S. TAUBE. 2002. Hippocampal spatial representations require vestibular input. Hippocampus 12: 291–303.
7. RUSSELL, N.A., A. HORII, P.F. SMITH, et al. 2003. The long-term effects of permanent vestibular lesions on hippocampal spatial firing. J. Neurosci. 23: 6490–6498.
8. LIN, P., Y. ZHENG, J. KING, et al. 2003. Long-term changes in hippocampal N-methyl-D-aspartate receptor subunits following unilateral vestibular changes in rat. Neuroscience 117: 965–970.

9. GLASAUER, S., M.A. AMORIM, E. VITTE & A. BERTHOZ. 1994. Goal-directed linear locomotion in normal and labyrinthine-defective subjects. Exp. Brain Res. **98:** 323–335.
10. GLASAUER, S., M.A. AMORIM, I. VIAUD-DELMON & A. BERTHOZ. 2002. Differential effects of labyrinthine dysfunction on distance and direction during blindfolded walking of a triangular path. Exp. Brain Res. **145:** 489–497.
11. HAMILTON, D.A., I. DRISCOLL & R.J. SUTHERLAND. 2002. Human place learning in a virtual Morris water task: some important constraints on the flexibility of place navigation. Behav. Brain Res. **129:** 159–170.
12. HAMILTON, D.A., P. KODITUWAKKU, R.J. SUTHERLAND & D.D. SAVAGE. 2003. Children with fetal alcohol syndrome are impaired in place learning but not cued navigation in a virtal Morris water task. Behav. Brain Res. **143:** 85–94.

The Human Horizontal Vestibulo-Ocular Reflex in Response to Active and Passive Head Impulses after Unilateral Vestibular Deafferentation

G.M. HALMAGYI,[a] R.A. BLACK,[a] M.J. THURTELL,[a] AND I.S. CURTHOYS[b]

[a]*Department of Neurology, Royal Prince Alfred Hospital, Sydney, Australia*
[b]*School of Psychology, University of Sydney, Sydney, Australia*

ABSTRACT: We studied the compensatory eye movements made by subjects with unilateral vestibular deficits in response to passive (unpredictable, manually generated) and active (predictable, self-generated) head impulses. A typical head impulse is a brief, low-amplitude (15–20°), high-velocity (150–350°/s), high-acceleration (4000–6000°/s^2), yaw head-on-trunk rotation. In the initial 75 ms of the response, the vestibulo-ocular reflex gain was significantly higher during active head impulses to both ipsilesional and contralesional sides, than during passive impulses. Mean gains were 0.15 (ipsilesional passive), 0.44 (ipsilesional active), 0.5 (contralesional passive), and 0.76 (contralesional active). Differences between active and passive head impulses were present from near the onset of head rotation. The mechanism for producing this behavior is unclear, but the findings could be related to enhanced sensitivity of second-order neurons during active head impulses. However, even with active movements, there is still a large and statistically significant asymmetry in the eye-movement responses for ipsilesional as opposed to contralesional head rotations. After 75 ms, rapid corrective eye movements often were generated to reduce any remaining gaze error.

KEYWORDS: human; active; passive; vestibulo-ocular reflex; head movement

INTRODUCTION

The function of the vestibulo-ocular reflex (VOR) is to stabilize gaze during head rotations. When tested with rapid head "impulses" in yaw and pitch, VOR gain, calculated as the ratio of instantaneous eye to head velocity, is near unity in normal subjects.[1] After unilateral vestibular deafferentation (uVD), VOR gain remains close to normal in response to passively generated yaw head impulses toward the intact side, although VOR gain is severely and permanently reduced in response to passively generated yaw impulses toward the lesioned side in humans as well as in animals.[2–8]

Address for correspondence: G.M. Halmagyi, Department of Neurology, Royal Prince Alfred Hospital, Camperdown, NSW 2050, Sydney, Australia. Voice: 0011 61 2 9515 8300; fax: 0011 61 2 9515 8347.
michael@icn.usyd.edu.au

When tested with sinusoids, horizontal VOR gain is higher in response to actively than in response to passively generated stimuli in normal subjects,[9] bilateral vestibular impaired subjects,[10] and in uVD subjects.[5,11] However, the VOR in response to active head impulses has not been studied in uVD subjects. Our hypothesis was that VOR gain would be higher in response to active than in response to passive head impulses, just as it is higher in response to active than passive sinusoids. To test the hypothesis, we compared the VOR in response to actively generated yaw head impulses with the VOR in response to passively generated yaw head impulses in uVD subjects.

METHODS AND MATERIALS

Subjects

We studied four subjects 1 year or more after each had undergone surgery to remove an acoustic neuroma. The study was performed with the understanding and written consent of each subject, and with approval of the CSAHS Human Ethics Committee.

Recording System

Eye and head positions in three-dimensional space were measured using the magnetic search-coil technique,[12,13] with subjects seated in the center of 1.9 × 1.9 × 1.9–m magnetic field coils (CNC Engineering, Seattle, WA). Eye position was recorded with a dual search coil (Skalar, Delft, the Netherlands) placed on the left eye. Head position was recorded with a dual search coil secured to the nosepiece of a lightweight spectacle frame and with a mouth-guard. The spectacle frame was very tightly coupled to the head in an attempt to reduce slippage. The mouth-guard was composed of dental impression material (President putty; Coltene/Whaledent Inc, Cuyahoga Falls, OH) in a tray onto which a search coil was fixed. There were marked differences between the data from the spectacle frame and mouth-guard. FIGURE 1 shows representative yaw head-velocity data during active and passive head impulses. The yaw head velocity derived from the spectacle frame consistently led that of the mouth-guard during passive head impulses. The experimenter's hands moving the subject's scalp may have introduced the artifact by moving the spectacle frame relative to the skull or by moving it directly. When the experimenter's hands were removed from the subject's scalp, as during active head impulses, data from the spectacle frame and mouth-guard were very similar. Because the mouth-guard was firmly clenched by the subject's teeth, it is unlikely to have been perturbed by the experimenter and therefore is considered a reliable measure of head movement. All head-in-space and eye-in-head data are derived from the mouth-guard search coil in the present study.

The four signals from each search coil were recovered by phase detection (CNC Engineering, Seattle, WA) and passed through a custom-made antialiasing filter with a passband of 0–100 Hz. All signals were acquired at 1 kHz with a 16-bit analogue-digital converter. Before each test, the head and eye search coils were calibrated *in vitro* with a Plexiglas Fick gimbal positioned in the center of the magnetic fields (as in Aw *et al.*[1] and Thurtell *et al.*[14]). It was assumed that the gains and offsets of the search coils were the same *in vivo* as they were during the *in vitro* calibration.[1,15]

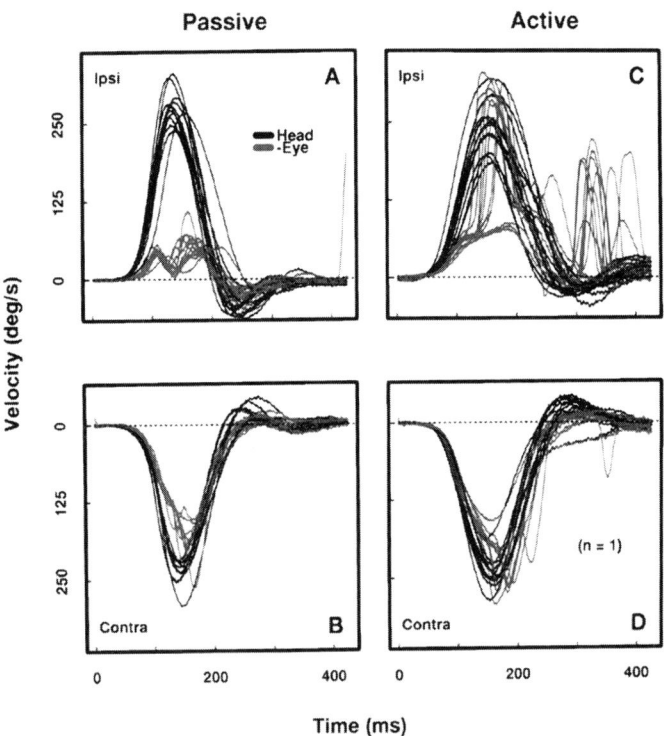

FIGURE 1. The first column shows a set of overlaid time series plots of head-in-space (head) velocity stimuli (black) and eye-in-head (eye) velocity responses (grey) during (**A**) passive ipsilesional and (**B**) contralesional impulses. The second column shows a set of overlaid time series plots of head-velocity stimulus and eye-velocity responses during (**C**) active ipsilesional and (**D**) contralesional impulses. Eye data have been inverted to aid comparison with head data. Head rotation direction is indicated on each plot. All data are from a single representative subject. During active ipsilesional impulses, increased slow-phase velocities and a rapid corrective eye movement enhance the poor compensatory eye response observed during passive ipsilesional impulses. The compensatory slow-phase eye movement of passive contralesional impulses is also enhanced during active contralesional impulses. Rapid corrective eye movements may also occur after the head has stopped moving to reduce any remaining gaze error.

A fixation target was provided by a red laser dot, which was rear projected onto a 2 × 1.5m Plexiglas screen located exactly 94cm from the front of the subject's cornea. The fixation spot was positioned in the center of the tangent screen and at the level of the subject's left eye.

Experimental Protocol

All subjects were tested under two conditions in each session. In the first, the response to passive yaw head impulses[2,16] was investigated. The passive yaw head impulse is an unpredictable, low-amplitude (15–20°), high-acceleration (4000–6000°/s^2) horizontal head rotation with a peak velocity of 150–350°/s. In the second condition, the head rotation stimulus was an active (self-generated) yaw head impulse.[14] Subjects were required to maintain fixation on the earth-fixed target during the impulses. Subjects were given the opportunity to practice before the experiment, because they were required to match the displacement, velocity, and acceleration characteristics of the passive head impulses. The head velocities and accelerations for ipsilesional and contralesional passive and active head impulses were found to be significantly different over the period of interest ($P < 0.05$). Subjects generated higher head velocities and accelerations during active head impulses than during passive impulses.

In vivo calibration data were gathered while the subject was fixating the target. During this calibration (and before the onset of each active and passive head impulse), the subject's head was positioned so that the yaw, pitch, and roll signals from the head search coil (head-in-space) were in a software window of $\pm 1°$ from the zero position of the head. The *in vivo* calibration was repeated at regular intervals during the test. In the active head impulse condition, the experimenters removed their hands once the subject's head was positioned in the software window. Subjects were required to maintain the starting position for several seconds, before rotating their heads to the predetermined side. Data acquisition commenced approximately 1 s before the onset of a head impulse and ceased several seconds after the impulse ended. Trials were discarded when the subjects: (1) moved their heads outside the $\pm 1°$ window before the head impulse; (2) initially rotated their heads in the opposite direction to the predetermined direction; or (3) generated a saccade before the head impulse.

Data Analysis

The eye and head data were analyzed off-line using C, Matlab 4.1, and Splus under Ultrix. The same analysis procedures were used for both experiments.

The Fick angles representing eye and head position, with reference to a right-handed space-fixed coordinate frame, were calculated from the raw data and the search-coil gains.[17,18] The Fick angles were used to calculate the rotation matrices representing eye and head rotations in three-dimensional space. The data from the *in vivo* calibrations were used to correct for misalignment of the search coil on the eye (as in Tweed *et al.*[19]). The rotation vectors representing eye and head position were derived from the corrected matrices. The velocities of head-in-space, eye-in-space, and eye-in-head were calculated from the rotation vectors,[20] and the accelerations were derived using the formula of Savitzky and Golay.[21] Head velocity for a head-fixed coordinate frame was calculated using the methods of Aw *et al.*[1]

Previous work on head impulses has restricted the period of analysis to the first 100 ms of the response, to exclude the influence of long latency, non-VOR systems such as pursuit and the cervicoocular reflex.[1,2,14] The current analysis was taken over the initial 75 ms of the response, because rapid corrective eye movements were generated after this period.

The gain of the VOR was calculated by finding the gradient of a line fitted to the mean of eye velocity plotted as a function of head velocity, from 30 to 75 ms after the onset of head movement. If eye velocity equalled head velocity during this part of the analysis period, the gradient of the fitted line and, hence, the gain of the VOR would be unity. Similar methods for calculating gain have been reported in other studies.[22,23] In the current study, the line was fitted using a linear least squares regression algorithm. The square of the multiple correlation coefficient (R^2) for the regression analysis was ≥ 0.99 in all subjects, indicating a good linear fit.

Means ± two-tailed 95% confidence intervals were computed for the eye-in-head and head-in-space velocities. Means ± standard deviations were computed for VOR gains. A standard two-sample t-test was performed to establish the existence of a significant difference or otherwise between two samples.[24] The P value was set at 0.05 and the null hypothesis was that the difference between the means of the two samples was equal to zero.

RESULTS

The time series of head-in-space (head) and eye-in-head (eye) velocity during passive and active yaw head impulses, in a representative uVD subject, is shown in FIGURE 1A–D. A passive ipsilesional impulse results in failure of eye velocity to match head velocity (FIG. 1A). The eye initially follows the head-velocity profile quite well but decreases at about peak head acceleration. Thereafter, eye velocity decreases as head velocity increases. Eye velocity almost ceases at peak head acceleration but then increases to its previous peak as head velocity decreases. A large corrective saccade, followed by smaller saccades, is typically generated after the end of head rotation to compensate for eye and head position mismatch. These saccades occur just outside the time interval shown. During a passive contralesional head impulse, the eye velocity does not quite match the head velocity throughout the response (FIG. 1B). Midway through the increase in head velocity (at approximately peak head acceleration), the difference between eye and head velocity is most obvious. Thereafter, eye velocity increases as head velocity reaches a maximum, and then both decrease toward zero. Any gaze error developed during the period of low eye velocity is corrected by a saccade after the head has stopped moving.

The active ipsilesional head impulse is characterized by initial failure of the eye-in-head to match head velocity. The eye velocities approximate head velocities after a rapid, corrective eye movement that typically occurs at about peak head acceleration (FIG. 1C). In this subject, there are several instances in which the corrective eye movement does not occur until just after the head movement has ceased, as is seen in passive head impulses. However, the initial eye response is similar during all active head movements, irrespective of the point at which the subsequent rapid corrective eye movement occurs. During the active contralesional head impulse, eye velocity approximately matches head velocity throughout the period of head rotation (FIG. 1D).

Differences between active and passive impulses to the ipsilesional and contralesional sides are apparent from near the onset of head rotation (FIG. 2). Passive ipsilesional impulses result in no compensatory eye movement followed by a small compensatory response at approximately 30 to 35 ms after the onset of head rotation (vertical dotted line). However, active ipsilesional impulses are associated with a compensatory movement from the outset. The compensatory eye velocity is initially low and, at approximately 30 ms after the onset of head rotation, increases monotonically but at a lower rate than head velocity.

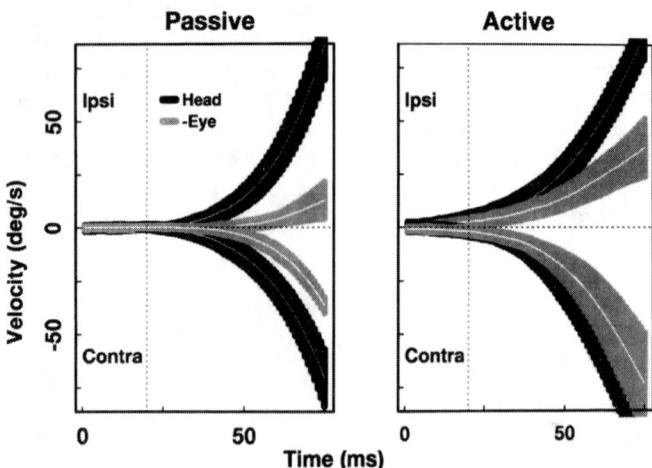

FIGURE 2. The means ± two-tailed 95% confidence intervals of head and eye velocities in the initial 75 ms of active and passive head impulses from all subjects. The eye data have been inverted to aid comparison with head data. Head rotation direction is indicated on each plot. The onset of head rotation is indicated by the vertical dotted line. Marked differences exist between active and passive head impulses in both the ipsilesional and contralesional directions.

During passive contralesional head rotations the eye velocity follows the head velocity quite well. Active contralesional head rotations are associated with an eye-movement response that approximates head movement more closely than during passive contralesional rotations. However, the eye-movement response is less than unity in both ipsilesional and contralesional head impulses and a small rapid corrective eye movement was typically observed at the end of both types of head impulse (outside the time interval shown).

Analysis of eye as a function of head velocity confirms the marked differences between active and passive head impulses. The responses from the other uVD subjects, like those from the representative subject (FIG. 1), were very repeatable. The mean ± 95% confidence intervals of eye as a function of head velocity, over all subjects, are shown in FIGURE 3. The mean gains ± standard deviations are listed in TABLE 1. The mean gains were found to be significantly higher for active compared with passive head impulses to the ipsilesional side ($P \ll 0.01$). There was also a significant difference between mean gains for active compared with passive head impulses to the contralesional side ($P < 0.05$).

Because the correcting saccade is driven by gaze position error, we simulated retinal image stabilization using the eye position data acquired during active and passive head impulses (FIG. 4). In the simulation, the fixation point is projected onto the inner surface of a hemisphere representing the central 30° of retina of one eye, and the movement of the fixation target image throughout an active or passive head impulse is plotted. The dimensions of the retina and fovea are anatomically proportional and the target image was initially at the fovea. The gaze error which accrues

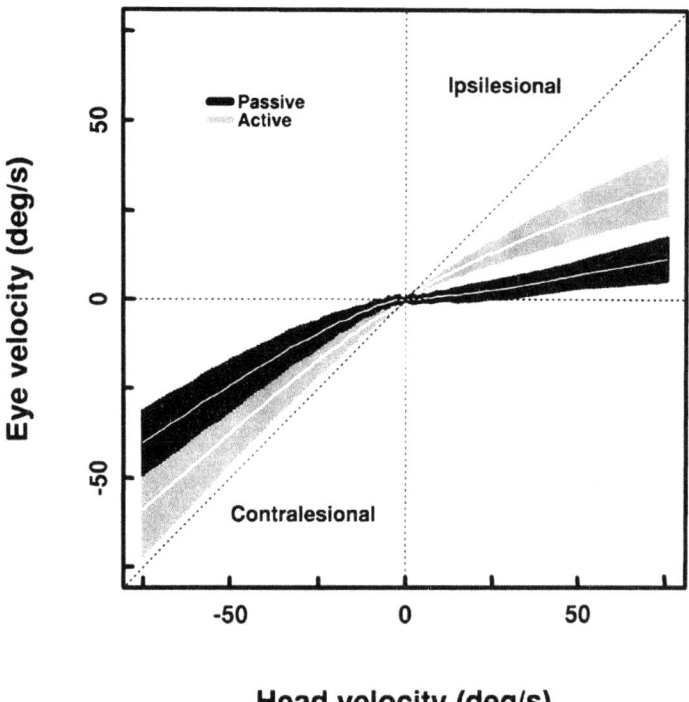

FIGURE 3. The means ± two-tailed 95% confidence intervals of horizontal eye velocity as a function of head velocity during active and passive ipsilesional and contralesional head impulses. There are significant differences between active and passive impulses in both directions of head rotation that are apparent from the onset of head rotation.

TABLE 1. VOR gain during active and passive ipsilesional and contralesional head impulses (mean ± standard deviation)

	Subjects ($n = 4$)	
	Passive	Active
Ipsilesional	0.15 ± 0.07	0.44 ± 0.12
Contralesional	0.50 ± 0.13	0.76 ± 0.16

during a passive head impulse causes the target image to shift 10° or more off the fovea (FIG. 4A); the correcting saccade then relocates the target back on the fovea. In contrast, during an active head impulse the target remains close to the fovea throughout the head movement (FIG. 4B); although there is an initial shift of the target image off the fovea, a saccade returns the target image almost immediately.

Retinal Slip

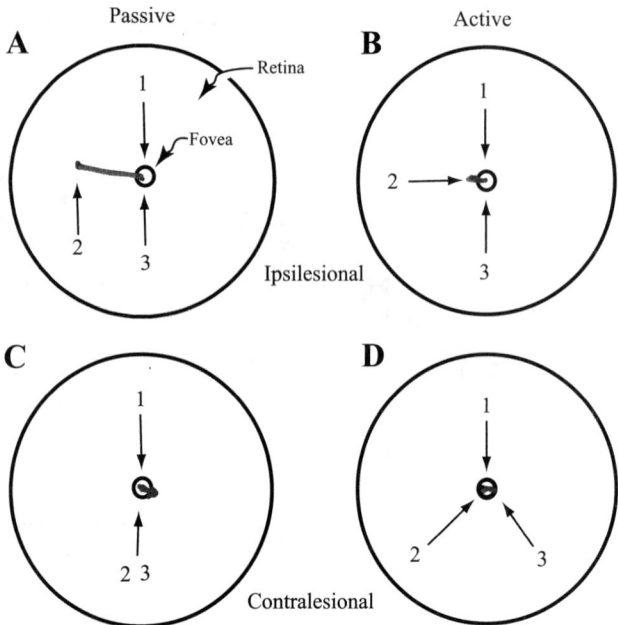

FIGURE 4. A computer simulation of the retinal slip obtained from representative active and passive head impulses to the ipsilesional and contralesional sides over a period of 550 ms. The view is anteroposterior, toward the rear of the subject's retina. The numbered *arrows* indicate the same events as in FIGURE 2. The target image is located at the center of the fovea at the onset of head rotation (*arrow 1*). (**A**) In response to a passive ipsilesional head rotation, the target image slips out of the fovea and well into the retina as a large gaze error is accrued. When the rapid corrective eye movement occurs (*arrow 2*), the image is returned to the fovea (*arrow 3*). (**B**) In response to an active ipsilesional head impulse, there are only a few degrees of retinal image slip. The image is maintained close to the fovea. (**C**) Similarly, in response to a passive contralesional head impulse, the image is maintained close to the fovea. As expected, the direction of retinal slip is opposite to that of the ipsilesional head impulse because the head impulses are in opposite directions. (**D**) During active contralesional head impulses, the target image remains within the bounds of the fovea throughout the head impulse.

DISCUSSION

The main finding of this study is that even with active predictable head movements, there is still a large and statistically significant asymmetry in the eye-movement responses for ipsilesional as opposed to contralesional rotations. Active ipsilesional head impulses result in higher initial VOR gain than do passive ipsilesional impulses. Similarly, active contralesional impulses result in higher initial VOR gain than do passive contralesional head impulses.

The finding of a mean VOR gain of 0.15 during passive head impulses to the ipsilesional side is within the ranges reported for uVD subjects. In previous studies, mean ipsilesional gains have ranged from 0.14 to 0.59.[2–4,11,25] The associated mean contralesional gains from these studies ranged from 0.58 to 0.94. Mean contralesional gain was 0.5 in the current study. Differences between values may be attributed to variability between subjects, stimuli, experimental protocols, and methods of calculating gain.

Contralesional head impulses produce ampullopetal deflection of the intact lateral semicircular canal cupula and thereby increased activity in the associated vestibular nucleus.[26] Greater head velocities produce faster compensatory eye movements at least up to head velocities less than 350°/s.[27] We found that in the initial 75-ms active contralesional impulses had significantly higher velocities and accelerations than did passive contralesional impulses, so that the greater gain from active than from passive contralesional impulses might have been caused by greater excitation of the contralesional vestibular nucleus. In normal subjects, increasing head accelerations result in increasing initial (75 ms) VOR gain.[6] Surprisingly, mean gain during active contralesional head impulses was only 0.76. A unity gain might be expected because of the combined effects of enhanced vestibular drive due to increased activity of type 1 neurons on the contralesional side and because active head rotation provides an opportunity for a preprogrammed response.[26,28,29] Perhaps the loss of the input from the lesioned side afferents, which would normally act to enhance gain on the contralesional side, is not adequately compensated for by central preprogramming, and the result is a VOR gain of less than unity.

High-velocity and acceleration head rotations toward the ipsilesional side result in inadequate compensatory eye movements and reduced VOR gain. The reduced VOR gain is caused by ampullofugal disfacilitation of the intact contralesional horizontal semicircular canal and is present in even the lowest head velocities.[2] We found that in the initial 75 ms after stimulus onset, active ipsilesional head impulses had significantly higher velocities and accelerations than did passive ipsilesional impulses. The early VOR gain during ipsilesional passive head rotations has been shown to be higher with lower head accelerations.[6] When comparing passive and active impulses, we found the opposite to be so. Consequently, some other mechanism must be at work to counter, and indeed reverse, the effect of ampullofugal disfacilitation of the intact lateral semicircular canal by higher head velocities and accelerations during active ipsilesional head impulses. It has been shown that the sensitivity of secondary vestibular neurons can be modified by central and presynaptic and postsynaptic mechanisms.[28,30,31] The sensitivity of vestibular neurons has been found to be *reduced* during active head movements and *enhanced* during passive head movements.[31,32] During active head movements, the head-velocity signal carried by type I pure vestibular neurons is markedly attenuated irrespective of whether an animal is redirecting or stabilizing gaze, immediately after a gaze shift.[33] However, these authors also note that the vestibular neurons that mediate the VOR (e.g., PVP-I) convey information between end-organ and motoneurons in a manner that depends on the "current gaze strategy (stabilization vs. redirection)" and that vestibular signals can be modified as a function of behavioral goal and context.[34,35] In our paradigm, high VOR gain and compensatory eye movements are required *throughout* the head rotation rather than toward the end of head rotation as in the gaze redirection tasks that have been reported to date. Our subjects were required to maintain their gaze during head rotation rather than refix it. The gain increases we obtained might be explained by increased sensitivity of second-order neurons to head rotation during active head impulses. Our results could predict that neuronal recordings, during active and passive head impulses, would demonstrate *enhanced* activity during active head movements when the goal is gaze maintenance during a rapid head rotation. Because significant differences exist between active and passive ipsilesional head impulses from the onset of head rotation in this study, whatever mechanism is used to achieve these differences must be functional from the onset of head rotation. This conclusion is consistent with that of McCrea *et al.*[31] who noted that the ability to distinguish between externally applied and self-generated movements is critical for sensory processing and is made at an early stage in the vestibular system.

The low initial VOR gain during active ipsilesional head impulses does not persist for the length of the stimulus. After the period described in the current study, a rapid compensatory eye movement is generated, followed by a period in which the eye velocity matches the head velocity. We have evidence that these rapid eye movements are saccades, because they lie on a main sequence and obey Listing's law.[36]

ACKNOWLEDGMENTS

The authors acknowledge M.J. Todd and Dr. S.T. Aw for their helpful suggestions. This study was supported by the National Health and Medical Research Council and by the RPAH Neurology Department Trustees.

REFERENCES

1. AW, S.T., T. HASLWANTER, G.M. HALMAGYI, *et al.* 1996. Three-dimensional vector analysis of the human vestibuloocular reflex in response to high-acceleration head rotations. I. Responses in normal subjects. J. Neurophysiol. **76:** 4009–4020.
2. HALMAGYI, G.M., I.S. CURTHOYS, P.D. CREMER, *et al.* 1990. The human horizontal vestibulo-ocular reflex in response to high-acceleration stimulation before and after unilateral vestibular neurectomy. Exp. Brain Res. **81:** 479–490.
3. AW, S.T., G.M. HALMAGYI, T. HASLWANTER, *et al.* 1996. Three-dimensional vector analysis of the human vestibuloocular reflex in response to high-acceleration head rotations. I. Responses in subjects with unilateral vestibular loss and selective semicircular canal occlusion. J. Neurophysiol. **76:** 4021–4030.
4. TABAK, S., H. COLLEWIJN, L.J. BOUMANS & J. VAN DER STEEN. 1997. Gain and delay of human vestibulo-ocular reflexes to oscillation and steps of the head by a reactive torque helmet. II. Vestibular deficient subjects. Acta Otolaryngol. **117:** 796–809.
5. FOSTER, C.A., J.L. DEMER, M.J. MORROW & R.W. BALOH. 1997. Deficits of gaze stability in multiple axes following unilateral vestibular lesions. Exp. Brain Res. **116:** 501–509.
6. CRANE, B.T. & J.L. DEMER. 1998. Human horizontal vestibulo-ocular reflex initiation: effects of acceleration, target distance, and unilateral deafferentation. J. Neurophysiol. **80:** 1151–1166.
7. GILCHRIST, D.P.D., I.S. CURTHOYS, A.D. CARTWRIGHT, *et al.* 1998. High acceleration impulsive rotations reveal severe long-term deficits of the horizontal vestibulo-ocular reflex in the guinea-pig. Exp. Brain Res. **123:** 242–254.
8. LASKER, D.M., T.E. HULLAR & L.B. MINOR. 2000. Horizontal vestibuloocular reflex evoked by high-acceleration rotations in the squirrel monkey. III. Responses after labyrinthectomy. J. Neurophysiol. **83:** 2482–2496.

9. JELL, R.M., C.W. STOCKWELL, G.T. TURNIPSEED & F.E. GUEDRY. 1988. The influence of active versus passive head oscillation, and mental set on the human vestibulo-ocular reflex. Aviat. Space Environ. Med. **59:** 1061–1065.
10. HOSHOWSKY, B., D. TOMLINSON & J. NEDZELSKI. 1994. The horizontal vestibulo-ocular reflex gain during active and passive high-frequency head movements. Laryngoscope **104:** 140–145.
11. DELLA SANTINA, D.C., P.D. CREMER, J.P. CAREY & L.B. MINOR. 2002. Comparison of head thrust test with head autorotation test reveals that the vestibulo-ocular reflex is enhanced during voluntary head movements. Arch. Otolaryngol. Head Neck Surg. **128:** 1044–1054.
12. ROBINSON, D.A. 1963. A method of measuring eye movements using a scleral search coil in a magnetic field. IEEE Trans. Biomed. Eng. BME **10:** 137–145.
13. COLLEWIJN, H., J. VAN DER STEEN, L. FERMAN & T.C. JANSEN. 1985. Human ocular counterroll: assessment of static and dynamic properties from electromagnetic scleral coil recordings. Exp. Brain Res. **59:** 185–196.
14. THURTELL, M.J., R.A. BLACK, G.M. HALMAGYI, et al. 1999. Vertical eye position-dependence of the human vestibuloocular reflex during passive and active yaw head rotations. J. Neurophysiol. **81:** 2415–2428.
15. HASLWANTER, T., I.S. CURTHOYS, R.A. BLACK, et al. 1996. The three-dimensional human vestibulo-ocular reflex: response to long duration yaw angular accelerations. Exp. Brain Res. **109:** 303–311.
16. HALMAGYI, G.M. & I.S. CURTHOYS. 1988. A clinical sign of canal paresis. Arch. Neurol. **45:** 737–739.
17. HASLWANTER, T. 1995. Mathematics of three-dimensional eye rotations. Vision Res. **35:** 1727–1739.
18. BRUNO, P. & A.V. VAN DEN BERG. 1997. Torsion during saccades between tertiary positions. Exp. Brain Res. **117:** 251–265.
19. TWEED, D., W. CADERA & T. VILIS. 1990. Computing three-dimensional eye position quaternions and eye velocity from search coil signals. Vision Res. **30:** 97–110.
20. HEPP, K. 1990. On Listing's Law. Commun. Math. Phys. **132:** 285–292.
21. SAVITZKY, A. & M.J.E. GOLAY. 1964. Smoothing and differentiation of data by simplified least squares procedures. Anal. Chem. **36:** 1627–1639.
22. MINOR, L.B., D.M. LASKER, D.D. BACKOUS & T.E. HULLAR. 1999. Horizontal vestibuloocular reflex evoked by high-acceleration rotations in the squirrel monkey. I. Normal responses. J. Neurophysiol. **82:** 1254–1270.
23. COLLEWIJN, H. & J.B. SMEETS. 2000. Early components of the human vestibulo-ocular response to head rotation: latency and gain. J. Neurophysiol. **84:** 376–389.
24. WINER, B.J., D.R. BROWN & K.M. MICHELS. 1991. Statistical Principles in Experimental Design. 3rd edit. McGraw-Hill. New York.
25. TIAN, J., B.T. CRANE & J.L. DEMER. 2000. Vestibular catch-up saccades in labyrinthine deficiency. Exp. Brain Res. **131:** 448–457.
26. LEIGH, R.J. & D.S. ZEE. 1999. The Neurology of Eye Movements. 3rd edit. F.A. Davis Co. Philadelphia.
27. PULASKI, P.D. & D.S. ZEE. 1983. The behavior of the vestibulo-ocular reflex at high velocities of head rotation. Brain Res. **222:** 159–165.
28. BARR, C.C., L.W. SCHULTHEIS & D.A. ROBINSON. 1976. Voluntary, non-visual control of the human vestibulo-ocular reflex. Acta Otolaryngol. **81:** 365–375.
29. KASAI, T. & D.S. ZEE. 1978. Eye-head coordination in labyrinthine defective human beings. Brain Res. **144:** 123–141.
30. STRAKA, H., S. BIESDORF & N. DIERINGER. 1997. Canal-specific excitation and inhibition of frog second order vestibular neurons. J. Neurophysiol. **78:** 1363–1372.
31. MCCREA, R.A., G.T. GDOWSKI, R. BOYLE & T. BELTON. 1999. Firing behavior of vestibular neurons during active and passive head movements: vestibulo-spinal and other non-eye-movement related neurons. J. Neurophysiol. **82:** 416–428.
32. BOYLE, R., T. BELTON & R.A. MCCREA. 1996. Responses of identified vestibulospinal neurons to voluntary eye and head movements in the squirrel monkey. Ann. N.Y. Acad. Sci. **781:** 244–263.

33. CULLEN, K.E. & J.E. ROY. 1999. Modulation of vestibular neuron activity: active versus passive head movements. Arch. Ital. Biol. **137** (Suppl.): 16–17.
34. ROY, J.E. & K.E. CULLEN. 2001. Selective processing of vestibular reafference during self-generated head motion. J. Neurosci. **21:** 2131–2142.
35. CULLEN, K.E., J.E. ROY & P.A. SYLVESTRE. 2001. Signal processing by vestibular nuclei neurons is dependent on the current behavioral goal. Ann. N.Y. Acad. Sci. **942:** 345–363.
36. BLACK, R.A., M.J. THURTELL, G.M. HALMAGYI, *et al.* 1999. Characteristics of corrective eye movements made in response to active and passive head impulses in subjects with vestibular loss. Soc. Neurosci. Abstr. **25:** 264.8.

Evaluating Small Eye Movements in Patients with Saccadic Palsies

SIOBHAN GARBUTT,[a] MARK R. HARWOOD,[b] ARUN N. KUMAR,[a] YANNING H. HAN,[a] AND R. JOHN LEIGH [a]

[a]*Neurology Service, Veterans Affairs Medical Center and Case Western Reserve University, Cleveland, Ohio, USA*

[b]*City College of the City University of New York, New York, USA*

ABSTRACT: Slow saccades are an important diagnostic feature of a range of degenerative, metabolic, and genetic diseases of the nervous system. Many affected patients have difficulty initiating saccades, and the movements themselves may be small, making it difficult to make comparisons with control subjects. A large-field optokinetic stimulus may elicit quick phases of nystagmus in patients who cannot initiate voluntary saccades, but these movements may also be small. We show that it is still possible to compare amplitude-duration and amplitude-peak velocity relations with controls if data are fit with a power function (rather than an exponential equation). When analyzed this way, the dynamic properties of small saccades and quick phases from patients with progressive supranuclear palsy (PSP) could be differentiated from fast movements made by patients with idiopathic Parkinson's disease or controls. Normal saccades show a fairly constant ratio: peak velocity/mean velocity (Q ~1.6 for vertical saccades). This ratio was abnormally high (Q >3) for some larger saccades made by patients with PSP, suggesting that either these movements were not entirely saccadic or that they were composed of a series of small saccades.

KEYWORDS: saccades; quick phases; Parkinson's disease; progressive supranuclear palsy

INTRODUCTION

Voluntary saccades are the rapid eye movements by which we shift our line of sight between objects of interest. During self-rotation, which stimulates vestibular and optokinetic (OK) compensatory movements, quick phases of nystagmus move the eyes in the orbit in the same direction as that of head rotation to enable perusal of the oncoming visual scene. Both voluntary saccades and quick phases of OK and vestibular nystagmus are generated by the same premotor circuitry that comprises brainstem burst and omnipause neurons.[1] Horizontal saccades are generated by burst neurons in the paramedian pontine reticular formation (PPRF),[2] and vertical saccades by burst neurons in the midbrain rostral interstitial nucleus of the medial lon-

---

Address for correspondence: R. John Leigh, Neurology Service, Veterans Affairs Medical Center and Department of Neurology, University Hospitals, 11100 Euclid Avenue, Cleveland, OH 44106-5040. Voice: 216-844-3190; fax: 216-231-3461.

rjl4@po.cwru.edu

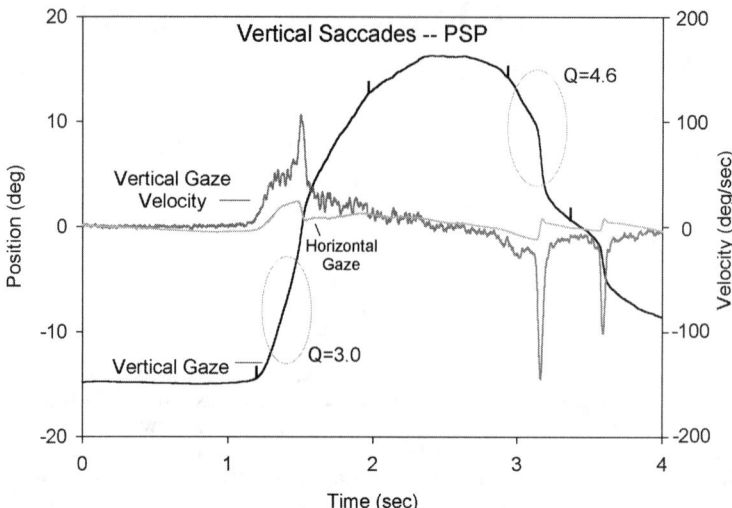

FIGURE 1. Representative record of slow vertical saccades in PSP. Upward deflections indicate upward eye rotations. The upward movement that commences at 1.2 s is 27.1° amplitude, lasts 764 ms (indicated by small vertical marks), and has a peak velocity of 106.4°/s; its Q value is 3.0. Note the small horizontal saccade that occurs during the course of the large vertical movement and corresponds to the peak vertical velocity. The downward saccade that commences at 2.9 s is 13.5° amplitude, lasts 434 ms (indicated by small vertical marks), and has a peak velocity of –145.0°/s. Its Q value is 4.6. See text for discussion.

gitudinal fasciculus (riMLF).[3] Activity in both populations of burst neurons is gated by omnipause neurons in the pontine nucleus raphe interpositus.[4] The dynamic properties of saccades and quick phases show similarities that reflect this shared brainstem substrate, and certain differences that reflect different inputs to brainstem burst and omnipause neurons.

Slow saccades are a cardinal feature of certain degenerative, genetic, and metabolic disorders. One example is progressive supranuclear palsy (PSP), which causes slow vertical saccades early in the course of the disease (FIG. 1).[5] Horizontal saccades are usually hypometric in PSP, and also become slow as the disease progresses. Most disorders that cause slow saccades usually also cause difficulty in initiating saccades as well as hypometria; voluntary saccades are often small. In some patients who have difficulties initiating saccades (especially children with genetic disorders such as Gaucher's disease), it is still possible to evoke quick phases using a large OK stimulus.[6] However, quick phases of OK nystagmus—even in healthy control subjects—may be small (typically 2°, vertically). Distinguishing normal and slow saccades is relatively easy if affected patients can still make large movements; the distinction becomes more difficult to make if saccades are small. This paper addresses the difficulties of analyzing small saccades and quick phases of nystagmus and attempts to provide an approach that could be diagnostically useful as well as providing some insights into the pathogenesis of the saccadic disturbance.

METHODS

Subjects

We analyzed saccades and OK nystagmus from 12 patients studied in our laboratory over the past five years who showed abnormally slow vertical saccades and were diagnosed as probable PSP.[1,7] Their ages ranged from 64–77 years, and duration of illness was from 2–7 years. We also studied control subjects with normal vertical saccades, including a group of 7 healthy elderly subjects (age range 62–75 years) that we have previously reported,[8] a younger group of 10 healthy subjects (age range 23–64 years), and 5 patients diagnosed with idiopathic Parkinson's disease (PD) (age range 56–80 years, and duration of illness 2–14 years). After explanation of the protocol, which had been approved by our Institutional Review Board, all patients and subjects gave written, informed consent in accordance with the Declaration of Helsinki.

Recording Methods and Visual Stimuli

Horizontal and vertical gaze and head rotations were measured using the magnetic search-coil technique with six-foot field coils (CNC Engineering, Seattle, WA), as previously described.[8,9] The OK stimulus was rear-projected onto a semitranslucent tangent screen at a viewing distance of 1 m. The stimulus subtended 72° horizontally and 60° vertically. The OK stimuli were generated by a Cambridge Research Systems VSG2/5 visual stimulus generator and projected using an Epson Powerlite 9100i video projector. The stimulus consisted of alternating black-and-white stripes, with luminance of 0.7 and 13.7 cd/m^2, respectively. The spatial frequency of the stimulus was 0.04 cycles/°. The display was carefully aligned so that stimulus motion was either earth-vertical or earth-horizontal. The visual stimuli moved at 10, 20, 30, 40, and 50°/s for 20 s, upward, downward, to the left, and to the right. The screen was blanked for 10 s between stimuli. The speed and direction of the OKN stimulus were randomized. The stimulus for eliciting reflexive saccades was a red laser spot presented on a semitranslucent screen. Saccades of 5, 10, 15, 20, 25, 30, 35, and 40° eccentricity, to the left, right, upward, and downward were elicited.

Data Analysis

To avoid aliasing, coil signals were passed through Krohn-Hite Butterworth filters (bandwidth 0–150 Hz) before digitization at 500 Hz with 16-bit resolution. These digitized coil signals were then passed through an 80-point Remez FIR (bandwidth 0–140 Hz), and differentiated to yield eye velocity.[9] All measurements were checked interactively, and eye movements associated with blinks were rejected. A saccade or OKN quick phase (fast eye movement [FEM]) was detected when the velocity was continuously above 10°/s for at least 5 points. The peak velocity of each FEM was then determined. FEM onset and offset were then defined as the last points either side of the peak velocity before which the velocity fell below 10°/s. These points were used to calculate the amplitude and duration of the FEMs.

We plotted and analyzed the data in two separate ways. First, we plotted duration (D) versus amplitude (A), and peak velocity (PV) versus amplitude on linear scales. For the saccades between 4° and 40°, recorded from normal subjects, the D-A data were fitted with a linear regression, and the PV-A data were fitted with an equation of the form:

$$PV = V_{max} * (1 - e^{-A/C}) \qquad (1)$$

where Vmax is the asymptotic peak velocity, and C is a constant defining the exponential rise. Because the D-A relationship of fast eye movements is nonlinear for saccades <4°, and many of the movements we recorded were in this range, it was not possible to fit the data for small fast eye movements with a linear equation;[6,10] furthermore, an exponential equation similar to equation 1 gave a poor fit for some subjects. Therefore, we also constructed logarithmic (base 10) plots of peak velocity against amplitude and performed linear regressions for saccades or quick phases for each data set from each eye to calculate the intercept and slope. Thus, the data of these log-log plots were fit with an equation of the form:

$$\log PV = m^* \log A + c \qquad (2)$$

$$\log D = n^* \log A + d \qquad (3)$$

where m and n are the slopes, and c and d are the intercepts. These equations used to fit the log-log data are equivalent to power functions:

$$PV = K^* A^m \qquad (4)$$

$$D = L^* A^n \qquad (5)$$

where K and L are 10^c and 10^d (unlogged values), respectively. This form of power function was proposed by Yarbus in 1967 for amplitude-duration relationships of saccades[11] and has received experimental and theoretical support.[12,13]

In addition, we measured the relationship between peak velocity and mean velocity (MV), calculating the ratio:

$$Q = PV/MV \qquad (6)$$

This ratio, Q, has been reported to be fairly constant not only for saccades,[10,14–16] but also for eye blinks[17] and perhaps for ballistic limb movements.[17,18] We were interested to determine whether Q remained similar to normal subjects for the abnormal vertical saccades made by PSP patients. Because MV = A/D, it follows that Q = (PV * D)/A, and we estimated Q from linear fits of plots of PV * D versus A.[14,16]

RESULTS

Application of Exponential Fits to Amplitude-Peak Velocity Data Plots

The potential problems arising from using exponential fits of amplitude versus peak velocity to identify abnormal saccades are illustrated in FIGURE 2. The upper two panels separately plot upward and downward saccades from PSP patients as data points, and also provide an exponential fit of the form of equation 1 (plus 95% prediction intervals)

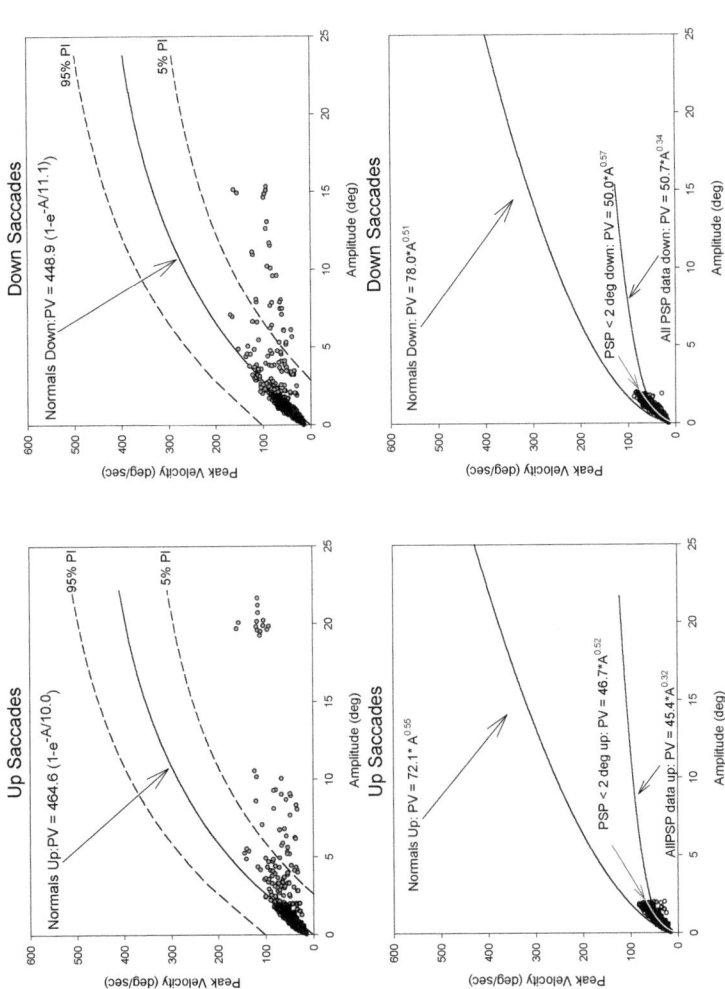

FIGURE 2. Plots of peak velocity versus amplitude for 6 patients with PSP, previously reported.[19] The *top two panels* show upward and downward saccade, comparing PSP saccades with 95% prediction intervals from age-matched control subjects. Note how larger saccades (shown in *gray*) are clearly slower than control subjects, but saccades < 2° lie within normal subjects' prediction intervals. In the *lower two panels*, peak velocity is plotted as a power function of amplitude. Note that whether the complete data set of PSP saccades or the data < 2° are fitted by this power function, there are substantial differences in the scaling factor (K of Eq. 4) compared with that of normal subjects.

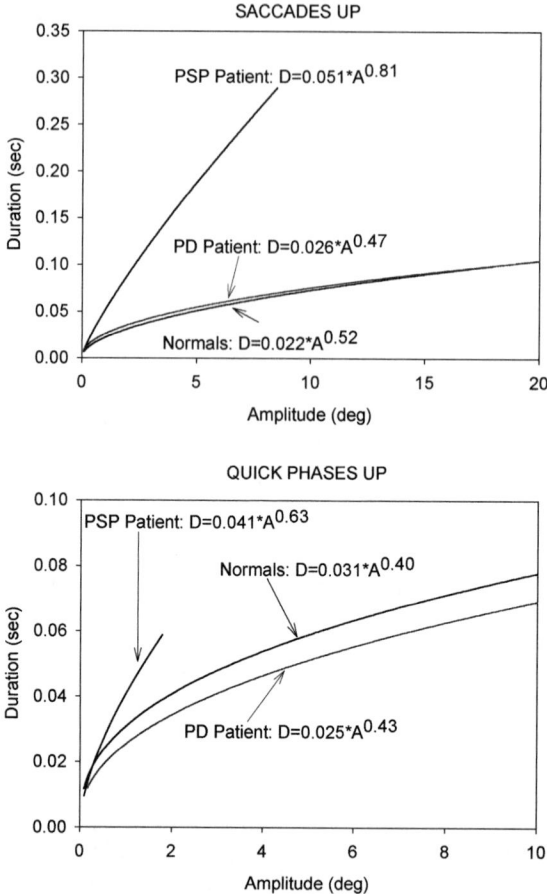

FIGURE 3. Examples of power function fits of duration versus amplitude plots for the group of normal subjects, as well as for one patient with PSP and one with PD. In the *upper panel*, upward saccades are shown. In the *lower panel*, upward quick phases are shown. The parameters of the fits for the patient with PD are similar to control subjects, but parameters for the PSP patient differ substantially.

for the control subjects. It is evident that it is the larger saccades (gray data points) that are abnormal, lying outside the prediction intervals for normal subjects. If these large saccades are removed from the data set, then the remaining small saccades, and all saccades < 2°, lie within the prediction intervals for normal subjects, as we have previously reported.[19] If, however, the data set of saccades < 2° are fit with a power function (as shown in the lower panels), the parameters remain different from the normal subjects—especially the scaling factor K in equation 4 (which corresponds to the intercept, c, on log-log plots).

When we plotted amplitude versus duration and fit the data with a curve based on equation 5, PSP patients showed parameter values that differed from either controls or patients with PD; examples are shown in the upper panel of FIGURE 3.

Comparison of Quick Phases of Nystagmus in Patients and Normal Subjects

We found that our OK stimulus was an effective method to elicit quick phases of nystagmus in PSP and PD patients. PSP patients often showed small horizontal components to these movements, making their trajectory oblique; this finding will be the subject of a future paper. In addition, PSP patients tended to show a tonic deviation of their gaze in the direction of slow phases (stimulus direction), although they usually continued to make quick phases. Using the approach of log-log plots of quick-phase data, we estimated the parameter values for equations 4 and 5 and found that all parameters (K and m for velocity and L and n for duration) for the PSP group differed substantially from control subjects or PD patients. Examples for the duration-amplitude relationship are shown in the lower panel of FIGURE 3. We also noted no significant difference between quick phases made by PD patients and our group of 10 younger control subjects.

Measurements of the Ratio of Peak Velocity/Mean Velocity (Q)

Our younger group of 10 control subjects showed a mean Q value ± standard deviation) of 1.52 ± 0.31 for upward saccades and 1.60 ± 0.32 for downward saccades, which are similar values to those reported for horizontal saccades. In general, PD patients showed similar values, but patients with PSP sometimes did not, with mean values exceeding 3.0. Prior reports of measurements of Q for horizontal saccades in disease states have indicated that they were not much different from controls, even if saccades were slowed due to olivopontocerebellar degeneration.[15,20] Inspection of raw data suggested some possible explanations for our surprising result. Thus, in FIGURE 1, the large upward saccade (amplitude 27°) lasts 764 ms (mean speed 35.4°/s) and has a peak velocity of 106°/s—yielding a Q ratio of 3.0. However, careful inspection reveals an unusual velocity profile, with the peak velocity occurring 304 ms into the movement, and corresponding to the time of a small horizontal saccade that corrects for a small horizontal drift of the eye during the first part of the vertical saccade. A similar explanation accounts for the slow downward saccade that follows in FIGURE 1, with a Q value of 4.6. One possible interpretation of this behavior is that the movement was not one, but a series of small saccades. Support for this explanation comes from the trend shown by PSP patients of showing their largest Q values for large saccades (FIG. 4). It is also possible that part of the vertical movement is nonsaccadic in origin (see DISCUSSION).

DISCUSSION

We set out to identify methods to elicit and analyze saccades that could be applied to patients with a range of neurological disorders that impair the ability to make fast eye movements. For these purposes we selected data from a group of patients with PSP who showed varying degrees of vertical saccadic palsy. We found that large-field OK stimulation was a useful way to elicit quick phases in patients who had some difficulty in initiating voluntary saccades. We also found that using a power function to fit the relationship between the amplitude and duration or peak velocity of fast eye movements was an effective way of identifying the abnormal vertical saccades and quick phases in patients with PSP. This was the case even if small saccades or quick phases (which tend to be <2°) were analyzed. We suggest that a power-

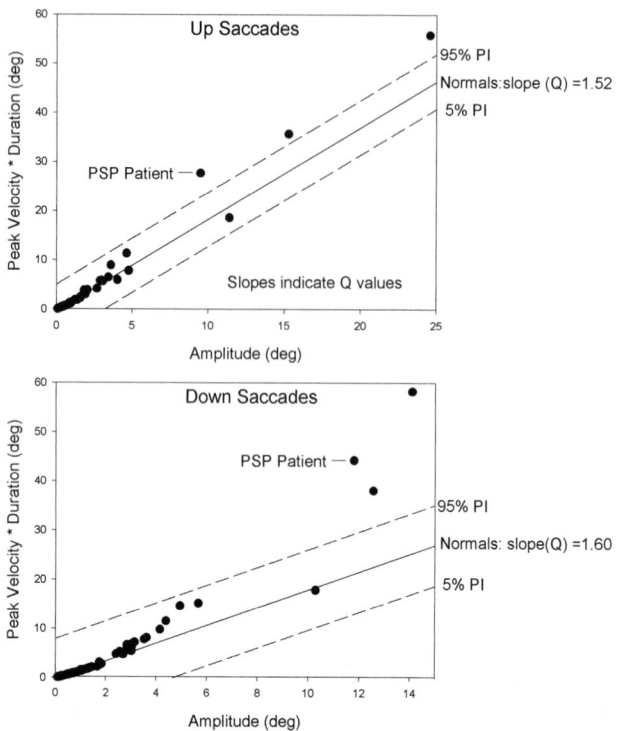

FIGURE 4. An example of the dependence of the ratio Q (peak velocity/mean velocity) on saccade amplitude in a patient with PSP (same as in FIG. 1). It is the slope that defines Q in this plot of peak velocity * duration versus amplitude. The linear fit and prediction intervals for the group of normal subjects are also shown. Note that with progressively larger saccades, especially downward, data points of the PSP patient greatly exceed the slope of normals, corresponding to large Q values.

function approach is more likely to be useful in identifying saccadic abnormalities in disorders such as PSP than the conventionally used exponential equation. Baloh and colleagues pointed out that the shortcoming of a power-function fit is that it does not account for the "soft" saturation of peak velocity that is apparent in normal subjects for movements greater than about 15°.[21] However, in many disorders that interfere with saccade generation, saccades become both small and slow and, in these cases, a power function appears to be a superior approach. Although a power function has been accepted as a useful approach to summarizing the relationship between amplitude and duration (because of the nonlinearity of the relationship for small saccades),[11,12] we suggest that this same approach is useful for amplitude-peak velocity plots in the range 0–10°.

An unexpected finding was that our PSP patients made saccades with values for the ratio peak velocity/mean velocity which exceed the range reported in normals.[10,14–16] Close inspection of our data (FIG. 1) showed that such deviations from the normal range mainly affected larger saccades (and did not apply to quick phases of nystagmus). This finding has bearing on several hypotheses concerning the pathogenesis of slow saccades in PSP and a range of other neurological disorders. First, it has been postulated that slow saccades in PSP are due primarily to dysfunction of omnipause neurons.[22] This hypothesis rests partly on the experimental finding that inactivation of omnipause neurons in monkey causes slow horizontal and vertical saccades.[23] Against this hypothesis is the finding that vertical saccades are slowed much more than horizontal movements early in the course of PSP.[5] However, it remains possible that large, slow saccades such as those shown in FIGURE 1, may in fact constitute a series of closely spaced, small saccades. Normal subjects are reported to show "discrete decelerations" during large saccades,[24] and both phenomena might be explained by some omnipause neurons temporarily recommencing discharge. Alternatively, vertical saccades may be slow because of diseased vertical burst neurons in the midbrain; during such long movements, a small horizontal saccade (e.g., FIG. 1) might, via connections between the PPRF and riMLF, momentarily increase the discharge rate of vertical burst neurons. If the latter were the case, then perhaps the small horizontal saccadic intrusions (square-wave jerks) that are common in PSP,[1] are adaptive, serving the function of transiently increasing the discharge of riMLF neurons through their shared circuitry (possibly by silencing omnipause neurons). It is well known that PSP patients often make saccadic trajectories that are curved ("round the houses")[25] when they attempt to look between two targets separated in the vertical plane. A similar phenomenon is described in Niemann-Pick type C disease.[26] More work is needed to clarify the way that horizontal saccades influence gaze shifts in patients with vertical saccadic palsies.

ACKNOWLEDGMENTS

This work was supported by Office of Research and Development, Medical Research Service, Department of Veterans Affairs; National Institutes of Health grant EY06717; Evenor Armington Fund (to R.J.L.); Iris Fund; Help a Child to See (to S.G.); and to Dr. David E. Riley for referring some of the patients studied.

REFERENCES

1. LEIGH, R.J. & D.S. ZEE. 1999. The Neurology of Eye Movements. Third edit. Oxford University Press. New York.
2. HORN, A.K.E. *et al.* 1997. Histological identification of premotor neurons for horizontal saccades in monkey and man by parvalbumin immunostaining. J. Comp. Neurol. **359:** 350–363.
3. HORN, A.K.E. & J.A. BÜTTNER-ENNEVER. 1998. Premotor neurons for vertical eye-movements in the rostral mesencephalon of monkey and man: the histological identification by parvalbumin immunostaining. J. Comp. Neurol. **392:** 413–427.
4. BÜTTNER-ENNEVER, J.A. *et al.* 1988. Raphe nucleus of pons containing omnipause neurons of the oculomotor system in the monkey, and its homologue in man. J. Comp. Neurol. **267:** 307–321.
5. BHIDAYASIRI, R. *et al.* 2001. Pathophysiology of slow saccades in progressive supranuclear palsy. Neurology **57:** 2070–2077.
6. GARBUTT, S., M.R. HARWOOD & C.M. HARRIS. 2001. Comparison of the main sequence of reflexive saccades and the quick phases of optokinetic nystagmus. Br. J. Ophthalmol. **85:** 1477–1483.

7. LITVAN, I. et al. 2002. Research goals in progressive supranuclear palsy. Movement Disord. **15:** 446–458.
8. ROTTACH, K.G. et al. 1996. Dynamic properties of horizontal and vertical eye movements in parkinsonian syndromes. Ann. Neurol. **36:** 129–141.
9. RAMAT, S. et al. 1999. Conjugate ocular oscillations during shifts of the direction and depth of visual fixation. Invest. Ophthalmol. Visual Sci. **40:** 1681–1686.
10. BECKER, W. 1989. Metrics. *In* The Neurobiology of Saccadic Eye Movements. R.H. Wurtz & M.E. Goldberg, Eds.: 13–67. Elsevier. Amsterdam.
11. YARBUS, A.L. 1967. Eye Movements and Vision. Plenum Press. New York.
12. LEBEDEV, S., P. VAN GELDER & W.H. TSUI. 1996. Square-root relations between main sequence parameters. Invest. Ophthalmol. Visual Sci. **37:** 2750–2758.
13. HARWOOD, M.R. & C.M. HARRIS. 2002. Time-optimality and the spectral overlap of saccadic eye movements. Ann. N. Y. Acad. Sci. **956:** 414–417.
14. VAN OPSTAL, A.J. & J.A.M. VAN GISBERGEN. 1987. Skewness of saccadic velocity profiles: a unifying parameter for normal and slow saccades. Vision Res. **27:** 731–745.
15. INCHINGOLO, P., M. SPANIO & M. BIANCHI. 1987. The characteristic peak velocity – mean velocity of saccadic eye movements in man. *In* Eye Movements: From Physiology to Cognition. J.K. Regan & A. Levy-Schoen, Eds.: 17–26. Elsevier. Amsterdam.
16. HARWOOD, M.R., L.E. MEZEY & C.M. HARRIS. 1999. The spectral main sequence of human saccades. J. Neurosci. **15:** 9098-9106.
17. EVINGER, C. et al. 1984. Blinking and associated eye movements in humans, guinea pigs, and rabbits. J. Neurophysiol. **52:** 323–339.
18. FREUND, H.J. & H.J. BUDINGEN. 1978. The relationship between speed and amplitude of the fastest voluntary contractions of human arm muscles. Exp. Brain Res. **18:** 1–12.
19. AVERBUCH-HELLER, L. et al. 2002. Small vertical saccades have normal speeds in progressive supranuclear palsy (PSP). Ann. N.Y. Acad. Sci. **956:** 434–437.
20. BALOH, R.W. et al. 1975. The saccade velocity test. Neurology **25:** 1071–1076.
21. BALOH, R.W. et al. 1975. Quantitative measurement of saccade amplitude, duration, and velocity. Neurology **25:** 1065–1070.
22. REVESZ, T., H. SANGHA & S.E. DANIEL. 1996. The nucleus raphe interpositus in the Steele-Richardson-Olszewski syndrome (progressive supranuclear palsy). Brain **119:** 1137–1143.
23. KANEKO, C.R.S. 1996. Effect of ibotenic acid lesions of the omnipause neurons on saccadic eye movements in rhesus macaques. J. Neurophysiol. **75:** 2229–2242.
24. ABEL, L.A., S. TRACCIS, B.T. TROOST & L.D. DELL'OSSO. 1987. Saccadic trajectories change with amplitude, not time. Neuro-ophthalmol. **7:** 309–314.
25. QUINN, N. 1996. The "round the houses" sign in progressive supranuclear palsy. Ann. Neurol. **39:** 368–377.
26. ROTTACH, K.G. et al. 1997. Evidence for independent feedback control of horizontal and vertical saccades from Niemann-Pick type C disease. Vision Res. **37:** 3627–3638.

Incomitance of Ocular Rotation Axes in Trochlear Nerve Palsy

KONRAD P. WEBER,[a] ANTONELLA PALLA,[a] KLARA LANDAU,[b] THOMAS HASLWANTER,[a] AND DOMINIK STRAUMANN[a]

[a]*Department of Neurology, Zurich University Hospital, Zurich, Switzerland*

[b]*Department of Ophthalmology, Zurich University Hospital, Zurich, Switzerland*

ABSTRACT: Strabismus due to palsy of a single muscle in one eye is always incomitant, which is a consequence of Hering's law of equal innervation. We asked whether this law had similar consequences on the orientation of ocular rotation axes. Patients with unilateral trochlear nerve palsy were oscillated about the nasooccipital (= roll) axis (±35°, 0.3 Hz), and monocularly fixed on targets on a head-fixed Hess screen. Both the covered and uncovered eyes were measured with dual search coils. The rotation axis of the covered eye (paretic or healthy) tilted more nasally from the line of sight when gaze was directed toward the side of the healthy eye. The rotation axis of the viewing eye (paretic or healthy), however, remained roughly aligned with the line of sight. We conclude that incomitance due to eye muscle palsy extends to ocular rotation axes during vestibular stimulation.

KEYWORDS: strabismus; eye movements; vestibuloocular reflex; kinematics; three-dimensional

INTRODUCTION

Strabismus due to palsy of a single muscle in one eye is always incomitant; that is, the deviation between the two eyes increases when gaze is moved in the pulling direction of the paretic muscle. A direct consequence of Hering's law of equal innervation[1] is that for a specific position of one eye, the deviation between two eyes is equal, regardless of which eye is covered.[2] Therefore, the squint angle between the two eyes is smaller when the healthy eye fixes upon a given target (primary deviation) than when the paretic eye fixes upon the very same target (secondary deviation).[3]

In trochlear nerve palsy the force exerted by the superior oblique muscle is reduced. Hence, the line of sight of the covered eye no longer points toward the target, but deviates extorsional-upward or extorsional-downward when the paretic or healthy eye is covered, respectively. As a consequence of Hering's law, this torsional-vertical deviation increases when neural signals associated with ocular counterroll try to activate the paretic superior oblique muscle. Based on this obser-

---

Address for correspondence: D. Straumann, M.D., Neurology Department, Zürich University Hospital, CH-8091 Zürich, Switzerland. Voice: 41-1-255-5564; fax: 41-1-255-4507.

dominik@neurol.unizh.ch

vation, Bielschowsky and Hofmann described the head-tilt test for diagnosing trochlear nerve palsy.[4]

We asked whether Hering's law had similar consequences on the orientation of ocular rotation axes as on the position of the eyes. Specifically, we speculated that in patients with trochlear nerve palsy the angle between the rotation axes of the two eyes were incomitant during Bielschowsky head-tilt testing. To determine the orientations of rotation axes, we used continuous sinusoidal vestibular stimulation about the nasooccipital axis while one eye was covered and the other was fixing upon targets on a Hess screen.

METHODS

We tested 12 patients (age 15–57 years, 2 female) with non-operated unilateral trochlear nerve palsy. The comparison group consisted of 11 healthy subjects (age 21–40 years, 6 female). The protocol was approved by a local ethics committee and was in accordance with the ethical standards laid down in the Declaration of Helsinki for research involving human subjects.

Subjects were seated upright on a turntable with three servocontrolled motor driven axes (prototype built by Acutronic, Jona, Switzerland). The head was restrained with an individually molded thermoplastic mask (Sinmed BV, Reeuwijk, The Netherlands). Movements of both eyes were recorded with dual search coils in three dimensions[5] (horizontal, vertical, torsional) on the turntable. Subjects monocularly fixed upon nine laser dots projected on a spherical screen at a distance of 1.4 m, whereas the other eye was covered. The dots were located straight ahead and at eight eccentric head-fixed positions (0° and ±20° horizontal and vertical, square grid). During monocular fixation, subjects were oscillated about the nasooccipital (= roll) axis (±35°, 0.3 Hz). Eye and chair position signals were digitized with 16-bit accuracy. All data were sampled at 1 kHz and analyzed off-line with Matlab software (The MathWorks, Inc., Natick, MA).

Three-dimensional eye positions in the magnetic coil frame were expressed as rotation vectors.[6] From these rotation vectors, the corresponding gaze direction was calculated. In addition, the corresponding angular velocity vectors $\vec{\omega}$ were derived to determine "ocular rotation axes," that is, the direction of $\vec{\omega}$.[7] The length of $\vec{\omega}$ is proportional to the rotational speed. To relate the ocular rotation axes to the corresponding gaze trajectories on the same Hess screen chart, we projected them stereographically. Data from patients with left-sided trochlear nerve palsies were mirrored to the right side.

RESULTS

FIGURE 1 summarizes the locations of the rotation axes during monocular fixation of the nine cardinal gaze directions in patients and healthy subjects. The paretic right eyes of the patients, when covered (FIG. 1B, gray ellipses), showed rotation axes that, on average, were shifted nasally compared with the eyes of healthy subjects (black ellipses). This horizontal deviation increased with adduction of the covered paretic eye. The healthy left eyes of patients, when covered (FIG. 1A, gray ellipses), showed

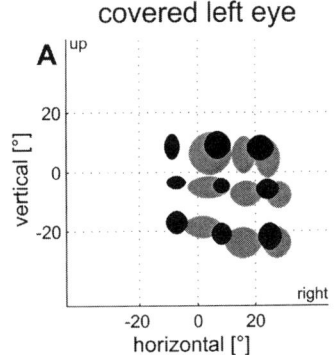 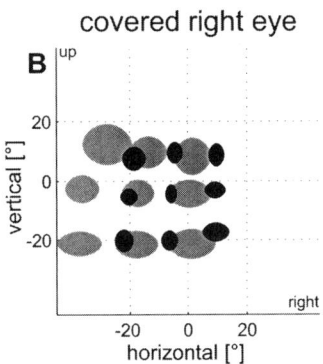

FIGURE 1. Orientation of ocular rotation axes (stereographic projection onto Hess screen). Ellipses: average (center) ±1 SD (horizontal and vertical radius). Healthy subjects (*black*); patients (*gray*). Intersections of dotted lines indicate location of visual targets. (**A**) Left eye during right eye viewing. (**B**) Right eye during left eye viewing.

a nasal shift of the rotation axes as well, but, in contrast to the paretic eyes, the deviation increased with abduction. The rotation axes of the viewing eyes in patients and healthy subjects matched closely (not shown); that is, the rotation axes in both groups of subjects were near the line of sight, when fixation was maintained by the respective eye.

To test whether the eye position–dependent angle between the rotation axes of both eyes follows the same principle as the incomitant squint angle, we used the graphical method to analyze strabismus proposed by Zee *et al.*[2] but plotted the absolute horizontal angle of ocular rotation axes of both eyes, instead of their horizontal gaze position, against each other (FIG. 2). Data points of axes moving in parallel would lie on a line with zero intercept and a slope of one (dashed line). Data points below this line represent convergent axes and data points above the line represent divergent axes. A slope of one always indicates that axes are comitant; otherwise, they are incomitant. Data points of healthy subjects with either eye covered were located on a regression line with a slope of almost one, indicating comitance (FIG. 2, squares). Thus, analogous to binocular eye positions, binocular axes were comitant in healthy subjects, indicating that Hering's law of equal innervation extends to the orientation of rotation axes. Consistent with the fact that axes normally show a slight convergence,[8] data points were situated below the dashed line.

The slopes of regression lines in patients (triangles: average of pooled data from fixations along the horizontal meridian) were larger than one, demonstrating incomitance between the rotation axes of both eyes. As in healthy subjects, the fitted lines through the data with either eye covered (filled: paretic right eye covered = primary axis deviation, open: healthy left eye covered = secondary axis deviation) were similar. In other words, for a given axis orientation of one eye, the angle between the ocular rotation axes was almost the same, independent of which eye was covered. Note, however, that, for a given orientation of an ocular rotation axis in one eye, the deviation of the axis of the fellow eye was larger when the former eye was the

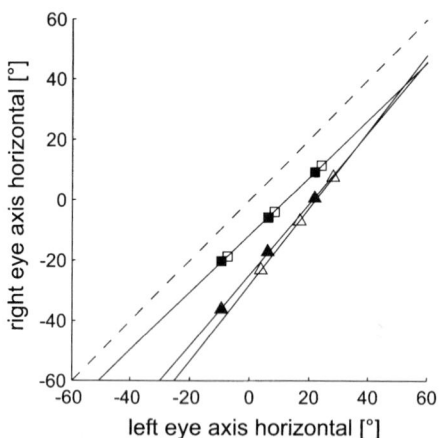

FIGURE 2. Comitance and vergence of ocular rotation axes during fixations along horizontal meridian. Orientations of rotation axes of both eyes plotted against each other. *Triangles:* Average data in patients; *squares:* average data in healthy subjects; *open symbols:* right eye viewing condition; *filled symbols:* left eye viewing condition; *dashed line*: absolute comitance and no vergence between both eyes; *solid lines:* first-order linear regression. Data points below dashed line: convergence. Slope >1: increasing convergence of axes with left gaze.

healthy one. Thus, the primary axis deviation was larger than the secondary axis deviation. This is exactly opposite of what one observes for eye positions with the primary squint angle being smaller than the secondary squint angle.

DISCUSSION

Our data reveal that in patients with trochlear nerve palsy Hering's law has similar consequences on the orientation of ocular rotation axes as on eye positions. During torsional vestibular stimulation about the nasooccipital axis, ocular rotation axes are incomitant. In the covered condition the rotation axis of both the paretic and healthy eye moves nasally; its deviation from the rotation axis of the viewing eye, however, increases when the patient looks in the direction of the healthy eye.

A detailed geometrical explanation for the incomitance of rotation axes will be given elsewhere (Weber *et al.*, in preparation). Intuitively, however, this phenomenon can be understood for the situation when the paretic eye is covered: the larger the vertical component of the superior oblique (SO) muscle is in a given eye position, the more a paresis will lead to a deviation of the ocular rotation axis from the line of sight. Because the vertical component of the SO muscle pulling direction increases with adduction, we can expect a larger deviation of the ocular rotation axis in this gaze direction.

To explain the incomitance of rotation axes when the healthy eye is covered, one must apply Hering's law of equal innervation to conjugate torsion. This can be done by assuming equal distribution of innervation between two muscle *pairs*, not just single muscles. Specifically, superior oblique and superior rectus muscles of one eye are yoked with inferior oblique and inferior rectus muscles of the other eye, respectively. If the SO muscle becomes paretic and the subject fixates with the ipsilateral eye, there will be hyperinnervation in the healthy eye along a vector parallel the vector of the paretic SO. This in turn will lead to incomitance of ocular rotation axes along the horizontal direction (geometrical details: Weber *et al.*, in preparation).

In conclusion, the concept of incomitance in the presence of eye muscle palsy includes not only binocular positions, but also binocular rotation axes during concurrent vestibular stimulation.

ACKNOWLEDGMENTS

The authors thank Chris Bockisch, Albert Züger, and Tanja Schmückle for their assistance. This work was supported by Swiss National Science Foundation 32-51938.97 SCORE A/31-63465.00 and Betty and David Koetser Foundation for Brain Research.

REFERENCES

1. HERING, E. 1868. Die Lehre vom binocularen Sehen. Verlag von Wilhelm Engelmann, Leipzig.
2. ZEE, D.S., F.C. CHU, L.M. OPTICAN, *et al.* 1984. Graphic analysis of paralytic strabismus with the Lancaster red-green test. Am. J. Ophthalmol. **97:** 587–592.
3. VON NOORDEN, G.K. 1996. Binocular Vision and Ocular Motility. 5th edit. Mosby. St. Louis, MO.
4. BIELSCHOWSKY, A. & F.B. HOFMANN. 1900. Die Verwerthung der Kopfneigung zur Diagnostik von Augenmuskellähmungen aus der Heber- und Senkergruppe. [The evaluation of head inclination for the diagnosis of pareses of ocular muscles from the group of elevators and depressors.]. Graefes Arch. Ophthalmol. **51:** 174–185.
5. BERGAMIN, O., D.S. ZEE, D.C. ROBERTS, *et al.* 2001. Three-dimensional Hess screen test with binocular dual search coils in a three-field magnetic system. Invest. Ophthalmol. Visual Sci. **42:** 660–667.
6. HAUSTEIN, W. 1989. Considerations on Listing's law and the primary position by means of a matrix description of eye position control. Biol. Cybern. **60:** 411–420.
7. HEPP, K. 1990. On Listing's law. Commun. Math. Phys. **132:** 285–292.
8. BERGAMIN, O. & D. STRAUMANN. 2001. Three-dimensional binocular kinematics of torsional vestibular nystagmus during convergence on head-fixed targets in humans. J. Neurophysiol. **86:** 113–122.

Eye Movements and Balance

MICHAEL STRUPP, STEFAN GLASAUER, KLAUS JAHN, ERICH SCHNEIDER, SIEGBERT KRAFCZYK, AND THOMAS BRANDT

Department of Neurology, University of Munich, Klinikum Grosshadern, Munich, Germany

KEYWORDS: retinal slip; vestibulo-ocular reflex; eye movement; head motion

INTRODUCTION

It is a basic and common experience that vision improves postural balance. Ever since the early 1940s, this effect of vision has been a subject of investigation.[1–3] It is still not known what serves as the cue for visual stabilization of posture. It generally is assumed that postural sway causes the image of the visual scene to move on the retina in the opposite direction to that of head sway. This so-called retinal slip is utilized as feedback to compensate for body sway. A comparison of posture in darkness with stable, room-fixed targets to posture with full-field vision revealed that vision significantly increased stability (e.g., Paulus et al.[4]). Large-field, moving visual scenes were found to cause body sway in the same direction as stimulus motion.[2,5–7] There is, however, a problem with using the amount of retinal slip as a cue to control posture. If a subject fixates a stationary target, there is almost no retinal slip. This is caused by the vestibulo-ocular reflex (VOR) and visual smooth pursuit, which keep the gaze in space and on target constant. Thus, with fixation, eye movements rather than retinal slip reflect head motion in space.[8–10]

On the basis of this rationale, we addressed the following question: does visual stabilization of postural balance depend on retinal slip or on extraocular signals, namely, ocular motor input provided by efferent or reafferent (proprioceptive) signals. Two series of experiments were performed. In the first, postural sway was measured in patients with acute vestibular neuritis (VN) with and without visual suppression of spontaneous nystagmus (SPN).[11] In the second, postural sway was measured and retinal error (slip) was calculated in healthy subjects with and without smooth pursuit during fixation (S. Glasauer et al., unpublished).

PATIENTS AND METHODS

In the first series, 10 patients with VN participated. Patients were tested 2 to 6 days after symptom onset. Horizontal and vertical eye positions were measured with infrared videooculography integrated in a head-fixed mask that prevented perception of ambient light and visual orientation as described previously.[11] A mask-integrated and thereby also head-fixed light-emitting diode (LED) could be turned on in two modes: dimmed light or bright light for fixation. To determine postural sway, we measured anteroposterior (AP) and right-left sway velocity and root mean square (RMS) values by posturography, while the subject was standing on a foam-rubber padded force measuring platform. Four conditions were tested: (1) standing in darkness, (2) looking at the dimmed head-fixed LED (as one of the control conditions because this should not suppress SPN), (3) fixation of the bright head-fixed LED (this should suppress SPN), and (4) fixation of a bright space-fixed LED (the second control condition).

In the second series of experiments, postural sway was measured in healthy subjects with and without smooth pursuit with a stationary background at a distance of 0.7 m (S. Glasauer *et al.*, unpublished). To disentangle the relative contributions of retinal slip and eye movement to postural stability, body sway, head position in space, target in space, and gaze direction in head were measured. From the data, eye position in space, gaze direction in space, target in head coordinates, and retinal error were calculated. The following four conditions were tested in 15 healthy subjects, standing heel-to-toe: 1) standing in darkness, 2) fixation of a stationary space-fixed target, 3) smooth pursuit with a stationary visual background, and 4) smooth pursuit without a visual background in darkness.

RESULTS

Intensity of Spontaneous Nystagmus in Vestibular Neuritis and Postural Imbalance

Compared with the condition of complete darkness, fixation of the bright head-fixed LED caused a significant suppression of the SPN and a decrease of sway velocity. This is illustrated by an original recording of the horizontal eye position and sway velocity of a patient with right-sided VN with and without fixation of the bright head-fixed LED in FIGURE 1. As shown in FIGURE 2, fixation of the bright head-fixed LED significantly reduced the mean peak slow-phase velocity (PSPV) of the horizontal component of SPN from $13.5 \pm 5.6°/s$ to $4.3 \pm 2.4°/s$ (ANOVA, $P < 0.05$). In parallel, the RMS values for sway also decreased: RMS significantly decreased from 25.2 ± 7.6 to 16.2 ± 7.7 mm (right-left RMS values (ANOVA, $P < 0.05$). Thus, although there was no space-fixed visual target, the suppression of SPN per se improved balance. Under the second control condition, looking at the dimmed, head-fixed LED, the sway RMS did not change, despite the highest value for retinal slip. Plotting the RMS values against mean PSPV of SPN showed that there was a clear correlation between body sway and intensity of nystagmus ($r = 0.64$, $P < 0.05$, FIG. 3), that is, the higher the PSPV of SPN, the greater the postural imbalance or sway.

Smooth Pursuit and Postural Imbalance

In the second series of experiments, postural sway was dependent on whether smooth pursuit was performed or not. FIGURE 4 shows an example of the raw data

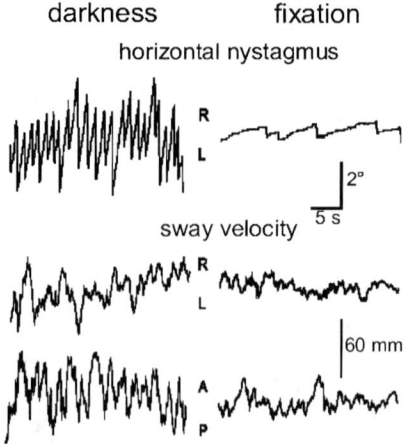

FIGURE 1. Original registrations of horizontal eye movements, RL and AP sway path in darkness and during fixation of the head-stationary LED. When spontaneous nystagmus was suppressed, postural sway was also reduced. Scaling is the same for both experimental conditions (from Jahn et al.[11]).

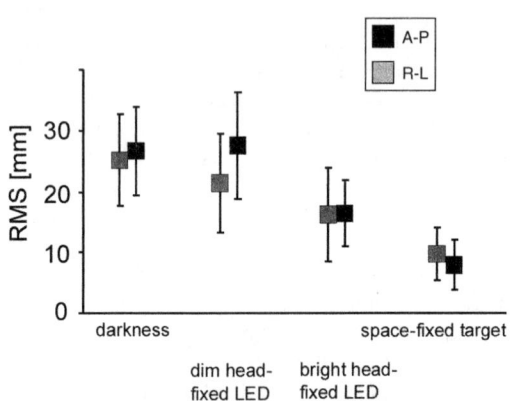

FIGURE 2. Body sway of patients with vestibular neuritis under different visual conditions. Mean and SD RMS values on foam rubber (*squares*). Lateral (*gray symbols*) and fore-aft sway (*black symbols*) are shown. Fixation of a bright head-fixed LED only reduced sway when subjects stood on foam rubber. Attempted fixation of a dim LED with minor suppression of spontaneous eye movements had no significant effect (from Jahn et al.[11]).

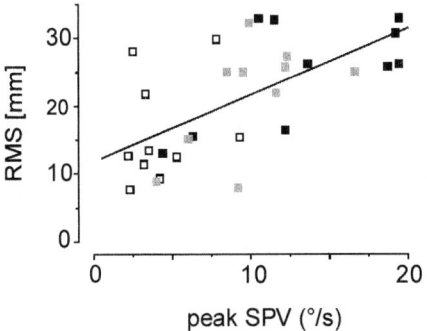

FIGURE 3. Correlation of mean peak slow-phase velocity (SPV) and total postural sway (RMS). There was a correlation of eye and body movements ($r = 0.64$, $P < 0.05$). Symbols represent nystagmus in darkness (*black*), during fixation of a dim head-fixed LED (*gray*), and during fixation of a bright head-fixed LED (*open white*) (from Jahn et al.[11]).

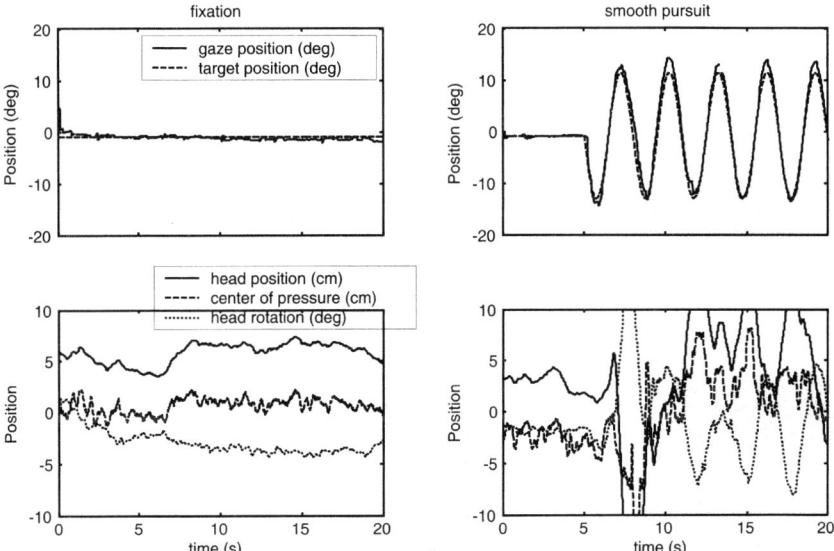

FIGURE 4. Example of raw data for one subject for two conditions without visual background. (*left*) Fixation of a stationary target. (right) Smooth pursuit of a moving target. (*top plots*) Gaze and target. (*bottom plots*) Head position and center of pressure. Even though the subject tracks the target almost perfectly during smooth pursuit, a significant sway develops after about 5 s of smooth pursuit onset (Glasauer *et al.*, unpublished).

for a subject under the two conditions: (1) fixation of a stationary space-fixed target, and (2) smooth pursuit of a moving target without a visual background. Even though the subject tracked the target almost perfectly during smooth pursuit, and thus retinal slip was minimal, a significant sway developed after about 2 s of smooth pursuit onset. The results of this series of experiments are summarized in FIGURE 5. The highest postural stability was measured when subjects fixated a space-fixed target. Smooth pursuit significantly increased postural sway in unstable stance, even in the presence of a stable background and with minimal retinal slip (Glasauer *et al.*, unpublished).

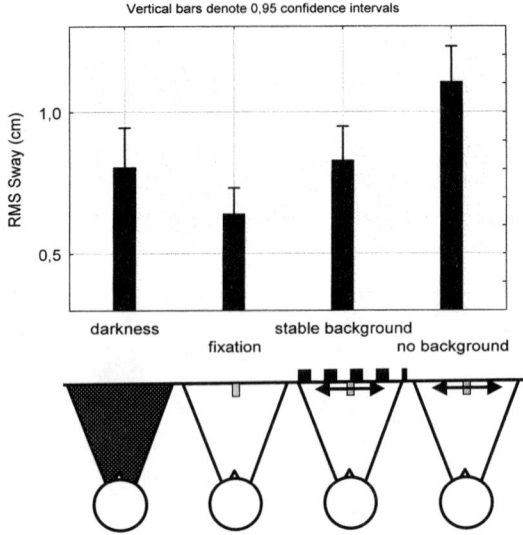

FIGURE 5. Mean sway data (in cm) for "fixation" (*left*) and "eye movement" (*right*) conditions. The error bars give 95% confidence intervals of means. The pictograms illustrate the different experimental conditions; the numbers refer to the experimental condition. For statistical analysis, the conditions were grouped so that "fixation" versus "eye movement" could be tested. A repeated-measures ANOVA revealed significant effects of "fixation" versus "eye movement" ($P = 0.005$) and the paired conditions but no interaction. The highest postural stability was measured when subjects fixated a space-fixed target. Smooth pursuit significantly increased postural sway in unstable stance, even in the presence of a stable background and with minimal retinal slip (Glasauer *et al.*, unpublished).

DISCUSSION

The major question addressed by this study was whether visual stabilization of postural balance depends on retinal slip or on extraocular signals. From the first series of experiments, we can conclude that high retinal slip with head-fixed target does not improve postural stability, but suppression of nystagmus per se improves balance. Furthermore, because in these experiments a head-fixed target was used to suppress SPN (a condition which suppresses eye movements but does not provide any additional visual information for postural control), we can also conclude that ocular motor signals rather than afferent visual input are used for balance stabilization, at least in this experimental paradigm.[11] These data agree with findings in an earlier study on the effects of nicotine on nystagmus and postural imbalance. That study showed a high correlation between the intensity of the nicotine-induced nystagmus and the increase in total sway path; the correlation coefficient was 0.78.[12] As in the case of patients with VN, fixation of a bright head-fixed LED caused visual suppression of nicotine-induced nystagmus as well as a significant decrease of postural sway. These results also fit earlier reports of a correlation between eye movements and postural sway.[13–15] All in all, the second series of experiments also provided ev-

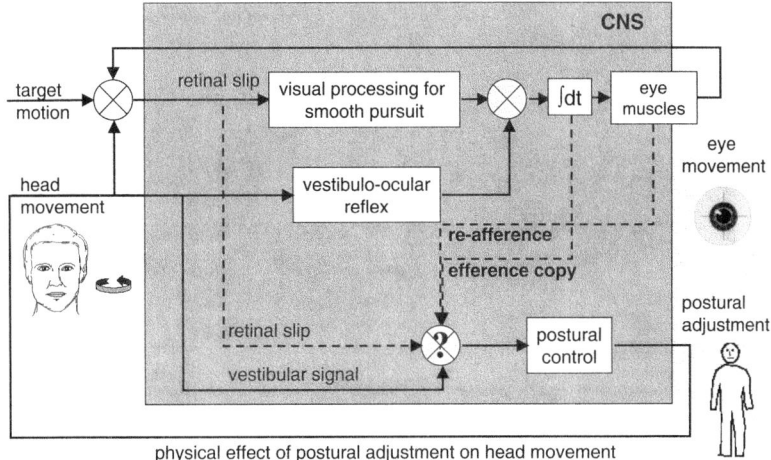

FIGURE 6. Simplified schematic flow of information for eye movements and postural control. The postural control system (*lower right corner*) receives information from the vestibular system about head motion, from the somatosensory system about body motion (omitted in the figure for clarity), and from the visuoocularmotor system. A possible visuoocularmotor information is retinal slip; another one is an efference copy or a reafference of eye movements. In this scheme, it is assumed that the head is stable on the body so that the vestibular signal reflects body movement as does the somatosensory system. Provided fixation of a space-fixed target, the efference copy reflects the movement of the head (and body) for the space-fixed target and thus is suited for postural control. Even in darkness, the efference copy still reflects head motion via the VOR. If, however, the target is moving, the efference copy is no longer a good signal for body stabilization and thus will cause increased body sway (Glasauer *et al.*, unpublished).

idence that in conditions of unstable stance, ocular motor rather than visual signals are used for postural stability.

The data of both series of experiments can be represented by a schematic flow of information for eye movements and postural control as illustrated in FIGURE 6 (S. Glasauer, unpublished). Two factors in this diagram should be pointed out: (1) the reafference signal, and (2) the ocular motor efference copy. In patients with SPN the reafference signal as well as the efference copy can contribute to postural instability. Visual suppression of SPN, on the other hand, reduces both disturbing signals and may thereby improve postural stability. If, as in the second series of experiments, the eyes follow a moving target, the reafference signal and or efference copy may cause increased body sway. This model can also explain other phenomena; for example, in downbeat nystagmus, the correlation between the simultaneous increase of nystagmus and body sway during lateral gaze.[13]

CONCLUSION

Contrary to common belief, these experiments suggest that visual stabilization of postural control depends on extraocular signals (efference copy and/or reafferent signals) rather than retinal slip. Why are ocular motor signals useful for postural control? While fixating a target, retinal slip is close to zero because of the combined capacity of VOR, smooth pursuit, and the fixation that drives the eyes to move in their orbits in the opposite direction to that of head motion with the same velocity and amplitude. Thus, to use visual information to compensate for head and body sway during fixation, information on eye velocity or position is the reliable cue. During fixation, efference copy or reafferent (proprioceptive) signals about eye movements may be equally good indicators of body sway, and, hence, both are possible candidates for carrying out the sensorimotor task.

ACKNOWLEDGMENTS

We are grateful to J. Benson for copyediting the manuscript. The work was supported by the Deutsche Forschungsgemeinschaft (STR 384/4-2).

REFERENCES

1. TRAVIS, R.C. 1945. An experimental analysis of dynamic and static equilibrium. J. Exp. Psychol. **35:** 216–234.
2. EDWARDS, A.S. 1946. Body sway and vision. J. Exp. Psychol. **36:** 526–535.
3. LEE, D.N. & J.R. LISHMAN. 1974. Visual proprioceptive control of stance. J. Hum. Mov. Stud. **1:** 87–95.
4. PAULUS, W., A. STRAUBE & T. BRANDT. 1984. Visual stabilization of posture. Physiological stimulus characteristics and clinical aspects. Brain **107:** 1143–1163.
5. DICHGANS, J., K.H. MAURITZ, J.H.J. ALLUM & T. BRANDT. 1976. Postural sway in normals and atactic patients: analysis of stabilizing and destabilizing effects of vision. Agressologie **17:** 15–24.
6. LESTIENNE, F., J. SOECHTING, & A. BERTHOZ. 1977. Postural readjustments induced by linear motion of visual scenes. Exp. Brain Res. **28:** 363–384.
7. BERTHOZ, A., M. LACOUR, J. SOECHTIG & P. VIDAL. 1979. The role of vision in the control of posture during linear motion. *In* Progress in Brain Research. R. Granit & O. Pompeiano, Eds.: 197–210. Elsevier. New York.
8. ROLL, J.P., J.P. VEDEL & R. ROLL. 1989. Eye, head and skeletal muscle spindle feedback in the elaboration of body references. Prog. Brain Res. **80:** 113–123.
9. WOLSLEY, C.J., D. BUCKWELL, V. SAKELLARI & A.M. BRONSTEIN. 1996. The effect of eye/head deviation and visual conflict on visually evoked postural responses. Brain Res. Bull. **40:** 437–441.
10. GUERRAZ, M., V. SAKELLARI & A.M. BRONSTEIN. 2000. Influence of motion parallax in the control of spontaneous body sway. Exp. Brain Res. **131:** 244–252.
11. JAHN, K., M. STRUPP, S. KRAFCZYK, *et al.* 2002. Suppression of eye movements improves balance. Brain **125:** 2005–2011.
12. PEREIRA, C.B., M. STRUPP, T. HOLZLEITNER & T. BRANDT. 2001. Smoking and balance: correlation of nicotine-induced nystagmus and postural body sway. Neuroreport **12:** 1223–1226.
13. BÜCHELE, W., T. BRANDT & D. DEGNER. 1983. Ataxia and oscillopsia in downbeat nystagmus/vertigo syndrome. Adv. Otorhinolaryngol. **30:** 291–297.
14. BRANDT, T., W. PAULUS & A. STRAUBE. 1986. Vision and posture. *In* Disorders of Posture and Gait. W. Bles & T. Brandt, Eds.: 157–176. Elsevier. Amsterdam.
15. HUNTER, M.C. & M.A. HOFFMAN. 2001. Postural control: visual and cognitive manipulations. Gait Posture **13:** 41–48.

The Critical Role of Velocity Storage in Production of Motion Sickness

BERNARD COHEN,[a] MINGJIA DAI,[a] AND THEODORE RAPHAN[b]

[a]*Department of Neurology, Mount Sinai School of Medicine, New York, New York 10029, USA*

[b]*Department of Computer and Information Sciences, Brooklyn College of the City University of New York, Brooklyn, New York 11210, USA*

ABSTRACT: We propose that motion sickness is mediated through the orientation properties of velocity storage in the vestibular system that tend to align eye velocity produced by the angular vestibulo-ocular reflex (aVOR) with gravito-inertial acceleration (GIA). (GIA is the sum of the linear accelerations acting on the head. In the absence of translational accelerations, gravity is the GIA.) We further postulate that motion sickness produced by cross-coupled vestibular stimulation can be characterized by a metric composed of the disparity between the axis of eye rotation and the GIA, the strength of the response to angular motion, and the response duration, as determined by the central vestibular time constant, that is, by the time constant of velocity storage. The nodulus and uvula of the vestibulocerebellum are likely to be the central sites where the disparity is sensed, where the vestibular time constants are habituated, and where links are made to the autonomic system to produce the symptoms and signs.

KEYWORDS: head movements; nystagmus; vestibular; vertigo; roll while rotating; nodulus; uvula; vestibulocerebellum

INTRODUCTION

Motion sickness has plagued humans since the dawn of recorded history,[1] but the specific mechanisms that lead to the sensation of motion sickness and its treatment are still not well understood. Both visual and vestibular stimuli produce motion sickness, and nausea and vomiting also have been produced by manipulation of the eye muscles during ocular surgery. Seasickness is a well-known variant, as is space motion sickness, which occurs in approximately 60% of astronauts when they make active pitch or roll head movements, shortly after insertion into space.

The cause of motion sickness usually is attributed to a sensory conflict,[2–4] but as yet the precise nature of the conflict and what is sensed is still obscure. Some things are well established, however. Motion sickness cannot be evoked after the vestibular labyrinths have been destroyed or damaged,[5] showing that vestibular processing is

---

Address for correspondence: Bernard Cohen, Department of Neurology, Mount Sinai School of Medicine, New York, NY 10029. Voice: 212-241-7068; fax: 212-831-1610.
bernard.cohen@mssm.edu

critical for its production. Because motion sickness also can be produced by visual stimuli in the absence of vestibular activation, it is not necessary to activate vestibular receptors to generate motion sickness. This implies that the critical processing takes place in the central vestibular system. Nevertheless, the processing chain by which activity from the peripheral labyrinth reaches centers in the medulla that control autonomic reactions, including nausea and vomiting, is still unknown.[6]

Bles et al.[7] have redefined the sensory rearrangement theory of motion sickness, based on a subjective vertical conflict model developed by Oman,[4] as "all situations which provoke motion sickness are characterized by a condition in which the sensed vertical as determined on the basis of integrated information from the eyes, the vestibular system, and nonvestibular proprioceptors is at variance with the subjective vertical as predicted on the basis of previous experience." Whether the sensed vertical actually is compared with the subjective vertical based on previous experience is difficult to prove, and the central processing that might evaluate this disparity and project disparity information to portions of the autonomic system responsible for motion sickness are also unknown (see Yates et al.[6] for review).

Active pitch or roll of the head while rotating around a vertical axis, which we define as cross-coupled vestibular stimulation, has been a robust method for producing severe vertigo, nausea, and vomiting. Consequently, it has been used in several studies to test the efficacy of drugs on motion sickness[8–15] and to study its habituation.[7,13,15–20] By repetitive exposure, most individuals adapt to the cross-coupled stimulus, and the vertigo and motion sickness abate.[9,15,21–26] The stimulus induced by tilting the head while rotating often has been referred to as "Coriolis cross-coupling," although the magnitude of the Coriolis force is small and unlikely to cause such severe symptoms.[11,27] Rather, head tilt while rotating generates angular acceleration along the axes of canals as they move into and out of the plane of rotation. The otoliths on the other hand signal a head movement around the roll or pitch axis of the head relative to the upright position. The difference between the head movement signaled by the canals and otoliths is a potential conflict that could be responsible for the symptoms.

Alternatively, because both the yaw and pitch stimuli occur during constant velocity rotation, the changes in head position would excite the canals and activate velocity storage. The consequence would be that per- and/or postrotatory nystagmus are generated around a third axis that long outlasts the head roll. The latter suggests that activation of velocity storage might be important for the production of motion sickness. There is considerable evidence to substantiate this view. It is known, for example, that repetitive vestibular stimulation habituates the central vestibular time constant (see Cohen et al.[28] for review), which reflects the state of velocity storage.[29] Consequently, figure skaters, dancers, acrobats, and fighter pilots whose vestibular time constants have been habituated can perform almost any head movement while in motion without inducing motion sickness. Thus, the duration of caloric nystagmus, which is, in part, dependent on the velocity storage time constant[30] and motion sickness declined concurrently in figure skaters.[31] In addition, the incidence of space motion sickness was less in Russian cosmonauts who went through a program of adaptation to pitching during constant rotation at high velocity (180°/s) than in American astronauts who did not.[32] Such exposure probably would have resulted in a shorter angular vestibulo-ocular reflex (aVOR) time constant, but the time constants of the subjects were not measured. Many recent studies also support the hypothesis that there is a connection between velocity storage and motion sickness,[33,34] with relatively few contrary views.[35] To our knowledge, there is no study that specifically addresses the comparative rates of adaptation of sensitivity to motion sickness and that attempts to link susceptibility to motion sickness to the central vestibular time constant. This was one purpose of this study.

We further questioned what aspect of velocity storage besides the length of the time constant might be important for producing motion sickness. As is well known,[7,34,36] rotation about axes tilted from the vertical are much more provocative than vertical axis rotation. This implies that discordance between gravity and the axis of rotation might be a critical conflict for producing motion sickness. From this, we postulated that the conflict is related to aspects of the orientation properties of velocity storage.[37] In favor of this postulate, motion sickness susceptibility was abolished or substantially diminished in dogs by destruction of nodulus and uvula,[38–40] which involved regions of the cerebellum that are responsible for the orientation property of velocity storage.[41–45] Precisely how the spatial orientation properties of velocity storage are linked to the conflicting canal–otolith interaction and to motion sickness is not known, however. An investigation of this was another purpose of this study.

METHODS

Sixteen normal healthy subjects (4 females and 12 males; mean age, 22.3 years) participated in this study, which involved tilting the head 45° over approximately 2 s in roll while rotating at a velocity of 138°/s in darkness about a spatial vertical axis. We first utilized roll of the head to lateral positions and back to the upright position while rotating to test whether promethazine, a commonly used antiemetic drug would protect subjects against development of motion sickness. We also wished to determine whether the drug affected the rate of habituation to provocative stimuli. A complete description of the techniques and methods of analysis is given elsewhere,[37] and only essential details are provided here. The test procedure was explained to the subjects beforehand and all gave informed consent. The study was approved and conformed to the guidelines set by the institutional review board of the Mount Sinai School of Medicine.

Experimental Design

The experimental protocol was a double-blind, crossover design that was first used to study the effects of promethazine on the sensation of nausea and on the rate of habituation. One group received placebo and the second group received 25 mg of promethazine orally. A single test on each day was called a test session. A set of test sessions on four consecutive days defined an experimental series. Subjects were tested in two series one month apart. Subjects were told about the stressful motion sickness and "apparent" disorientation that they would encounter during the test. Then, they were trained to make appropriate roll head movements while stationary. They were instructed to sit upright, tilt the head laterally over 2 s to approximately 45°, and then to hold their head in this position until instructed to return the head back to the upright position over the same time course. This head tilt then was repeated on the other side. After training, subjects were seated in a standard vertical-axis rotation chair (Neurokinetics). A three-point seat belt held their trunk firmly. A sur-

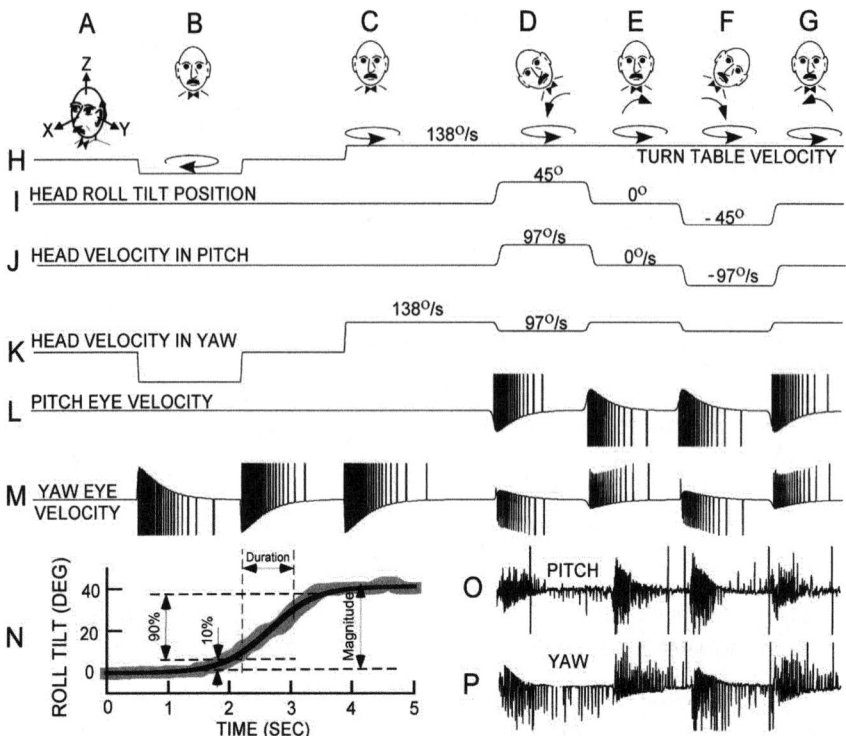

FIGURE 1. (**A**) Coordinate system; (**B–G**) head positions used in the experimental paradigms; (**H**) turntable velocity, which in this study was 138°/s, first to the subject's right and then to the left; (**I**) head roll tilt position recording. The head was tilted 45° left, center, and 45° right. (**J, K**) Head velocities in pitch (**J**) and yaw (**K**) generated by the head position changes in **D–G**. (**L, M**) Model simulations of eye velocities in pitch (**L**) and yaw (**M**). (**N**) Parameters of mean head roll tilt obtained by fitting the head-movement data by a sigmoidal function. (**O, P**) Eye velocities in pitch (**O**) and yaw (**P**) from one subject during the four head roll tilts made while rotating.

veillance camera was used to monitor the subjects and chair operation throughout the experiment.

Coordinate Frame

Head coordinates were defined by a right-hand rule (FIG. 1A). The +Z (yaw) axis was upward, the +Y (pitch) axis was along the interaural axis to the left, and the +X (roll) axis was along the forward nasooccipital axis. Horizontal and vertical positions of the right eye were recorded by videooculography (ISCAN) at 60 Hz. Subjects viewed targets that subtended visual angles of ±20° horizontally and 15° upward from the midposition for calibration. In the recordings, eye position and slow phase eye velocities to the left and down are positive.

Test Protocol

The test paradigm is shown in FIGURE 1B–G. Subjects were rotated in darkness from 0°/s to 138°/s with an angular acceleration of 180°/s² (FIG. 1B, H). This generated perrotatory horizontal nystagmus. When the perrotatory nystagmus had declined close to zero, the chair was stopped, producing postrotatory nystagmus, which was used to establish baseline measurements of the gain and time constant of the horizontal aVOR. The chair then was rotated in the opposite direction (FIG. 1C). After the nystagmus elicited by this rotation had dissipated, subjects were instructed to tilt their head (FIG. 1D) and hold it there for as long as horizontal and vertical nystagmus was present, usually for approximately 10–40 s. The head subsequently was returned to the upright position (FIG. 1E), tilted to the left (FIG. 1F), and returned to the upright position again (FIG. 1G). In each instance, the subjects held their head in position until the operator determined that the nystagmus had completely disappeared. They then were instructed to move to a new position. Subjects followed this sequence of head movement until they were no longer able to continue. The rotatory chair then was stopped, producing postrotatory horizontal nystagmus in an upright position.

Measures of Motion Sickness

Dizziness and nausea were precipitated immediately by head tilt while rotating but generally subsided to a stable level within 30 s. The level of motion sickness 10–30 s after head movement was scaled from 1 to 20.[25,26] In brief, 1 was no reaction, 10 was a moderate gastrointestinal reaction and dizziness, and 20 was a sense of being about to vomit or becoming too dizzy to continue. The endpoint of the test was either a score of 20 or after the subjects had made 50 head movements. When an endpoint was reached, the chair was returned to rest with the head upright. All 16 subjects who formed the database for this study completed both series of tests.

Analysis of Head and Eye Movements

The stimulus to the semicircular canals is shown in head coordinates in FIGURE 1H–K for the head tilts to and away from the axis of rotation. With the subjects rotating around a vertical axis at 138°/s to the left (+Z in space coordinates), yaw head velocity decreased when the head was tilted away from the axis of rotation (FIG. 1D, F) and pitch head velocity increased (FIG. 1J, K), according to the cosine and sine of the angle of head tilt, respectively. For a head tilt of 45° (FIG. 1D), pitch head velocity increased by 97°/s in the downward direction (+Y in head coordinates) and decreased 41°/s along the yaw axis (–Z in head coordinates). The stimulus velocity vector was –41°/s in yaw and 97°/s in pitch, causing a stimulus vector of –41, 97°/s in head coordinates, which can be represented in polar coordinates with a magnitude and angle of 105°/s, 113°. The angle of 113° is the location of the stimulus velocity vector relative to the head yaw axis. With the head tilted 45°, the vector in spatial coordinates can be given in polar form as 105°/s, 67°, representing a tilt of the stimulus vector of 67° relative to the spatial vertical axis. Similarly, when the head was tilted from lateral positions to the upright position (FIG. 1E, G), yaw head velocity increased by 41°/s, whereas pitch decreased by 97°/s (FIG. 1J, K), giving a velocity vector of 41, −97°/s, which is 105°/s, −67° in polar coordinates. Because the head was upright, the angle of the stimulus velocity was 67° relative to the spatial vertical, but was the mirror image of that when the head was tilted.

To predict the expected eye velocities from these head movements, we determined the trajectory of eye velocity after each head tilt from plots of yaw versus pitch eye velocity. The trajectory is dependent on the initial eye-velocity vector as well as the eigenvalues (inverse of time constants) and yaw eigenvector of velocity storage.[46–48] To estimate this change in head velocity, we measured the roll movements of the head during the experiments and fit them with a sigmoidal function (FIG. 1N; see Dai et al.[37] for the equation). A three-dimensional model of the aVOR[49] then was utilized to predict the expected eye velocities in pitch and yaw in response to the roll tilt of the head in the rotating frame (FIG. 1L, M). The duration of the roll movement, D, was defined as the time that it took for the head to go from 10% to 90% of its amplitude (FIG. 1N).

The sigmoidal fit to a representative head movement with a Marquardt algorithm, shown in FIGURE 1N, was used as the roll input to the model and generated the horizontal and vertical head and eye velocities shown in FIGURE 1L and M, which were similar to the actual eye velocities (FIG. 1O, P). Using the predicted pitch and yaw head velocities for a head roll tilt with the profile in FIG. 1N, we found that the peak acceleration of the head in pitch was approximately 56°/s^2. The angle of head roll tilt varied from 35°, corresponding to a pitch-yaw stimulus velocity expressed in spatial polar coordinates of 83°/s, 72° to 70°, corresponding to a pitch-yaw head velocity of 158°/s, 55°. The stimulus velocity varied considerably over this range of tilts. Approximately 85% of 2,780 analyzed head movements fell in a range of 40° (94°/s, 70°) to 50° (116°/s, 65°), in which the maximum variation in the stimulus pitch-yaw head velocity magnitude and angle relative to gravity was 22°/s and 5°. To promote comparison of the trajectory of eye-velocity axis induced by head tilt, we analyzed only those eye movements associated with head roll tilts between 40° and 50° in the first and second test of Series I and the final test of Series II. These corresponded to most of the active head movements. Over this range, the average angle of head roll tilt was close to 45°, and all of the stimulus velocities could be treated as being roughly equivalent.

Analysis of the Axis of Eye Velocity

Eye positions in pitch and yaw recorded in a head frame were differentiated to obtain pitch and yaw eye velocities. To determine the axis of eye velocity for gravity, we took slow phase velocities from the point at which the head had reached 90% of its final position (FIG. 1N) to where the velocity of the horizontal nystagmus approached zero; the yaw eye velocity (ordinate) then was plotted against pitch eye velocity (abscissa) to form a trajectory of the axis of eye velocity. The magnitude of eye velocity was calculated from the square root of the sum of squares of horizontal and vertical eye velocities from the initial 1–2 s of the data. Gains of pitch and yaw eye velocities were obtained by dividing the averaged peak eye velocity by the stimulus velocities in head pitch and yaw, respectively. The angle of the axis of eye velocity for gravity was the cotangent of the pitch eye velocity divided by yaw eye velocity. The value of the initial deviation was averaged over 1–2 s from the beginning of the trajectory. The slope of the trajectory was taken from linear fits to the point at which the pitch eye velocity was close to zero.

Analysis of VOR Gain and Time Constant

Horizontal VOR gains and time constants were determined from the per- and postrotatory nystagmus induced by steps of velocity when the subject was upright before any roll head movements were made. The gain of the horizontal VOR was the ratio of peak eye velocity relative to the head stimulus velocity in yaw (138°/s). The central horizontal vestibular time constant was extracted from fits of slow phase eye velocity using the two time constant model of velocity storage.[50] The gains and time constants of vertical nystagmus were calculated from the 45° head position from the first three to five head movements into the side-down position. Vertical gains were determined from the peak vertical eye velocity, obtained immediately after head had stopped tilting, divided by the head stimulus velocity in pitch, for example, 97°/s for a tilt of 45°.

RESULTS

Head Movements and General Subjective Sensation

The average roll tilt of the head for the 2,780 head movements made by the 16 subjects while rotating about a spatial vertical axis was 44.7° ± 6.2°, and the average time for the head tilt was 1.9 ± 0.9 s. Promethazine had no effect on the amplitude, direction, or velocity of the head movements. There were also individual differences in the subjective spatial disorientation and motion sickness that were produced by

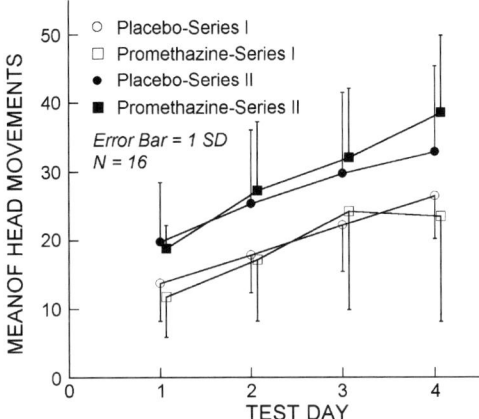

FIGURE 2. Average number of head movements made in test Series I and II for placebo (*circles*) and promethazine groups (*squares*). The number of head movements made in successive sessions increased progressively, and the number of head movements made in Series II were significantly greater than that made in Series I. There was no difference of number of head movements made between the two groups. The *vertical bars* represent one SD.

tilting the head while rotating. In general, the dizziness and vertigo peaked immediately after a head tilt and then subsided to a stable level in from several seconds to approximately 30 s. By the last test of Series II, both the placebo and promethazine group had habituated to the stimulus, and several subjects made 50 head movements with a motion sickness score of only 4 (slight malaise). Therefore, in agreement with previous studies, there was substantial habituation of motion sickness during the repeated trials.

Promethazine and the Number of Head Movements

Subjects in each group adapted over time and were able to make more head movements before becoming nauseated. There was no statistical difference between the placebo and promethazine groups in either series of tests (FIG. 2). Thus, promethazine neither interfered with nor hastened the adaptation, nor was there a protective effect of the drug on the symptoms produced by the provocative vestibular stimuli.

Yaw aVOR Gains and Time Constants

Consistent with previous data from the monkey,[28] yaw aVOR gains did not change over the course of the experiments. However, there was a highly significant reduction in time constant for each series and for both series together ($P < 0.0001$). Because there was no statistical difference between the changes in time constants of the horizontal aVOR between promethazine and placebo groups, these changes were grouped and are shown together in FIGURE 3. The overall reduction in time constant

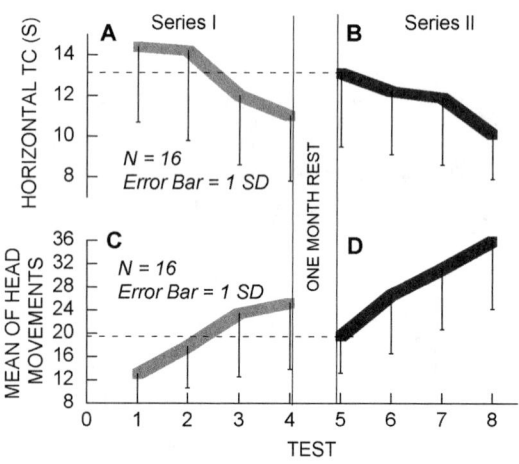

FIGURE 3. Yaw time constants (horizontal TC; *top two graphs*) and the number of head movements (*bottom two graphs*) made in the two series of tests. In each test, the decrease in time constant over time was mirrored by an increase in the number of head movements. The *dashed lines* show the level of retention both of the reduction in horizontal time constant and of the increase in number of head movements made by the subjects in the first test of Series II. The *vertical bars* represent one SD.

was 29%. The horizontal time constant was closely correlated with the number of head movements made on each test day by a strong inverse relationship. Over the entire sequence, a decrease of each second in time constant was associated with an increase of roughly five head movements.

Vertical aVOR Gains and Time Constants

The mean vertical gain in Series I was 0.61 ± 0.06, slightly less than a previously reported gain of 0.67,[51] but not significantly different from the gain of 0.59 ± 0.07 in Series II. As for the yaw component, there was a significant reduction (32%; $P = 0.001$) in the average vertical time constants, which went from 5.8 ± 0.8 s on day 2 of Series I to 3.8 ± 0.3 s on day 4 of Series II. The percentage of reduction in the vertical time constant was comparable to the percentage of decrease in the horizontal

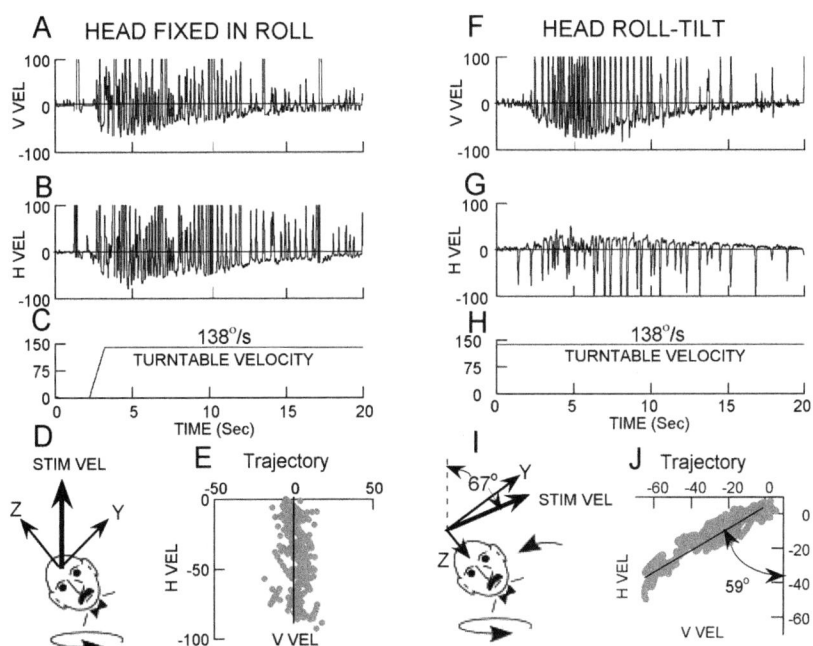

FIGURE 4. Comparison of the axis trajectory of eye velocity in space for a rotation with a fixed head in roll (**A–E**) and for a head roll tilt during the rotation (**F–J**). From *top to bottom* are shown pitch (V VEL; **A, F**) and yaw (H VEL; **B, G**) eye velocity in head coordinates, turntable velocity (**C, H**), head stimulus velocity in pitch (Y) and yaw (Z) and the sum (STIM VEL; **D, I**), as well as the axis trajectory of eye velocity in space (trajectory; **E, J**). Eye velocities are in °/s. (**A**) When the head was fixed in roll 45° before and during rotation (**A–E**), the sum of stimulus velocities was along gravity as was the trajectory of eye velocity. The subjects reported neither motion sickness nor disorientation to this stimulus. When the head was roll tilted 45° during rotation (**F–J**), the sum of the stimulus velocities was away from gravity (67°) as was the trajectory (59°), and the subject reported both motion sickness and disorientation. Note that the linear fit of the trajectory declined close to the origin, so that it could be approximately used as the average axis of eye velocity.

time constant. The vertical time constant of 5.8 s was shorter than the time constant of the vertical VOR (7.3 s) reported by Tweed *et al.*[52] This is likely because the head was tilted only 45° in our study, whereas subjects were in 90° side-down positions in the study of Tweed *et al.* The latter aligns the axis of eye velocity with the spatial vertical, maximizing the vertical VOR time constant.[53,54]

Axis of Eye Velocity and Motion Sickness

To demonstrate the effect of active and passive head position on the eye velocities and the motion sickness that were induced, we compared the axis of eye velocity during perrotatory nystagmus in six subjects in two conditions: with the head fixed 45° in roll (FIG. 4A–E) and with the head actively roll-tilted 45° during rotation FIG. 4F–I). With the head fixed during the perrotatory stimulus, the axis of eye velocity was along the spatial vertical (FIG. 4D), and approximately equal eye velocities were induced in head coordinates in pitch and yaw (FIG. 4A, B). Eye velocity in space started at approximately 80°/s and fell continuously toward zero. The eye-velocity trajectory in space, fitted with a least squares line, paralleled the spatial vertical along gravity and went through the origin of the coordinate frame, i.e., the spatial vertical axis (FIG. 4E). Thus, it was an eigenvector of velocity storage.[47] In this head-fixed paradigm, subjects accurately reported that they had been rotated around the spatial vertical and had no dizziness, disorientation, or nausea.

In contrast, when subjects roll-tilted their heads actively to the right during constant velocity rotation to the same final 45° position (FIG. 4I), the sum of the stimulus vectors in pitch (Y) and yaw (Z) was quite different, deviating 67° from gravity (FIG. 4J). In response, the induced horizontal eye velocity was reversed (FIG. 4G) relative to the horizontal eye velocity when the head was fixed (FIG. 4B). This caused a reversal of the velocity along the Z-axis of the head, and the eye-velocity trajectory was deviated from gravity (FIG. 4J). The initial axis of eye velocity in space was deviated 59° from the spatial vertical (FIG. 4J), and the trajectory in space declined along an approximately straight path in space toward the origin, close to the direction of the stimulus velocity. In response, all six subjects reported substantial disorientation and motion sickness during this trial. Because the eye-velocity vector approximately followed the stimulus velocity vector in this trial, we inferred that it was not the deviation of the axis of eye velocity from the axis of the stimulus that had induced the disorientation, but rather the deviation of the axis of eye velocity from gravity.

It was a general finding in all 16 subjects that head movements made from the left lateral position to the upright position during leftward rotation (FIG. 1G) or from the right lateral position to the upright position during rightward rotation caused much more dizziness, disorientation, and nausea than any of the other head tilts. The period of the most intense dizziness and nausea only lasted for approximately 3–10 s. However, the symptoms associated with these head movements often exceeded a motion sickness scale of 20 during that period, as reported by the subjects after the peak nausea and disorientation had subsided. The subjects did not report the same extent of dizziness, disorientation, or nausea from any of the other head maneuvers. The disparity in subjective sensations produced by the different head maneuvers became less prominent with further testing, and in the last several tests, most of the subjects did not differentiate in the level of dizziness between the different head tilts.

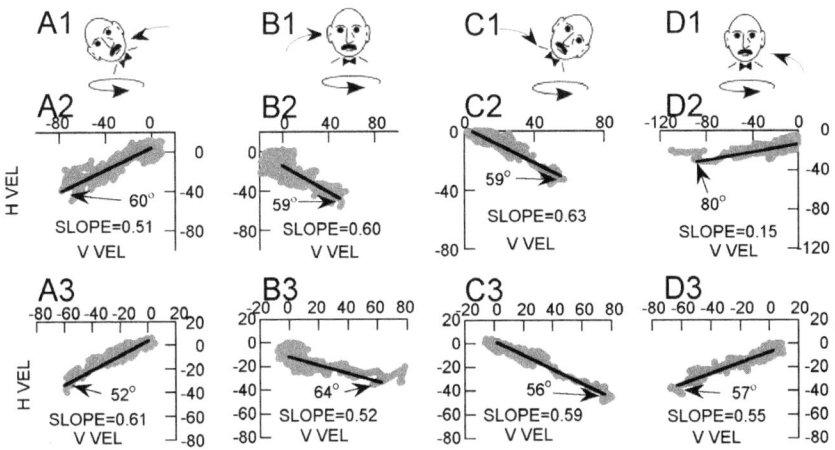

FIGURE 5. Comparison of the trajectories of the axes of eye velocity elicited by four different head roll tilts during rotation in the first test of Series I (**A2, B2, C2, D2**) and from the final test of Series II (**A3, B3, C3, D3**). Both recordings were from the same subject. The head tilts and directions of rotation are shown in **A1, B1, C1**, and **D1**. The heavy lines in **A2–D3** indicate a linear fit of the trajectory plot. The slopes of the trajectories for gravity are given below each trajectory plot. The numbers with the arrows show the angle of the initial axis of eye velocity from gravity. In **D2**, the trajectory had an initial angle of 80° and was deviated the farthest from gravity (trajectory slope: 0.15). The subject experienced distinctly more dizziness in this than the other head roll tilts in tests 1 and 2 of Series I. **A3–D3** show a comparison of the trajectories of the eye-velocity axes from head roll tilts during rotation in the last test of Series II for the same subject as that shown in **A2–D2**. Note that in **D3** the trajectory did not deviate as much as in **D2** and had approximately the same angle as the other head tilts (**A3–C3**). The subject also did not sense a distinct difference in the dizziness generated by this head tilt, as in the first test. The subject was able to make only 16 head tilts in the first test but could make 33 head movements in the final test.

The intense subjective sensations of motion sickness associated with the various head tilts were compared to the axes of eye velocity associated with those tilts. There was no difference in the rate or amplitude of head movement in the head tilts made in Tests 1, 2, and 8. Head tilts in Tests 1 and 2 of about 45° from the upright to the right lateral position to the upright and from the upright to the left lateral position (FIG. 5A1, B1, C1) were associated with tilts of the initial eye-velocity vector of 60°, 59°, and 59° away from gravity, respectively (FIG. 5A2, B2, C2), and the slopes of the trajectories of the induced nystagmus were similar (0.51, 0.60, and 0.63). The averaged initial deviations of eye-velocity axis and the slopes of the trajectories of the induced nystagmus were similar (0.51, 0.60, and 0.63). The averaged initial deviations of eye velocity axis and the slopes of the trajectories for these three tilts were also approximately the same.

In contrast, a tilt from the left lateral position to the upright during rotation to the left in the first tests (FIG. 5D1) was associated with a larger deviation of the eye velocity vector from the upright (80°; FIG. 5D2) and a smaller slope of the eye velocity trajectory (0.15). This was a general phenomenon and the averaged initial deviations of the eye velocity axes from gravity in 13 subjects were 79.5 ± 6.5° slopes of 0.14 ± 0.25, both of which were significantly different from the values for the other head tilts. The reason for the large eye-velocity axis shift away from gravity produced by this head movement was that the horizontal component only reached 14°/s in both head and spatial coordinates, while the vertical component was 100°/s. Consequently, the gain of horizontal velocity was reduced, from an average value of 0.74 to 0.26, as opposed to an increase in the vertical gain from 0.61 to 0.71.

As the subjects became more adapted by repetitive testing, the average deviation of the eye-velocity vectors from gravity decreased so that the axis of eye velocity was not significantly different in any of the head tilts. Associated with this, subjects complained less when making similar head movements in the last test. Head tilts of approximately 45° in Test 8 for a similar set of movements as in Tests 1 and 2 were associated with tilts of the initial eye-velocity vector away from gravity of 52°, 64°, 56°, and 57°, respectively (FIG. 5A3, B3, C3, D3), and the slopes of the trajectories of the induced nystagmus were also not different (0.61, 0.52, 0.59, and 0.55). Reflecting these data, by Test 8, there was no difference in the average deviation of the axis of eye velocity from gravity between the various tilts (55.3 ± 3.9°; 54.6 ± 7.2°; 55.2 ± 5.6°; 57.4 ± 5.5°), and the slopes were also not different for these head tilts (0.54 ± 0.91; 0.62 ± 0.17; 0.57 ± 0.13; 0.52 ± 0.19). Thus, the head movement from the side to the upright position in the direction of rotation did not induce different eye velocities from the other head tilts in the last test, and there was no difference in the dizziness and nausea in any of these conditions. These findings support the hypothesis that the trials associated with the largest tilts of the eye-velocity trajectories from gravity were associated with the greatest disorientation, dizziness, and nausea.

We considered whether promethazine had affected the initial values of the axis of eye velocity. There was no difference in the average values of the axis of eye rotation or slopes in any of the tests for the groups receiving promethazine or placebo. Promethazine also did not alter either the initial velocity or the slope of the trajectory of eye velocity associated with these tests, nor did it affect the vertigo.

DISCUSSION

Data in this study support the hypothesis that there is an important link between motion sickness and velocity storage,[29] the process in the vestibular system that is responsible for the dominant time course of the eye velocity response and its spatial orientation.[46,47,49] Motion sickness evoked by a provocative vestibular stimulus, rolling the head while rotating (RWR), habituated on repeated testing in close association with a reduction in the dominant time constant of the aVOR, that is, with habituation of velocity storage.[28] In addition, the nausea, disorientation, and dizziness, that is, the motion sickness produced by RWR, were greatest in conditions in which the eye-velocity trajectory deviated farthest from the spatial upright position. From this, we propose that the motion sickness elicited by rolling the head while rotating is related to the difference between the yaw axis eigenvector of velocity storage, which is close to the spatial vertical, and the trajectory of the induced eye velocity after the head tilt.

Habituation of Head-Movement–Induced Motion Sickness, aVOR Time Constants, and Promethazine

The data show that promethazine did not significantly reduce the nausea and dizziness provoked by RWR and that both drug and placebo groups adapted to the test situation at the same rate. Promethazine has found extensive use in orbital space flight, because it is effective in reducing motion sickness and vertigo after entry into microgravity.[55–57] If promethazine had reduced the nausea associated with RWR, as reported under somewhat different conditions,[24] subjects might have been able to make more head movements that would promote habituation. Contrary to our expectations, however, both the promethazine and placebo groups habituated at the same rate, and there was a progressive reduction in motion sickness over time due to repeated testing, as indicated by the increased number of roll head movements that subjects were able to make for each day of the test. This habituation occurred regardless of whether subjects had received promethazine or placebo, and the rate of habituation was the same with or without the drug. Thus, promethazine neither reduced the nausea associated with roll while rotating nor affected habituation to this nauseogenic vestibular stimulus.

Lackner and Graybiel[24] found a mild protective effect of promethazine in subjects who made more than 800 movements in a test session. The number of head movements made by subjects in their study far exceeded the 12–40 head movements made on average in the present series before reaching a full level of nausea. This difference is likely due to differences in methodology; their subjects made paced head movements every 2 s, which is well within the time constant of the cupula (4 s[50,58,59]), whereas our subjects held their heads stationary in position for up to 1 min after each head movement. The 2-s paced head movements would have activated predominantly direct aVOR pathways[29] and would not activate velocity storage. In contrast, our subjects had a full period of per- and/or postrotatory nystagmus after each head movement. Consequently, velocity storage was fully excited each time the head was moved. On the basis of these results, we propose that activation of velocity storage is the critical element in activation of the neural mechanisms for motion sickness and that the direct pathways are unlikely to have much input.

There is considerable indirect evidence to support a relation between susceptibility to motion sickness and the time constant of velocity storage, but to our knowledge this is the first direct demonstration of such a link. As shown by our data, if subjects were compared with themselves, susceptibility to motion sickness decreased as the vestibular time constant got shorter with repeated exposure to motion stimuli. These results correspond well to the data of Clément et al.[15] in which the duration of horizontal nystagmus was reduced by 20–30% after vestibular training of cosmonauts.

Relation of the Axis of Eye Velocity with regard to Gravity to Induction of Motion Sickness

A key outcome of this study was that the maximal vertigo and disorientation occurred after a head movement that induced an eye-velocity trajectory that was deviated maximally from the spatial vertical. Presumably, the sense of dizziness associated with this was caused by the perception that the subject was pitching forward, which induced a sense of falling for a critical time. The farther the axis of rotation was from the spatial vertical and the longer it stayed deviated, the more disturbing the sense of dizziness and disorientation was and the greater the nausea, that is, the level of motion sickness. Thus, the subjective symptoms could be related to the angular displacement of the average eye-velocity trajectory from the spatial vertical: the greater the deviation of the eye-velocity trajectory from the spatial vertical, the more severe the vertigo.

Utilizing OKN, OKAN, and vestibular nystagmus, it has been shown that velocity storage orients eye velocity toward the spatial vertical or GIA.[47,48,60,61] By altering vestibular and OKAN time constants, velocity storage also codes temporal aspects of the orientation response.[29,43,47,62] The trajectory of the eye velocity embodies both aspects. It contains information about the initial eye-velocity vector relative to the spatial vertical and the angle of the vector at various points along its trajectory. It also contains temporal information about how fast the trajectory reaches the eigenvector of velocity storage, which is the internal representation of the spatial vertical. Thus, when one plots the trajectory of the eye-velocity decay after vestibular stimulation in state space, the spatial aspects are quite obvious, but the temporal aspects of the response are implicit and are measures of how long it takes a trajectory to reach the eigenvector, which is governed by the time constants of the various components of the response.[47] A shallower trajectory indicates that more time was spent with a stronger pitch than yaw component, consistent with the idea that the amount of time spent from the eigenvector during nystagmus, the more likely it is for the stimulus to produce motion sickness.

From this, we propose that a weighted average of the factors inherent in the trajectory is a crucial metric for determining the degree of nausea and vertigo during the cross-coupled vestibular stimulation and that the degree and length of time that the eye-velocity trajectory is removed from the spatial vertical and the strength of stimulation determine the intensity of the vertigo and nausea. Promethazine had very little effect on these properties, but this could be expected, because promethazine has no effect on either vestibular gain or time constant.

There is much indirect evidence that supports this theoretic formulation. Rotation about a vertical axis with the head fixed does not induce motion sickness (FIG. 4A–E).[34,63] On the other hand, many well-known stimuli produce stimulus vectors that are not aligned with gravity, and uniformly these induce motion sickness and habituation of the aVOR time constant. These include tests of head movement during circularvection induced by optokinetic stimulation,[64] caloric stimulation, in which eye velocities are induced about a spatial-horizontal axis while subjects are supine, off-vertical axis rotation, where compensatory eye velocity is generated around an axis tilted from gravity,[34,65] and head-to-heel rotation.[52] Data in this report are consistent with this formulation.

Findings in orbital and parabolic flight are particularly significant in evaluating whether the orientation properties of velocity storage have a critical role in producing nausea associated with head movements in a rotating frame. Astronauts performed serial pitch head movements while rotating around a yaw axis in the M131 experiment during the Skylab flights.[66] Remarkably, several days after injection into microgravity, the astronauts were unaffected by the same stimulus in space that had produced severe disorientation, vertigo, and nausea on Earth. We interpret this as being caused by the absence of a gravitational vector in microgravity, which could not be compared with the axis of eye velocity, precluding a disparity that triggered motion sickness. The occurrence of "dumping" of velocity storage was further evaluated during parabolic[67] and orbital space flight.[68,69] Postrotatory nystagmus slow phase velocity also was not "dumped" by pitch head movements in the lack of the gravitational field in parabolic or orbital flight.[68]

The nodulus and uvula have been shown to control the orientation vectors and time constants of velocity storage,[43,45] as well as habituation of the time constants,[28,41,70] all of which are critical factors in the production of motion sickness. We further postulate that the nodulus and uvula play an important role in the production of motion sickness. Consistent with this hypothesis, motion sickness was reduced or could no longer be elicited in highly susceptible dogs after removal of the nodulus and uvula.[38–40] Whether the nodulus and uvula couple directly to the autonomic system or indirectly through pathways in the vestibular nuclei is unknown. Projections from the nodulus and uvula to posterior portions of the vestibular nuclei,[71] which, in turn, project to the autonomic system, could provide the link between the two.[6,72]

Our hypothesis also can be related to the most widely accepted theory of motion sickness, the sensory rearrangement theory. Reason and Brand[2] proposed that motion sickness is induced as a result of a sensory rearrangement in which the motion signals transmitted by the eyes, the vestibular system, and nonvestibular proprioceptors are at variance with one another or with what is expected from previous experience. On the basis of a subjective vertical conflict model developed by Oman,[4] Bles[36] proposed that motion sickness is produced when the sensed vertical is at variance with the subjective vertical. Our results, which tie motion sickness to the yaw axis orientation vector, the associated time constants, and the trajectory of eye velocity, extend the notion that the subjective vertical conflict is the major source of motions sickness by identifying the central mechanisms responsible for producing the imbalance and by adding a temporal component. This links motion sickness to a specific vestibular mechanism, which is also a focus for integrating visual, vestibular, and proprioceptive information regarding motion.[47,73] How linear motion might contribute to motion sickness is currently unknown to us.

In summary, we have demonstrated that moderate doses of promethazine, that is, 25 mg by the oral route, had no effect on relieving the motion sickness caused by roll head movements during constant velocity rotation, nor did the drug affect habituation. There was concurrent reduction in aVOR time constants with progressive habituation of motion sickness, suggesting that velocity storage is closely linked to the production of motion sickness. We propose that there is a critical interaction between velocity storage and spatial orientation that is responsible for producing motion sickness, and that the spatial parameters related to deviation of the axis of eye velocity from gravity, the strength of the stimulus, and the temporal parameters of the trajectory of eye velocity toward the eigenvector and to the GIA are responsible for the generation of motion sickness in response to cross-coupled vestibular stimuli.

ACKNOWLEDGMENTS

The authors are grateful to the subjects for their dedication and endurance throughout the experiments. Thanks are also extended to Drs. Laurence Young and

Heiko Hecht of MIT for sharing their expertise on production and coding of motion sickness. This work was supported by National Space Biomedical Research Institute grants NCC 9–58–25 (M.D.) and NCC9–58 (T.R.), and National Institutes of Health grants DC05222 (T.R.), DC03284 (B.C.), DC05204 (B.C.), and EY01867.

REFERENCES

1. BALABAN, C.D. & R.G. JACOB. 2001. Background and history of the interface between anxiety and vertigo. J. Anxiety Disord. **15:** 27–51.
2. REASON, J.T. & J.J. BRAND. 1975. Motion Sickness. Academic Press. London.
3. TRIESMAN, M. 1977. Motion sickness: an evolutionary hypothesis. Science **197:** 493–495.
4. OMAN, C.M. 1982. A heuristic mathematical model for the dynamics of sensory conflict and motion sickness. Acta Otolaryngol. (Suppl.) **392:** 4–44.
5. MONEY, K.E. 1972. Motion sickness. Physiol. Rev. **50:** 1–39.
6. YATES, B.J., A.D. MILLER & J.D. LUCOT. 1998. Physiological basis and pharmacology of motion sickness: an update. Brain Res. Bull. **47:** 395–406.
7. BLES, W., J.E. BOS, B. DE GRAAF, et al. 1998. Motion sickness: only one provocative conflict? Brain Res. Bull. **47:** 481–487.
8. PURKINJE, J.E. 1820. Beiträge zur näheren Kenntnis des Schwindels aus heutognostischen Daten. Med. J.B. (Wien) **6:** 79–125.
9. GRAYBIEL, A., B. CLARK & J.J. ZARRIELLO. 1960. Observations of human subjects living in a "slow rotation room" for periods of two days. Arch. Neurol. **3:** 55–73.
10. MILLER, E.F. & A. GRAYBIEL. 1973. Experiment M-131—human vestibular function. Aerosp. Med. **44:** 593–608.
11. GUEDRY, F.E. 1974. Psychophysics of vestibular sensation. In Handbook of Sensory Physiology. H.H. Kornhuber, Ed.: 3–154. Springer Verlag. Berlin, Heidelberg, New York.
12. YOUNG, L.R. 1983. Perception of the body in space: mechanisms. In Handbook of Physiology. In The Nervous System III. J.M. Brookhart, V.B. Mountcastle, and H.W. H. W. Magoun, Eds.: 1023–1066. American Physiological Society. Bethesda, MD.
13. GUEDRY, F.E., A.R. RUPERT & M.F. RESCHKE. 1998. Motion sickness and development of synergy within the spatial orientation system. A hypothetical unifying concept. Brain Res. Bull. **47:** 475–480.
14. YOUNG, L.R. 1999. Artificial gravity consideration for a Mars exploration mission. Ann. N.Y. Acad. Sci. **871:** 367–378.
15. CLÉMENT, G., O. DEGUINE, M. PARANT, et al. 2001. Effects of cosmonaut vestibular training on vestibular function prior to spaceflight. Eur. J. Appl. Physiol. **85:** 539–545.
16. SCHUBERG, G. 1932. Die physiologischen Auswirkungen der Coriolisbeschleunigungen bei Flugzeugsteuerung. Arch. Ohr. Nas. Heilk. **30:** 595–604.
17. GRAYBIEL, A., C.W. WOOD, E.F. MILLER, et al. 1968. Diagnostic criteria for grading the severity of acute motion sickness. Aerosp. Med. **39:** 4453–4455.
18. GUEDRY, F.E. & A.J. BENSON. 1978. Coriolis cross-coupling effects: disorienting and nauseogenic or not? Aviat. Space Environ. Med. **49:** 29–35.
19. LACKNER, J.R. & A. GRAYBIEL. 1980. Elicitation of motion sickness by head movements in the microgravity phase of parabolic flight maneuvers. Aviat. Space Environ. Med. **55:** 513–520.
20. FITGER, C. & T. BRANDT. 1982. Posturography of ataxia induced by Coriolis and Purkinje effects. Aviat. Space Environ. Med. **53:** 153–161.
21. GUEDRY, F.E., A. GRAYBIEL & W.E. COLLINS. 1962. Reduction of nystagmus and disorientation in human subjects. Aerosp. Med. **33:** 1356–1360.
22. GUEDRY, F.E., W.E. COLLINS & A. GRAYBIEL. 1964. Vestibular habituation during repetitive complex stimulation: a study of transfer effects. J. Appl. Physiol. **19:** 1005–1015.
23. GUEDRY, F.E. 1965. Habituation to complex vestibular stimulation in man: transfer and retention of effects from twelve days of rotation at 10 rpm. Percept. Mot. Skills. **21:** 459–481.

24. LACKNER, J.R. & A. GRAYBIEL. 1994. Use of promethazine to hasten adaptation to provocative motion. J. Clin. Pharmacol. **34:** 644–648.
25. HECHT, H., J. KAVELAARS, C.C. CHEUNG, et al. 2001. Orientation illusions and heart-rate changes during short-radius centrifugation. J. Vestib. Res. **11:** 115–127.
26. YOUNG, L.R., H. HECHT, L. LYNE, et al. 2001. Artificial gravity: head movements during short-radius centrifugation. Acta Astronaut. **49:** 215–226.
27. HOWARD, I.P. & W.B. TEMPLETON. 1966. Human Spatial Orientation. Wiley. New York.
28. COHEN, H., B. COHEN, T. RAPHAN, et al. 1992. Habituation and adaptation of the vestibulo-ocular reflex: a model of differential control by the vestibulo-cerebellum. Exp. Brain Res. **90:** 526–538.
29. RAPHAN, T., V. MATSUO & B. COHEN. 1979. Velocity storage in the vestibulo-ocular reflex arc (VOR). Exp. Brain Res. **35:** 229–248.
30. ARAI, Y., S.B. YAKUSHIN, J.-I. SUZUKI, et al. 2002. Spatial orientation of caloric nystagmus in canal plugged monkeys. J. Neurophysiol. **88:** 914–928.
31. MCCABE, B.E. 1960. Vestibular suppression in figure skaters. Trans. Am. Acad. Ophthalmol. Otol. **64:** 264–268.
32. DAVIS, J.R., J.M. VANDERPLOEG, P.A. SANTY, et al. 1988. Space motion sickness during 24 flights of the space shuttle. Aviat. Space Environ. Med. **59:** 1185–1189.
33. DIZIO, P. & J.R. LACKNER. 1991. Motion sickness susceptibility in parabolic flight and velocity storage activity. Aviat. Space Environ. Med. **62:** 300–307.
34. BOS, J.E., W. BLES & B. DE GRAAF. 2002. Eye movements to yaw, pitch, and roll about vertical and horizontal axes: adaptation and motion sickness. Aviat. Space Environ. Med. **73:** 436–444.
35. QUARCK, G., O. ETARD, M. OREEL, et al. 2000. Motion sickness occurrence does not correlate with nystagmus characteristics. Neurosci. Lett. **287:** 49–52.
36. BLES, W. 1988. Coriolis effects and motion sickness modeling. Brain Res. Bull. **47:** 543–549.
37. DAI, M.J., M. KUNIN, T. RAPHAN & B. COHEN. 2003. The relation of motion sickness to the spatial-temporal properties of velocity storage. Exp. Brain Res. May 29 [Epub ahead of print].
38. BARD, P. 1945. Committee on aviation medicine. National Research Council. Washington, DC.
39. TYLER, D.B. & P. BARD. 1949. Motion sickness. Physiol. Rev. **29:** 311–369.
40. WANG, S.C. & H.I. CHINN. 1956. Experimental motion sickness in dogs. Importance of labyrinth and vestibular cerebellum. Am. J. Physiol. **185:** 617–623.
41. WAESPE, W., B. COHEN & T. RAPHAN. 1985. Dynamic modification of the vestibulo-ocular reflex by the nodulus and uvula. Science **228:** 199–201.
42. SOLOMON, D. & B. COHEN. 1994. Stimulation of the nodulus and uvula discharges velocity storage in the vestibulo-ocular reflex. Exp. Brain Res. **102:** 57–68.
43. WEARNE, S., T. RAPHAN & B. COHEN. 1998. Control of spatial orientation of the angular vestibuloocular reflex by the nodulus and uvula. J. Neurophysiol. **79:** 2690–2715.
44. SHELIGA, B.M., S.B. YAKUSHIN, A. SILVERS, et al. 1999. Control of spatial orientation of the angular vestibulo-ocular reflex by the nodulus and uvula of the vestibulocerebellum. Ann. N.Y. Acad. Sci. **871:** 94–122.
45. COHEN, B., P. JOHN, S.B. YAKUSHIN, et al. 2002. The nodulus and uvula: source of cerebellar control of spatial orientation of the angular vestibulo-ocular reflex. Ann. N.Y. Acad. Sci. **978:** 28–45.
46. DAI, M., T. RAPHAN & B. COHEN. 1991. Spatial orientation of the vestibular system: dependence of optokinetic after nystagmus on gravity. J. Neurophysiol. **66:** 1422–1438.
47. RAPHAN, T. & D. STURM. 1991. Modelling the spatiotemporal organization of velocity storage in the vestibuloocular reflex by optokinetic studies. J. Neurophysiol. **66:** 1410–1420.
48. RAPHAN, T., M. DAI & B. COHEN. 1992. Spatial orientation of the vestibular system. Ann. N.Y. Acad. Sci. **656:** 140–157.
49. RAPHAN, T. & B. COHEN. 2002. The vestibulo-ocular reflex (VOR) in three dimensions. Exp. Brain Res. **145:** 1–27.
50. DAI, M., A. KLEIN, B. COHEN, et al. 1999. Model-based study of the human cupular time constant. J. Vestib. Res. **9:** 293–301.

51. TWEED, D., D. SIEVERING, H. MISSLISCH, *et al.* 1994. Rotational kinematics of the human vestibuloocular reflex I. Gain matrices. J. Neurophysiol. **72:** 2467–2479.
52. TWEED, D., M. FETTER, D. SIEVERING, *et al.* 1994. Rotational kinematics of the human vestibuloocular reflex II. Gain matrices. J. Neurophysiol. **72:** 2480–2489.
53. MATSUO, V. & B. COHEN. 1984. Vertical optokinetic nystagmus and vestibular nystagmus in the monkey: up-down asymmetry and effects of gravity. Exp. Brain Res. **53:** 197–216.
54. RAPHAN, T. & B. COHEN. 1988. Organizational principles of velocity storage in three dimensions: the effect of gravity on cross-coupling of optokinetic after-nystagmus. Ann. N.Y. Acad. Sci. **545:** 74–92.
55. GRAYBIEL, A. & J. KNEPTON. 1977. Evaluation of a new antinauseant drug for the prevention of motion sickness. Aviat. Space Environ. Med. **48:** 867–871.
56. GRAYBIEL, A. & J.R. LACKNER. 1987. Treatment of severe motion sickness with antimotion sickness drug injections. Aviat. Space Environ. Med. **58:** 773–776.
57. BAGIAN, J.P. & D.F. WARD. 1994. A retrospective study of promethazine and its failure to produce the expected incidence of sedation during space flight. J. Clin. Pharmacol. **34:** 649–651.
58. GOLDBERG, J.M. & C. FERNANDEZ. 1971. Physiology of peripheral neurons innervating semicircular canals of the squirrel monkey. I. Resting discharge and response to angular accelerations. J. Neurophysiol. **34:** 635–660.
59. BÜTTNER, U. & W. WAESPE. 1981. Vestibular nerve activity in the alert monkey during vestibular and optokinetic nystagmus. Exp. Brain Res. **41:** 310–315.
60. GIZZI, M., T. RAPHAN, S. RUDOLPH, *et al.* 1994. Orientation of human optokinetic nystagmus to gravity: a model based approach. Exp. Brain Res. **99:** 347–360.
61. RAPHAN, T., S. WEARNE & B. COHEN. 1996. Modeling the organization of the linear and angular vestibulo-ocular reflexes. Ann. N.Y. Acad. Sci. **781:** 348–363.
62. COHEN, B., V. MATSUO & T. RAPHAN. 1977. Quantitative analysis of the velocity characteristics of optokinetic nystagmus and optokinetic after-nystagmus. J. Physiol. (Lond.). **270:** 321–344.
63. PETERKA, R.J., F.O. BLACK & M.B. SCHOENHOFF. 1987. Optokinetic and vestibulo-ocular reflex responses to an unpredictable stimulus. Aviat. Space Environ. Med. **58:** A180–A185.
64. DE GRAAF, B., W. BLES & J.E. BOS. 1999. Roll motion stimuli: sensory conflict, perceptual weighting and motion sickness. Brain Res. Bull. **47:** 489–495.
65. BENSON, A.J. & M.A. BODIN. 1966. Interaction of linear and angular accelerations on vestibular receptors in man. Aerosp. Med. **37:** 144–154.
66. GRAYBIEL, A., E.F. MILLER & J.L. HOMICK. 1977. Experiment M-131. Human vestibular function. *In* Biomedical Results from Skylab. Section II. R.S. Johnston & L.F. Dietlein, Eds.: 74–103. US Government Printing Office (NASA SP-77). Washington, DC.
67. LACKNER, J.R. & A. GRAYBIEL. 1986. The effective intensity of Coriolis, cross-coupling stimulation is gravitoinertial force dependent: implications for space motion sickness. Aviat. Space Environ. Med. **57:** 229–235.
68. DIZIO, P. & J.R. LACKNER. 1988. The effects of gravitoinertial force level and head movements on post-rotational nystagmus and illusory after-rotation. Exp. Brain Res. **70:** 485–495.
69. OMAN, C.M. & M.D. BALKWILL. 1993. Horizontal angular VOR, nystagmus dumping, and sensation duration in Spacelab SLS-1 crewmembers. J. Vestib. Res. **3:** 315–330.
70. SINGLETON, G.T. 1967. Relationships of the cerebellar nodulus to vestibular function: a study of the effects of nodulectomy on habituation. Laryngoscope **77:** 1579–1620.
71. BARMACK, N.H., R.W. BAUGHMAN, F.P. ECKENSTEIN, *et al.* 1992. Secondary vestibular cholinergic projection to the cerebellum of rabbit and rat as revealed by choline acetyltransferase immunohistochemistry, retrograde and orthograde tracers. J. Comp. Neurol. **317:** 250–270.
72. YATES, B.J. & A.D. MILLER. 1998. Physiological evidence that the vestibular system participates in autonomic and respiratory control. J. Vestib. Res. **8:** 17–25.
73. SOLOMON, D. & B. COHEN. 1992. Stabilization of gaze during circular locomotion in darkness. II. Contribution of velocity storage to compensatory eye and head nystagmus in the running monkey. J. Neurophysiol. **67:** 1158–1170.

Visually Guided Saccade Adaptation: Transfer to Averaging Saccades Elicited by Double Visual Stimuli

NADIA ALAHYANE AND DENIS PÉLISSON

"Espace et Action" INSERM U534, IFR19 Institut Fédératif des Neurosciences de Lyon, 16 avenue du doyen Lépine, 69500 Bron, France

KEYWORDS: eye movement; human; adaptation; saccade averaging; double target

INTRODUCTION

Several studies have analyzed the adaptive mechanisms which control the amplitude of saccadic eye movements, using the double-step target paradigm pioneered by McLaughlin.[1] It was found that the adaptation of automatic visually guided saccade (VGS) toward a suddenly presented visual target does not transfer to voluntary saccades (like scanning saccades toward permanent targets or memory-guided saccades), indicating that the adaptation of these different saccade types relies on partly separated mechanisms.[2–4] Concerning automatic VGS, adaptive mechanisms have been shown to rely on the medial part of the cerebellum, but the levels along the visuosaccadic pathways where oculomotor commands are modified during adaptation are still debated (see discussion in Desmurget *et al.*[5]).

In the current study, we tested in human subjects the transfer of automatic horizontal VGS adaptation to saccades elicited by the simultaneous presentation of two visual targets vertically separated and located symmetrically around the position where the target of trained VGS had been presented. We were particularly interested in the averaging saccades which were directed toward an intermediate position between the two stimuli and which described a vector similar to that of the horizontal trained VGS. The rationale is illustrated in FIGURE 1 (panels A–C). If the adaptation of VGS modifies the visuosaccadic pathways at a level at which the two oblique saccadic components directed toward each of the two targets presented separately are encoded, upstream of the level of integration into a single motor command (hypothesis 1), then the transfer to averaging saccades should equal the mean of amplitude modifications of the two *oblique* VGS. Conversely, if adaptation acts downstream (hypothesis 2), then the transfer should equal the amplitude modification of the *horizontal* VGS.

Address for correspondence: Dr. Denis Pélisson, "Espace et Action" INSERM U534, 16 avenue du doyen Lépine, 69500 Bron, France. Voice: 33 (0)472 91 34 14; fax: 33 (0)472 91 34 01.
pelisson@lyon.inserm.fr; alahyane@lyon.inserm.fr

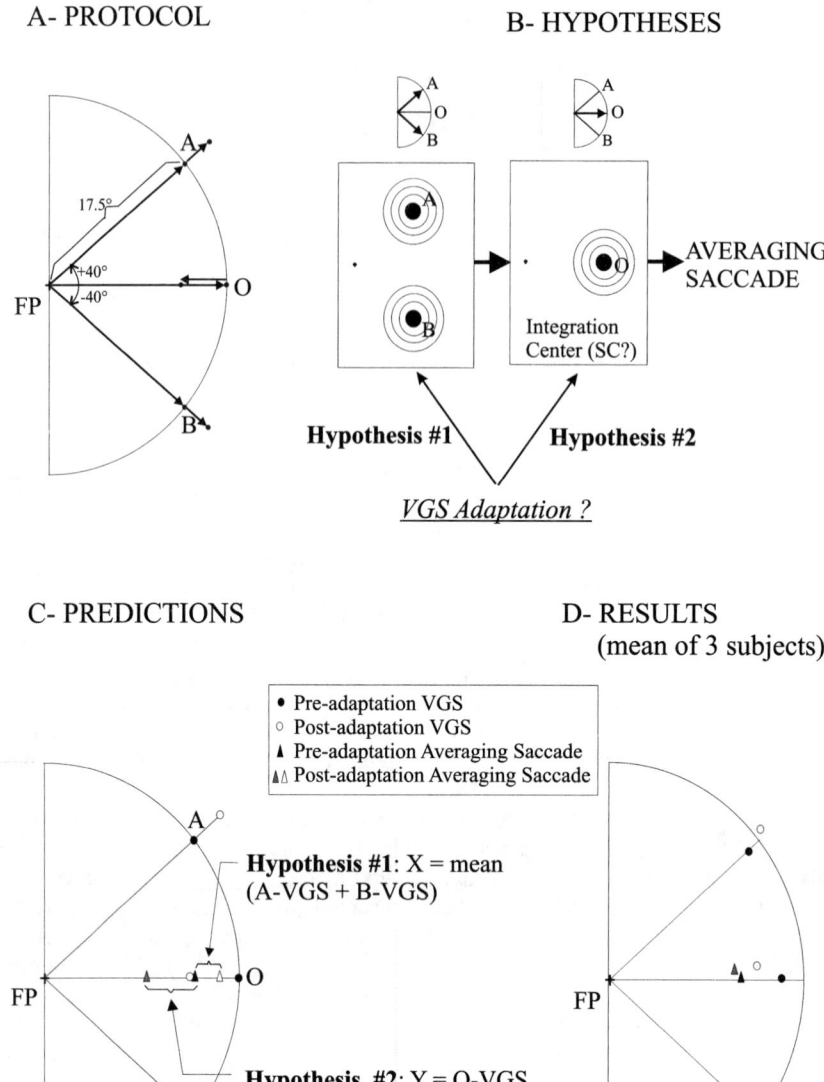

FIGURE 1. (**A**) Dual adaptation protocol: backward and forward double steps were used in a single session to both decrease the amplitude of O-VGS (0°) and increase that of oblique A-VGS and B-VGS (+40° and −40°), respectively. (**B**) The upstream (#1) and downstream (#2) hypotheses on the site of saccadic adaptation relative to averaging saccade programming. (**C**) Predicted end points of pre- and postadaptation saccades (*filled and open*

MATERIALS AND METHODS

Three subjects have been tested, the two authors and one naive subject. They sat in a dimly illuminated room, with their head immobilized by a chin rest, and looked at red light–emitting diodes (targets) located on a concave spherical target board (distance 1.1 m). At the beginning of a trial, the fixation point (FP) located at the center of the board was replaced by a target presented at a single eccentricity of 17.5° and along different directions relative to the azimuth (step 1). During the adaptation condition (FIG. 1A), three targets, A, O, B (directions of +40°, 0°, and −40°, respectively), were used for step 1. The target stepped again during the saccade (step 2) to elicit both a decrease of the 0° saccade (5° = 28% backward training) and an increase of the ±40° oblique saccades (2.5° = 14% forward training). Two hundred fifty-six backward trials for the 0° direction and 128 forward trials for each oblique direction were interleaved in a random order. This adaptation condition was preceded and followed by a test condition (pre- and posttest, respectively). During the test condition, a single target was presented along nine different directions (0°, ±10°, ±20°, ±30°, and ±40°), and sometimes targets A and B (+40° and −40°) were presented simultaneously to elicit averaging saccades. In all test condition trials, the target was switched off during the saccadic response. For each pre- and posttest condition, a total of 144 single (16 for each direction) and 24 double-target trials were randomly presented. Other information regarding the recording and analyses of eye movements can be found in Alahyane and Pélisson, this volume.

RESULTS AND DISCUSSION

Adaptation of VGS

In pilot experiments, we found that submitting only the O-VGS to a 24% backward training produced a significant decrease of the amplitude of that saccade (12.5%, $n = 2$ subjects) as well as that of all oblique VGS, including the A- and B-VGS (mean decrease = 11.8%). Because of this unexpected (according to the notion of vector-specific saccade adaptation; see, e.g., Deubel[6]; Frens et al.[7]) generalization of adaptation to different saccade directions, we used in the main experiment the dual adaptation protocol described in MATERIALS AND METHODS. This protocol successfully led to a selective training of the O-VGS relative to A- and B-VGS. Indeed, the O-VGS amplitude was significantly reduced (−13.1%, $n = 3$ subjects, t-test : $P < 0.001$), whereas the A- and B-VGS showed an opposite, although not statistically significant, change of amplitude (mean = +8.4%, t-test: $P = 0.2$).

---

symbols, respectively) for VGS (*circles*) directed toward targets A, O, and B and for averaging saccades (*triangles*) elicited by the simultaneous presentation of targets A and B. X and Y = amplitude changes of averaging saccades predicted from hypotheses 1 and 2, respectively. (**D**) The actual mean responses pooled across three subjects are plotted in the same format as in panel C.

Transfer to Averaging Saccades

The mean data from our group of three subjects are depicted in FIGURE 1D. It can be seen that the change of averaging saccade amplitude after the dual adaptation session is in the same direction as that of the O-VGS but in the opposite direction relative to the amplitude changes of the A- and B-VGS. We quantitatively compared the percentage of change of averaging saccade amplitude after adaptation [100*(posttest − pretest)/pretest] to the predicted amplitude changes according to hypothesis 1 (predicted change X = mean of percentage of changes of A-VGS and of B-VGS) and to hypothesis 2 (predicted change Y = percentage of change of the O-VGS). We found that the amplitude change of the averaging saccade (−5.6%) differs significantly from the X-value (8.4%; paired t-test, $P < 0.01$) but not from the Y-value predicted from hypothesis 2 (−13.1%, paired t-test, $P = 0.3$).

In conclusion, our results indicate that *horizontal* VGS adaptation transfers to averaging saccades, which is not consistent with hypothesis 1. However, the limited transfer rate (43%) from horizontal VGS adaptation to averaging saccades is also inconsistent with hypothesis 2 which predicts a *complete* transfer, although this difference could not be established statistically on our small subject group. Further recordings and analyses thus will be necessary to confirm that the data are not consistent with either of these two mutually exclusive hypotheses. This will allow us to infer the level(s) of VGS adaptation, based on the hypothesis that the programming of averaging saccades may occur at the level of the superior colliculus motor map or upstream.[8,9]

ACKNOWLEDGMENTS

We thank subject A.K. for his participation in this study. We also thank Marcia Riley and Christian Urquizar for designing the data replay/parameter extraction software. Research was supported by INSERM U534.

REFERENCES

1. MCLAUGHLIN, S.C. 1967. Parametric adjustment in saccadic eye movements. Percept. Psychophys. **2:** 359–362.
2. ERKELENS, C.J. & J. HULLEMAN. 1993. Selective adaptation of internally triggered saccades made to visual targets. Exp. Brain Res. **93:** 157–164.
3. DEUBEL, H. 1995. Separate adaptive mechanisms for the control of reactive and volitional saccadic eye movements. Vision Res. **35:** 3529–3540.
4. FUJITA, M., A. AMAGAI, F. MINAKAWA & M. AOKI. 2002. Selective and delay adaptation of human saccades. Cogn. Brain Res. **13:** 41–52.
5. DESMURGET, M., D. PÉLISSON, J.S. GRETHE, et al. 2000. Functional adaptation of reactive saccades in humans: a PET study. Exp. Brain Res. **132:** 243–259.
6. DEUBEL, H. 1987. Adaptivity of gain and direction in oblique saccades. *In* Eye Movements: From Physiology to Cognition. J.K. O'Regan & A. Levy-Schoen, Eds.: 181–190. Elsevier/North-Holland. New York.
7. FRENS, M.A. & A.J. VAN OPSTAL. 1994. Transfer of short term adaptation in human saccadic eye movements. Exp. Brain Res. **100:** 293–306.
8. GLIMCHER, P.W. & D.L. SPARKS. 1993. Representation of averaging saccades in the superior colliculus of the monkey. Exp. Brain Res. **95:** 429–435.
9. EDELMAN, J.A. & E.L. KELLER. 1998. Dependence on target configuration of express saccade-related activity in the primate superior colliculus. J. Neurophysiol. **80:** 1407–1426.

Saccade Disconjugacy and Adaptation in Strabismic Monkeys

VALLABH E. DAS,[a,b] LAI NGOR FU,[a] SEIJI ONO,[a] RONALD J. TUSA,[a,b] AND MICHAEL J. MUSTARI[a,b]

[a]*Division of Visual Science, Yerkes National Primate Research Center, Emory University, Atlanta, Georgia 30322, USA*

[b]*Department of Neurology, Emory University, Atlanta, Georgia 30322, USA*

KEYWORDS: sac cade disconjugacy; *Macaca mulatta*; strabismus; binocular coordination

In our work with animals reared with sensory forms of strabismus, we have described horizontal saccade disconjugacy in monkeys with large horizontal misalignment.[1] The goals of this study were to determine whether the double-step paradigm[2] could induce saccade adaptation during monocular viewing in animals with large horizontal misalignment and to compare the adaptation induced in the two eyes. Some of the results have been published in preliminary form.[3]

Behavioral data were collected from three strabismic (S1, S2, S3) and one normal juvenile rhesus monkey (N1) (*Macaca mulatta*) weighing 3–7 kg. Monkeys with strabismus were reared at the Yerkes National Primate Research Center using visual sensory deprivation methods for the first 4–6 months of life.[1] We chose to study animals with large angles of strabismus (16–29°), no measurable latent nystagmus, and no amblyopia. The goal of the backward adaptation paradigm was to adaptively reduce saccade gain. In this paradigm, a trial began with the animal monocularly fixating a stationary target at primary position (i.e., straight ahead). The target then randomly jumped to a location either 10° or 15° to the right of primary gaze. A saccade to this new target location was detected by the computer and this triggered a backward jump equal to 30% of initial target movement. Trials were presented repeatedly until it appeared that the animal was consistently making saccades to the final target location rather than the initial target location. The four animals were each tested once with either the left or right eye viewing resulting in a total of eight adaptation sessions. In monkey S3, we also induced an increase in saccade gain by triggering a forward jump equal to 30% of initial target movement. Saccade gain was calculated as the ratio of eye amplitude (difference between eye position at saccade offset and eye position at saccade onset) to target amplitude. In all analyses, the saccade gain that is described is for the first saccade and the initial target step.

Address for correspondence: Vallabh E. Das, Ph.D., Division of Visual Sciences, Yerkes National Primate Research Center, Emory University, 954 Gatewood Road, Atlanta, GA, 30322. Voice: (404)-727-9906; fax: (404)-727-7729.
vdas@rmy.emory.edu

TABLE 1. Exponential fit parameters

Subject/ Viewing Condition	No. of saccades analyzed	G_0		A		λ		Goodness of fit (r^2)	
		VE	NVE	VE	NVE	VE	NVE	VE	NVE
S1/LEV	473	0.64 ± 0.06	0.67 ± 0.09	0.23 ± 0.06	0.23 ± 0.09	425 ± 184	481 ± 280	0.40	0.28
S1/REV	379	0.66 ± 0.02	0.68 ± 0.01	0.32 ± 0.02	0.26 ± 0.02	153 ± 21	116 ± 19	0.50	0.40
S2/LEV	335	0.83 ± 0.02	0.70 ± 0.02	0.10 ± 0.02	0.17 ± 0.03	56 ± 54	60 ± 32	0.06	0.10
S2/REV	340	0.77 ± 0.03	0.81 ± 0.03	0.25 ± 0.03	0.21 ± 0.03	99 ± 35	97 ± 45	0.18	0.12
S3/LEV	315	0.60 ± 0.01	0.56 ± 0.01	0.10 ± 0.01	0.10 ± 0.01	137 ± 39	121 ± 33	0.13	0.14
S3/REV	492	0.86 ± 0.01	0.75 ± 0.01	0.19 ± 0.01	0.18 ± 0.01	134 ± 17	133 ± 17	0.40	0.36
N1/LEV	269	0.65 ± 0.15	0.67 ± 0.08	0.31 ± 0.14	0.36 ± 0.07	272 ± 185	217 ± 90	0.34	0.48
N1/REV	737	0.63 ± 0.03	0.67 ± 0.03	0.33 ± 0.02	0.28 ± 0.02	543 ± 80	524 ± 96	0.58	0.56
S3/REV (increase)	815	0.87 ± 0.01	0.95 ± 0.01	0.29 ± 0.03	0.30 ± 0.05	514 ± 125	632 ± 221	0.35	0.27

VE, viewing eye; NVE, nonviewing eye; LEV, left eye viewing; REV, right eye viewing; S1, S3, animals with exotropia; S2, animal with esotropia; N1, normal animal; equation of fit for backward adaptation: $G = G_0 + A*e^{(-n/\lambda)}$; equation of fit for forward adaptation (last row of table): $G = G_0 + A*(1 - e^{(-n/\lambda)})$; G_0, asymptotic gain estimated by fit for backward adaptation and critical gain estimated by fit for forward adaptation; A, change in gain estimated by fit; λ, time constant of adaptation. Values in the table indicate the parameter estimate ± standard error of the estimate.

FIGURE 1 shows that both normal animals and animals with strabismus adapt their saccades during monocular viewing. Furthermore, animals with strabismus adapt saccadic gain in both their viewing and their nonviewing eyes. We characterized saccade adaptation by fitting an exponential function to the saccadic gain and order number of the saccades. Examples of the exponential fits to the viewing and nonviewing eye in S3 are shown in FIGURE 1E–H. The parameters of the fit and the goodness of fit (estimated by the r^2 value) are shown in TABLE 1 for all the conditions tested. The variability in goodness of fit is similar to reports by other investigators.[2] Statistical analysis showed no significant differences between the time constant of adaptation in the viewing and the nonviewing eye (in 9/9 conditions in the strabismic and normal animals), suggesting that progression of saccade adaptation was similar in the two eyes. Panels in FIGURE 1 also show that the preadaptation saccade gain is unequal in the two eyes. We were able to partially account for this preexisting disconjugacy by examining percentage changes in gain due to adaptation. The asymptotic percentage decrease in gain ranged from 11.12% to 33.92% (mean 24.32 ± 8.35%) in the viewing eye and 14.97% to 35.15% (mean 24.12 ± 6.25%) in the nonviewing eye for the backward adaptation conditions. The percentage change of sac-

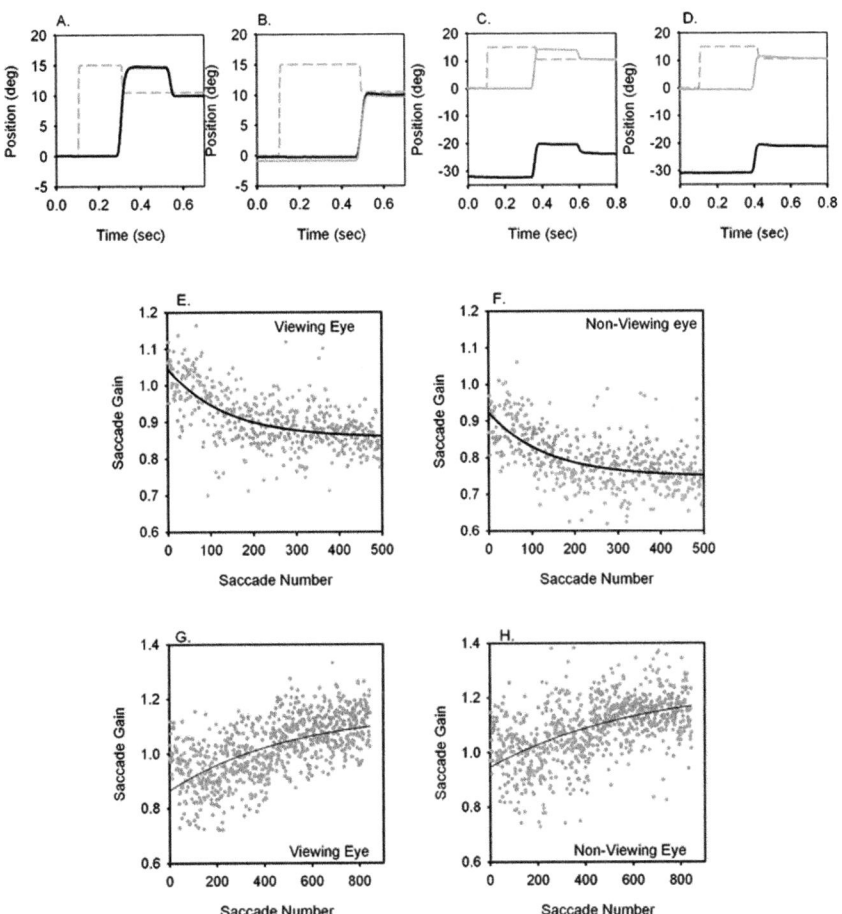

FIGURE 1. (**A–D**) Single saccade trials illustrating saccade adaptation in both eyes during monocular viewing in a normal monkey (**A** and **B**) and in monkey S3 with exotropia (**C** and **D**). During initial trials (**A** and **C**), the animals make a saccade to the initial target location and then make a corrective backward saccade. After repeated trials (**B** and **D**), the animals make a saccade directly to the final target location. (*gray solid line*) Right eye; (*black solid line*) left eye; (*gray dashed line*) target. Gain adaptation in the strabismic monkey (**C** and **D**) appears qualitatively similar to adaptation in the normal monkey (**A** and **B**). (**E** and **F**) Gradual decrease of saccade gain elicited by the backward gain adaptation paradigm in exotropic monkey S3. Each data point represents the gain of a single saccade plotted against the trial number. The panels show that saccade gain reduces exponentially and reaches asymptotic values. Adaptation occurs in both the viewing and nonviewing eye. (**G** and **H**) Gradual increase of saccade gain elicited by the forward gain adaptation paradigm in exotropic monkey S3. Again adaptation occurs in both the viewing and the nonviewing eyes.

cadic gain in the viewing and nonviewing eye was not statistically significantly (paired t-test for the whole group; $P = 0.88$).

In summary, we have shown that the double-step paradigm induces saccade adaptation (either increase or decrease) in both eyes during monocular viewing conditions in normal and strabismic monkeys. We have also shown that adaptation in the viewing and the nonviewing eye is equal (equal time constant and equal percentage change in gain). Our data therefore show that even animals with large strabismus retain the ability to elicit a conjugate adaptation of saccades using this mechanism. It appears that a single central representation of positional retinal error (positional error in the viewing eye) drives adaptation for both eyes. So what is the source of saccade disconjugacy in some animals and humans with large angles of strabismus? We suggest that saccade disconjugacy is not caused by a generalized failure of the adaptive process. The underlying cause of disconjugacy could be related to the specific inability to adapt disconjugately to asymmetries in the oculomotor plant[4] or could be related to other motor aspects associated with strabismus (e.g., a miscalibrated neural integrator, aspects of torsional control, oculomotor muscle pulleys).

ACKNOWLEDGMENTS

This work was supported by National Institutes of Health grants EY06069, RR00165, and NS07480.

REFERENCES

1. TUSA, R.J., M.J. MUSTARI, V.E. DAS & R.G. BOOTHE. 2002. Animal models for visual deprivation-induced strabismus and nystagmus. Ann. N.Y. Acad. Sci. **956:** 346–360.
2. STRAUBE, A., A.F. FUCHS, S. USHER & F.R. ROBINSON. 1997. Characteristics of saccadic gain adaptation in rhesus macaques. J. Neurophysiol. **77:** 874–895.
3. DAS, V.E., S. ONO, R.J. TUSA & M.J. MUSTARI. 2002. Saccade gain daptation in monkeys with strabismus. ARVO Abstr. 2653.
4. BUCCI, M.P., Z. KAPOULA, T. EGGERT & L. GARRAUD. 1997. Deficiency of adaptive control of the binocular coordination of saccades in strabismus. Vision Res. **37:** 2767–2777.

Analysis of Saccades to Stationary and Moving Targets in the Monkey

YANFANG GUAN, THOMAS EGGERT, OTMAR BAYER, AND ULRICH BÜTTNER

Department of Neurology, Ludwig-Maximilians University, D 81377 Munich, Germany

KEYWORDS: saccade dynamics; rhesus monkey

INTRODUCTION

According to classical models,[1] the retinal position error is the main driving factor that guides saccades accurately to a *stationary* target, which is assumed to be sampled approximately 80 ms before the start of a saccade. If the amplitude of a saccade to a *moving* target would also and exclusively be guided by the retinal position error, such a saccade would always miss the target. Therefore, it has to be supposed that additional information about target velocity is needed to make such a "catch-up" saccade to a moving target accurate. Both the superior colliculus (SC)[2–5] and the cerebellar fastigial nucleus (FOR)[6–8] with the oculomotor vermis make saccades accurate by modulating the output of the brainstem saccade generator.[9] The role of the SC is to encode saccades in retinal coordinates that suffice to make saccades land accurately on stationary targets.[10,11] Recently, Optican and Quaia[12] proposed a theoretical model in which the FOR provides the additional neuronal information (about target velocity) needed to adjust saccades to moving targets. Here, the specific features of saccades to stationary targets are compared experimentally with those of "catch-up" saccades to moving targets.

METHODS

Experiments were performed on Rhesus monkeys, which had been trained to make saccades to stationary targets as well as to targets that moved with a velocity of 10°/s both forward and backward after an initial target step of 5.8° or 9.2°. Steps were chosen in such a way that the moving targets were always at the same eccentricity (at 7.2°) when a saccade started, assuming average saccade latency of approximately 200 ms (FIG. 1). In addition to the step-ramp stimuli pure steps without subsequent target motion and with amplitudes of ±3.0° and ±12° were applied. As a result of our paradigm, the moving targets will, in addition to a saccade, evoke a

---

Address for correspondence: Ulrich Büttner, Department of Neurology, Klinikum Grosshadern, Marchioninistrasse 15, 81377 Munich, Germany. Voice: 49-89-7095-2560; fax: 49-89-70-95-5561.

ubuettner@brain.nefo.med.uni-muenchen.de

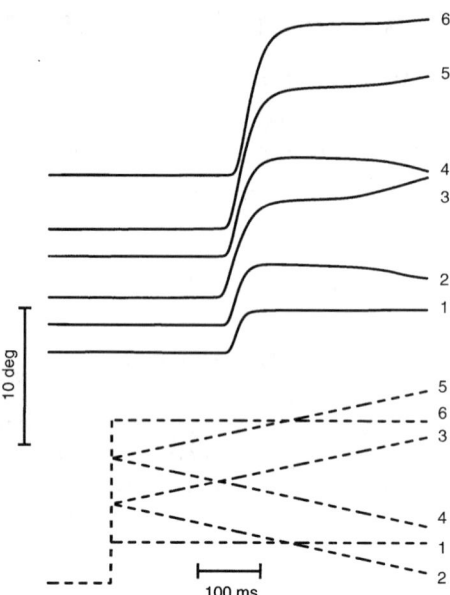

FIGURE 1. Eye position (*solid lines*) and target position (*dashed lines*) for the step-ramp stimuli (2–5) and the two different stationary target steps (1, 6). For stimuli 3 and 4, the primary target steps were chosen to converge after 200 ms at the same position (7.2°). Saccades to the left side were mirrored. Saccades made to moving targets are followed by SPEM. Note that there is no indication for the occurrence of pursuit before the saccades. Averaged data from one monkey.

smooth pursuit eye movement (SPEM), which is known to be added to the saccadic component during sustained SPEM.[13] To free saccade parameters from SPEM components, we subtracted the SPEM velocity, obtained by extrapolation of the smooth pursuit velocity before and after the saccade, from the original velocity data, resulting in a "pure" saccadic velocity profile.

RESULTS

By analyzing saccades, the following four saccade properties were characterized.

Effect of Target Velocity on Duration and Peak Velocity of Saccades

When comparing saccades to forward and backward-moving targets with identical amplitude (7.2°), the average peak velocity of backward saccades was higher than that of forward saccades. The duration of forward saccades was longer than that of backward saccades (FIG. 2). Thus, target velocity influences the main sequence.

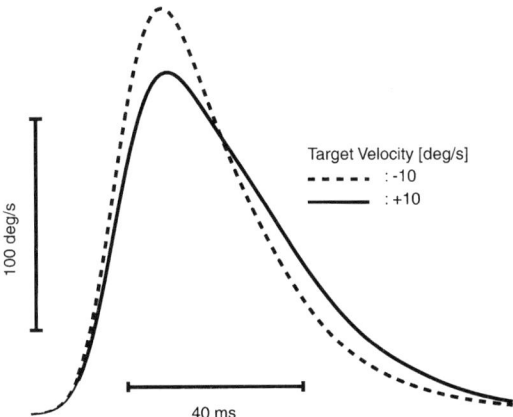

FIGURE 2. Mean velocity profiles of saccades to backward- (*dashed line*) and forward-moving targets (*solid line*) with the same amplitude (7.2°). Data obtained from saccades made to stimulus 3 and 4 are shown in FIGURE 1. Forward saccades are slower and last longer than backward saccades.

Latency

Latencies of saccades varied between 90 and 300 ms. For saccades to moving targets, the amplitude was linearly related to latency. For forward saccades, a latency increase of 100 ms led to larger saccades by 1.5°, whereas backward saccades showed a decrease in amplitude by 1.0°.

Retinal Position Error

For saccades to moving targets, the retinal error depends on the latency and the sampling time. Thus, dependency of saccade amplitude on latency may be explained by the retinal position error alone. An explicit use of target velocity information may not be necessary. However, the sampling time of the retinal position error implicit in such an explanation was found to be too short or sometimes negative; that is, sampling would have occurred after saccade onset. In contrast, the peak velocities can be explained by a retinal error sampled 80 ms before saccade onset. Therefore, target velocity will affect a saccade mainly after the peak velocity, that is, during the deceleration phase of the saccade.

The results lead to the following conclusions.

1. Saccades to forward- and backward-moving targets are on different main sequences.

2. Latency enhancement increases the amplitude of saccades to forward-moving targets but decreases the amplitude of saccades to backward-moving ones.

3. Saccades to moving targets are not (exclusively) determined by the retinal position error but (also) by the target velocity.

These observed differences between saccades to stationary and moving targets, as well as the differences between saccades to forward- and backward-moving targets, provide experimental support for the theoretical model for saccade generation by Optican and Quaia.[12]

ACKNOWLEDGMENT

This work was supported by the Deutsche Forschungsgemeinschaft.

REFERENCES

1. BECKER, W. 1989. Metrics. *In* The Neurobiology of Saccadic Eye Movements, Reviews of Oculomotor Research. Vol. III. R.H. Wurtz and M.E. Goldberg, Eds.: 13–67. Elsevier. Amsterdam.
2. LEE, C., W.H. ROHRER & D.L. SPARKS. 1988. Population coding of saccadic eye movements by neurons in the superior colliculus. Nature **332:** 357–360.
3. SPARKS, D.L. & R. HARTWICH-YOUNG. 1989. The deep layers of the superior colliculus. *In* The Neurobiology of Saccadic Eye Movements, Reviews of Oculomotor Research. Vol. III. R.H. Wurtz & M.E. Goldberg, Eds.: 213–256. Elsevier. Amsterdam.
4. FRENS, M.A. & A.J. VAN OPSTAL. 1997. Monkey superior colliculus activity during short-term saccadic adaptation. Brain Res. Bull. **43:** 473–483.
5. QUAIA, C., P. LEFÈVRE & L.M. OPTICAN. 1999. Model of the control of saccades by superior colliculus and cerebellum. J. Neurol. **82:** 999–1018.
6. YAMADA, J. & H. NODA. 1987. Afferent and efferent connections of the oculomotor cerebellar vermis in the macaque monkey. J. Comp. Neurol. **265:** 224–241.
7. FUCHS, A.F., F.R. ROBINSON & A. STRAUBE. 1993. Role of the caudal fastigial nucleus in saccade generation. I. Neuronal discharge patterns. J. Neurophysiol. **70:** 1723–1740.
8. HELMCHEN, C., A. STRAUBE & U. BÜTTNER. 1994. Saccade-related activity in the fastigial region of the macaque monkey during spontaneous eye movements in light and darkness. Exp. Brain. Res. **98:** 474–482.
9. ROBINSON, F.R. & A.F. FUCHS. 2001. The role of the cerebellum in voluntary eye movements. Annu. Rev. Neurosci. **24:** 981–1004.
10. KELLER, E.L., N.J. GANDHI & P.T. WEIR. 1996. Discharge of superior collicular neurons during saccades made to moving targets. J. Neurophysiol. **76:** 3573–3577.
11. KLIER, E.M., H. WANG & J.D. CRAWFORD. 2001. The superior colliculus encodes gaze commands in retinal coordinates. Nat. Neurosci. **4:** 627–632.
12. OPTICAN, L.M. & C. QUAIA. 2002. Distributed model of collicular and cerebellar function during saccades. Ann. N.Y. Acad. Sci. **956:** 164–177.
13. DE BROUWER, S., M. MISSAL, G. BARNES & P. LEFÈVRE. 2002. Quantitative analysis of catch-up saccades during sustained pursuit. J. Neurophysiol. **87:** 1772–1780.

Accounting for Saccade Dysmetria after Cerebellar Lesion: A Modeling Approach

ANSGAR KOENE AND LAURENT GOFFART

INSERM U534, Bron, France

> KEYWORDS: saccade; dysmetria; modeling; cerebellum; fastigial nucleus; lesion

INTRODUCTION

The caudal fastigial nucleus (cFN) is a major output nucleus by which the cerebellum influences the generation of saccades.[1] In the head-restrained monkey, the unilateral inactivation of cFN by muscimol injection severely impairs the accuracy of all saccades. Horizontal saccades with a direction ipsilateral to the inactivated side are hypermetric, whereas contralesional saccades are hypometric. Vertical saccades are biased horizontally toward the inactivated side even though a horizontal displacement is not required.[2–4]

Despite the large amount of data showing an involvement of cFN in the control of saccade accuracy, there is no general consensus on how to incorporate this contribution into models of saccade generation (SG). Some of the few models that have included the cFN input to the SG are the models proposed by Dean[5] and Quaia *et al.*[6] Unfortunately, Dean's model does not consider the effect of cFN inactivation on vertical saccades and Quaia's model does not account for the contralesional hypometria.

To determine how the dysmetria after cFN inactivation fits into our current understanding of the saccadic system, we decided to use a generic local feedback-based saccade generator model (i.e., a model with the standard pulse generator, feedback integrator, etc. elements) and try to find which model parameters would need to be affected by the cFN lesion to reproduce the postlesional saccade dysmetria.

METHODS

The saccade generator model used in this study is shown in FIGURE 1. To differentiate the parameter values between the ipsi- and contralesional sides, we modeled the SG paths leading to the medial and lateral rectus (MR and LR) muscles separately as in Scudder[7] and Gancarz and Grossberg.[8] To incorporate the dynamical changes in neural activity, we modeled the pulse generator with an S-function type I/O

Address for correspondence: Ansgar Koene, PhD, INSERM u534, 16 avenue Doyen Lépine, 69500 Bron, France.

koene@lyon.inserm.fr

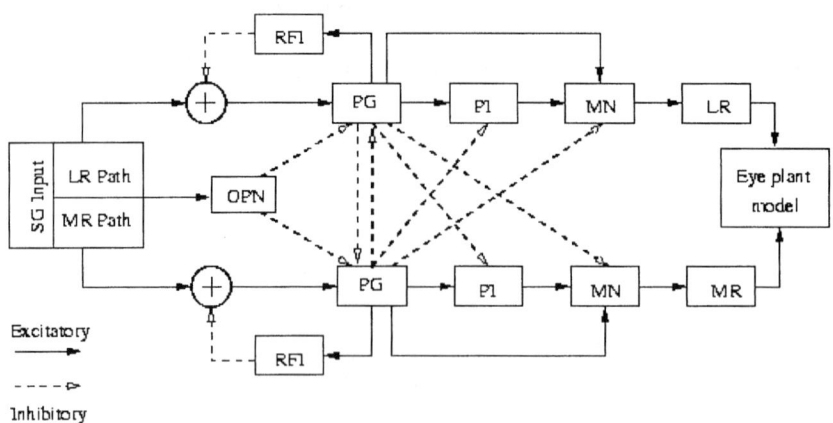

FIGURE 1. Generic saccade generator model. PG, pulse generator; RFI, resettable feedback integrator; PI, pulse integrator; MN, motoneurons; LR/MR, lateral/medial rectus muscles; OPN, omnipause neurons.

relationship (equation 1), whereas all other SG elements were modeled as leaky integrators (equation 2). The leak time constants of the resetable feedback integrator and the pulse integrator were assumed to be infinite.

$$Y(t) = B*[1/\{1 + \exp(-A\ (\Sigma_i\ [w_i * X_i\{t\}] + C)\}] \quad (1)$$

where $Y(t)$ is the output at time t, B is maximum burst frequency, A determines the steepness of the S-function, w_i is the connection weight of input i, $X_i\{t\}$ is the value of the input i at time t, and C shifts the function so that $Y(t) = 0$ if $\Sigma[w_i*X_i\{t\}] = 0$.

$$Y(t) = \int (L * Y[t] + \Sigma_i\ [w_i * X_i\{t\}])dt \quad (2)$$

where $Y[t]$ is the output at time t, L is the leak, w_i is the connection weight of input i, and $X_i\{t\}$ is the input value at time t of input i.

The eye plant model that was used for the results shown here was the model by Quaia and Optican.[9] Simulations using other eye plant models yielded qualitatively similar results (not shown).

To determine if specific changes in model parameters could qualitatively reproduce the effects of cFN inactivation, we focused on the following results that were observed by Goffart et al.[4] (and in preparation). (1) Unilateral cFN inactivation causes horizontal deviation of vertical saccades toward the ipsilesional side. (2) Horizontal ipsiversive saccades are hypermetric and associated with a decrease in the deceleration rate (acceleration and maximum velocity are not affected). (3) Horizontal contraversive saccades are hypometric and associated with a decrease in maximum velocity, which is not completely compensated, by a decrease in deceleration rate. (4) The magnitude of the dysmetria increases with saccade size.

RESULTS

Horizontal Deviation toward Ipsilesional Side during Vertical Eye Movements

To replicate this result with our SG model, we found that vertical saccades must be accompanied by an activation of the horizontal saccade generator. As long as the excitatory input from the ipsilateral pulse generator to the pulse integrator and motoneurons is just as strong as the inhibitory input from the contralateral pulse generator the signals cancel each other. Thus, a balanced bilateral activation of the LR and MR SG paths during vertical saccades will not lead to any horizontal displacement. The ipsilesional movement of the eye during saccades toward vertically displaced targets therefore indicates that lesioning the cFN increases the relative strength of the signals on the ipsilesional side for the signals on the contralesional side.

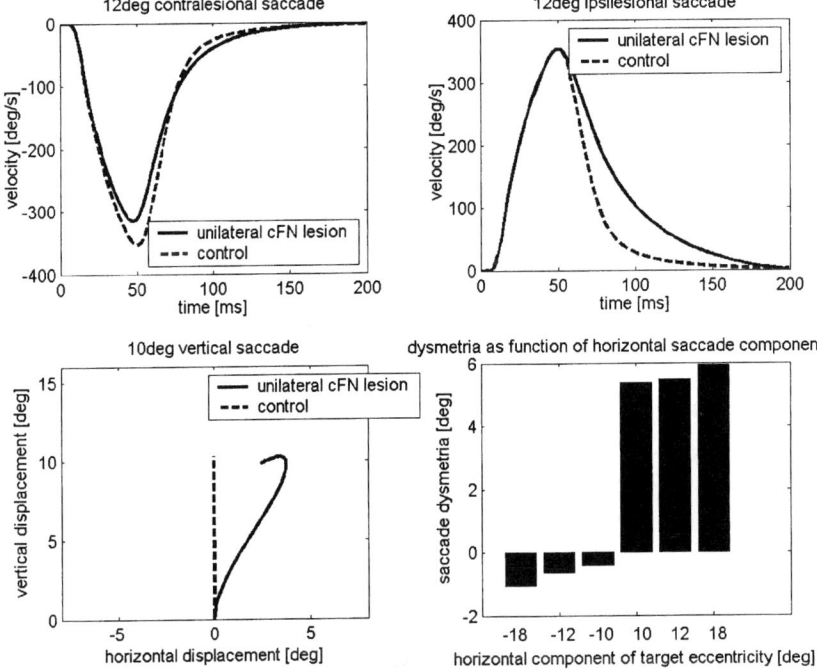

FIGURE 2. Simulation results of our saccade generator model with and without simulated cFN lesion. The *top two panels* show the velocity profiles for an 18° saccade to the contralesional (*left*) and ipsilesional (*right*) side. The bottom left panel shows the position profile of a 10° vertical saccade (positive horizontal direction corresponds to ipsilesional side). *Bottom right panel* shows the change in saccade dysmetria with saccade size (+ hypermetria, − hypometria).

Dysmetria of Horizontal Saccades

Because the results in the Goffart *et al.* (this volume) study are caused by a unilateral cFN lesion, the changes in model parameters simulating the lesion should be restricted to the side that the lesioned part of the cFN projects to (i.e., the contralesional side).

The effects of simulated lesions were as follows. (1) Changes to the pulse integrator and/or motoneurons of the contralesional side: Because the pulse integrator and motoneurons are involved in the acceleration of ipsilesional saccades, any change to the characteristics of the pulse integrator and/or motoneurons will also change the acceleration of ipsilateral saccades which is not in accordance with the experimental data. (2) Change in pulse generator: Because of the local feedback loop, this would not result in saccade dysmetria. It will, however, change the rate of acceleration and deceleration. (3) Change in the feedback integrator: Because the input to the contralesional side does not increase with larger ipsilesional saccades, changes in the feedback integrator would not cause ipsilesional hypermetria to increase for larger saccades. (4) Change in the input to the contralesional side: For the saccade dysmetria to increase with saccade size, the cFN lesion-induced change would have to increase with saccade size. The simplest way to achieve this is a leak. A leak, causing the input signal to gradually reduce over time would be almost equivalent to a saccade duration-dependent offset.

CONCLUSION

An analysis of our simple model of the SG revealed that to successfully reproduce the qualitative effects of cFN lesion, we need only to introduce a fixed bilateral bias (for the horizontal deviation during vertical saccades) together with a leak in the contralesional input (causing dysmetria that increases with saccade size and decreased deceleration rate of ipsilesional saccades), and we weaken the strength (w_i) of the inhibitory connection from the contralesional to the ipsilesional pulse generator and the excitatory connection from the contralesional pulse generator to the contralesional pulse integrator and motoneurons (causing reduced acceleration and deceleration rates during contralesional saccades; FIG. 2). All of these parameter changes are static. They change neither during a saccade nor as function of saccade size. (To paraphrase Shakespeare,[10] they are like true love which is an ever-fixed mark that does not alter when it alteration finds.)

REFERENCES

1. ROBINSON, F.R. & A.F. FUCHS. 2001. The role of the cerebellum in voluntary eye movements. Annu. Rev. Neurosci. **24:** 981–1004.
2. ROBINSON, F.R., A. STRAUBE & A.F. FUCHS. 1993. Role of the caudal fastigial nucleus in saccade generation. II. Effects of muscimol inactivation. J. Neurophysiol. **70:** 1741–1758.
3. IWAMOTO, Y. & K. YOSHIDA. 2002. Saccadic dysmetria following inactivation of the primate fastigial oculomotor region. Neurosci. Lett. **325:** 211–215.
4. GOFFART, L., L.L. CHEN & D.L. SPARKS. 2003. Saccade dysmetria during functional perturbation of the caudal fastigial nucleus in the monkey. Ann. N.Y. Acad. Sci. **1004:** this volume.

5. DEAN, P. 1995. Modelling the role of the cerebellar fastigial nuclei in producing accurate saccades: the importance of burst timing. Neuroscience **68:** 1059–1077.
6. QUAIA, C., P. LEFÈVRE & L.M. OPTICAN. 1999. Model of the control of saccades by superior colliculus and cerebellum. J. Neurophysiol. **92:** 999–1018.
7. SCUDDER, C.A. 1988. A new local feedback model of the saccadic burst generator. J. Neurophysiol. **59:** 1455–1475.
8. GANCARZ, G. & S. GROSSBERG. 1998. A neural model of the saccade generator in the reticular formation. Neural Netw. **11:** 1159–1174.
9. QUAIA, C. & L.M. OPTICAN. 1998. Commutative saccadic generator is sufficient to control a 3-D ocular plant with pulleys. J. Neurophysiol. **79:** 3197–3215.
10. SHAKESPEARE, W. Sonnet CXVI.

Characteristics of a Range Effect for Vergence Movements

ARUN N. KUMAR, YANNING H. HAN, AND R. JOHN LEIGH

Departments of Biomedical Engineering and Neurology,
Veterans Affair Medical Center, Case Western Reserve University,
Cleveland, Ohio, USA

KEYWORDS: vergence; saccades; eye position; memory

INTRODUCTION

A range effect for saccadic eye movements, in which the small saccades overshoot, and large saccades undershoot the target, has been reported.[1,2] The range effect reduces errors to approximately zero near the center of the range of targets, at the expense of errors at both edges. It also appears during the first trials, indicating that the effect is established as soon as subjects realize that a range of targets exists.[2] The range effect has also been reported with memory-guided saccades.[3] Most natural shifts of the point of visual fixation are between targets lying in different directions and at different distances, calling for combined saccade-vergence movements. We investigated whether a range effect exists for the vergence components of rapid shifts of the direction and distance of the fixation point. The main questions addressed in this preliminary study are as follows. (1) Is there a range effect for vergence eye movements? (2) Is this effect different for convergence and divergence? (3) Does it depend on the starting vergence position of the eye? (4) Does it apply to memory-guided saccade-vergence movements? (5) Does motion of the eye during the memory period affect the response?

METHODS

We studied four healthy normal subjects (age range, 20–54 years); two were naive to the purpose of the experiments. All subjects gave informed, written consent, and the study was conducted in accordance with the tenets of the Declaration of Helsinki and approved by our institutional review board. Horizontal and vertical movements of each eye were measured using the magnetic search-coil technique, as previously described.[4] Subjects viewed a red laser spot (the "primary target") that was projected

Address for correspondence: R. John Leigh, Departments of Biomedical Engineering and Neurology, Veterans Affairs Medical Center, Case Western Reserve University, Department of Neurology, University Hospitals, 11100 Euclid Avenue, Cleveland, OH 44106-5040. Voice: 216-844-3190; fax: 216-231-3461.

rjl4@po.cwru.edu

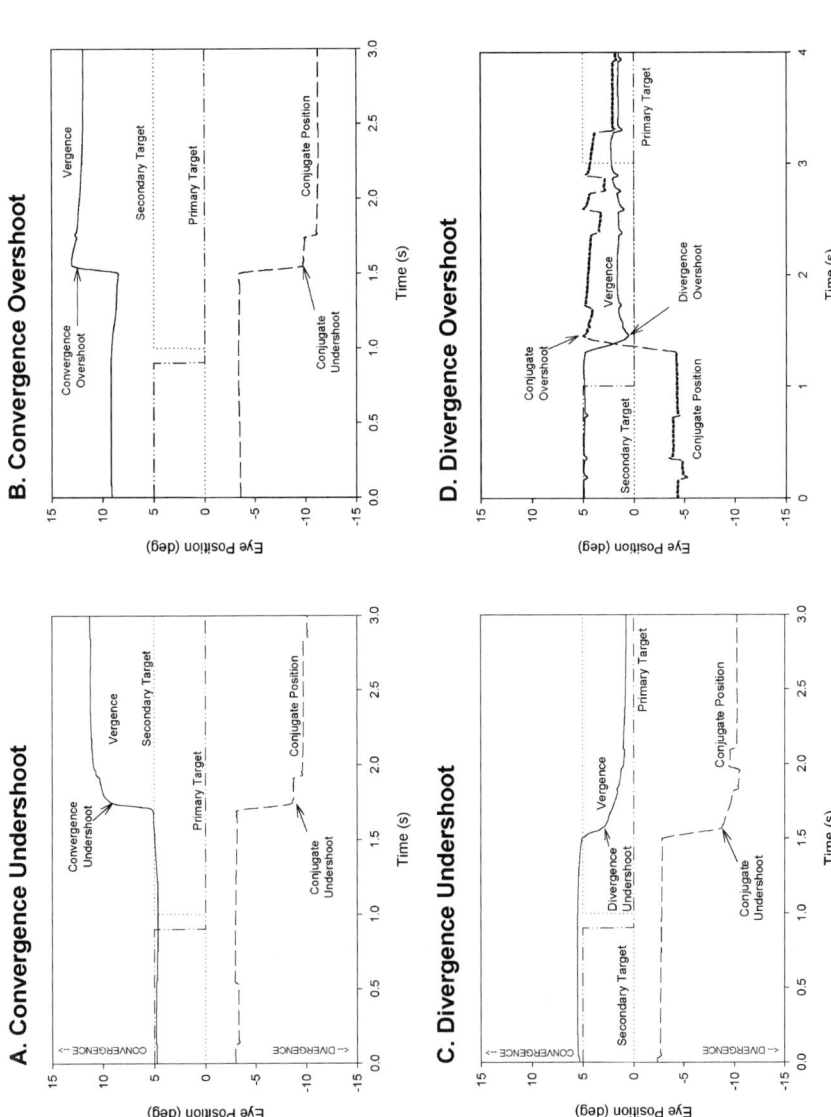

FIGURE 1. Representative records of **(A)** convergence undershoot, **(B)** convergence overshoot, **(C)** divergence undershoot, and **(D)** divergence overshoot.

from above onto a nearly horizontal plank of wood under the control of MiniSax servo controllers (GSI Lumonics, Inc.). A green laser spot (the "secondary target") was similarly projected onto the horizontal plank. We employed three test paradigms. The general instruction was to look at the primary target until it was turned off and then to look at the secondary target (or its remembered location). Instructions were given for each test paradigm, and some practice was allowed before search coils were inserted and data collection began.

Visually Guided Saccades during Fixation (GAP/FIX)

Subjects fixated the primary target located at one of three distances: 23.5, 33, or 51 cm, lying in the subject's midline. After 2.4 s, the primary target was turned off, and 100 ms later the secondary target was illuminated ("gap" paradigm). The secondary target was located at one of seven locations, over a distance range of 20.5 to 83 cm, with a constant direction of left 10°. The subject was instructed to look at the secondary target as soon as it became visible. The secondary target remained illuminated for 2.5 s.

Memory-Guided Saccades during Fixation (MEM/FIX)

Subjects fixated the stationary primary target located in the midline at either 23.5 or 70 cm. After 2.4 s, the secondary target flashed for 100 ms, being located at 30 or 60 cm, on either side of the midline requiring a saccade of 15°. The subject was instructed to continue to fixate the primary target. After an additional 7 s (the memory period), the primary target was extinguished (complete darkness), and the subject was asked to make an eye movement to where the flashed secondary target had been located. After another 2 s (allowing time for corrective eye movements in darkness), the secondary target reappeared and the subject looked at it, allowing a further 2 s to correct for any errors.

Memory-Guided Saccades to Target Presented during Pursuit (MEM/SP)

This paradigm was similar to the MEM/FIX paradigm except that subjects tracked the primary target that moved either purely in depth (aligned along the midline) or along an axis that required a change in both version and vergence. The primary stimulus moved sinusoidally, at 0.15 Hz.

Data were digitized and filtered as previously described.[4] We measured the size of the initial "vergence pulse" that occurred with the saccade-vergence response. The onset of the saccade was defined as the time at which gaze velocity exceeded 15°/s, and the end of the saccade was defined as time at which gaze velocity decreased to less than 15°/s. We made the assumption that the start and end of the initial vergence movement coincided with the start and end of the initial saccade.

RESULTS

Subjects showed idiosyncratic differences and some variability of their vergence responses. Convergence undershoots, convergence overshoots, divergence undershoots, and divergence overshoots were all encountered (FIG. 1). In general, small

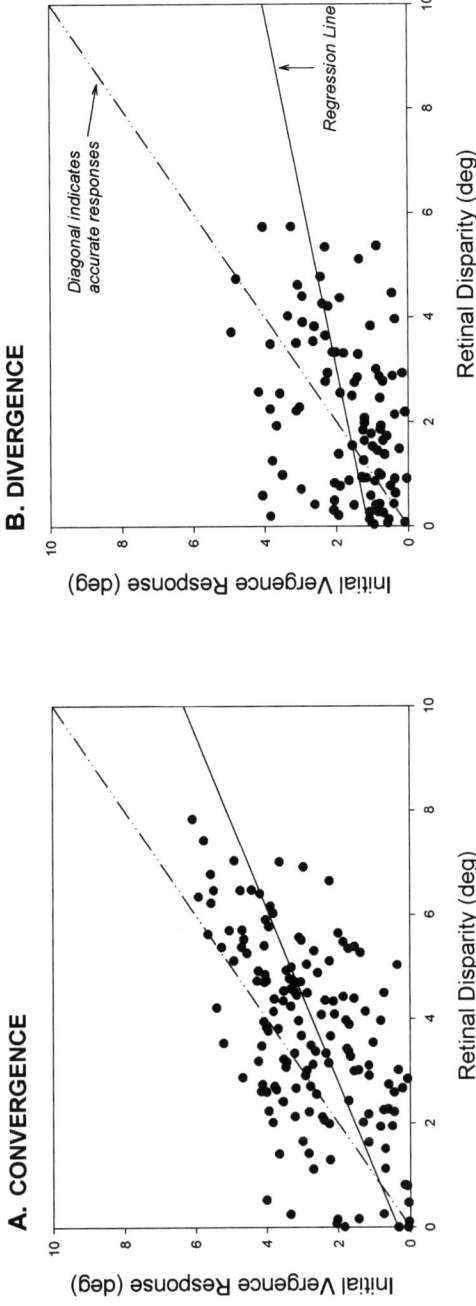

FIGURE 2. Plot of initial vergence response versus the retinal disparity (required vergence movement) for (**A**) convergence and (**B**) divergence. Points lying above the diagonal indicate overshoots (more evident for small retinal disparities) and points lying below the diagonal indicate undershoots (more evident for large retinal disparities).

disparity stimuli (<3°) elicited overshoots, whereas larger disparity stimuli elicited undershoots for all paradigms. The range effect was more marked for divergence movements. FIGURE 2 shows the range effect for the GAP/FIX stimulus. The range effect was also present for divergence movements during memory-guided (MEM/FIX) trials. Responses during the MEM/SP trials depended on the amount of vergence movement during the memory period; if the eye was at the same position at the end of the memory period as at secondary target presentation, a range effect was apparently similar to MEM/FIX. In two subjects, we performed multiple linear regressions on responses to the GAP/FIX trials, to compare the relative effects of retinal disparity and initial vergence angle; we found that retinal disparity exerted about twice as big an effect as initial vergence angle on the response.

We concluded from these preliminary studies that a range effect for vergence is apparent in some subjects and is more pronounced for divergence movements. It is also evident during memory-guided movements. Motion of the eye during the memory period does not affect the vergence response if the eye is at the same position at the end of the memory period as at the time of target presentation. In addition to retinal disparity, the initial vergence angle influences the response. It remains to be determined whether the range effect for vergence movements is correlated with the saccadic component of combined saccadic-vergence movements.

ACKNOWLEDGMENTS

This work was supported by National Institutes of Health grant EY06717, the Office of Research and Development, Medical Research Service, Department of Veterans Affairs, and Evenor Armington Fund.

REFERENCES

1. KAPOULA, Z. 1985. Evidence for a range effect in the saccadic system. Vision Res. **25:** 1155–1157.
2. KAPOULA, Z. & D.A. ROBINSON. 1986. Saccadic undershoot is not inevitable: saccades can be accurate. Vision Res. **26:** 735–743.
3. ISRAEL, I. 1992. Memory-guided saccades: what is memorized? Exp. Brain Res. **90:** 221–224.
4. KUMAR, A.N. *et al.* 2002. Properties of anticipatory vergence responses. Invest. Ophthal. Visual Sci. **43:** 2626–2632.

The Role of DLPN and NRTP in Visual-Vestibular Behavior

SEIJI ONO,[a] V.E. DAS,[a,b] AND M.J. MUSTARI[a,b]

Division of Visual Science, [a]Yerkes National Primate Research Center, and [b]Department of Neurology, Emory University, 954 Gatewood Road N.E., Atlanta, Georgia 30022, USA

KEYWORDS: pursuit; VOR; pontine nucleus; eye movement

During locomotion, the vestibular ocular reflex (VOR) produces compensatory eye movements to stabilize image motion on the retina. This stabilization is essential for preservation of high-acuity vision during locomotion. Residual visual motion or error signals during the VOR drive visual optokinetic or pursuit mechanisms to produce full compensation for head movements over a broad frequency range. The dorsolateral pontine nucleus (DLPN) and nucleus reticularis tegmenti pontis (NRTP) are major components of the cortico-ponto-cerebellar pathway[1–3] that carry retinal image motion and signals essential for smooth pursuit[4–7] and for visual-vestibular behavior. The aim of this study was to characterize the potential role of DLPN and NRTP in relation to eye movements during visual-vestibular testing.

We have examined the response properties of DLPN and NRTP neurons during smooth pursuit, passive whole-body rotation, and visual stimulation. Three normal *Macaca mulatta* monkeys were used in this study. Eye movements were measured (CNC Engineering, Seattle) with an electromagnetic method employing scleral search coils. Unit activity was recorded from the DLPN and rostral smooth pursuit related region of the NRTP using glass-coated tungsten electrodes. Eye, head, and target signals were sampled at 1 kHz. Single-unit spike times were detected with a window discriminator and time stamped with high temporal resolution. During single-unit recording, neurons were tested with large-field visual motion during smooth pursuit and during vestibular testing. Four vestibular testing paradigms were used including sinusoidal rotation in darkness (VORd), sinusoidal rotation in light while viewing an earth-stationary target during (VORl), VOR cancellation (VOR×0) and VOR enhancement, produced by having the monkey track a target that moved counterphase to the chair (VOR×2). Neurons that only responded during large-field visual motion were also tested in the VORd condition.

We tested 51 DLPN neurons that responded during smooth pursuit or during motion of a large-field stimulus. The majority of smooth-pursuit–related neurons in

Address for correspondence: Seiji Ono, Division of Visual Science, Yerkes National Primate Research Center, Emory University, 954 Gatewood Road N.E., Atlanta, GA 30022. Voice: 404-727-8218; fax: 404-727-7729.
 sono@rmy.emory.edu

Ann. N.Y. Acad. Sci. 1004: 399–403 (2003). © 2003 New York Academy of Sciences.
doi: 10.1196/annals.1303.040

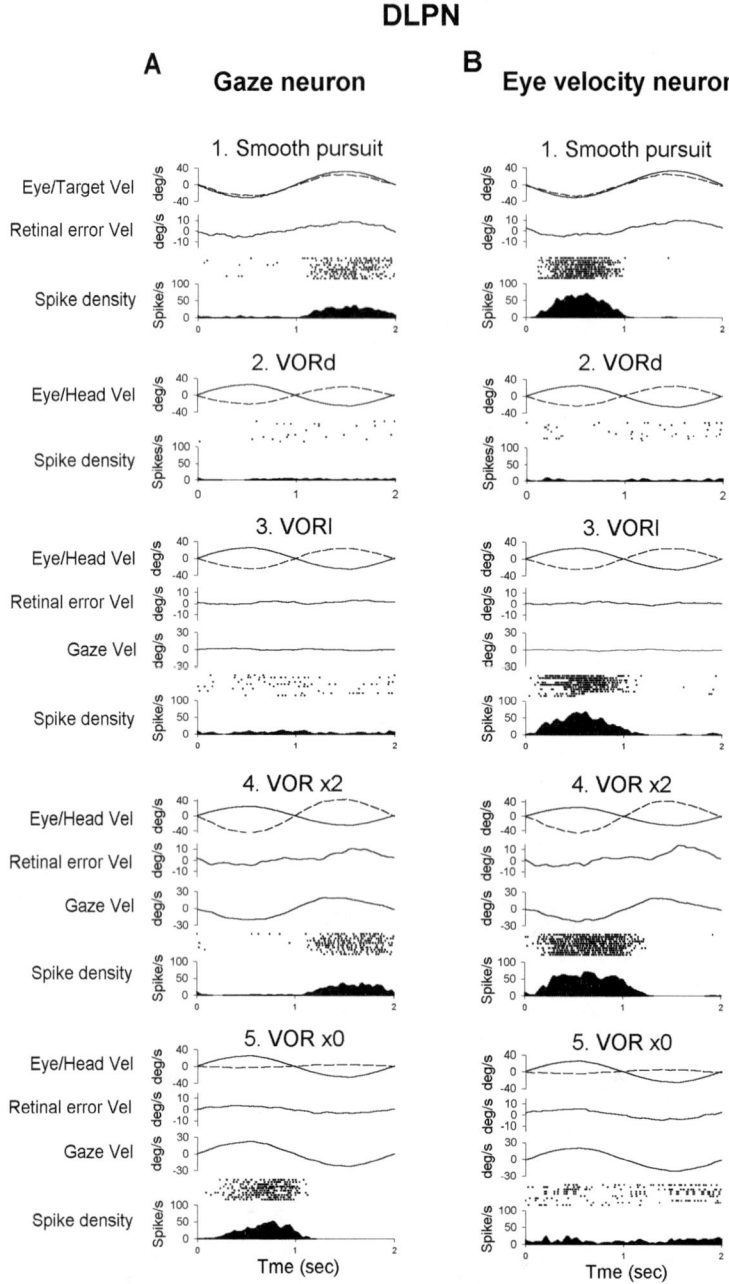

FIGURE 1. Response properties of representative gaze neuron (**A**) and eye velocity neuron (**B**) in DLPN during five different behavioral conditions. Each trace shows 10 cycle averages. *Dashed lines* indicate eye velocities after desaccading the data.

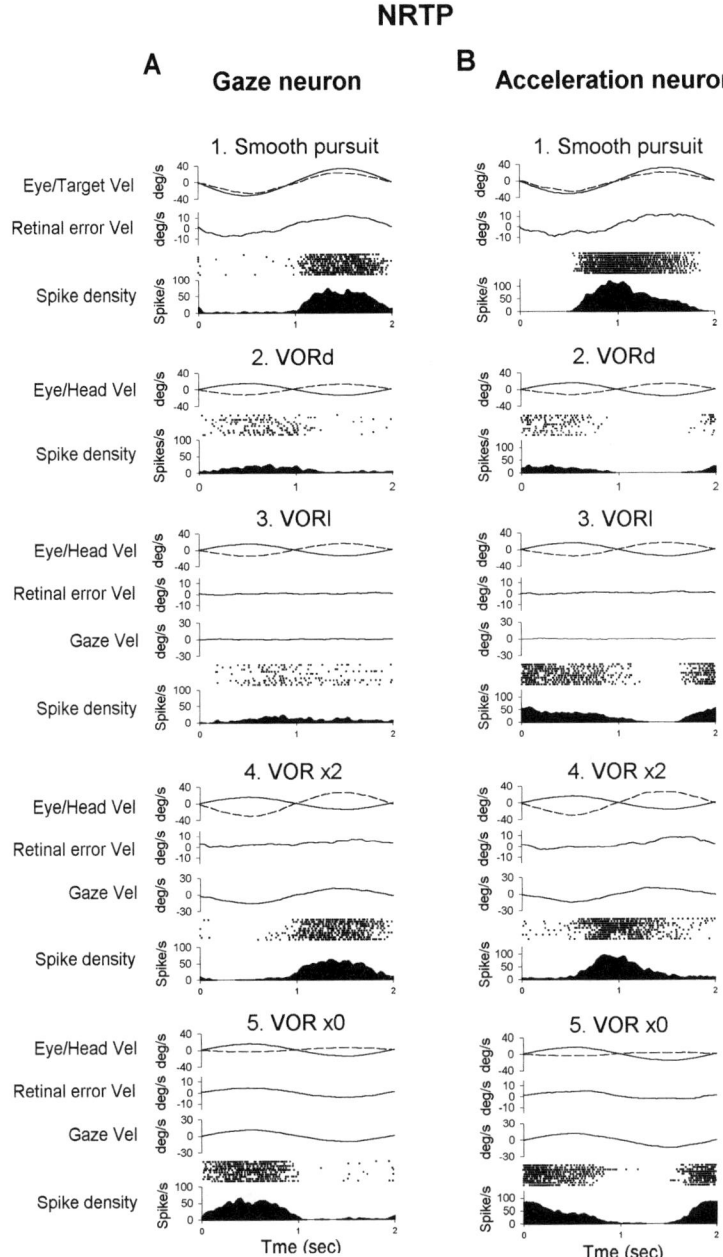

FIGURE 2. Response properties of representative gaze neuron (**A**) and acceleration neuron (**B**) recorded from the rostral smooth pursuit region of NRTP during five different behavioral conditions. Traces as in FIGURE 1.

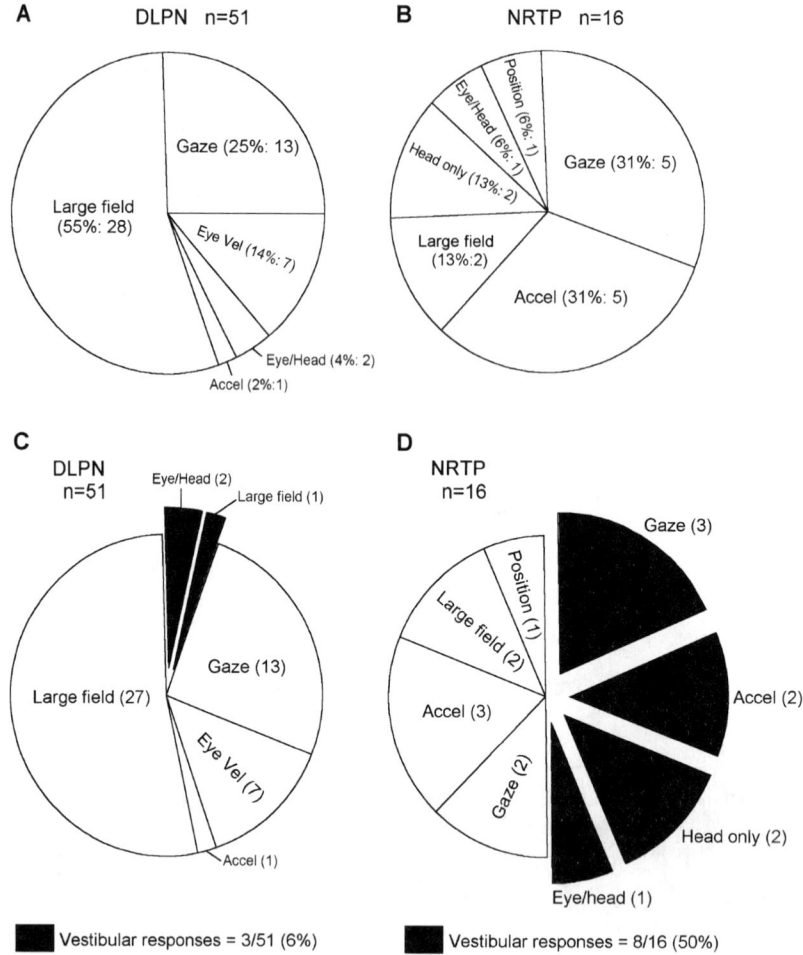

FIGURE 3. Proportional distribution of different types of neurons in DLPN (**A**) and NRTP (**B**). Smooth-pursuit–related neurons were classified as gaze, eye velocity (Eye Vel), acceleration (Accel), eye and head (Eye/Head), and position. *Filled areas* of **C** and **D** show VORd responses in DLPN and NRTP, respectively.

DLPN were classified as gaze or eye velocity neurons during visual-vestibular behavior. DLPN gaze neuron modulation during the VOR×2 condition was in the same direction as smooth pursuit, but was in the opposite direction during VOR×0 (FIG. 1A). Gaze neurons were not well modulated during the VOR1 because gaze is stable. Eye-velocity neurons are modulated in the same direction during VOR1 and VOR×2 conditions (FIG. 1B). However, no significant modulation was present during VOR×0.

More than half of DLPN neurons responded only during large-field visual motion (FIG. 3A). Only a small percentage of DLPN neurons responded during VORd (FIG. 3C).

Sixteen neurons recorded from the rostral smooth-pursuit region of NRTP responded during smooth pursuit or motion of a large-field stimulus. The majority of smooth-pursuit–related neurons in NRTP were classified as gaze or acceleration sensitive. NRTP gaze neuron modulation during VOR×2 was in same direction as smooth pursuit and in the opposite direction during VOR×0 (FIG. 2A). At least half of our NRTP gaze neurons were also modulated during VORd (FIG. 2B). We found NRTP neurons often had apparent eye acceleration sensitivity, which can be seen in several conditions including VOR×2, VOR×0 (gaze acceleration phase), and during VORd (FIG. 2B). Only a small proportion of NRTP neurons respondedto motion of a large-field stimulus (FIG. 3D).

Our results suggest that the DLPN and NRTP have different functional roles in visual-vestibular behavior. These different functional roles may in part reflect different balances of cortical-pontine inputs[3,8] and pontine efferents to the vestibulocerebellum.[2] The DLPN is known to receive strong inputs from the middle temporal and medial superior temporal areas. In contrast, the NRTP may receive a biased input from other cortical areas such as the frontal eye fields. Further studies are required to define the precise roles played by the DLPN and NRTP in visual-vestibular.

REFERENCES

1. MAY, J.G. & R.A. ANDERSEN. 1986. Different patterns of corticopontine projections from separate cortical fields within the inferior parietal lobule and dorsal prelunate gyrus of the macaque. Exp. Brain Res. **63:** 265–278.
2. GLICKSTEIN, M., N. GERRITS, I. KRALJ-HANS, et al. 1994. Visual pontocerebellar projections in the macaque. J. Comp. Neurol. **349:** 51–72.
3. DISTLER, C., M.J. MUSTARI & K.P. HOFFMANN. 2002. Cortical projections to the nucleus of the optic tract and dorsal terminal nucleus and to the dorsolateral pontine nucleus in macaques: a dual retrograde tracing study. J. Comp. Neurol. **444:** 144–158.
4. SUZUKI, D.A. & E.L. KELLER. 1984. Visual signals in the dorsolateral pontine nucleus of the alert monkey: their relationship to smooth-pursuit eye movements. Exp. Brain Res. **53:** 473–478.
5. MUSTARI, M.J., A.F. FUCHS & J. WALLMAN. 1988. Response properties of dorsolateral pontine units during smooth pursuit in the rhesus macaque. J. Neurophysiol. **60:** 664–686.
6. THIER, P., W. KOEHLER & U.W. BUETTNER. 1988. Neuronal activity in the dorsolateral pontine nucleus of the alert monkey modulated by visual stimuli and eye movements. Exp Brain Res. **70:** 496–512.
7. SUZUKI, D.A., T. YAMADA, R. HOEDEMA & R.D. YEE. 1999. Smooth-pursuit eye-movement deficits with chemical lesions in macaque nucleus reticularis tegmenti pontis. J. Neurophysiol. **82:** 1178–1186
8. STANTON, G.B., M.E. GOLDBERG & C.J. BRUCE. 1988. Frontal eye field efferents in the macaque monkey. II. Topography of terminal fields in midbrain and pons. J. Comp. Neurol. **271:** 493–506.

Influence of Head Restraint on Visually Triggered Saccades in the Rhesus Monkey

JULIE QUINET AND LAURENT GOFFART

INSERM U534, Bron, France

KEYWORDS: saccade; head; unrestrained; latency; monkey

INTRODUCTION

The sudden appearance of an object in the visual field elicits a rapid orienting gaze shift toward the object's location. This orienting response is ensured by a saccadic eye movement and can be accompanied by a concurrent orienting movement of the head.

In the cat, saccades produced with the unrestrained head have been shown to have higher peak velocities than saccades of similar amplitudes performed in the head-restrained condition.[1,2] In contrast, most studies in the monkey indicate a reduction in gaze peak velocity for head-unrestrained gaze shifts with amplitude larger than 20°.[3–5] In humans, one study reported that gaze shifts with the head unrestrained were faster and shorter in duration than gaze shifts of the same size with the head restrained, irrespective of whether head movements were small or substantial.[6] Based on these observations, Collewijn *et al.*[6] proposed that "the oculomotor system does not work naturally, or near capacity, when the head is prevented from moving" and that "attempts to resist the natural tendency to move the head and the eyes could inhibit saccadic commands to some degree."

In this study, we searched for evidence that restraining the head in the monkey could affect the generation of saccades toward a visual target. We demonstrate that restraining the head is indeed influencing the initiation of visually triggered saccades.

METHODS

Animal Preparation

Two rhesus monkeys (B and E) were used in the current study. All experimental protocols complied with the guidelines from the French Ministry of Agriculture (87/848) and from the European Community (86/609/EEC). A light titanium head post (weight <7 g), secured by stainless steel screws and bone cement, was placed on the skull for immobilizing the head. A Teflon-coated coil was sutured to the sclera of the

Address for correspondence: Laurent Goffart, PhD, INSERM U534, 16 avenue Doyen Lépine, 69500 Bron, France. Voice: 33 472 91 34 01; fax: 33 472 91 34 03.
goffart@lyon.inserm.fr

left eye. A similar coil was glued to a flat piece of plastic and embedded in the bone cement on the skull. These two coils served to measure gaze (eye-in-space) and head orientation with a phase-angle detection system (CNC Engineering, Seattle, WA).

Behavioral Training and Experimental Procedures

During all training and experimental sessions, each animal was placed in a primate chair that prevented movements of the body. Experiments were conducted in a dimly illuminated room. The monkey was facing a spherical board of 1454 light-emitting diodes (LEDs) that were all located at a distance of 110 cm from the glabella (midpoint between both eyes) and was trained to perform a saccade task that shifted gaze from a central fixation LED (located straight ahead) toward a peripheral brief target LED (duration, 100 ms). The target LED was flashed 200 ms after the fixation LED was extinguished (gap paradigm). Its location was pseudorandomly selected among several preselected positions (11 or 49) along the horizontal and vertical meridians. Reward was delivered for fixating within a spatial window around the target LED (2° and 2–4° for the head-restrained and head-unrestrained conditions, respectively). In the current study, our analysis is restricted to saccades aimed at targets located at ±16° and ±8° along the horizontal and vertical meridians. The onset and offset of saccades and head movements were defined on a velocity threshold (15°/s). Every trial was examined individually and saccades that were accompanied by a concurrent head movement were discarded from analysis (34% and 46% for monkey B and E, respectively) to have head-restrained and head-unrestrained saccades absolutely comparable. Data recorded in the head-restrained (13 and 12 sessions for monkey B and E, respectively) and the head-unrestrained (10 and 15 sessions for monkey B and E, respectively) conditions were collected on different days.

RESULTS

FIGURE 1 shows for each monkey the average amplitude (A), maximum velocity (B), duration (C), and latency (D) of saccades generated with the head restrained (white histograms) and unrestrained (black histograms). For both monkeys and irrespective of the head-restraint condition, the amplitude of saccades matched well with the target eccentricity. The paired comparison of the average amplitude did not exhibit any statistically significant difference between the head-restrained and head-unrestrained conditions (Wilcoxon test, $P > 0.05$; differences = 0.1° ± 0.3° and 0.2° ± 0.4° for monkey B and E, respectively). Similarly, the average value of maximum velocity was not influenced in a consistent way by the head restraint (B). The paired comparison did not reveal any statistically significant difference between the head-restrained and head-unrestrained conditions ($P > 0.05$; differences = 9° ± 43°/s and 6° ± 36°/s for monkey B and E, respectively). For each monkey, the average duration of saccades (C) did not consistently and significantly change between the two head-restraint conditions ($P > 0.05$; differences 0 ± 2 ms and 0 ± 8 ms for monkey B and E, respectively). Concerning the latency of saccades (D), the paired comparison of the latency revealed a statistically significant reduction in latency when the head was unrestrained ($P < 0.05$, differences = −34 ± 25 ms and −12 ± 10 ms for monkey B and E, respectively). *Post hoc* analysis showed that the latency changes observed in

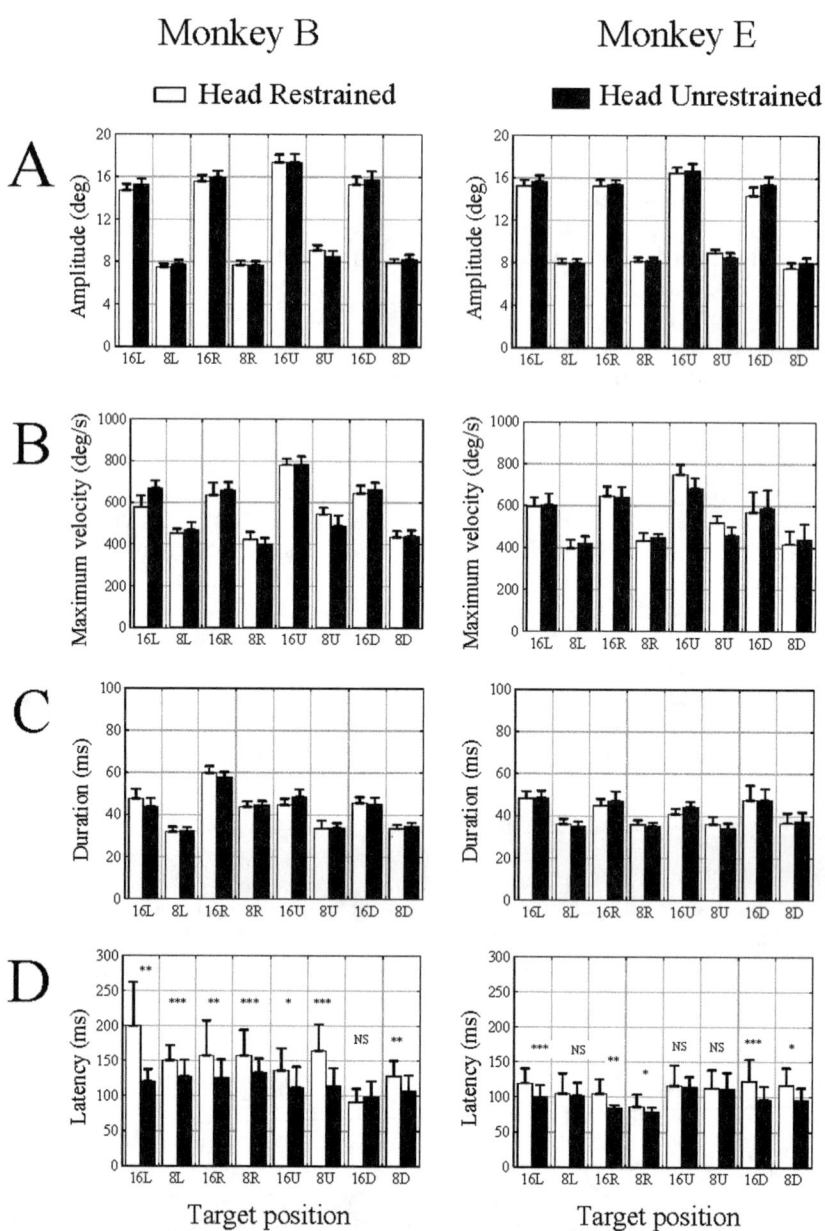

FIGURE 1. Average values of amplitude (**A**), maximum velocity (**B**), duration (**C**), and latency (**D**) of saccades recorded in two monkeys (B and E) with the head restrained (*white histograms*) and unrestrained (*black histograms*). The target LEDs were located 16° and 8° to the left (16L and 8L), to the right (16R and 8R) and above (16U and 8U) or below (16D and 8D) the central fixation LED. Only those saccades that were not accompanied with a concurrent head movement were considered (see METHODS). The error bar corresponds to the standard deviation. NS = $P > 0.05$; *$P < 0.05$; **$P < 0.01$; ***$P < 0.001$ (Mann–Whitney U test).

monkey B were statistically significant for seven of eight targets, whereas in monkey E, they were statistically for five targets (Mann–Whitney U test, $P < 0.05$). The smaller range of average saccade latencies in monkey E may account for this less frequent statistically significant difference.

DISCUSSION

Our results show that the accuracy, peak velocity, and duration of saccades toward slightly eccentric visual targets did not differ between the head-restrained and head-unrestrained conditions. However, the latency of saccades was significantly smaller when the head was unrestrained.

The lack of changes in the peak velocity and duration of saccades is compatible with most studies performed in the monkey.[3-5] In our testing conditions, we did not observe a consistent higher peak velocity in head-unrestrained saccades as might be expected from the study of Collewijn et al.[6] in human subjects. These authors report that the initial acceleration of gaze was substantially higher with the head unrestrained than with the head restrained. On the basis of these observations, they suggested that "the oculomotor system does not work naturally, or near capacity, when the head is prevented from moving" and that "attempts to resist the natural tendency to move the head and the eyes could inhibit saccadic commands to some degree." The implications of this hypothesis are very important because most of the knowledge in oculomotor neurophysiology has been gathered in the head-restrained preparation and may correspond to a "distorted picture of normal oculomotor capacities."[6]

This hypothesis led us to discover an influence of the head motor context on the initiation of saccades. The latency of saccades generated with the head-unrestrained was shorter than the latency of saccades performed with the head restrained. Two more conservative hypotheses can be proposed to account for this result. According to the first one, the reduced latency may result from an increase in target-related retinal image motion cues when the head is unrestrained as compared with when the head is restrained.[7] Motion cues indeed have been shown to facilitate the generation of express saccades.[8] According to the second one, the brainstem saccade generator may be facilitated by the activation of head-related premotor neurons such as the reticulospinal neurons.[9]

ACKNOWLEDGMENTS

We thank Drs. David L. Sparks and Paul Glimcher for graciously providing us with their analysis program (Eyemove) and data acquisition program (Gramalkn). We also thank Kathy Pearson for her invaluable software programming support, Christian Urquizar for helping in building the experimental setup, and Marie Line Loyalle for taking care of the animals.

REFERENCES

1. BLAKEMORE, C. & M. DONAGHY. 1980. Co-ordination of head and eyes in the gaze changing behaviour of cats. J. Physiol. **300**: 317–335.

2. GUITTON, D., R.M. DOUGLAS & M. VOLLE. 1984. Eye-head coordination in cats. J. Neurophysiol. **52:** 1030–1050.
3. TOMLINSON, R.D. & P.S. BAHRA. 1986. Combined eye-head gaze shifts in the primate. I. Metrics. J. Neurophysiol. **56:** 1542–1557.
4. PHILLIPS, O.J., L. LING, A.F. FUCHS, *et al.* 1995. Rapid horizontal gaze movement in the monkey. J. Neurophysiol. **73:** 1632–1652.
5. FREEDMAN, E.G. & D.L. SPARKS. 1997. Eye-head coordination during head-unrestrained gaze shifts in rhesus monkeys. J. Neurophysiol. **77:** 2328–2348.
6. COLLEWIJN, H., R.M. STEINMAN, C.J. ERKELENS, *et al.* 1992. Binocular gaze control under free-head conditions. *In* Vestibular and Brain Stem Control of Eye, Head and Body Movements. H. Shimazu & Y. Shinoda, Eds.: 203–220. S. Karger. Basel.
7. STEINMAN, R.M. & H. COLLEWIJN. 1980. Binocular retinal image motion during active head rotation. Vision Res. **20:** 415–429.
8. MCPEEK, R.M. & P.H. SCHILLER. 1994. The effects of visual scene composition on the latency of saccadic eye movements of the rhesus monkey. Vision Res. **17:** 2293–2305.
9. GRANTYN, A., V. ONG-MEANG JACQUES & A. BERTHOZ. 1987. Reticulo-spinal neurons participating in the control of synergic eye and head movements during orienting in the cat. II. Morphophysiological properties as revealed by intra-axonal injections of horseradish peroxidase. Exp. Brain Res. **66:** 355–377.

Distribution of HSV-1 in Human Geniculate and Vestibular Ganglia: Implications for Vestibular Neuritis

V. ARBUSOW,[a] D. THEIL,[a] P. SCHULZ,[a] M. STRUPP,[a] M. DIETERICH,[b] E. RAUCH,[c] AND T. BRANDT[a]

[a]*Department of Neurology, Klinikum Grosshadern, University of Munich, D-80337 Munich, Germany*

[b]*Department of Neurology, University of Mainz, Mainz, Germany*

[c]*Institute of Forensic Medicine, University of Munich, D-80337 Munich, Germany*

KEYWORDS: HSV-1; human geniculate ganglion; vestibular ganglion; vestibular neuritis

Vestibular neuritis (VN) is the third most common cause of peripheral vestibular vertigo. Epidemic occurrence of the condition, postmortem studies, and the demonstration of latent HSV-1 in human vestibular ganglia suggest that the cause of the disease might be reactivation of latent HSV-1 in the vestibular ganglion (VG).[1] VN is a partial rather than a complete paresis with predominant involvement of the anterior and horizontal semicircular canals and the utricle.[2] Anatomical studies have shown an anastomosis between the intermediate nerve and the superior portion of the vestibular nerve,[3] which led us to the hypothesis that after primary viral infection of the ganglion geniculi (GG) via chorda tympani, migration of HSV-1 to the superior portion of the VG along this facio-vestibular anastomosis is possible (FIG. 1). Reactivation of HSV-1 then would cause selective inflammation of the superior vestibular nerve and the dysfunction of the anterior and horizontal semicircular canals (SCCs), typical for VN. To determine HSV-1 distribution between the GG and VG and within the different parts of the VG, we examined 35 human temporal bones for HSV-1–specific DNA by nested polymerase chain reaction.

MATERIALS AND METHODS

The study was performed with the consent of the ethics committee of the Medical Faculty of the University of Munich. Thirty-five temporal bones were obtained from the Institute of Forensic Medicine of the University of Munich at the time of autopsy.

Address for correspondence: Dr. V. Arbusow, Department of Neurology, University of Munich, Klinikum Grosshadern, Marchioninistrasse 15, D-81377 Munich, Germany. Voice: +49-89-7095-2571; fax: +49-89-7095-8883.
varbusow@nro.med.uni-muenchen.de

Ann. N.Y. Acad. Sci. 1004: 409–413 (2003). © 2003 New York Academy of Sciences.
doi: 10.1196/annAls.1303.042

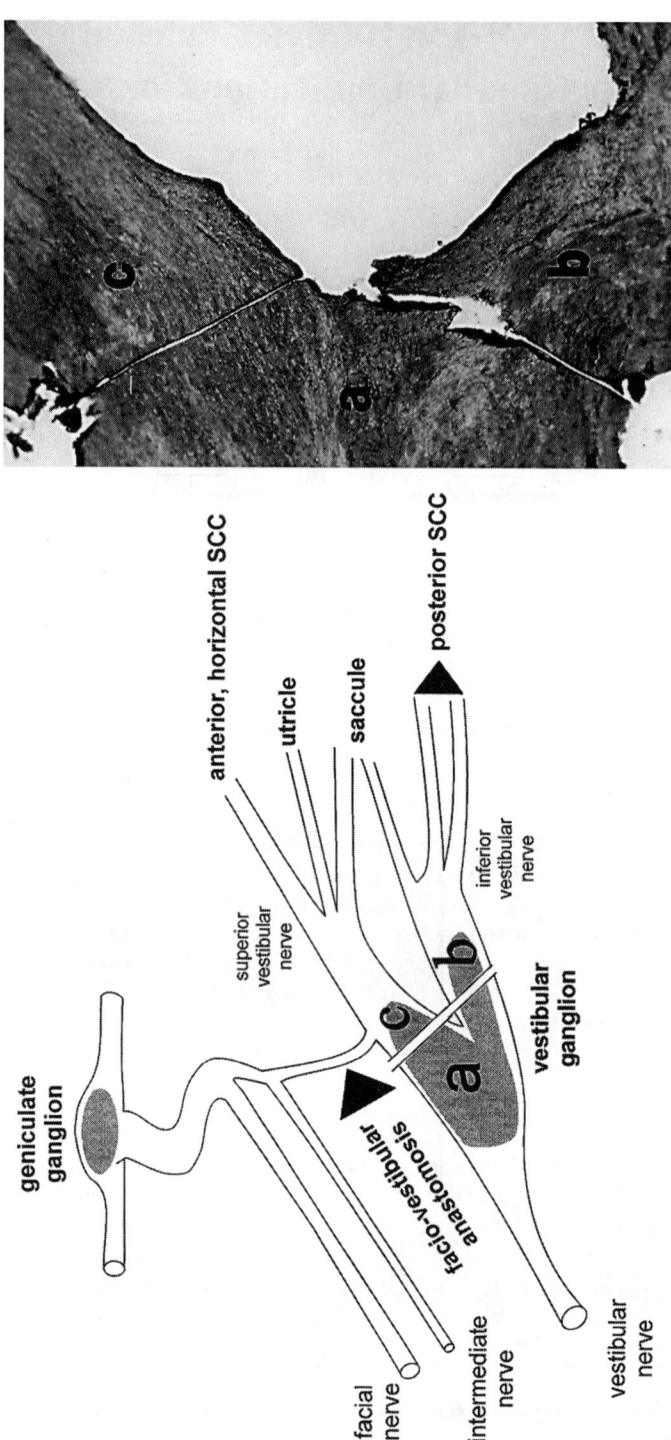

FIGURE 1. Schematic drawing of geniculate ganglion, vestibular ganglion, and the superior and inferior vestibular nerves (*left*). A facio-vestibular anastomosis connects the facial (intermediate) nerve with the superior vestibular nerve. Bipolar neurons of the VG extend in the proximal superior and inferior vestibular nerves. An accessory posterior ampullary nerve branches off the posterior ampullary nerve. Sections of the vestibular ganglion indicate the preparation for separation into (**a**) stem; (**b**) inferior portion; and (**c**) superior portion of the vestibular ganglion. Longitudinal cryosection (30 μm) through a human vestibular ganglion stained with cresyl violet (*right*). The very proximal parts of the superior (**c**) and the inferior (**b**) vestibular nerves containing neurons of the VG were separated from the ganglion stem (**a**) by transversal cuts and analyzed individually for HSV-1 latency. SCC, semicircular canal.

The cause of death was unrelated to cranial nerve dysfunction in all cases. Age distribution ranged from 3 months to 74 years with a median of 44 years (13 males and 5 females). Geniculate and vestibular ganglia were prepared free of bone and connective tissue and cryosectioned. Slides (30 µm) were separated in three parts under an inverted microscope with a microstilette: stem of the ganglion and the very proximal parts of superior and inferior portion of the vestibular nerve. After DNA extraction, nested polymerase chain reaction for HSV-1 was conducted according to the method described by Aurelius et al.[4]

RESULTS

In 29 of 35 human temporal bones, HSV-1 was found in at least one of the investigated ganglia. GG was affected in 55% (23/35) and VG in 50% (21/35). Distribution of HSV-1 among of the vestibular ganglia was as follows: stem only 5/21 (24%), superior portion only 5/21 (29%), inferior portion only 3/21 (14%), and combined infections of two or three examined parts 7/21 (33%).

DISCUSSION

Although multiple neighboring cranial nerve ganglia may be HSV-1 infected, experience shows that clinical manifestation of viral reactivation is restricted to singular nerves. The vestibular ganglion has three portions: the *stem* and the ganglion cells in the *proximal superior and inferior vestibular nerves* (FIG. 1). Based on this anat-

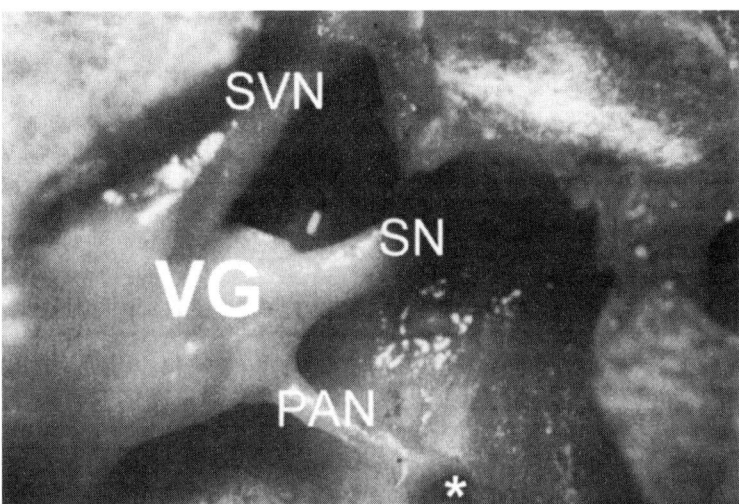

FIGURE 2. Microscopic preparation (×10) of a human vestibular ganglion and nerves. VG, vestibular ganglion; SVN, superior vestibular nerve; SN, saccular nerve; PAN, posterior ampullary nerve. *Separate bony canal of the PAN.

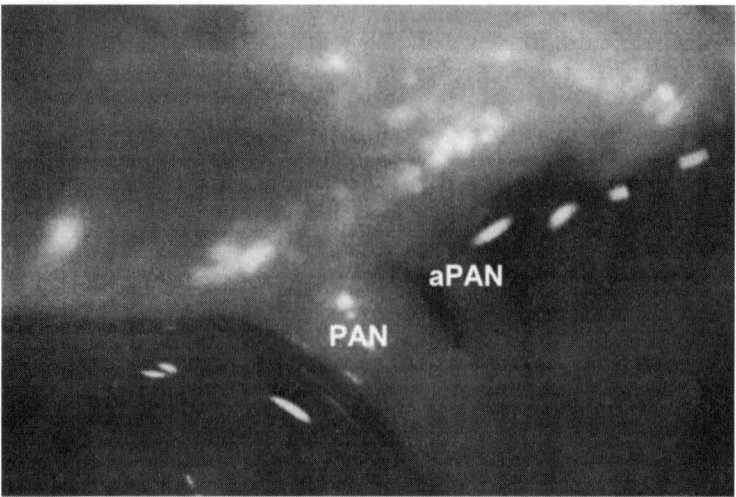

FIGURE 3. Amplification of the posterior ampullary nerve (×40) that reveals the common accessory posterior ampullary nerve. PAN, posterior ampullary nerve; aPAN, accessory posterior ampullary nerve.

omy, theoretically three different types of VN are possible. (1) Entire VG inflammation (stem) that causes complete loss of unilateral vestibular dysfunction with ocular tilt reaction and rotatory spontaneous nystagmus toward the nonaffected ear: this has been described for herpes zoster oticus.[1] (2) Inferior vestibular nerve inflammation that causes complete loss of posterior canal and partial loss of saccular function: this, to our knowledge, has not yet been described. (3) Superior vestibular nerve inflammation that causes complete paresis of the anterior and horizontal canals, the utricle and partial paresis of the saccule: this is the typical clinical pattern of VN.[1,2] However, despite the simplicity and attractiveness of the hypothesis of viral migration along this facio-vestibular anastomosis to the ganglion cells of the superior vestibular nerve, it is not supported by our data. Therefore, regular preservation of posterior canal function in VN requires an alternative explanation. This could be offered by an anatomical variant of the innervation of the posterior semicircular canal. Anatomical studies in vertebrates with sections through the posterior ampulla revealed a small vestibular end organ in the floor of the posterior recess of the utricle, the so-called crista neglecta,[5] which is innervated by a small accessory nerve that originates from the posterior ampullary nerve.[3,5] In humans, this accessory cupula organ is rarely detectable,[5] but the posterior SCC is still innervated by two distinct nerves that reach the posterior cupula in a separate bony canal (FIGs. 2 and 3), as demonstrated by Montandon *et al.* in more than 500 human temporal bone specimens.[5] In our temporal bone preparations, 27 of 35 (77%) exhibited double innervation of the posterior ampulla (FIGs. 2 and 3). This double innervation by two ampullary nerves running in a separate bony canal provides two plausible explanations for sparing posterior SCC function in VN. (1) If the neuronal pools of both branches were located separately in the VG, one pool might be spared in viral inflammation. (2) The course of both posterior ampullary nerves through a separate bony canal makes it possible that they are less afflicted by inflammatory swelling of the perineural tissue of the vestibular nerve encapsulated within the intrameatal duct.

REFERENCES

1. BRANDT, T. 1999. Vestibular neuritis. *In* Vertigo: Its Sensorimotor Syndromes. 2nd edit. 57–81. Springer. London.
2. BÜCHELE, W. & T. BRANDT. 1988. Vestibular neuritis—a horizontal semicircular canal paresis? Adv. Otorhinolaryngol. **42:** 157–151.
3. BERGSTRÖM, B. 1973. Morphology of the vestibular nerve. II. The number of myelinated vestibular nerve fibers in man at various ages. Acta Otolaryngol. (Stockh.) **75:** 173–179.
4. AURELIUS, E., B. JOHANSSON, B. SKÖLDENBERG, *et al.* 1991. Rapid diagnosis of herpes simplex encephalitis by nested polymerase chain reaction assay of cerebrospinal fluid. Lancet **337:** 189–192.
5. MONTANDON, P., R.R. GACEK & R.S. KIMURA. 1970. Crista neglecta in the cat and human. Ann. Otol. Rhinol. Laryngol. **79:** 105–112.

Twitch and Non-Twitch Motoneurons of Extraocular Muscles Have Different Histochemical Properties

ANDREAS C. EBERHORN, ANJA K.E. HORN, AHMED MESSOUDI, AND JEAN A. BÜTTNER-ENNEVER

Anatomische Anstalt, Lehrstuhl III, LMU München, 80336 München, Germany

KEYWORDS: abducens nucleus; perineuronal nets; SMI32

INTRODUCTION

The extraocular muscles of vertebrates show a highly complicated organization. Their muscle fibers can be classified into two main categories: singly innervated "twitch" fibers (TMF), resembling those of skeletal muscle, and multiply innervated "non-twitch" fibers (non-TMF). The motoneurons of extraocular muscles lie in three brainstem nuclei: the oculomotor nucleus, the trochlear nucleus, and the abducens nucleus. Recent work in the macaque monkey showed that the motoneurons innervating non-TMFs are located in separate subgroups, which lie around the borders of the classic nuclei.[1]

In the current study, we investigated whether TMF and non-TMF motoneurons differ in their histochemical properties, using combined tract-tracing and immunofluorescence methods.

METHODS

Animal care and experimental procedures conformed to the state and university regulations on Laboratory Animal Care and were approved by their Animal Care Officers and Institutional Animal Care and Use Committees. Under general anaesthesia, a retrograde tract tracer (cholera toxin subunit B [CTb] 15 µL, 1%; List, Campbell, CA) was injected into the distal myotendinous junction of the lateral rectus eye muscle. After 3 days' survival time, the animals were killed by an overdose of anaesthesia and perfused transcardially with saline, followed by 4% paraformaldehyde in 0.1 M phosphate buffer (PB) and 10% sucrose in 0.1M PB at pH 7.4. Forty micrometers of frozen-cut free-floating frontal brain sections were first processed for tracer detection by immunofluorescence (goat anti-choleragenoid, 1:5000; List)

Address for correspondence: Andreas Eberhorn, Anatomische Anstalt, Lehrstuhl III, LMU München, Pettenkoferstrasse 11, D-80336 München, Germany. Voice: 49-89-5160-4824/4876; fax: 49-89-5160-4857.

andreas.eberhorn@anat.med.uni-muenchen.de

Ann. N.Y. Acad. Sci. 1004: 414–417 (2003). © 2003 New York Academy of Sciences.
doi: 10.1196/annals.1303.043

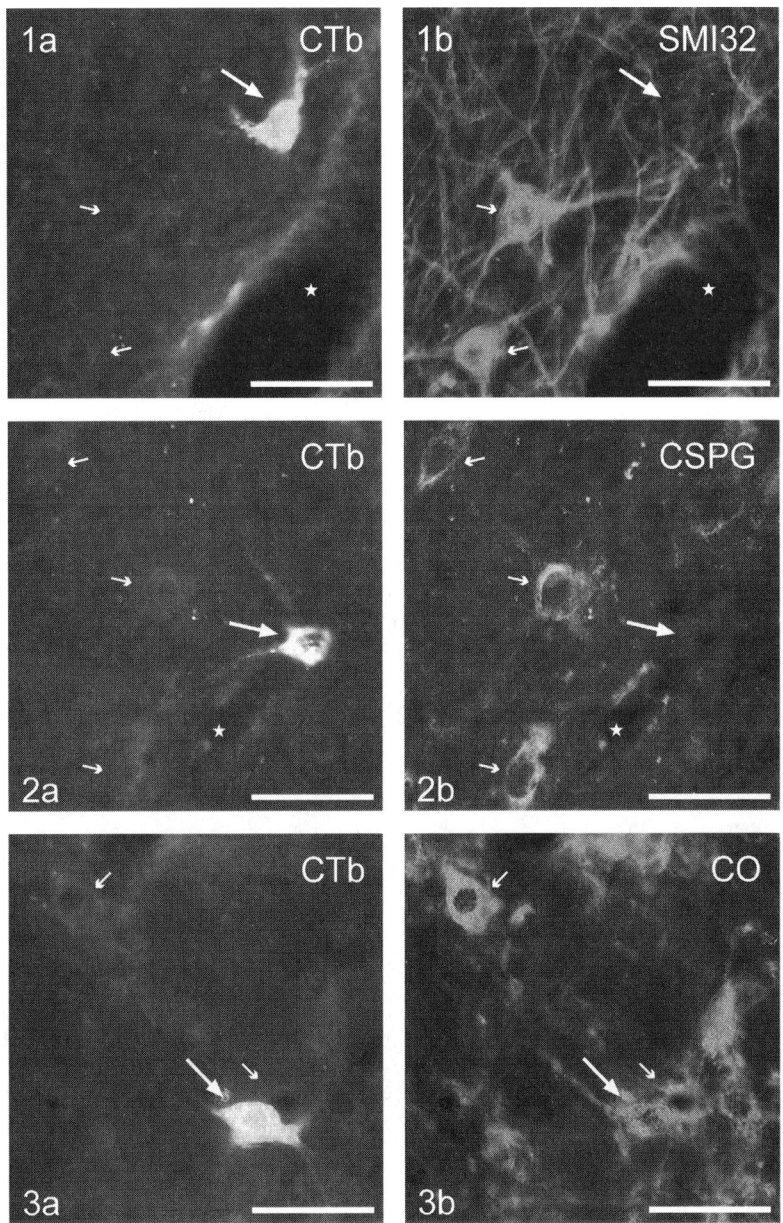

FIGURE 1–3. High-power magnification of retrogradely labeled CTb-positive (Cy2-tagged antibody) non-TMF motoneurons in **1a, 2a, 3a** (*big arrows*) combined with immunofluorescence (Cy3-tagged antibody) using SMI32 antibodies (**1b**), CSPG antibodies in **2b** and CO antibodies in **3b**. Note that in contrast with neurons within the abducens nucleus the retrogradely labeled non-TMF motoneurons do not express SMI32 immunolabeling (**1a, 1b**, *small arrows*) and are not ensheathed by perineuronal nets detected by CSPG immunolabeling (**2a, 2b**). CO immunoreactivity is present in non-TMF motoneurons and neurons within the abducens nucleus (**3a, 3b**). Scale bar is 20 μm.

and then treated with a second immunofluorescence protocol for one of the following antibodies: anti-chondroitin sulfate proteoglycans (mouse anti-CSPG; 1:100; Chemicon) as a label for perineuronal nets,[2] SMI32 (mouse SMI32, 1:900; Sternberger Monoclonals) for nonphosphorylated neurofilaments, anti-parvalbumin (mouse anti-PV, 1:1000; Swant), and anti-cytochromeoxidase (mouse anti-CO, 1:100; Molecular Probes).

RESULTS

The tracer injections (CTb) into the distal tip of lateral rectus muscle labeled neurons which lie almost exclusively around the borders of the classic abducens nucleus, representing non-TMF motoneurons. The SMI32 antibody, which is proved to be a reliable motoneuron marker in the brainstem across many mammalian species,[3] labels cell somata, dendrites, and axons. Double-labeling experiments with SMI32 antibodies revealed that none of the CTb-positive motoneurons showed SMI32 immunoreactivity, whereas virtually all neurons within the classic abducens nucleus were strongly labeled (FIG. 1a,b). Double-labeling experiments with anti–PV antibodies showed a similar result, though a low number of CTb-positive cells showed light PV immunoreactivity.

Anti–CSPG antibodies label the so-called perineuronal nets, which surround neurons as lattice-like structures and presumably are associated with fast-spiking neurons.[4] The double-labeling experiments revealed that, like PV and SMI32, none of the CTb-positive motoneurons showed CSPG immunoreactivity (FIG. 2a,b), whereas virtually all neurons within the abducens nucleus display prominent perineuronal nets. In contrast, double-labeling with anti–CO antibodies stained both TMF motoneurons within and most of the CTb-positive non-TMF motoneurons in the periphery (FIG. 3a,b).

CONCLUSIONS

The present data provide first evidence that TMF and non-TMF motoneurons of the macaque monkey differ in their histochemical properties. The TMF motoneurons within the abducens nucleus exhibit strong SMI-32, PV, and CSPG immunoreactivity, whereas the retrogradely labeled non-TMF motoneurons in the periphery of the abducens nucleus do not show PV and SMI32 immunoreactivity, and they lack CSPG-positive perineuronal nets. CO immunoreactivity was more or less present in both TMF and non-TMF motoneurons. The "negative" markers PV, SMI32, and CSPG may help to identify the homologue non-TMF motoneurons in other species, including humans.

ACKNOWLEDGMENTS

This work was supported by the Deutsche Forschungsgesellschaft (SFB 462/B3) and the Graduiertenkolleg (Andreas Eberhorn): Sensory interaction in biological and technical systems (GRK 267).

REFERENCES

1. BÜTTNER-ENNEVER, J.A. *et al.* 2001. Motoneurons of twitch and nontwitch extraocular muscle fibres in the abducens, trochlear, and oculomotor nucleus of monkeys. J. Comp. Neurol. **438:** 318–335.
2. CELIO, M.R. & I. BLÜMCKE. 1994. Perineuronal nets—a specialized form of extracellular matrix in the adult nervous system. Brain Res. Rev. **19:** 128–145.
3. TSANG, Y.M. *et al.* 2000. Motor neurons are rich in non-phosphorylated neurofilaments: cross-species comparison and alterations in ALS. Brain Res. **861:** 45–58.
4. HÄRTIG, W. *et al.* 1999. Cortical neurons immunoreactive for the potassium channel Kv3.1b subunit are predominantly surrounded by perineuronal nets presumed as a buffering system for cations. Brain Res. **842:** 15–29.

Plasticity in Brainstem Motor Systems When Innervating a New Muscle in Adult Mammals

AGNÈS GRUART,[a] MICHAEL STREPPEL,[b] ORLANDO GUNTINAS-LICHIUS,[b] D. N. ANGELOV,[b] WOLFRAM F. NEISS,[c] AND JOSÉ M. DELGADO-GARCÍA[a]

[a]*Laboratorio Andaluz de Biología, Universidad Pablo de Olavide, 41013 Sevilla, Spain*

[b]*Klinik für Hals-, Nasen- und Ohrenheilkunde, Universität zu Köln, Köln, Germany*

[c]*Institut I für Anatomie, Universität zu Köln, Köln, Germany*

KEYWORDS: anastomosis; blinks; corneal reflex; facial motor system; hypoglossal nucleus; motor learning; neural plasticity; classic conditioning; reinnervation

INTRODUCTION

Because motoneurons represent the final common site where neuronal motor commands are integrated and executed, it seems interesting to determine to what extent motoneuronal pools are able to modify those motor commands when reinnervating a new muscle. Years ago, Sperry[1] suggested that motor centers in adult mammals lack the capacity to reorganize their firing to accomplish the functional requirements of new motor targets. The successful reproduction in rats[2] and cats[3,4] of the classic hypoglossal-facial and facial-facial anastomoses used in humans for the treatment of some types of facial paralysis prompted us to perform a physiological study on the capability of different brainstem motoneuron pools to fulfil the specific tasks of the upper eyelid during the performance of reflex and patterned motor responses.

THE EXPERIMENTAL MODEL

Experiments were conducted on adult female cats, following the specific recommendations of the European Union (86/609/EU) for the use of experimental animals in chronic experiments. Under general anesthesia (sodium pentobarbital 35 mg/kg and atropine sulfate 0.5 mg/kg), animals were implanted with metal coils for the recording of eyelid movements with the search coil in a magnetic-field technique and with bipolar electrodes for electromyographic (EMG) recordings of the orbicularis oculi muscle. Animals were also implanted with a head-holding system to allow chronic recordings of eyelid position and EMG activity. The following nerve manip-

---

Address for correspondence: Prof. José M. Delgado-García, M.D., Ph.D., Laboratorio Andaluz de Biología, Universidad Pablo de Olavide, Ctra. de Utrera, KM. 1, Sevilla 41013, Spain. Voice: 34-954-349374; fax: 34-954-349375.

jmdelgar@dex.upo.es

ulations were performed: (1) a transection, 180° rotation, and resuture of the zygomatic branch of the facial nerve plexus (zygomatic nerve rotation); (2) a transection and crossed suture of the proximal buccal to the distal zygomatic stump of these facial nerve branches (buccal-zygomatic anastomosis); and (3) a hypoglossal-facial anastomosis. Recording sessions were conducted up to 1 yr after surgery. Functional recovery of eyelid motorics on the anastomosed side was checked every 10–15 days by the presentation of eyelid- and mouth-evoking stimuli (puffs of air, flashes of light, tones, and drops of milk applied to the tongue). Further details of this chronic preparation have been presented elsewhere.[2–4]

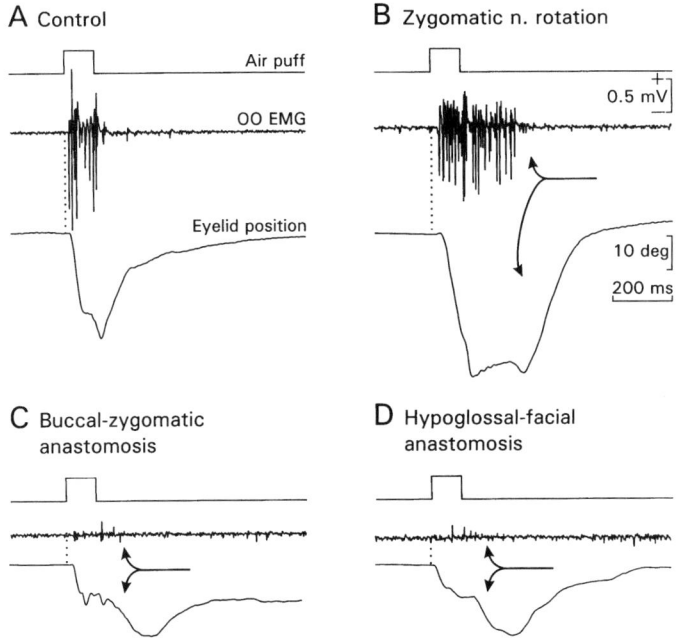

FIGURE 1. Blinks evoked by air puffs presented to the cornea and periorbital skin ipsilateral to the anastomosed side. Recordings were conducted 9 months after surgery. (**A–D**) From top to bottom are illustrated the stimulus presented (an air puff of 3 kg/cm² lasting for 100 ms), the electromyographic activity of the orbicularis oculi muscle (OO EMG) and the eye position for control (**A**), and after zygomatic nerve transection, 180° rotation, and resuture (**B**), buccal-zygomatic anastomosis (**C**), and hypoglossal-facial anastomosis (**D**). The double-headed arrow in **B** points to the presence of late downward eyelid movements in the absence of EMG activity in the OO muscle. Double-headed arrows in **C** and **D** point to the presence of downward eyelid movements in response to air-puff presentation in the absence of any noticeable EMG activity of the OO muscle. Note that EMG and eyelid responses were larger than in control after zygomatic nerve rotation (**B**) and smaller after buccal-zygomatic (**C**) and hypoglossal-facial (**D**) anastomoses. Calibrations in **B** are also for **A**, **B**, and **D**. (Traces in **A–C** were taken and modified from FIG. 2B in Gruart et al.[4]).

RESULTS AND CONCLUSIONS

Animals with a zygomatic nerve rotation recovered spontaneous and reflex eyelid responses approximately 6–8 weeks after surgery. However, they presented evident (and permanent) alterations in eyelid kinematics due to the improper regional distribution of orbicularis oculi motor units after zygomatic nerve rotation and resuture. A significant (bilateral) hyperreflexia was observed in animals with zygomatic nerve rotation (FIG. 1B). This hyperreflexia was able to evoke the activation of the retractor bulbi system, as evidenced by the presence of large blink responses to air-puff presentations in the absence of any noticeable EMG activity of the orbicularis oculi muscle, an occurrence not observed in controls (FIG. 1A, B). The hyperreflexia has a trigeminal origin, because it was not noticed after the presentation of blink-evoking stimuli of different sensory modalities (flashes, tones).

The EMG activity of the orbicularis oculi muscle was recovered in 6–8 weeks after the buccal-zygomatic anastomosis. Nevertheless, this muscle never presented a proper EMG response to blink-evoking stimuli for the time of the study. Eyelid downward displacements observed during air-puff presentations were produced by the activation of the retractor bulbi system (FIG. 1C). Animals with buccal-zygomatic anastomosis also presented hyperreflexic responses to trigeminal stimuli, as evidenced mainly in the EMG activity of the contralateral (nonoperated side) orbicularis oculi muscle (not illustrated, but see Gruart et al.[4]).

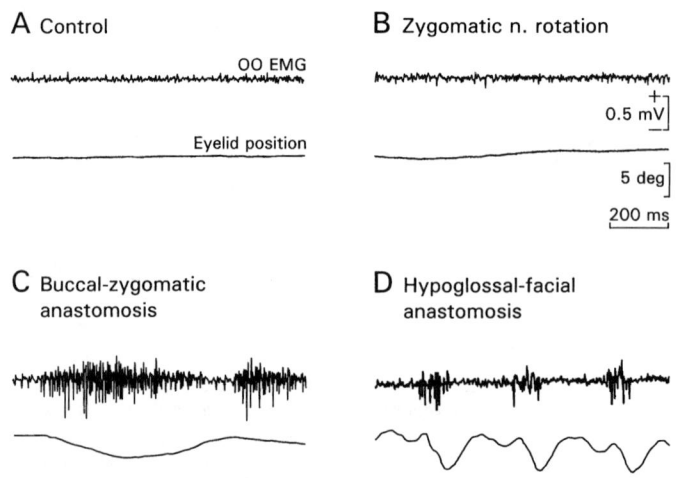

FIGURE 2. Electromyographic (EMG) activity of the orbicularis oculi (OO) muscle and eyelid movements during licking of a few drops of milk in a control (**A**) and after zygomatic nerve transection, 180° rotation, and resuture (**B**), buccal-zygomatic anastomosis (**C**), and hypoglossal-facial anastomosis (**D**). Note the absence of muscle activity and eyelid movement in **A** and **B**. In contrast, animals with buccal-zygomatic (**C**) or hypoglossal-facial (**D**) anastomosis presented a rhythmic activity during licking. Calibrations in **B** are also for A–C. (Traces in **D** were modified from FIG. 7B in Gruart et al.[3])

Animals with a hypoglossal-facial anastomosis also recovered the EMG activity of the orbicularis oculi muscle in 6–8 weeks but were never able to evoke a true blink response to air-puff presentations (FIG. 1D). Although the EMG activity of the orbicularis oculi muscle in response to corneal air puffs, flashes of light, or tones was not recovered in the 12 months of this study, reflex blinks were reestablished by the increased activity of the retractor bulbi motor system. Hyperreflexic eyelid responses were evident in the side contralateral to air-puff presentations, but not to flashes or tones (not illustrated, but see Gruart et al.[4]).

Mouth-related facial and hypoglossal motoneurons did not readapt their firing to the kinetic, timing, and oscillatory properties of the orbicularis oculi muscle fibers as shown during licking and eating (FIG. 2). Indeed, during licking a few drops of milk, animals with buccal-zygomatic (FIG. 2C) and hypoglossal-facial (FIG. 2D) anastomoses presented rhythmic eyelid displacements resembling those produced by mouth and tongue muscles.[3,4]

In conclusion, motor and immediately premotor facial circuits maintain their motor programs in adult cats when motoneurons are obliged to reinnervate a foreign muscle, or even a new set of muscle fibers.

REFERENCES

1. SPERRY, R.W. 1945. The problem of central nervous system reorganization after nerve regeneration and muscle transposition. Q. Rev. Biol. **20:** 311–369.
2. NEISS, W.F., O. GUNTINAS-LICHIUS, D.N. ANGELOV, et al. 1992. The hypoglossal-facial anastomosis as model of neural plasticity in the rat. Ann. Anat. **174:** 419–433.
3. GRUART, A., A. GUNKEL, W.F. NEISS, et al. 1996. Changes in eye blink responses following hypoglossal-facial anastomosis in the cat: evidence of adult motoneuron unadaptability to new motor tasks. Neuroscience **73:** 233–247.
4. GRUART, A., M. STREPPEL, O. GUNTINAS-LICHIUS, et al. 2003. Motoneuron adaptability to new motor tasks following two types of facial-facial anastomosis in cats. Brain **126:** 115–133.

Vestibulo-Oculomotor Behavior in Rats after a Transient Unilateral Vestibular Loss Induced by Lidocaine

ANNA K. MAGNUSSON[a,c] AND RICHARD THAM[b]

[a]*Department of Biomedicine and Surgery, Faculty of Health Sciences, SE-581 85 Linköping, Sweden*

[b]*Department of Neuroscience and Locomotion, Faculty of Health Sciences, SE-581 85 Linköping, Sweden*

KEYWORDS: vestibular compensation; labyrinthectomy; habituation

Hitherto, it has been impossible to investigate the vestibulo-oculomotor behavior during the first hours after a unilateral labyrinthectomy properly because of confounding factors such as anesthesia and postsurgical trauma. Chemical labyrinthectomies are also unsuitable for assessment of the initial behavioral consequences of a vestibular loss because the symptoms develop gradually over several hours.[1] A controlled intratympanic installation of lidocaine offers a possibility to study alert behaving animals in the very first period of compensation after a unilateral vestibular loss.[2] The aim of this investigation was to evaluate vestibulo-oculomotor symptoms, during and after a transient unilateral peripheral vestibular loss in pigmented rats caused by lidocaine. The vestibulo-oculomotor reflex was assessed with or without dynamic vestibular stimulations by recordings of horizontal eye movements.

Lidocaine caused an almost immediate functional labyrinthectomy, lasting for about 1 h. During this time, all the postural as well as vestibulo-oculomotor disturbances, which are related to a peripheral vestibular loss, could be demonstrated. After instillation of 4% lidocaine into the middle ear cavity, a vigorous spontaneous nystagmus (SN) was evident within 15 min. The slow-phase velocity (SPV) and the frequency increased rapidly to values up to 120°/s and 250–300 beats/min, respectively, after which SN abruptly failed, as if the system overloaded. This state lasted about 40 min when SN reappeared with about the same frequency and SPV as during the period before the failure. Once reappeared, the SN frequency gradually abated

Address for correspondence: Richard Tham, Department of Neuroscience and Locomotion, Faculty of Health Sciences, SE-581 85 Linköping, Sweden. Voice: 46-13-222516; fax: 46-13-222558.

ricth@inr.liu.se

[c]Present address: Max-Planck-Institute of Neurobiology, Am Klopferspitz 18a, D-82152 Martinsried, Germany.

and the gaze stabilized within 10 min. The SN failure could be avoided by providing visual feedback in between the recordings in darkness or by a contralateral instillation of 2.5% lidocaine.

After recovery from the acute lidocaine effect, when the SN had subsided, a reversed SPV gain asymmetry was observed during 0.2-Hz sinusoidal stimulation, that is, a decrease in SPV gain during rotation to the contralidocaine side and a normal or slightly increased SPV gain during rotation to the ipsilidocaine side. Likewise, a reduced time constant was observed with a step stimulus ($1000°/s^2$ up to a constant velocity of $120°/s$ toward the contralidocaine side, whereas the time constant during stimulation toward the ipsilidocaine side remained normal. A similar vestibulo-oculomotor behavior has been observed with unilateral repeated rotational stimulation causing unidirectional habituation.[3] It has also been demonstrated that vestibular habituation is related to the cerebellar nodulus.[4] In the current investigation, a previous nodulectomy significantly reduced the reversed gain asymmetry, as observed after the short-lasting lidocaine-induced vestibular loss. This finding further supports a notion that the reversed gain asymmetry is a manifestation of vestibular habituation.

In summary, this study shows that (1) the vestibulo-oculomotor system seems to overload shortly after a sudden unilateral vestibular loss; and (2) a mechanism to counteract the pronounced asymmetry in the vestibulo-oculomotor circuitry develops during the first hour after the loss. This mechanism, which might be related to the concept of vestibular habituation, is retained for many hours despite recovery of peripheral vestibular function.

REFERENCES

1. MAGNUSSON, A.K., M. ULFENDAHL & R. THAM. 2002. Early compensation of vestibulo-oculomotor symptoms after unilateral vestibular loss in rats is related to $GABA_B$ receptor function. Neuroscience **111:** 625–634.
2. JENKINS, H.A., B.S.V. HONRUBIA & P.H. WARD. 1969. Pharmacological labyrinthectomy. Ann. Otol. Rhinol. Laryngol. **78:** 562–574.
3. CLÉMENT, G., J.-H. COURJON, M. JEANNEROD & R. SCHMID. 1981. Unidirectional habituation of vestibulo-ocular responses by repeated rotational or optokinetic stimulations in the cat. Exp. Brain Res. **42:** 34–42.
4. COHEN, H., B. COHEN, T. RAPHAN & W. WAESPE. 1992. Habituation and adaptation of the vestibuloocular reflex: a model of differential control by the vestibulocerebellum. Exp. Brain Res. **90:** 526–538.

A Synaptic Mechanism on Prepositus Hypoglossi Neurons Underlying Eye Fixation

JUAN D. NAVARRO-LOPEZ,[a] JUAN CARLOS ALVARADO,[a,b] MIGUEL ESCUDERO,[c] JOSÉ M. DELGADO-GARCÍA, AND JAVIER YAJEYA[b]

[a]*División de Neurociencias, Laboratorio Andaluz de Biología, Universidad Pablo de Olavide, Sevilla 41013, Spain*

[b]*Instituto de Neurociencias de Castilla y León, Universidad de Salamanca, Salamanca 37007, Spain*

[c]*Departamento de Fisiología y Zoología, Facultad de Biología, Universidad de Sevilla, Sevilla 41012, Spain*

> ABSTRACT: We have studied *in vitro* and *in vivo* the origin of the persistent neuronal activity underlying eye positions of fixation after eye saccades in the horizontal plane. It is proposed that the tonic firing presented by prepositus hypoglossi neurons during eye fixations is the result of the combined action of eye-velocity signals arriving from excitatory burst neurons and the facilitative role of cholinergic terminals of reticular origin.
>
> KEYWORDS: cats; rats; oculomotor system; acetylcholine; glutamatergic receptors; neural persistent activity; eye fixation

It has been shown in alert cats that prepositus hypoglossi (PH) neurons encode pure eye position (or related position-velocity and velocity-position) signals.[1] Moreover, permanent electrolytic lesions and transient pharmacological inactivation have shown that PH neurons are necessary for eye fixation.[2,3] The main source of eye-velocity signals arriving at PH neurons is excitatory burst neurons (EBNs) located in the paramedian pontine reticular formation (PPRF), rostrally to the abducens motor nucleus.[4] It generally is accepted that a sort of neural integration takes place in the PH nucleus, to transform transient eye-velocity signals into persistent eye-position neural commands,[5] but the intrinsic neural processes involved in this integration are largely unknown. Recently, it has been convincingly demonstrated that neural integration taking place in hindbrain area I in goldfish is a synaptic process, independent of the passive or active membrane properties of neurons generating eye-position signals.[6] Here, we have studied both *in vitro* (in newborn rats) and *in vivo* (in alert cats) the synaptic mechanisms evoked in PH neurons by EBNs and by reticular cholin-

---

Address for correspondence: José M. Delgado-García, División de Neurociencias, Laboratorio Andaluz de Biología, Universidad Pablo de Olavide, Ctra. de Utrera, Km. 1, Sevilla 41013, Spain. Voice: 34-954-349374; fax: 34-954-349375.
 jmdelgar@dex.upo.es

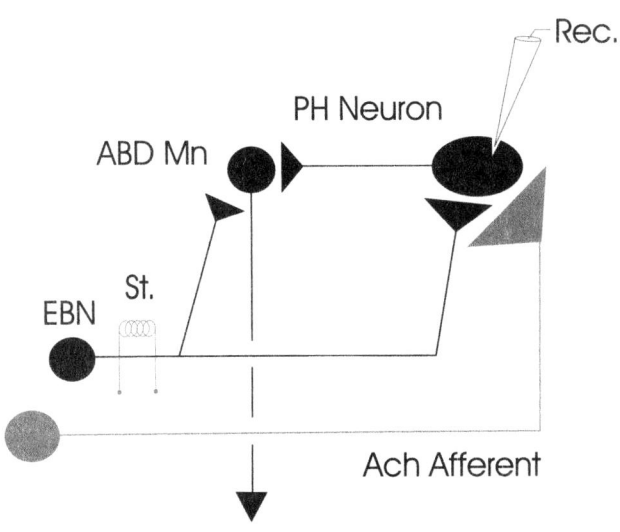

FIGURE 1. Experimental design. Sagittal brainstem slices obtained from 3–4-week-old rats were used in this study. Stimulation (St.) and recording (Rec.) sites are indicated Stimuli applied to the paramedian pontine reticular formation activated both excitatory burst neurons (EBN) and descending cholinergic axons from the pontomesencephalic area. Ach acetylcholine; PH, prepositus hypoglossi.

ergic axons, and the neurotransmitters involved in the generation of the persistent activity underlying eye fixation.

In vitro experiments were conducted in 3–4-week-old rats obtained from an official supplier. Brainstem sagittal slices (400 μm thick) including the PPRF and the PH nucleus were obtained after procedures described elsewhere.[7] Slices were maintained in a recording chamber bathed with artificial cerebrospinal fluid (ACSF). Intracellular records were obtained with glass microelectrodes (140–180 Mohms) filled with potassium acetate 3 M connected to a Bio-logic (Claix, France) recording amplifier. Only neurons with resting potentials greater than −55 mV were recorded. Synaptic potentials were elicited by stimulating the ipsilateral PPRF with a monopolar stainless steel electrode (2 Mohms). Single (100–200 μs) and train (100–200 μs, 100-ms trains, at 50–200 Hz) cathodal, square-wave pulses (100–500 μA) were applied to the BEN area (FIG. 1). Chemicals were applied by superfusion in the ACSF. Data were acquired with the help of a CED 1401 interface (Cambridge, England) and analyzed with the 5.2.1 Analysis Program from Synaptosoft (Decatur, GA, USA). Selected neurons were filled with biocytin and stained with the avidin-biotin-peroxidase procedure (ABC; Vectors Labs, Burlingame, CA, USA). Neurons were reconstructed with the help of a camera lucida from Nikon (Kawasaki, Japan). *In vivo* experiments were conducted in adult cats ($n = 2$) prepared for the chronic recording of eye movements (with the search-coil-in-a-magnetic-field technique) and of the electrical activity of PH neurons. Drug injections in the PH area were performed by means of glass pipettes filled with the corresponding chemical dissolved in phosphate buffer

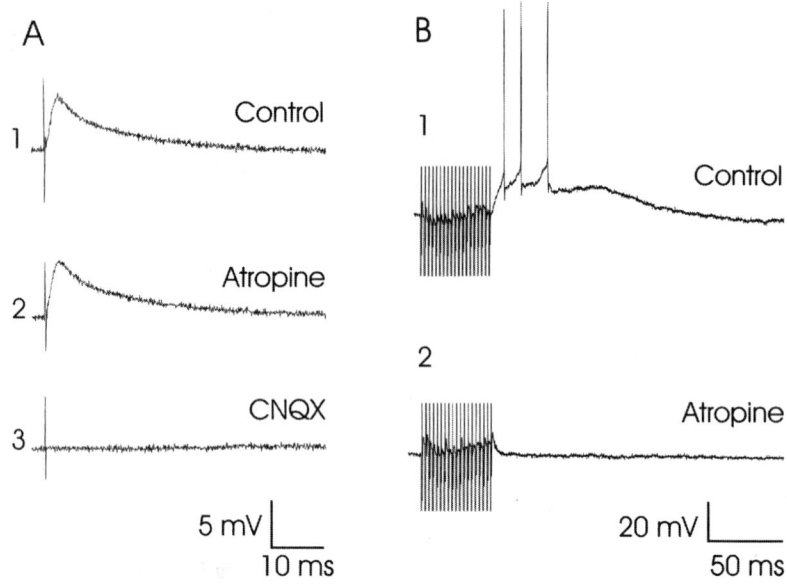

FIGURE 2. Different effects of single and train stimulation of paramedian pontine reticular formation (PPRF) on prepositus hypoglossi neurons *in vitro*. (**A**) An example of EPSP evoked in a prepositus hypoglossi (PH) neuron by a single (100 ms, 300 mA) pulse applied to the PPRF (**A1**) and the effects of atropine sulfate (**A2**; 1.5 mM) and CNQX (**A3**; 10 mM). (**B**) Effects of PPRF train (200 Hz, 250 mA) stimulation on the same PH neuron. Note the large, sustained depolarization following the end of the burst stimuli, including the presence of action potentials (**B1**). This sustained depolarization could not be evoked in presence of atropine sulfate (**B2**; 1.5 mM). Calibrations for **A** and **B** as indicated.

0.1 M, pH 7.4. Further details of this chronic preparation can be found elsewhere.[1,3] Experiments were conducted after the European Union directive (609/86/CEE) for the use of laboratory animals.

Single electrical pulses applied to the PPRF evoked excitatory postsynaptic potentials (EPSPs) in PH neurons ($n = 60$) with a mean latency of 2.54 ± 0.35 ms and a mean duration of 70.1 ± 18.9 ms (FIG. 2A). The EPSPs showed a graded nature, depending on the stimulus intensity, and were completely blocked by superfusion with CNQX (10 μM), a specific blocker of AMPA-kainate receptors. In the absence of CNQX, superfusion with APV (50 μM) or atropine sulfate (1.5 μM) had no effect on evoked EPSPs. Train stimulation of the PPRF evoked a sustained depolarization of PH neurons exceeding the end of the train by hundreds of milliseconds (FIG. 2B). This late depolarization had amplitude and duration linearly related ($r \geq 0.9$; $P \leq 0.01$) to stimulus frequency during the train, was impossible to evoke in the presence of atropine sulfate (FIG. 2B) or pirenzepine (0.5 μM), and was mimicked by superfusion of the slice with carbachol (25 μM).

An attempt was made to confirm the effects of cholinergic terminals on PH neurons *in vivo* (FIG. 3). Unilateral microinjections of pirenzepine (40 nL, 0.1 μM) in

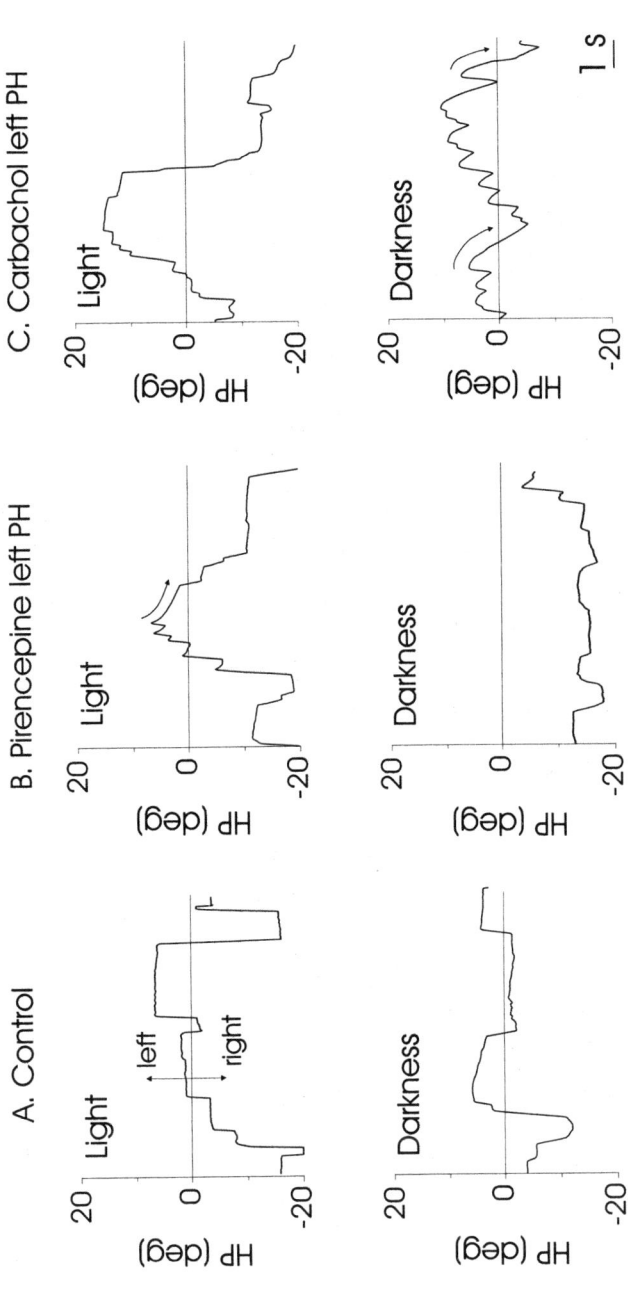

FIGURE 3. Horizontal eye movements recorded in alert-behaving cats. Recordings were conducted in controls and after microinjections of the indicated drugs in the left prepositus hypoglossi nucleus, in light conditions and in complete darkness. (**A**) Control records. (**B**) Eye movements 2 min after the microinjection of pirenzepine (40 nL, 0.1 mM) in light and darkness. (**C**) Eye movements 1 min after microinjection of carbachol (40 nL, 250 mM). The zero (0) line indicates the central position of the eye in the orbit. Vertical arrows indicate movement direction of the eye. Eye positions to the left were assigned positive values, whereas rightward eye positions were assigned negative values.

identified PH areas induced a contralateral deviation of the eyes and a noticeable ipsilateral gaze-holding deficit (FIG. 3B). The gaze-holding deficit was an exponential displacement of the eye to the center of the orbit after saccades toward the injected side. Deficits in a proper eye-fixation mechanism were more evident in light than in complete darkness. In contrast, microinjections of carbachol produced the most evident deficits in darkness, characterized by a nystagmus with slow phases toward the contralateral (noninjected) side.

In short, we have recorded in rat sagittal brainstem slices the activity of identified PH neurons evoked by direct current injections and by the electrical stimulation of the PPRF. It has been shown that the excitatory action of burst neurons on PH neurons is glutamatergic in nature, acting on AMPA-kainate receptors. Train stimulation of the PPRF evoked a sustained depolarization of PH neurons by the activation of reticular cholinergic axons, removed by superfusion with atropine sulfate (a cholinergic antagonist) and pirenzepine (a selective blocker of muscarinic M1 receptors), and mimicked by carbachol (a cholinergic agonist). *In vitro* studies were further confirmed by pirenzepine and carbachol microinjections in the PH nucleus during spontaneous eye movements in alert-behaving cats, suggesting a fundamental role of acetylcholine in the generation and maintenance of eye-position signals.

REFERENCES

1. ASKAY, E., G. GAMKRELIDZE, H.S. SEUNG, *et al.* 2001. *In vivo* intracellular recording and perturbation of persistent activity in a neural integrator. Nat. Neurosci. **4:** 184–193.
2. CHERON, G. & E. GODAUX. 1987. Disabling of the oculomotor neural integrator by kainic acid injections in the prepositus-vestibular complex in the cat. J. Physiol. (Lond.) **399:** 267–290.
3. DELGADO-GARCÍA, J.M., P.-P. VIDAL, C. GÓMEZ & A. BERTHOZ. 1989. A neurophysiological study of prepositus hypoglossi neurons projecting to oculomotor and preoculomotor nuclei in the alert cat. Neuroscience **29:** 291–307.
4. IGUSA, A., S. SASAKI & H. SHIMAZU. 1980. Excitatory premotor burst neurons in the cat pontine reticular formation related to the quick phase of vestibular nystagmus. Brain Res. **182:** 451–456.
5. MORENO-LÓPEZ, B., M. ESCUDERO, J.M. DELGADO-GARCÍA & C. ESTRADA. 1996. Nitric oxide production by brain stem neurons is required for normal performance of eye movements in alert animals. Neuron **17:** 739–745.
6. ROBINSON, D.A. 1981. The use of control system analysis in the neurophysiology of eye movements. Annu. Rev. Neurosci. **4:** 463–503.
7. YAJEYA, J., A. DE LA FUENTE, J.M. CRIADO, *et al.* 2000. Muscarinic agonistic carbachol depresses excitatory synaptic transmission in the rat basolateral amygdala in vitro. Synapse **38:** 151–160.

Spatial Convergence Pattern of Canal and Macular Nerve Afferent Signals in Frog Second-Order Vestibular Neurons

HANS STRAKA AND NORBERT DIERINGER

Physiologisches Institut, LMU München, Pettenkoferstrasse 12, 80336 München, Germany

KEYWORDS: semicircular canal; utricle; lagena; saccule; convergence pattern

INTRODUCTION

Linear and angular head accelerations are detected separately by the different macular and semicircular canal organs in the labyrinth. These signals are mediated by vestibular nerve afferent fibers to the vestibular nuclei, the brainstem reticular formation, and the cerebellum. Afferent nerve fibers from individual labyrinthine end-organs terminate in all major vestibular subnuclei and overlap to a large extent in frog[1] as in other vertebrate species.[2] The overlapping termination areas of vestibular nerve afferent fibers allow for a considerable convergence of afferent signals onto second-order vestibular neurons (2°VN). Thus, three questions arise. First, do afferent nerve signals from all three semicircular canals converge onto 2°VN (FIG. 1A) or do they remain largely separate at the first central synapse? Second, do afferent nerve signals from the macula organs converge onto 2°VN (FIG. 1B)? This question is particularly interesting because the saccule in frog is considered an acoustic sense organ,[3] and thus signals from this macula organ should be processed separately from linear head acceleration signals, mediated by utricular and lagenar afferent fibers. And third, do afferent nerve signals from canal and macula organs converge onto 2°VN (FIG. 1C), and, if so, are there distinct convergence patterns for particular organs?

METHODS

In vitro experiments were performed on isolated brains of grass frogs (*Rana temporaria*), with both VIIIth nerves attached. The convergence pattern of macular and canal nerve afferent inputs onto individual 2°VN was studied intracellularly by separate electrical stimulation of nerve branches from each of the three semicircular ca-

---

Address for correspondence: Dr. H. Straka, Physiologisches Institut, Pettenkoferstrasse 12, 80336 München, Germany. Voice: 49-89-5996-232; fax: 49-89-5996-216.
straka@wifomail.med.uni-muenchen.de

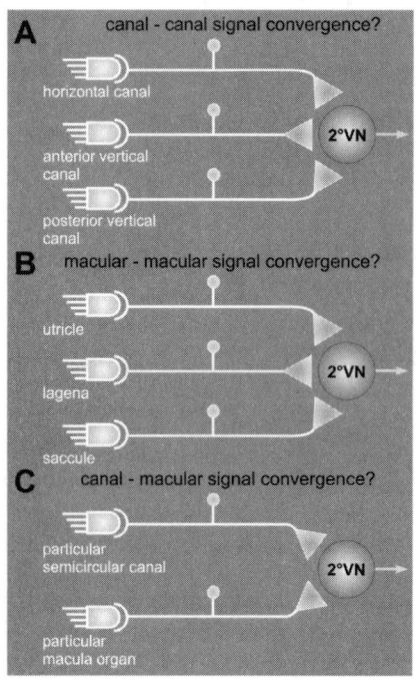

FIGURE 1. Schematic diagram depicting possible patterns of monosynaptic convergence of semicircular canal afferent signals (**A**), of macular afferent signals (**B**), and of afferent signals from particular canal and particular macula organs (**C**) onto 2°VN.

nals, the utricle (UT), the lagena (LA), or the saccule (SA). Monosynaptic responses evoked by stimulation of a particular labyrinthine nerve branch (FIG. 2A, B) served to identify 2°VN. These neurons were further subdivided into 2°canal, 2°macula, or 2°macular + canal neurons.[4,5] Furthermore, the presence of an antidromic spike after stimulation of the upper spinal cord and/or of the midbrain allowed a classification as projection neurons.

RESULTS

Most 2°VN (825 of 937 neurons; 88%) received a monosynaptic EPSP from only one of the three canal nerves (FIG. 3A). Some neurons received a monosynaptic EPSP from two (102 of 937 neurons; 11%) and very few from all three canal nerves (10 of 937 neurons; 1%). Because of the absence of a considerable canal–canal convergence, the spatial information extracted by the canals in the periphery is largely conserved at the first central synapse. After separate stimulation of the macular nerves, most 2°VN received an afferent signal from only one macular nerve branch (219 of 240 neurons; 91%). In the remaining 2°VN, afferent signals from two macula organs, respectively, converged (21 of 240 neurons; 9%). Interestingly, a convergence of UT and LA afferent signals predominated over a convergence of SA afferent signals with UT or LA afferent signals. Thus, macular afferent signals similar to semicircular canal signals remain largely separate at the level of 2°VN. Separate electrical stimulation of one macular nerve branch and all three canal nerves

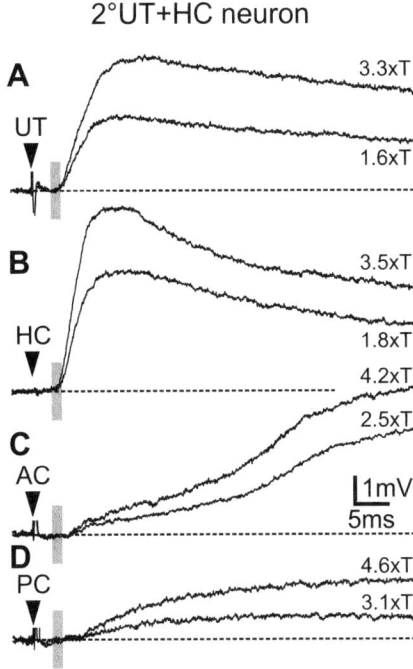

FIGURE 2. Utricular and canal nerve–evoked afferent inputs in a 2°VN. (**A–D**) monosynaptic EPSPs from the utricular (UT; A) and from the horizontal canal (HC) nerve (**B**) identified this neuron as a 2°UT + HC neuron. Oligosynaptic EPSPs were evoked from the anterior vertical (AC; **C**) and posterior vertical canal (PC; **D**) nerves, respectively. Stimulus intensity in multiples of the stimulus threshold intensity of the N_1 field potential. The *shaded vertical bars* indicate the mean ± SDs of the field potential onset after stimulation of the indicated nerve branch. *Dashed lines* indicate baselines; *arrowheads* mark stimulus onset. Each record represents the average of 24 responses.

(FIG. 2), respectively, indicated that UT or LA afferent signals converged with canal afferent signals in about 30% of 2°VN. UT nerve afferent signals (FIG. 2A) converged mainly with afferent horizontal canal (HC; FIG. 2B) signals (FIG. 3C). LA afferent signals converged only with anterior vertical (AC) or posterior vertical canal (PC) but not with HC afferent signals (FIG. 3D). This pattern of convergence correlates with a coactivation of particular combinations of canal and macula organs during natural head movements. A convergence of SA afferent and canal afferent signals was rare (3%; FIG. 3B). The paucity of SA afferent signals converging with canal afferent or other macular afferent signals is compatible with an auditory role of the frog's saccule. 2°VN mediating UT and/or canal afferent signals had ascending and/or descending axons, whereas 2°VN mediating LA or SA afferent signals had descending but no ascending axons.

DISCUSSION

The remarkable selectivity of 2°VN for afferent nerve inputs from particular vestibular sense organs is not unique for frogs but represents a more general organization principle. Available data from pigeon[6] and cat[7,8] support this hypothesis. The following comparison of the convergence patterns of afferent nerve signals in frog and cat 2°VN is made under the assumption that the saccule in cat and the lagena in frog play functionally equivalent roles.[3,9] The convergence of signals from the utri-

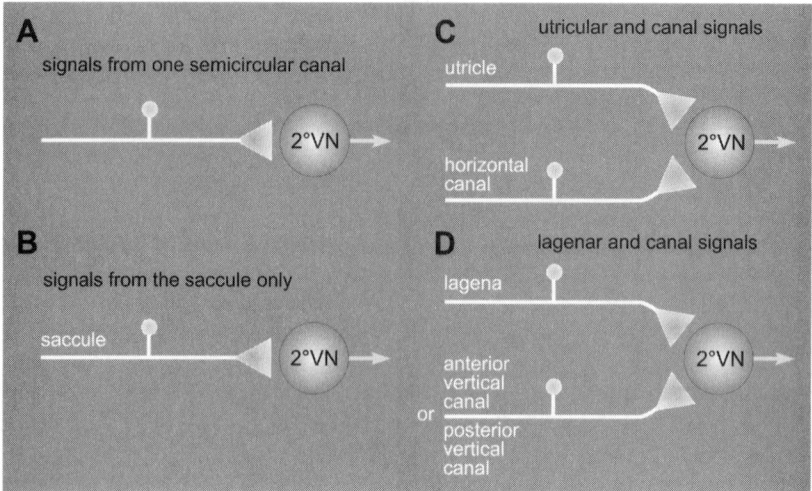

FIGURE 3. Schematic diagram summarizing the major convergence patterns of vestibular nerve afferent canal and macular signals. Afferent signals from particular semicircular canals (**A**) or from the saccule (**B**) remain largely separate. Afferent signals from the utricle converge mainly with those from the horizontal canal (**C**). Afferent signals from the lagena converge with those from the anterior vertical or posterior vertical canal (**D**).

cle and the vertical macula organ is rare in frogs but somewhat more common in cat.[8] The convergence of macula and canal afferent signals was studied in cat in different sets of experiments, in which a combination of two labyrinthine nerve branches was stimulated separately.[8] The results of these studies[8] were qualitatively similar but quantitatively different from corresponding results in frogs.[5] In general, the convergence of canal and macula afferent signals in cat appears to be much less common and spatially not as distinct as in frog.[5] Interestingly, similar proportions of 2°canal, 2°macular (about 25% each) and 2°canal + macular neurons (approximately 50%) were encountered in frog 2°VN after separate electrical stimulation of the three canal nerves, the utricle, and the lagena as in primate vestibular neurons after angular and linear head acceleration.[10] 2°VN mediating UT and/or canal afferent signals project to ocular motor and spinal targets and contribute to maculoocular as well as to spinal reflexes in frog[11] as in cat.[8] 2°VN with vertical otolith signals, however, did neither in frog nor in cat project to extraocular motoneurons.[11,12] Hence, the organization of maculoocular and of canal-ocular reflexes represents a general organization principle in species with a common bauplan.

REFERENCES

1. BIRINYI, A., H. STRAKA, C. MATESZ & N. DIERINGER. 2001. Location of dye-coupled second order and of efferent vestibular neurons labeled from individual semicircular canal or otolith organs in the frog. Brain Res. **921:** 44–59.
2. BÜTTNER-ENNEVER, J.A. 1992. Patterns of connectivity in the vestibular nuclei. Ann. N.Y. Acad. Sci. **656:** 363–378.

3. LEWIS, E.R. & P.M. NARINS. 1999. The acoustic periphery of amphibians: anatomy and physiology. *In* Comparative Hearing: Fish and Amphibians. Springer Handbook of Auditory Research. R.R. Fay & A.N. Popper, Eds.: 101–154. Springer. New York.
4. STRAKA, H., S. BIESDORF & N. DIERINGER. 1997. Canal-specific excitation and inhibition of frog second order vestibular neurons. J. Neurophysiol. **78:** 1363–1372.
5. STRAKA, H., S. HOLLER & F. GOTO. 2002. Patterns of canal and otolith afferent input convergence in frog second order vestibular neurons. J. Neurophysiol. **88:** 2287–2301.
6. WILSON, V.J. & L.P. FELPEL. 1972. Specificity of semicircular canal input to neurons in the pigeon vestibular nuclei. J. Neurophysiol. **35:** 253–254.
7. KASAHARA, M. & Y. UCHINO. 1974. Bilateral semicircular canal inputs to neurons in cat vestibular nuclei. Exp. Brain Res. **20:** 285–296.
8. UCHINO, Y. 2001. Otolith and semicircular canal inputs to single vestibular neurons in cats. Biol. Sci. Space **15:** 375–381.
9. HARADA, Y., S. KASUGA & S. TAMURA. 2001. Comparison and evolution of the lagena in various animal species. Acta Otolaryngol. **121:** 355–363.
10. DICKMAN, J.D. & D.E. ANGELAKI. 2002. Vestibular convergence patterns in vestibular nuclei neurons of alert primates. J. Neurophysiol. **88:** 3518–3533.
11. ROHREGGER, M. & N. DIERINGER. 2002. Principles of linear and angular vestibulo-ocular reflex organization in the frog. J. Neurophysiol. **87:** 385–398.
12. ISU, N., W. GRAF, H. SATO, *et al.* 2000. Sacculo-ocular reflex connectivity in cats. Exp. Brain Res. **131:** 262–268.

Acute Vestibular Nucleus Lesion Affects Cortical Activation Pattern during Caloric Irrigation in PET

SANDRA BENSE,[a,b] THOMAS STEPHAN,[b] PETER BARTENSTEIN,[c,d] MARKUS SCHWAIGER,[c] THOMAS BRANDT,[b] AND MARIANNE DIETERICH[a,b]

[a]*Department of Neurology, Johannes Gutenberg-University, Mainz, Germany*

[b]*Department of Neurology, Ludwig-Maximilians University, Munich, Germany*

[c]*Department of Nuclear Medicine, Technical University, Munich, Germany*

[d]*Department of Nuclear Medicine, Johannes Gutenberg-University, Mainz, Germany*

KEYWORDS: vestibular cortex; caloric stimulation; Wallenberg's syndrome; PET; activation study; hemispheric dominance

INTRODUCTION

In the last few years, cortical processing of vestibular information was analyzed in several functional imaging studies, PET and fMRI, in healthy volunteers.[1–4] Monaural caloric irrigation in healthy volunteers elicited significant increases of regional cerebral blood flow (rCBF) in a cortical and subcortical network within both hemispheres.[5] Activations were found in ocular motor centers such as the prefrontal cortex, frontal eye field, and parietal eye field, all of which are involved in the processing of caloric nystagmus. Further activations were located in several distinct vestibular areas bilaterally, especially at the posterior end of the insula and retroinsular regions corresponding to the multisensory parietoinsular vestibular cortex in monkeys (PIVC),[6,7] and the adjacent superior temporal gyrus and inferior parietal lobule, cingulum, vestibular thalamus, and anterior insula. Right-handed volunteers presented with a right hemispheric dominance for vestibular cortical structures.

Animal studies have shown that the afferent vestibular pathways run from the vestibular end-organs (semicircular canals and otoliths) and the vestibular nerve via the vestibular nuclei in the medullary brainstem to the thalamus and the cortical vestibular areas.[8,9] Several ascending pathways (such as the medial longitudinal fascicle, the ascending tract of Deiters, and the brachium conjunctivum) mediate vestibular information and cross at different brainstem levels. The aim of this PET study during caloric vestibular stimulation was to determine how an acute unilateral ischemic infarction of the lateral medulla oblongata (Wallenberg's syndrome) that

---

Address for correspondence: Dr. Sandra Bense, Department of Neurology, Johannes Gutenberg-University of Mainz, Langenbeckstrasse 1, D-55101 Mainz, Germany. Voice: + 49 6131 17 2510; fax: + 49 6131 17 5967.

bense@neurologie.klinik.uni-mainz.de

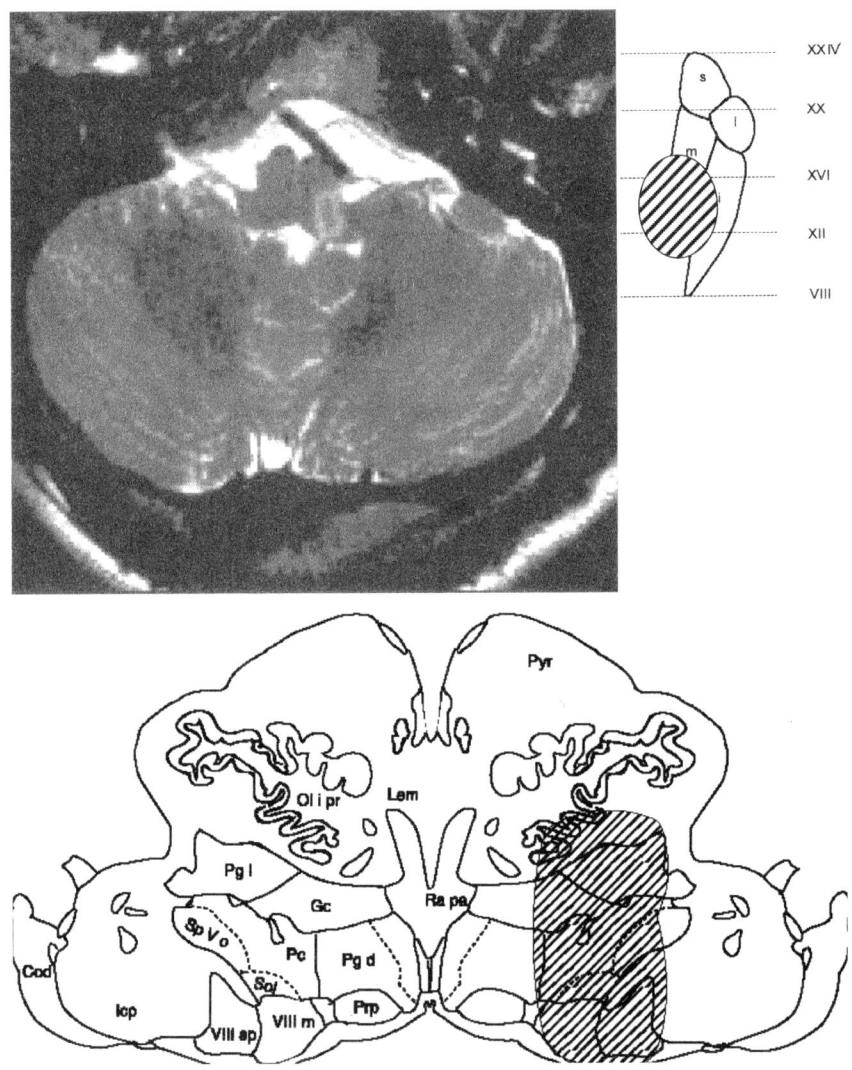

FIGURE 1. Axial slice of an anatomical MRI scan showing the unilateral ischemic infarction in the left lateral medulla oblongata of patient R.P. (**A**, *top left*). The overlay of the lesion onto the appropriate section of the brainstem atlas of Olszewski and Baxter (**B**, *bottom*), and the schematic drawing of the vestibular nucleus (**C**, *top right*) demonstrate that the lesion affects only parts of the medial (m) and spinal (sp) vestibular subnuclei.

affects one of the ascending vestibular pathways at its origin in the vestibular nucleus, alters the cortical activation pattern.

PATIENT AND METHODS

The right-handed male patient R.P. (35 years) had an acute lateral left-sided medullary infarction that affected parts of the medial and spinal vestibular subnuclei, as seen in the diffusion-weighted MRI scan (FIG. 1 A) and the superimposed projection of the ischemic lesion onto the appropriate section of the brainstem atlas of Olszewski and Baxter[10] (FIG. 1B). The patient presented with acute rotatory vertigo, vomiting, and gait deviation to the left. Clinical examination further revealed a Horner's syndrome on the left, a central facial and glossopharyngeal paresis on the left, hypesthesia of the right side of the face, sensorimotor hemiparesis on the right, and dysphagia with hypersalivation due to a Wallenberg's syndrome. Neuroophthalmologic examination in the acute phase further showed skew deviation associated with concomitant ocular torsion of 7.5° in fundus photography, and a significant ipsilateral tilt of 5° of the subjective visual vertical (SVV).[11] The patient had no history or complaints of earlier neurological or otoneurological dysfunction and took no drugs known to act on vestibular or ocular motor function.

^{15}O-labeled H_2O bolus PET scanning (Siemens 951 R/31 PET scanner; CTI, Knoxville, TN) was performed in three-dimensional mode on day 9 after the infarction. The procedure was similar to that used in an earlier PET study on healthy volunteers. PET scanning started after caloric vestibular stimulation with 100 mL water at 44°C of the right or left ear canals (eyes closed), whereas caloric nystagmus still persisted or during the rest condition without stimulation. For details of the experimental setup, especially vestibular stimulation, PET scanning, data acquisition, as well as image analysis, see Dieterich et al.[5] Volumes were realigned, spatially normalized, and smoothed before statistical single subject analysis by the Statistical Parametric Mapping Software (SPM99b; Wellcome Department of Cognitive Neurology, London, UK). The activation maps for the patient ($P = 0.01$ uncorrected) were compared with those during warm-water caloric vestibular stimulation in right-handed healthy volunteers.

RESULTS

Caloric vestibular stimulation of the ear contralateral to the infarcted left side yielded a *"normal"* activation pattern of the posterior insula and retroinsular region bilaterally, showing a typical predominance in the ipsilateral right hemisphere (right: x/y/z = 40/–20/–4, t-value = 5.24, 142 voxels, and x/y/z = 42/0/–2, t-value = 5.33, 278 voxels; left: z = –44/–10/4, t-value = 4.96, 149 voxels, and x/y/z = –42/–30/–2, t-value = 4.83, 33 voxels) (FIG. 2, first row). In addition, "vestibular" activations were located in the right thalamus, left cingulate gyrus (BA 24), and in the inferior parietal lobule bilaterally (BA 40; right: z = 70/–40/30, t-value = 7.76, 265 voxels; left: z = –70/–48/22, t-value = 3.84, 15 voxels), on the right side accompanied by activations of the adjacent superior temporal gyrus (BA 22 and BA 39). Further activations were found in the precentral gyrus bilaterally (BA 6), left superior (BA 9),

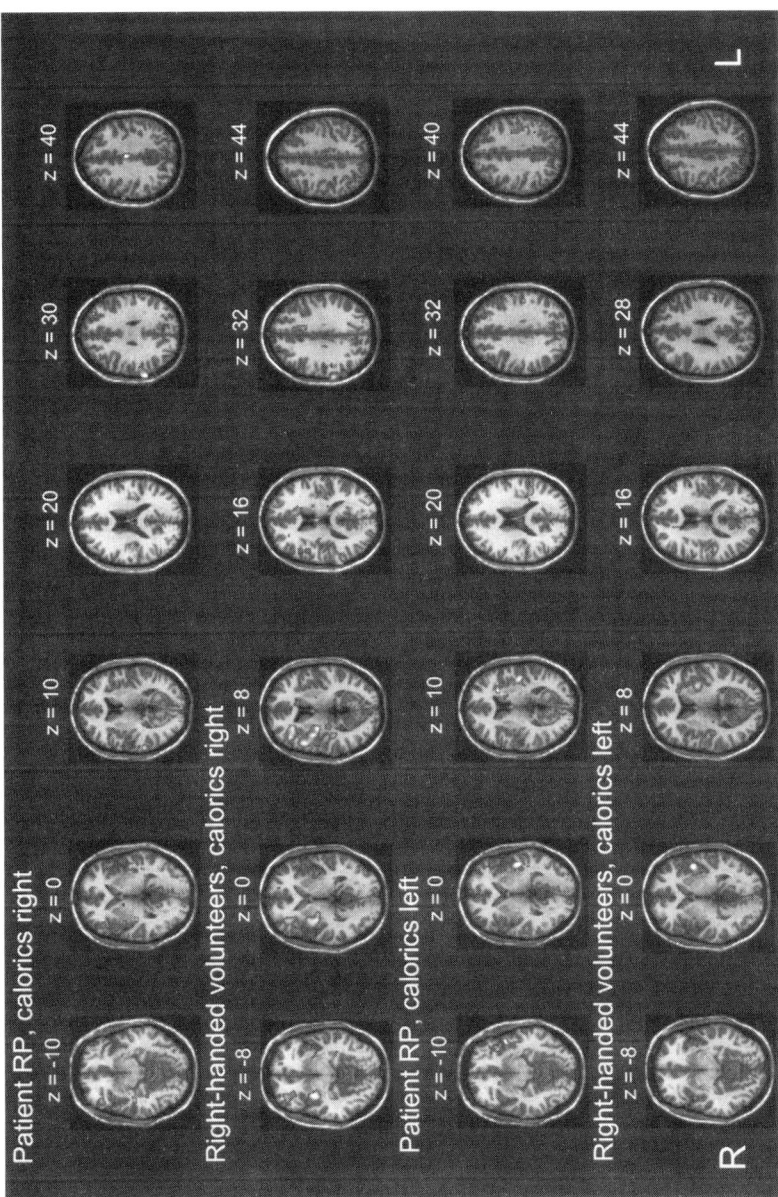

FIGURE 2. Activated areas during caloric stimulation of the right or left ear in a group of healthy volunteers and in the patient R.P. Caloric irrigation of the right ear (*first row*) caused "normal" bilateral PIVC activation in the posterior insula, also reflecting the typical dominance of the nondominant right hemisphere. Caloric irrigation of the left ear, ipsilateral to the infarction, showed activations in the ipsilateral left hemisphere only (*third row*). Contralateral activations, especially in the right posterior insula, were absent, although this is the hemisphere dominant for vestibular processing.

right middle (BA 6/8), and bilateral inferior frontal gyrus (BA 47/10), left superior temporal gyrus (BA 38), and in basal ganglia (left caudate nucleus; right putamen).

In contrast, caloric irrigation of the ear ipsilateral to the left-sided infarction showed strong activation only in the ipsilateral posterior insula (x/y/z = −46/−10/4, t-value 6.85, 1037 voxels), the adjacent superior parietal lobule (BA 40), and superior temporal gyrus (BA 22). There was no activation in the contralateral right hemisphere (especially not in the posterior insula) despite the right hemispheric vestibular dominance with right ear stimulation (FIG. 2, third row).

The further activated areas in the left hemisphere were located in the anterior cingulate gyrus (BA 24); caudate nucleus; superior (BA 6), middle (BA 9), and inferior frontal gyrus (BA 11/47); superior parietal lobule (BA 7); middle temporal gyrus (BA 39); central sulcus region (predominately precentrally, BA 4); and superior parietal lobule (BA 7). In the right hemisphere, minor activations were found only in the superior frontal gyrus (BA 9), superior parietal lobule (BA 7), and in frontal white matter.

The additional activated areas outside the temporoparietal region in the patient correspond to those found in healthy volunteers. They can be attributed especially to ocular motor (eye fields in the frontal cortex), vestibular (inferior parietal lobule, superior temporal gyrus, thalamus), and autonomic functions (cingulate gyrus).

DISCUSSION

Our preliminary PET study on one patient with an acute medullary infarction within one afferent vestibular pathway, running via the medial and spinal vestibular subnuclei into the medullary brainstem, supports the hypothesis of bilateral ascending pathways in the brainstem which spread out at medullary level. The activation pattern can be explained by the infarction that affects only the crossing fibers that ascend within the contralateral side to the contralateral hemisphere but spares the ipsilateral ascending pathway. This single case supports the assumption that there is no additional crossing of the fibers at a level above the medullary lesion, because stimulation of the ear ipsilateral to the affected left side caused only activation of the vestibular cortex within the "ipsilateral" left hemisphere. The activation pattern fits to animal data[8,9,12] that showed the ipsilateral ascending pathway travelling via the superior vestibular subnucleus, which apparently was not affected by the infarction of our patient, whereas crossing fibers to the medial longitudinal fascicle travel via the medial vestibular subnucleus that was lesioned in our patient. This also underlines the importance of the ipsilateral rather than contralateral pathways, as one of three determinants for the cortical activation pattern: (1) dominance of the hemisphere ipsilateral to the stimulation, (2) dominance of the nondominant hemisphere, and (3) direction of vestibular stimulation and nystagmus.

ACKNOWLEDGMENTS

We are grateful to Judy Benson for critically reading the manuscript. This work was supported by Deutsche Forschungsgemeinschaft (DI 379/4-1, BR 639/6-1) and the Wilhelm Sander-Stiftung (2001.084.1).

REFERENCES

1. BOTTINI, G. *et al.* 1994. Identification of the central vestibular projections in man: a positron emission tomography activation study. Exp. Brain Res. **99:** 164–169.
2. LOBEL, E. *et al.* 1998. Functional MRI of galvanic vestibular stimulation. J. Neurophysiol. **80:** 2699–2709.
3. BENSE, S. *et al.* 2001. Multisensory cortical signal increases and decreases during vestibular galvanic stimulation (fMRI). J. Neurophysiol. **85:** 886–899.
4. SUZUKI, M. *et al.* 2001. Cortical and subcortical vestibular response to caloric stimulation detected by fMRI. Cogn. Brain Res. **12:** 441–449.
5. DIETERICH, M. *et al.* 2003. Hemispheric dominance of the human multisensory vestibular cortex (a PET study). Cereb. Cortex.In press.
6. GRÜSSER, O.J., M. PAUSE & U. SCHREITER. 1990a. Vestibular neurons in the parieto-insular cortex of monkeys (*Macaca fascicularis*). Visual and neck receptor responses. J. Physiol. **430:** 559–583.
7. GRÜSSER, O.J., M. PAUSE & U. SCHREITER. 1990b. Localization and responses of neurons in the parieto-insular vestibular cortex of the awake monkeys (*Macaca fascicularis*). J. Physiol. **430:** 537–557.
8. GRAF, W., R.A. MCCREA & R. BAKER. 1983. Morphology of posterior canal-related secondary vestibular neurons in rabbit and cat. Exp. Brain Res. **52:** 125–138.
9. GRAF, W. & K. ENZURE. 1986. Morphology of vertical and canal related second order vestibular neurons in the cat. Exp. Brain Res. **63:** 35–48.
10. OLSZEWSKI, J. & D. BAXTER. 1982. Cytoarchitecture of the Human Brain Stem. 2nd edit. Karger. Basel.
11. DIETERICH, M. & T. BRANDT. 1993. Ocular torsion and tilt of the subjective visual vertical are sensitive brainstem signs. Ann. Neurol. **33:** 292–299.
12. MCMASTERS, R.E., A.H. WEISS & M.B. CARPENTER. 1966. Vestibular projections to the nuclei of extraocular muscles. Degeneration resulting from discrete partial lesions of the vestibular nuclei in the monkey. Am. J. Anat. **118:** 163–194.

Three Determinants of Vestibular Hemispheric Dominance during Caloric Stimulation

A Positron Emission Tomography Study

SANDRA BENSE,[a,b] PETER BARTENSTEIN,[c,d] STEFFI LUTZ,[c] THOMAS STEPHAN,[b] MARKUS SCHWAIGER,[c] THOMAS BRANDT,[b] AND MARIANNE DIETERICH[a,b]

[a]*Department of Neurology, Johannes Gutenberg-University, Mainz, Germany*

[b]*Department of Neurology, Ludwig-Maximilians University, Munich, Germany*

[c]*Department of Nuclear Medicine, Technical University, Munich, Germany*

[d]*Department of Nuclear Medicine, Johannes Gutenberg-University, Mainz, Germany*

KEYWORDS: vestibular cortex; iced water caloric stimulation; vestibular nystagmus; positron emission tomography (PET); brain activation study; hemispheric dominance

INTRODUCTION

Electrophysiological animal experiments[1-4] and functional imaging studies[5-10] have revealed that several parietotemporal areas are involved in cortical vestibular processing. Within this network, the posterior insula area is a kind of core region that contains the human homologue of the parietoinsular vestibular cortex in monkeys. A recent human positron emission tomography (PET) study during warm water caloric irrigation in right- and left-handed volunteers showed that two factors affect the cortical activation pattern: (1) the handedness of the subjects (that is, a vestibular dominance of the nondominant hemisphere) and (2) the side of the stimulation (that is, stronger activation occurs in the hemisphere ipsilateral to the stimulated ear).[10] The aim of this PET water activation study was to determine the influence of the direction of stimulation induced apparent self-motion and nystagmus on the cortical activation pattern. Therefore, right-handed volunteers were examined in PET after caloric irrigation with iced water. Iced water induces a nystagmus in which the quick phase occurs to the contralateral side, whereas warm water caloric irrigation induces a nystagmus to the ipsilateral side.

Address for correspondence: Dr. Sandra Bense, Department of Neurology, Johannes Gutenberg-University of Mainz, Langenbeckstrasse 1, D-55101 Mainz, Germany. Voice: +49 6131 17 2510; fax: +49 6131 17 5967.

bense@neurologie.klinik.uni-mainz.de

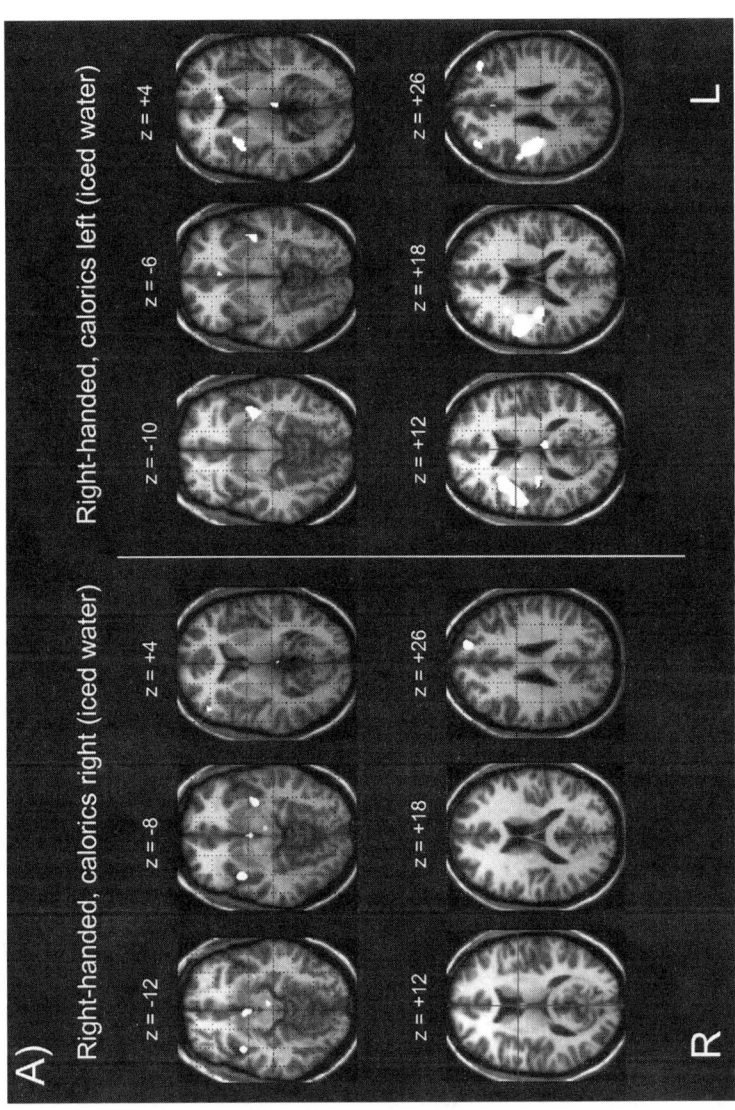

FIGURE 1. Activated areas after (**A**) iced water or (**B**) warm water caloric vestibular stimulation of the right or left ear in right-handed healthy volunteers projected onto a standard template brain. The activations can be attributed to vestibular (posterior insula and retroinsular region containing the human homologue of the parietoinsular vestibular cortex; vestibular thalamus), vestibular-autonomic (cingulate gyrus), and ocular motor functions (eye fields within the frontal cortex). The extent of vestibular cortex activation depends on the additive or subtractive effects of the three determinants: the nondominant hemisphere, the side of the stimulation, and the direction of vestibular motion sensation and nystagmus (quick phase).

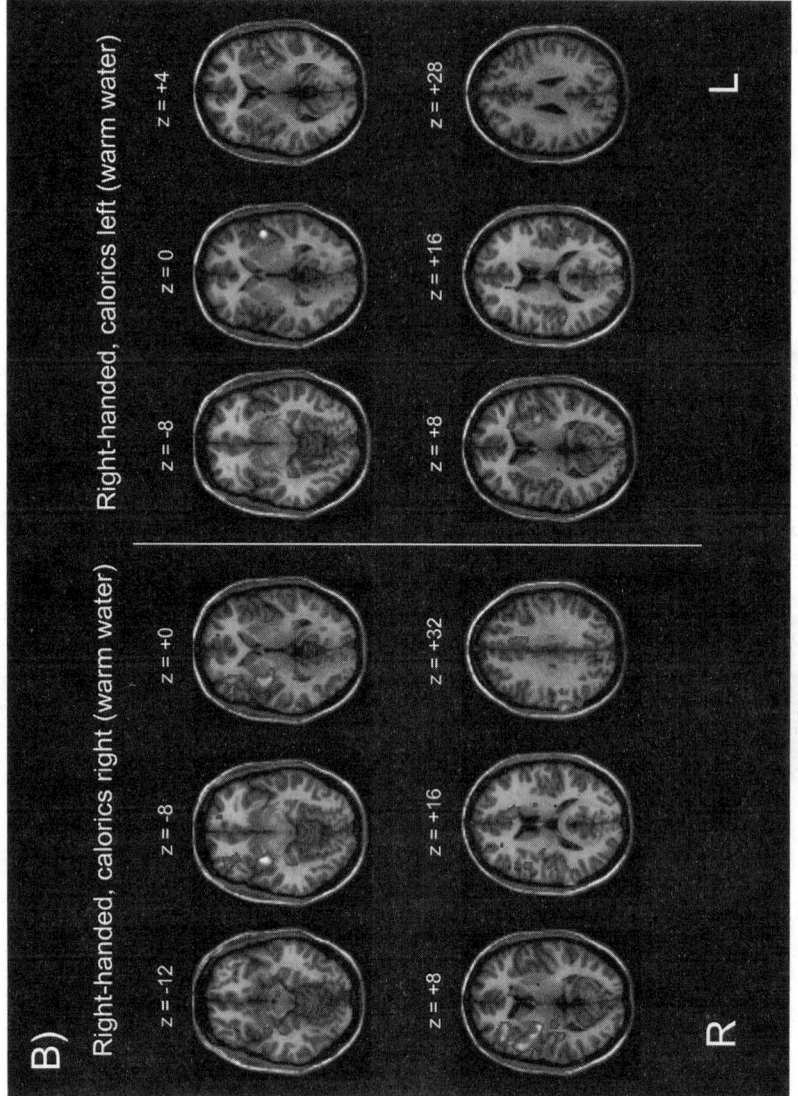

FIGURE 1. *Continued.*

TABLE 1.

Area	Function / BA	Coordinates [x, y, z]	Z-score	Cluster size
Caloric irrigation right ear				
Right posterior insula	PIVC	40, 6, −10	3.85	131
Left posterior insula	PIVC	−34, −6, −8	3.38	120
Left superior frontal gyrus	9	−20, −54, 30	3.85	331
Superior frontal gyrus	8	−14, 22, 56	3.38	81
Superior frontal gyrus	8/6	−46, 18, 50	3.14	51
Right hypothalamus		2, 4, −16	3.59	302
Left midbrain		−8, −20, −14	3.17	
Right inferior frontal gyrus	44/46	46, 42, 0	3.50	52
Left posterior cingulate gyrus/ paracentral lobule	24	−14, −22, 48	3.02	56
Left cingulate gyrus	24/23	−8, −12, 32	2.94	101
Left inferior parietal cortex	39/40	−50, −64, 36	2.73	46
Caloric irrigation left ear				
Right posterior insula	PIVC	44, −2, 20	3.97	2209
Precentral gyrus	6/44	54, 0, 22		
Postcentral gyrus	4	44, −12, 26		
Left posterior insula	PIVC	−38, 6, −12	3.19	181
Left middle frontal gyrus	8	−38, 36, 38	4.36	604
Superior frontal gyrus	8	−30, 46, 38		
Right middle frontal gyrus	9/46	36, 40, 30	4.36	384
Superior frontal gyrus	8/9	20, 46, 42		
Left paramedian thalamus		−4, −28, 8	3.27	135
Left anterior cingulate gyrus	32/24/6	−2, 6, 48	3.66	727
Right caudate nucleus		16, −2, 12	2.67	45
Left posterior cingulate gyrus	31/24/7	−4, −28, 44	2.82	167

METHODS

Eight right-handed healthy volunteers aged 27–39 years (mean age: 31.9 years; one woman, seven men) were examined by ^{15}O-labeled H_2O bolus PET (Siemens 951 R/31 Scanner; CTI, Knoxville, TN in two-dimensional mode with eyes closed after vestibular stimulation (by irrigation of the right or left ear canals with 100 mL of iced water solution for 50 s) or during the rest condition without stimulation. The vestibular effects were monitored by a horizontal direct current (DC) electrooculogram with the eyes closed. Volumes were realigned, spatially normalized, and smoothed prior to statistical fixed effects group analysis by the Statistical Parametric Mapping Software (SPM 96, Wellcome Department of Cognitive Neurology, London). For details on the experimental setup, especially vestibular stimulation, PET scanning, data acquisition, as well as image analysis, see Dieterich and colleagues.[10] The activation maps for the group ($P < 0.001$ uncorrected) were compared to those during warm water caloric vestibular stimulation. For illustrative purposes, voxels above a threshold of $P < 0.01$ are shown in FIGURE 1.

The laterality quotient for right-handedness according to the 10-item inventory of the Edinburgh test was +100 in seven volunteers, and +80 in one.[11]

RESULTS

Iced water caloric irrigation of the right ear caused nearly symmetric bilateral activation of the caudal posterior insula (right: $x/y/z = 40/6/–10$, z-value = 3.85, 131 voxels; left: $x/y/z = –34/–6/–8$, z-value = 3.38, 120 voxels). Parietotemporal activations were not found. Iced water vestibular stimulation of the left ear (nystagmus quick phase to the right) also caused bilateral posterior insular activation, but in different places and to different extents (TABLE 1). In the left hemisphere (opposite to nystagmus quick phase) a caudal posterior insular activation ($x/y/z = –38/–6/–12$, z-value 3.19, 181 voxels) was found, whereas in the right hemisphere (in the direction of nystagmus quick phase) a larger activation cluster (z-value = 3.97, 2209 voxels) was located in the posterior and anterior insula region, which extended to the parietotemporal cortex, including the superior temporal gyrus (Brodmann area 22, or BA 22) and inferior parietal lobule (BA 40), and spread into the central sulcus region (BA 40/42/43/44/6/4) (FIG. 1A, TABLE 1).

Furthermore, iced water stimulation of the right ear induced activation of the right inferior (BA 44/46), left superior (BA 9 and 8), and middle frontal gyri (BA 8/6); the left paracentral lobule and cingulate gyrus (BA 24/23); the left inferior parietal cortex (angular gyrus, BA 39/40); and the left mesencephalic brainstem, reaching the right subthalamic nucleus (FIG. 1A, left). Left caloric stimulation also showed frontal cortex activations bilaterally in the middle (right: BA 9/46; left: BA 8) and superior frontal gyri (right: BA 8/9; left: BA 8), in the left paramedian thalamus und right caudate nucleus, as well as in the left anterior (reaching the frontal diagonal gyrus; BA 32/24/6) and posterior cingulate gyrus (merging into the paracentral gyrus; BA 31/24/7) (FIG. 1A, right).

Thus, compared to warm water stimulation (FIG. 1B, TABLE 1), iced water stimulation in right-handed volunteers led to stronger activations in the right parietotemporal region during irrigation of the left ear, that is, when the nystagmus quick phase was parallel to the dominance of the nondominant right hemisphere.

DISCUSSION

This PET study provides evidence that besides the hemispheric dominance of the nondominant hemisphere and the side of the irrigation (stronger ipsilateral activation), the direction of the vestibular sensation of self-motion and nystagmus is a third determinant of vestibular hemispheric dominance. Stronger activation was found ipsilateral to the direction of the nystagmus quick phase. The extent of vestibular cortex activation depends on a combination of these three factors, which have either an additive or subtractive effect. Consequently, iced water stimulation of the left ear in right-handed volunteers showed the strongest activation in the right hemisphere, because two of the three factors occurred in parallel: dominance for the nondominant right hemisphere and direction of the induced nystagmus to the right side (FIG. 1A, z-level = 12–26). In contrast, during stimulation of the right ear when the hemispheric dominance for the nondominant right hemisphere and the side of irrigation are in parallel, the direction of nystagmus direction is to the left. These factors resulted in a "weaker" insular and parietotemporal activation compared to that during the left-ear stimulation. Thus, the direction of nystagmus appears to have more influence than the side of stimulation.

The additional activated areas outside the parietotemporal region were nearly identical for both stimulation sides during iced water caloric stimulation, and correspond to those found during warm-water caloric stimulation.[10] They can be attributed to ocular motor (eye fields in the frontal cortex), vestibular (vestibular thalamus), and autonomic functions (anterior cingulate gyrus).

ACKNOWLEDGMENTS

We are grateful to Judy Benson for critically reading the manuscript. This work was supported by Deutsche Forschungsgemeinschaft (DI 379/4-1, BR 639/6-1) and the Wilhelm Sander-Stiftung (2001.084.1).

REFERENCES

1. BÜTTNER, U. & U.W. BUETTNER. 1978. Parietal cortex area 2v neuronal activity in the alert monkey during natural vestibular and optokinetic stimulation. Brain Res. **153**: 392–397.
2. GRÜSSER, O.J., M. PAUSE & U. SCHREITER. 1982. Neuronal responses in the parieto insular vestibular cortex of alert Java monkeys (*Macaca fascicularis*). In Physiological and Pathological Aspects of Eye Movements. A. Roucoux & M. Crommelink, Eds.: 251–270.Junk W., The Hague.
3. GRÜSSER, O.J., M. PAUSE & U. SCHREITER. 1990. Vestibular neurons in the parieto-insular cortex of monkeys (*Macaca fascicularis*): visual and neck receptor responses. J. Physiol. **430**: 559–583.
4. GRÜSSER, O.J., M. PAUSE & U. SCHREITER. 1990b. Localization and responses of neurons in the parieto-insular vestibular cortex of the awake monkeys (*Macaca fascicularis*). J. Physiol. **430**: 537–557.
5. BOTTINI, G. *et al.* 1994. Identification of the central vestibular projections in man: a positron emission tomography activation study. Exp. Brain Res. **99**: 164–169.
6. WENZEL, R. *et al.* 1996. Deactivation of human visual cortex during involuntary ocular oscillations: a PET activation study. Brain **119**: 101–110.
7. LOBEL, E. *et al.* 1998. Functional MRI of galvanic vestibular stimulation. J. Neurophysiol. **80**: 2699–2709.
8. BENSE, S. *et al.* 2001. Multisensory cortical signal increases and decreases during vestibular galvanic stimulation (fMRI). J. Neurophysiol. **85**: 886–899.
9. SUZUKI, M. *et al.* 2001. Cortical and subcortical vestibular response to caloric stimulation detected by fMRI. Cogn. Brain Res. **12**: 441–449.
10. DIETERICH, M. *et al.* 2003. Dominance for vestibular cortex function in the non-dominant hemisphere. Cereb. Cortex **13**: 994–1007.
11. OLDFIELD, R.C. 1971. The assessment and analysis of handedness: the Edinburgh inventory. Neuropsychologia **9**: 97–113.

Brain Activation Patterns during Fixation of a Central Target

A Functional Magnetic Resonance Imaging Study

ANGELA DEUTSCHLÄNDER,[a] THOMAS STEPHAN,[a] ESTHER MARX,[a] HARTMUT BRÜCKMANN,[b] AND THOMAS BRANDT[a]

[a]*Center for Sensorimotor Research, Department of Neurology and*
[b]*Department of Neuroradiology, Klinikum Grosshadern, Ludwig-Maximilians University, Munich, Germany*

KEYWORDS: eye movement; fixation; fMRI; visual cortex; human

INTRODUCTION

An earlier functional magnetic resonance imaging (fMRI) study comparing the two conditions "eyes closed" and "eyes open" in complete darkness showed activations of ocular motor and attentional structures during "eyes open."[1] With the eyes open, blood oxygenation level-dependent (BOLD) signal increases that corresponded best to the frontal eye fields (FEFs), supplementary eye fields (SEFs), and parietal eye fields (PEFs) were seen as well as activations in the right prefrontal cortex and in the right posterior parietal cortex (PPC). These right-sided activations of frontal and posterior parietal regions most likely represent structures of the attentional system, which are also known to be involved in visuospatial tasks. In this fMRI study, we were interested in determining whether fixation of a stationary central target increases activity in ocular motor structures compared to the condition "eyes open" in total darkness.

METHODS

Subjects

Seven healthy volunteers (five females, two males; 23–32 years) participated in the study. Informed written consent was obtained from all subjects.

Address for correspondence: Angela Deutschländer, M.D., Department of Neurology, Klinikum Grosshadern, Marchioninistrasse 15, 81377 Munich, Germany. Voice: 0049-89/7095-4815; fax: 0049-89/7095-4805.
adeutsch@nro.med.uni-muenchen.de

Experimental Procedure

Subjects lay supine in the MRI scanner in a completely darkened room. A red light-emitting diode (LED) was placed at the end of the MRI bore above the subject's head at a distance of about 1.25 m from the subject's eyes. A mirror that was attached to the head coil reflected the light into the subject's eyes. Subjects were told to relax with eyes open and to avoid any eye movements. During the condition designated "FIX," subjects fixated the central LED in partial darkness. During the condition designated "REST," subjects lay still with eyes open in total darkness; no LED appeared.

Data Acquisition

Functional images were acquired on a 1.5 T standard clinical scanner (Siemens Vision, Erlangen, Germany) using echo-planar imaging with a T2*-weighted gradient-echo multislice sequence (TE = 60 ms; voxel size: $3.75 \times 3.75 \times 3.75$ mm^3; matrix: 64×64; interscan interval: 4.5 s). Thirty-two transversal slices covering the whole cerebrum and large parts of the cerebellum were acquired. Each scanning session comprised two successive series. The FIX condition was presented four times per subject and series and was always followed by the REST condition. Both conditions lasted for 22.5 s.

Data Analysis

Data processing was performed on UltraSPARC workstations (Sun Microsystems, Santa Clara, CA) using SPM99 implemented in MATLAB (Mathworks, Sherborn, MA). The first five images of each imaging series were discarded to eliminate spin saturation effects. Motion correction was performed by realigning each volume to the first one of each scanning session.[2] This processing step was performed with a binary image mask to exclude the region of the eyes from computations during parameter estimation.[3] Volumes were normalized to the template space defined by the Montreal Neurological Institute template and resampled to a resolution of $2 \times 2 \times 2$ mm^3. Data sets were smoothed with a 12-mm full-width half-maximum isotropic kernel. Group analysis was performed by collapsing repeated measures within subjects and experimental runs to allow inference to the general population. The resulting 14 condition images were compared among subjects, effecting a random effects model. Statistical parametric maps were generated using the general linear model and the theory of the Gaussian fields.[4] Activations exceeding a significance threshold of $P < 0.001$ were considered significant.

RESULTS

Five activation clusters were seen during fixation of the central LED. Two clusters were centered on the inferior occipital gyri (BA 18) bilaterally, and they extended into the middle occipital gyri. Two other clusters in the middle temporal gyri and middle occipital gyri, in Brodmann area (BA) 19/37, bilaterally most likely represented MT/V5, and one small cluster appeared in the right optic radiation (FIG. 1a, TABLE 1). Even at a lower significance threshold ($P < 0.01$), no activation cluster was observed that might have represented FEFs, SEFs, or PEFs, and no activation was seen in the PPC.

TABLE 1. Activations during fixation of a central LED (group analysis, $n = 7$, $P < 0.001$)

Brain area	Brodmann area	MNI coordinates (x,y,z)	voxels	t-value
left inferior/middle occipital gyrus	BA 18/(19/17)	-32,-96,-4	464	12.36
right inferior/middle occipital gyrus	BA 18/(19/17)	36,-92,-6	476	11.49
left middle temporal/middle occipital gyrus	BA 19/37	-42,-70,-6	60	4.76
right middle temporal/middle occipital gyrus	BA 19/37	42,-62,-4	89	4.73
right optic radiation		28,-28,-2	1	3.89

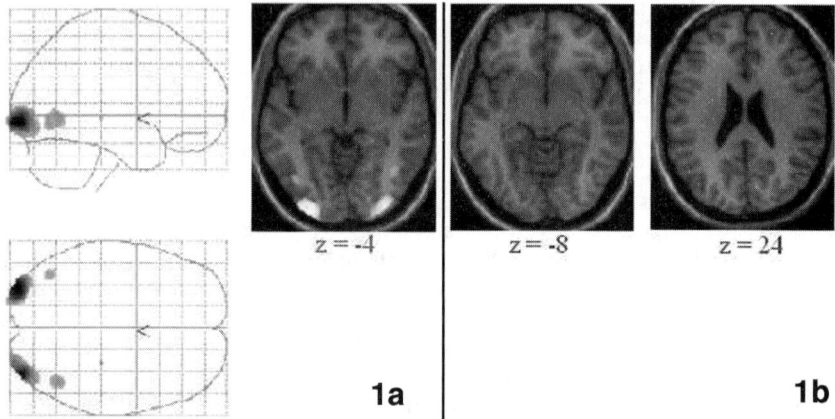

FIGURE 1. BOLD signal increases (**a**, *left*) and decreases (**b**, *right*) during fixation of a central stationary target compared to eyes open without fixation in total darkness ($N = 7$, $P < 0.001$). Projection of statistical parametric maps onto the Montreal Neurological Institute standard brain template and glass brain views.

Deactivations during fixation were seen bilaterally in the lingual gyri (BA 18), extending into the fusiform gyri (BA 19), and bilaterally in the upper cuneus (BA 19), bordering the parietooccipital sulcus (FIG. 1b, TABLE 2), that is, in occipital visual areas. Further deactivation clusters were seen in the right parahippocampal gyrus and in the left precentral gyrus (BA 4), extending into the left middle frontal gyrus (BA 6).

DISCUSSION

This fMRI study on human foveal fixation did not detect any differential activations of FEFs, PEFs, or SEFs, in the prefrontal cortex or in PPC areas, when central

TABLE 2. Deactivations during fixation of a central LED (group analysis, $n = 7$, $P < 0.001$)

Brain area	Brodmann area	MNI coordinates (x,y,z)	voxels	t-value
left precentral/middle frontal gyrus	BA 4/6	-24,-14,66	60	4.83
left lingual/fusiform gyrus	BA 18/19	-20,-72,-10	191	4.73
right parahippocampal gyrus		30,-52,0	30	4.70
right lingual/fusiform gyrus	BA 18/19	20,-72,-6	107	4.28
left cuneus (superior occipital gyrus)	BA 19	-10,-96,26	40	4.11
right cuneus (superior occipital gyrus)	BA 19	2,-94,26	1	3.65

fixation was compared with keeping eyes open and still without fixation in total darkness. BOLD signal increases found during central fixation were limited to the occipital and temporo-occipital regions, representing early visual areas. Activations of ocular motor (FEFs, PEFs, and SEFs) and attentional structures (right prefrontal cortex, right PPC) with the eyes open were reported in an earlier fMRI study comparing "eyes open" in total darkness to "eyes closed".[1] Therefore, BOLD signal increases of ocular motor and attentional structures may have occurred during the central fixation task, but did not significantly differ from putative activations during "eyes open" in complete darkness in our experimental set-up. One explanation for this finding may be that more spontaneous saccades were performed during the rest condition (no LED), which induced saccade-related activations that may have cancelled out fixation-related activations.

A region in the upper cuneus bordering the parietal lobe was found to be either deactivated during the fixation task or more strongly activated during eyes open in complete darkness than during fixation. This region may correspond to the parieto-occipital region (PO/V6), which is known to be involved in the spatial encoding of the extrapersonal visual space. PO contains neurons that are sensitive to eye positions, also in complete darkness.[5] These gaze-dependent neurons in PO are thought to be involved in the construction of an internal map of the visual environment by encoding spatial locations in the field of view in a head frame of reference, thereby allowing stability of visual perception during eye movements. Lesions of the superior parietal lobule (putative PO) in humans produce deficits in visual target localization. The regional cerebral blood flow (rCBF) decreases of PO have been described in patients with opsoclonus,[6] whereas increases were found to be related to the performance of voluntary saccades in the dark.[7] The visual areas in the lingual gyri also showed significantly stronger activation without the appearance of the LED in our study.

The results of three positron emission tomography (PET) studies on human central fixation have been published. Anderson and colleagues[8] compared central fixation with reflexive and remembered saccades in PET and found rCBF increases during fixation in the prefrontal cortex (ventromedial and anterolateral) and in the foveal visual cortex. Petit and colleagues[9] found activations in the FEFs, in the SEFs, and in the cingulate gyrus during the fixation of an imagined target in total darkness. Petit and colleagues[10] compared fixation of a central point to resting in complete darkness with open eyes in PET and found bilateral activations of the FEFs and the intraparietal sulcus as well as activations in the right frontal cortex (dorsolateral prefrontal cortex, inferior frontal gyrus, and precentral gyrus) during fixation, contrary to our results using fMRI. The authors also reported that a region in the precuneus showed a stronger activation bilaterally during eyes open without fixation than during the fixation task. Their cluster in the precuneus (506 voxels) may also represent PO; it is located only slightly more anterior to the clusters found in the upper cunei in our study. Differential activation of the lingual or fusiform gyri was not found in their study.

Our data are compatible with the findings of our earlier study on the differential effects of "eyes closed" and "eyes open" in total darkness. These data were interpreted to reflect two different states of mental activity: with the eyes closed, there was an "interoceptive" state, characterized by imagination and multisensory activity, and with the eyes open, an "exteroceptive" state, characterized by attentional and ocular motor activity. Thus, with the eyes open in darkness, fixation of a stationary LED was not necessarily expected to further increase activity in ocular motor centers.

REFERENCES

1. MARX, E. *et al.* 2003. Eye closure in darkness animates sensory systems. NeuroImage **19:** 924–934.
2. FRISTON, K. *et al.* 1995. Spatial registration and normalization of images. Hum. Brain Mapp. **2:** 165–189.
3. STEPHAN, T. *et al.* 2002. Lid closure mimics head movement in fMRI. NeuroImage **16:** 1156–1158.
4. WORSLEY, K.J. & K.J. FRISTON. 1995. Analysis of fMRI time-series revisited—again. NeuroImage **2:** 173–181.
5. GALLETTI, C., P.P. BATTAGLINI & P. FATTORI. 1995. Eye position influence on the parieto-occipital area PO (V6) of the macaque monkey. Eur. J. Neurosci. **7:** 2486–2501.
6. DE JONG, B.M., T.W. VAN WEERDEN & R. HAAXMA. 2001. Opsoclonus-induced occipital deactivation with a region-specific distribution. Vision Res. **41:** 1209–1214.
7. LAW, I. *et al.* 1998. Parieto-occipital cortex activation during self-generated eye movements in the dark. Brain **121:** 2189–2200.
8. ANDERSON, T.J. *et al.* 1994. Cortical control of saccades and fixation in man: a PET study. Brain **117:** 1073–1084.
9. PETIT, L. *et al.* 1995. Functional neuroanatomy of the human visual fixation system. Eur. J. Neurosci. **7:** 169–174.
10. PETIT, L. *et al.* 1999. PET study of the human foveal fixation system. Hum. Brain Mapp. **8:** 28–43.

Involvement of the Frontal Oculomotor Areas in Developmental Compensation for the Directional Asymmetry in Smooth-Pursuit Eye Movements in Young Primates

JUNKO FUKUSHIMA,[a] TEPPEI AKAO,[b] NORIHITO TAKEICHI,[b] CHRIS R.S. KANEKO,[c] AND KIKURO FUKUSHIMA[b]

[a]*College of Medical Technology and* [b]*Department of Physiology, School of Medicine, Hokkaido University, Sapporo, 060-8638, Japan*

[c]*Department of Physiology and Biophysics and Washington National Primate Research Center, University of Washington, Seattle, Washington 98195, USA*

ABSTRACT: The smooth pursuit system moves the eyes in space to accurately track objects of interest and maintain their images on the foveae while compensating for conflicting visual inputs from the moving background and/or vestibular inputs during head movements. Under demanding task conditions, young (but not mature) primates have difficulty with upward smooth gaze (eye in space) movement; pursuit breaks down, and they perform the task with saccades. Proper compensation matures later, after preadolescence. Chemical inactivation of the supplementary eye fields in compensated monkeys reproduced the directional asymmetry that had been compensated developmentally, suggesting that the supplemental eye fields may be involved in the compensation.

KEYWORDS: smooth pursuit; vestibulo-ocular reflex (VOR) cancellation; visual background; directional asymmetry; frontal eye fields; supplementary eye fields

INTRODUCTION

With the development of a high-acuity fovea in primates, visual information can be accurately obtained by maintaining target images on the foveae of both eyes. For small objects moving smoothly in frontal planes, the smooth pursuit system is used to move the eyes in space while compensating for visual inputs from the moving background and/or vestibular inputs during head movements.[1] Recently we have shown that children and young monkeys produce asymmetric eye movements during vertical pursuit across a textured (but not homogenous) background; upward pursuit was severely impaired and consisted mostly of catch-up saccades. Selective impair-

Address for correspondence: Kikuro Fukushima, Department of Physiology, Hokkaido University School of Medicine, West 7, North 15, Sapporo, 060-8638 Japan. Voice: +81-11-706-5038; fax: +81-11-706-5041.

kikuro@med.hokudai.ac.jp

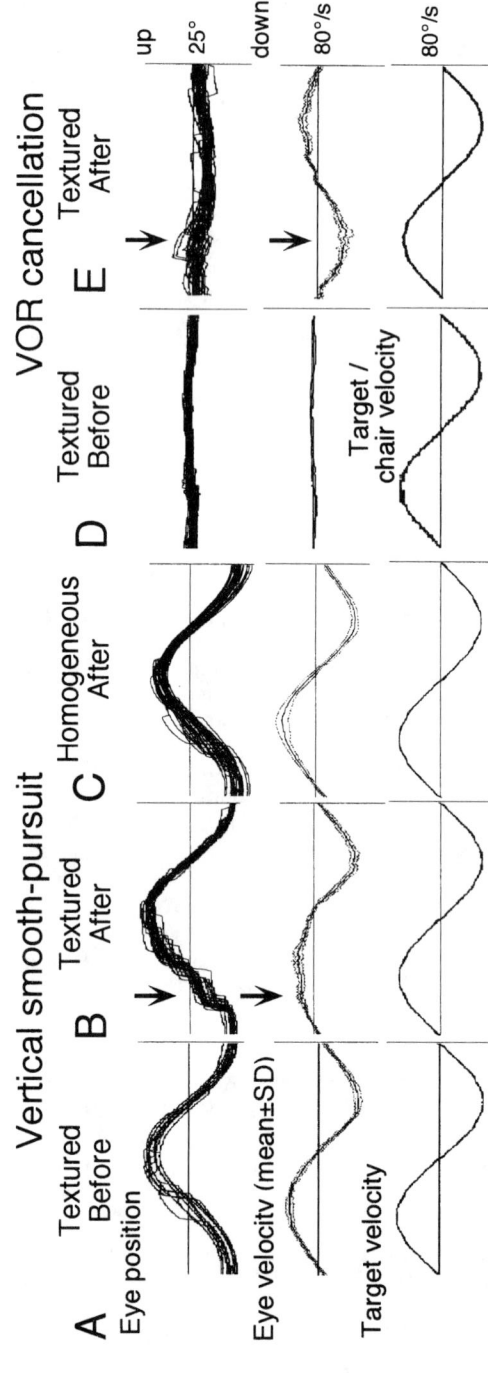

FIGURE 1. Effects of muscimol infusion into SEF (**A–E**) and major pathways related to smooth pursuit (**F**).[5] All eye velocity records in **A–E** were de-saccaded and averaged. Arrows in **B** and **E** indicate impaired smooth-gaze movements. VOR and ascending pathways are also shown in **F**. MT: middle temporal visual areas; MST: medial superior temporal visual areas. DLPN: dorsolateral pontine nuclei; DMPN: dorsomedial pontine nuclei; NRTP: nucleus reticularis tegmenti pontis; VPFL: ventral paraflocculus; DLFP: dorsal paraflocculus; IP: posterior interposed nucleus; INC: interstitial nucleus of Cajal; NPH: nucleus prepositus hypoglossi.

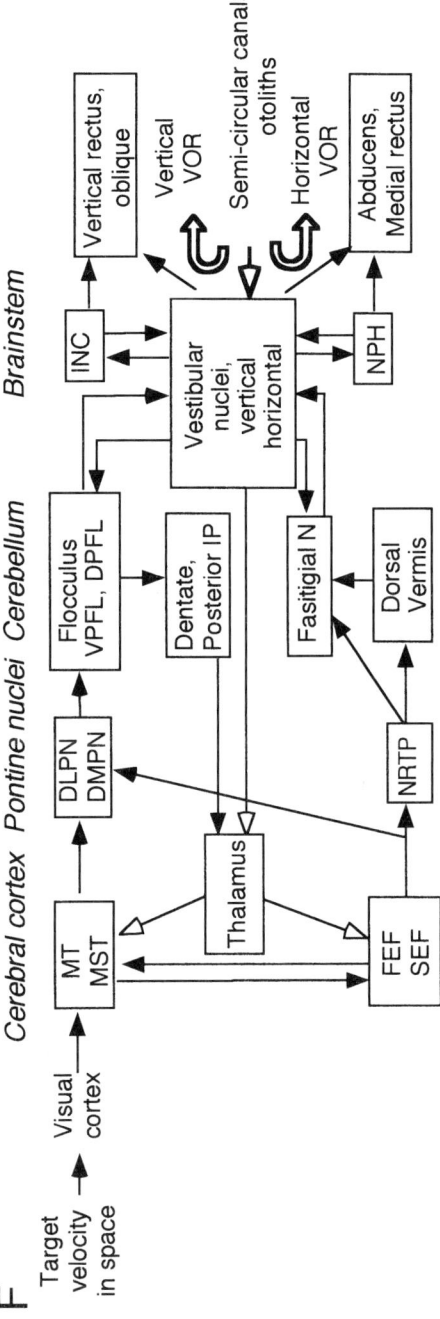

FIGURE 1. *Continued.*

ment of upward pursuit was correlated with impairment in cancellation of the downward vestibulo-ocular reflex (VOR) during nose-up, whole-body rotation.[2] Because proper compensation is still immature during preadolescence, the compensation may involve cortical mechanisms. In this study, we examined whether the frontal oculomotor areas (supplemental eye fields, SEFs, and frontal eye fields, FEFs) are involved in this compensation by chemical inactivation of these areas.

METHODS

Three monkeys (*Macaca fuscata*, 3.8–4.5 kg, 4–6 years old) were used. Two of them (~6 years old) were also used in previous studies.[2] All the procedures were evaluated and approved by the Animal Care and Use Committee of Hokkaido University School of Medicine. Our methods are described elsewhere in detail.[2,3] Briefly, monkeys were trained to fixate a 0.2° laser spot that was back projected on a tangent screen. Two different backgrounds, homogeneous and textured, were used. The mean luminance of the homogeneous background was 0.1 cd/m^2. The textured background was a random dot pattern that consisted of variable-size dots with mean luminance of dark and bright parts of 0.1 cd/m^2 and 25 cd/m^2, respectively. The target was moved sinusoidally (0.5 Hz, ±10°) either horizontally or vertically. Chair rotation was applied with the same amplitude, direction, and phase as the target so that the head-fixed monkey was required to cancel the VOR to track accurately. To locate the frontal oculomotor areas, extracellular recordings were made in the two older monkeys at A21–A24, L10–L15 and A21–A24, L3–L8 stereotaxic coordinates for the FEFs and SEFs, respectively. Once single neurons were isolated, standard tracking tasks were tested.[3] We examined the effects of the chemical inactivation of these areas next by injecting a GABA agonist muscimol (10–15 µg) dissolved in physiological saline (10 µg/µL) unilaterally into a single area where we recorded many pursuit-related neurons. The data were analyzed off-line as described previously.[2,3] Position signals were differentiated to obtain velocity by analogue circuits (DC to 100 Hz, –12 dB/octave). Saccades were removed using an interactive computer program.

RESULTS AND DISCUSSION

Consistent with our previous results,[2] a directional asymmetry was observed only for vertical pursuit across the textured background in a young monkey (~4 years old). This asymmetry was compensated in the two older monkeys (FIG. 1A) that had shown directional asymmetry in a previous test two years earlier.[2] Muscimol infusion into the SEFs resulted in selective impairment of upward pursuit across the textured—but not homogenous background (see FIG. 1B [arrow] vs. FIG. 1C). Mean eye velocity during pursuit decreased to nearly half, and catch-up saccades dominated. This impairment was correlated with selective impairment of cancellation of the downward VOR during up-pitch rotation across the textured background (compare FIG. 1A & B with FIG. 1D & E). Thus, selective impairment of upward smooth gaze (eye in space) tracking was reproduced by muscimol injection into the SEFs in the same monkey that had compensated previously. Pattern movement during fixation of the stationary spot induced only small effects (gain: <0.1), suggesting that an uncompensated optokinetic reflex alone during pursuit cannot explain the directional asymmetry. Muscimol infusion into the FEFs also impaired vertical pursuit across the textured background, but the effects were less selective, since similar impairment was observed across the homogeneous background (data not shown).[4]

This study indicates that selective impairment of upward pursuit across a textured background and the inability to cancel downward VOR during up-pitch were reproduced by chemical inactivation of the frontal oculomotor areas, including the SEFs. This suggests that the SEFs may be involved in normal compensation of these functions. To aid in the understanding of the neural mechanisms, FIGURE 1F summarizes the major pathways related to smooth pursuit.[5] Because neurons in the output pathways of the frontal oculomotor areas (that is, pontine nuclei, cerebellar dorsal vermis, fastigial nuclei) are known to carry omnidirectional pursuit signals,[1,5] selective impairment of upward pursuit induced by SEF inactivation (FIG. 1B) cannot be explained by inadequate control by the SEFs over the output pathways alone. Upward pitch rotation activates bilateral posterior canals.[1] Ito and colleagues[6] first showed that the cerebellar flocculus does not inhibit VOR relay neurons for the posterior canals in rabbits. This lack of floccular inhibition has been confirmed in other species as well.[1] Since vertical VOR and smooth pursuit share some of the floccular pathways,[1,5] selective impairment of upward smooth gaze movements may reflect this problem in young primates. Our results, which indicate that SEF inactivation reproduced this impairment in the compensated monkey, suggest that the SEFs are involved in the compensation of this problem. The cerebellar floccular lobe consists of the flocculus and ventral paraflocculus,[1] and the latter projects both to the vestibular nuclei and to the deep cerebellar nuclei that could furnish ascending signals.[7] It may well be that inadequate control of feedback from the floccular lobe to FEFs/SEFs is involved in the impairment of upward smooth gaze movement. Such possible feedback signals may be used for elaboration of binocular signals for upward pursuit to compensate for the floccular insufficiency during preadolescence.[8]

ACKNOWLEDGMENTS

This work was supported in part by the Japanese Ministry of Education, Culture, Sports, Science, and Technology and Marna Cosmetics.

REFERENCES

1. LEIGH, R.J. & D.S. ZEE. 1999. The Neurology of Eye Movements. 3rd edit. Oxford University Press. New York.
2. TAKEICHI, N., J. FUKUSHIMA, S. KURKIN, et al. 2003. Directional asymmetry in smooth ocular tracking in the presence of visual background in young and adult primates. Exp. Brain Res. **149:** 380–390.
3. SHINMEI, Y., T. YAMANOBE, J. FUKUSHIMA & K. FUKUSHIMA. 2002. Purkinje cells of the cerebellar dorsal vermis in the monkey: simple-spike activity during pursuit and passive whole body rotation. J. Neurophysiol. **87:** 1836–1849.
4. FUKUSHIMA, K., J. FUKUSHIMA & T. SATO. 1999. Vestibular-pursuit interactions: gaze velocity and target velocity signals in the monkey frontal eye fields. Ann. N.Y. Acad. Sci. **871:** 248–259.
5. FUKUSHIMA, K. 2003. Roles of the cerebellum in pursuit-vestibular interactions. Cerebellum **2:** 223–232.

6. ITO, M., N. NISHIMARU & M. YAMAMOTO. 1977. Specific patterns of neuronal connections involved in the control of the rabbit's vestibulo-ocular reflexes by the cerebellar flocculus. J. Physiol. **265:** 833–854.
7. NAGAO, S., T. KITAMURA, N. NAKAMURA, *et al.* 1997. Location of efferent terminals of the primate flocculus and ventral paraflocculus revealed by anterograde axonal transport methods. Neurosci. Res. **27:** 257–269.
8. KURKIN, S., N. TAKEICHI, T. AKAO, *et al.* Neurons in the caudal frontal eye fields of monkeys signal three-dimensional tracking. Ann. N.Y. Acad. Sci. **1004:** this volume.

Magnetoencephalography during Optokinetic and Vestibular Activation of the Posterior Insula

S. HEGEMANN,[a] M. PAWLOWSKI,[b] R. HUONKER,[b] J. HAUEISEN,[b] C. FITZEK,[c] AND M. FETTER[a]

[a]*Department of Neurology, Klinikum Karlsbad-Langensteinbach, Karlsbad, Germany*

[b]*MEG Center, Jena, Germany*

[c]*Institute of Diagnostic and Interventional Radiology, Jena, Germany*

KEYWORDS: magnetoencephalography (MEG); vestibular signal processing; posterior insula; caloric stimuli; optokinetic stimuli

INTRODUCTION

Cortical activity during caloric and optokinetic stimulation was demonstrated by several positron emission tomography (PET)[1] and functional magnetic resonance imaging (fMRI)[2] studies. According to these studies, the posterior insula and retroinsular region appear to be the human homologue of the parietoinsular vestibular cortex (PIVC) in monkeys that has been identified by single-cell recording as a cortical vestibular region.[3,4] This region seems to play a key role in processing vestibular signals and in generating spatial orientation.[5,6]

We wanted to know whether magnetoencephalography (MEG) is capable of measuring vestibular signal processing in the posterior insula during caloric and optokinetic stimuli. We also tried to obtain a better timely resolution of the activity in the vestibular cortex and looked for its correlation with the slow and fast phases of nystagmus.

METHODS

Nine volunteers (four women, five men) were positioned on their right side during measurements of the left hemisphere with a 31-channel SQUID Dewar positioned laterally as shown in FIGURE 1.

Address for correspondence: Dr. Stefan Hegemann, Klinik für Neurologie II, Klinikum Karlsbad-Langensteinbach, 76307 Karlsbad, Germany. Voice: 49-(0)7202-610; fax: 49-(0)7202-616180.

stefan.hegemann@kkl.srh.de

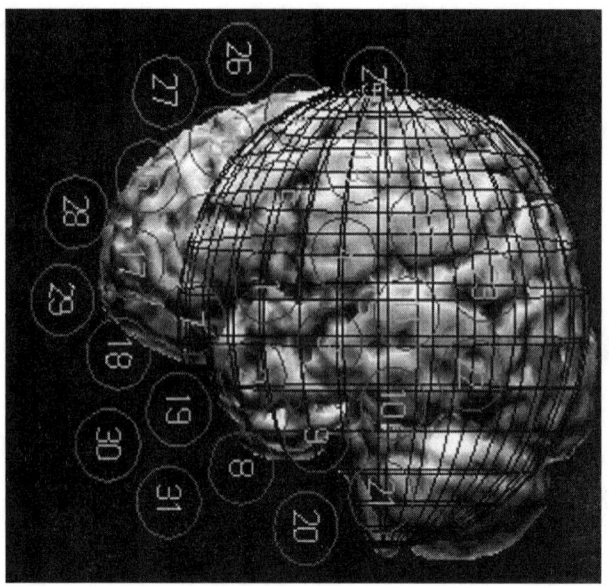

FIGURE 1. Individual MRI with coils and spherical model.

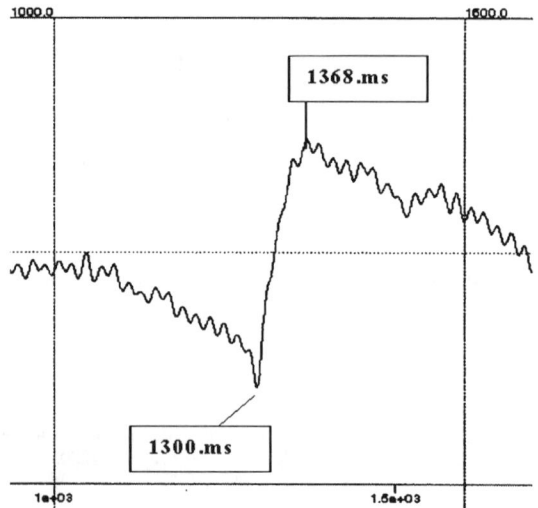

FIGURE 2. Horizontal electro-oculogram.

We elicited horizontal optokinetic nystagmus (OKN) for 5 min by rotating spotlights at a velocity of approximately 55°/s, back projected on a transparent white screen covering a visual field of about 150° horizontally (that is, in the direction of the interocular axis) and 60° vertically. Afterwards, we induced caloric nystagmus (eyes closed), rinsing the right ear with 20°C cold water for 5 min. Horizontal and vertical eye movements of one eye were recorded with a two-channel electro-oculogram (EOG). If no nystagmus was to be seen online, we repeated the measurement for one more time.

Because of the anatomical variation of the insula, we repeated the two measurements with a more posterior (about 5 cm) cryostat-to-head position. Subjects were totally free of pain for the duration of all measurements.

To improve the signal-to-noise ratio, we averaged off-line between 10 and 100 nystagmic beats supported by a Brainstar software written by U. Brandl, Jena, Germany. Markers were set either at the beginning or at the end of the saccades, with a maximum time range of approximately 2047 ms (about 1000 ms each time before and after the saccade).

After application of the common average reference (for example, using electroencephalography) and a 40-Hz low-pass filter in the Curry V4.5 software (Compumedics Germany, GmbH, Hamburg), we decomposed the magnetic activity in the selected time range using independent component analysis (ICA). The order of the components is dependent on the field strength, so the eye-artifact ICA component was listed mostly at the first position. FIGURE 2 shows an EOG-example of a typical nystagmus with the time interval selected for analysis and end points of the fast phase/saccade. FIGURE 3 shows the corresponding ICA components (3a) with a clear correlation of the first component to the EOG and a second component that is independent of the eye movement signal. The corresponding ICA pattern (FIG. 3b) reveals a dipole within the measured field only for the second component, not for the

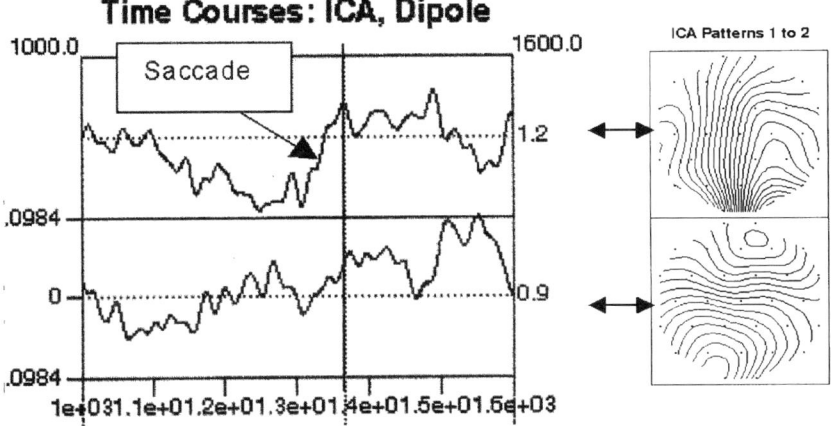

FIGURE 3. (**a**) First and second components and (**b**) corresponding patterns. For the source reconstruction, we used the spherical model. An individual T1-weighted MRI was used to fit the sphere.

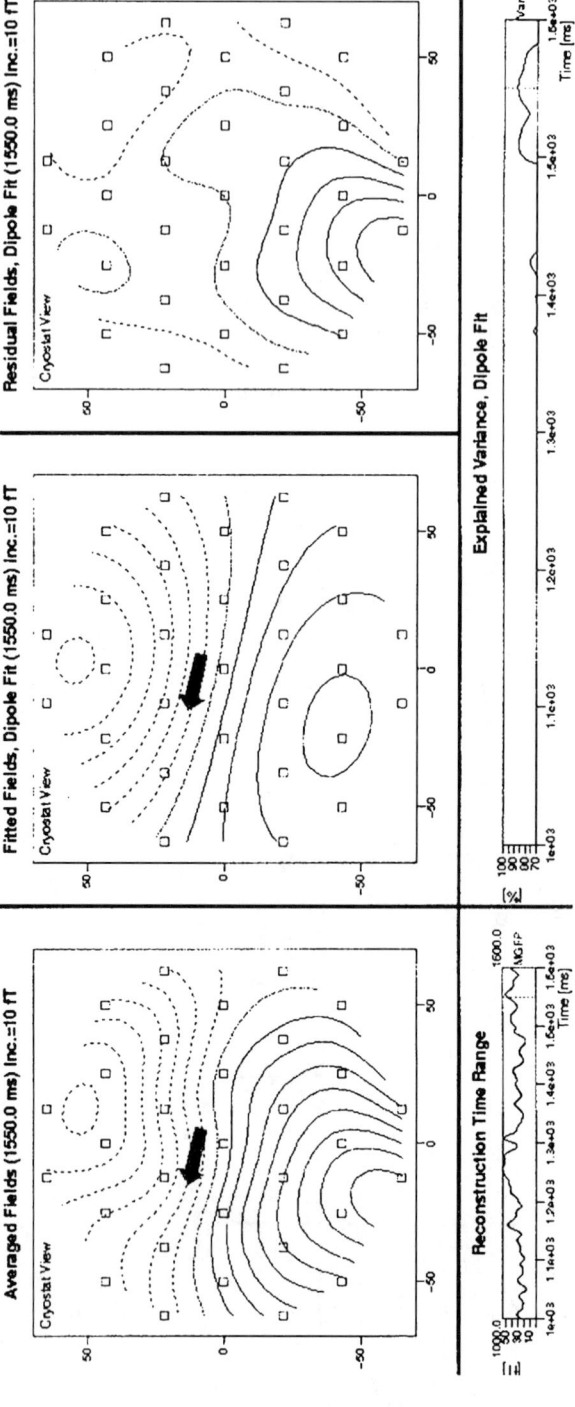

FIGURE 4. Averaged and fitted fields of the second ICA component with a peak at 200 ms after the saccade (1550 ms) during the time range of 600 ms (1000–1600 ms) with a dipole-localization in hPIVC.

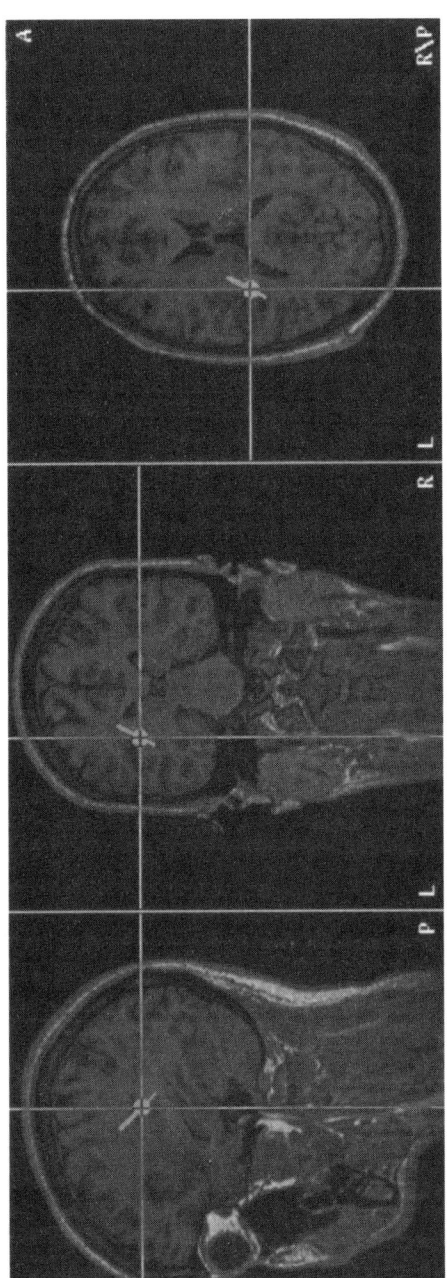

FIGURE 5. Caloric stimulation (10 averages; reconstruction time range: 2047 ms; first ICA component; maximum 100-fT field strength).

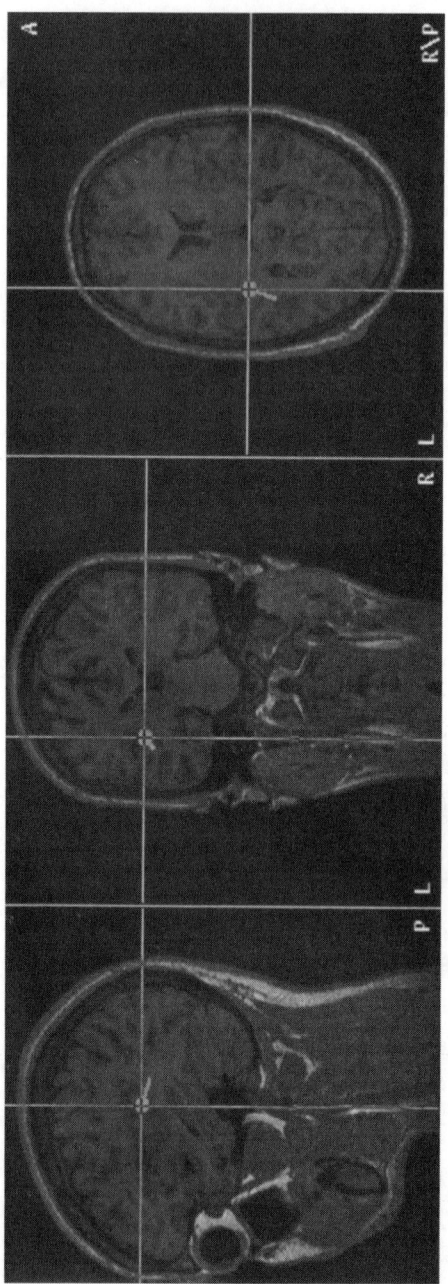

FIGURE 6. Optokinetic stimulation (52 averages; reconstruction time range: 506 ms; third ICA component: maximum 25-fT field strength).

eye artifact. FIGURE 4 shows how a single dipole is fitted from the pattern of the second ICA-component and what is left as residual fields. This fitted dipole is then matched with a high-resolution 3D MRI. Examples of such dipoles are shown for caloric (FIG. 5) and optokinetic (FIG. 6) stimulation.

RESULTS

In seven of nine volunteers—after caloric and optokinetic measurement—a typical dipolar pattern was found in one of the first three ICA components with a localization in the posterior insula. In two cases, we found a typical dipolar pattern with localization around the posterior insula without ICA during periods of minimal eye artifact (eyes close to primary position). It shows that even with less sophisticated dipole analysis there is a human PIVC (hPIVC) dipole detectable. The dipoles had a field strength between 20 and 170 fT and were located in the posterior insula for both caloric and optokinetic nystagmus by individual fitting to MRI. The group mean value of Tailarach coordinates was –33/22/15, which is also in the insula (Brodmann area 13; range: 5 mm).

Peak field strength occurred at about 200 ms after the saccade in 9 of 13 measurements, and at 250 ms in 3 of 13, one measurement could not be assessed because of technical problems. No significant differences could be observed between the left-beating caloric nystagmus and the right-beating OKN regarding dipole localization or polarization.

DISCUSSION

We were able to show for the first time that vestibular activation during caloric and optokinetic stimulation is detectable in the hPIVC using MEG. We found either an hPIVC localization during OKN and caloric-evoked nystagmus in individuals or none at all. This observation increases our confidence that the found dipoles are true. The first ICA component was clearly correlated with the EOG, so we are confident that it represents the eye artifact. The smaller the averaged amplitude of the saccade, the more probable it is that the hPIVC dipole has a stronger ICA component than the eye artifact.

Activation under both stimulus conditions corresponds well to previous fMRI studies and the multisensory function of the hPIVC. The uniform activity we measured during caloric and optokinetic stimulation was not modulated by the direction of nystagmus. Thus, the hPIVC seems not to be directly involved in sensing the direction of movement. We cannot say what exactly its function is. Interestingly, hPIVC activity seems to peak at a point in time related to the end of the fast phase of nystagmus. Because, to our knowledge, there is no hPIVC activity during pure saccadic tasks, we can only speculate about the underlying physiologic mechanism: A time delay of 200 ms could be due to processing of visual information that has to be integrated with vestibular and sensory afferents and is reset by each fast phase. Further studies have to resolve these open questions, but MEG seems to be a new and promising tool in vestibular and oculomotor research.

ACKNOWLEDGMENT

We thank Prof. U. Brandl, Jena, for supplying us with his "Brainstar" software.

REFERENCES

1. BOTTINI, G., R. STERZI, E. PAULESU, *et al.* 1994. Identification of the central vestibular projections in man: a positron emission tomography activation study. Exp. Brain Res. **99:** 164–169.
2. DIETERICH, M., S.F. BUCHER, K.C. SEELOS & TH. BRANDT. 1998. Horizontal or vertical optokinetic stimulation activates visual motion-sensitive, ocular motor and vestibular cortex areas with right hemispheric dominance: an FMRI study. Brain **121:** 1479–1495.
3. GRÜSSER, O.J., M. PAUSE & U. SCHREITER. 1990. Localization and responses of neurones in the parieto-insular vestibular cortex of awake monkeys (*Macaca fascicularis*). J. Physiol. (Lond.) **430:** 537–557.
4. GRÜSSER, O.J., M. PAUSE & U. SCHREITER. 1990. Vestibular neurones in the parieto-insular cortex of monkeys: visual and neck receptor responses. J. Physiol. (Lond.) **430:** 559–583.
5. BRANDT, TH., M. DIETERICH & A. DANEK. 1994. Vestibular cortex lesions affect the perception of verticality. Ann. Neurol. **35:** 403–412.
6. GULDIN, W. & O.J. GRÜSSER. 1996. The anatomy of the vestibular cortices of primates. *In* Le cortex vestibulaire. M. Collard, M. Jeannerod & Y. Christen, Eds.: 18–26. Ipsen. Boulogne.

Impaired Representation of Saccadic Eye Displacement after Posterior Parietal Lesions

Is It a Craniotopic or a Directional Deficit?

WOLFGANG HEIDE,[a] ANDREAS SPRENGER,[a] BARBARA SACKERER,[a] KLAUS G. ROTTACH,[b] CHRISTIAN GAEBEL,[c] AND DETLEF KÖMPF[a]

Departments of [a]Neurology and [c]Neuroradiology, University at Lübeck, Lübeck, Germany

[b]Neurological Outpatient Clinic, Kaufbeuren, Germany

KEYWORDS: spatial constancy; efference copy; double-step saccades; remapping

INTRODUCTION

Despite constant shifts of its retinal image, due to eye or head movements, we perceive space as stable. To maintain this amazing ability of spatial constancy, our brain cannot rely on retinal maps, but it needs nonvisual (extraretinal) information about eye or head movements. The most important source of this information is a copy of the motor signal ("efference copy") that is neuronally generated prior to each movement, such as a saccade, and fed back into the cortical visual pathways to compensate for the retinal image shift caused by the saccadic eye displacement.[1,2]

For saccadic eye movements, this can be investigated using the double-step task, where the locations of two successively flashed peripheral targets (for 140 and 100 ms, respectively) have to be fixated in darkness in the correct order. As there is a spatial dissonance after the first saccade between the retinal location of the second target and the required motor vector of the second saccade, the brain must update the spatial representation of the second target by using efference copy about current eye position or about the preceding saccadic eye displacement to achieve spatial accuracy for the second saccade. Patients with right posterior parietal lesions are specifically impaired in this task: The second saccade is grossly dysmetric (following the retinal vector of the target) whenever the first saccade is directed into the contralesional left hemifield[3].

Two alternative explanations may hold for this finding. These patients have no reliable extraretinal information about eye positions in left contralesional craniotopic hemispace, thus exhibiting a craniotopic deficit of maintaining spatial constancy

Address for correspondence: Prof. Wolfgang Heide, M.D., Department of Neurology, University at Lübeck, Ratzeburger Allee 160, D-23538 Lübeck, Germany. Voice: +49-451-500-3472; fax: +49-451-500-2489.

wolfgang.heide@akh-celle.de

Ann. N.Y. Acad. Sci. 1004: 465–468 (2003). © 2003 New York Academy of Sciences.
doi: 10.1196/annals.1303.053

a) <u>spatiotopic</u> model: b) <u>eye displacement</u> model:

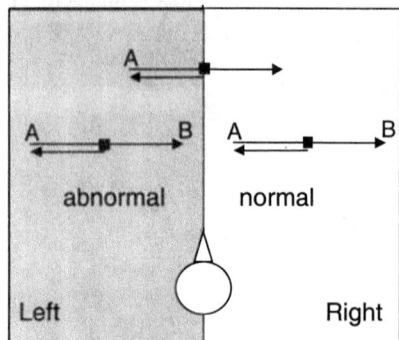 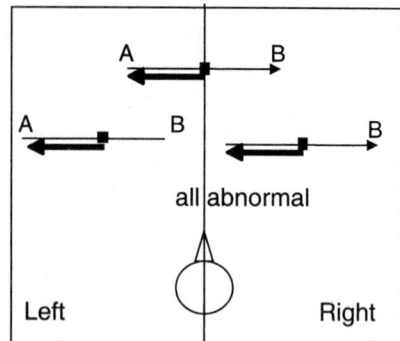

FIGURE 1. The two different models of how the parietal cortex codes the spatial location of a saccade goal. These models lead to contradictory predictions about the deficits of patients who have right parietal lesions and who perform the double-step task from different orbital positions.

across saccades in the double-step task, fitting to a *spatiotopic model* of coding a saccade goal in head- or world-centered coordinates.[4,5] Alternatively, they might be unable to update (remap) the spatial (retinotopic) representation of the second target in association with each leftward saccadic eye displacement, regardless of the hemifield in which this takes place, thus exhibiting a directional deficit of spatial constancy across saccades. This is based on the assumption (derived from monkey experiments[6,7]) that the parietal cortex codes a saccade goal in retinal or oculocentric coordinates that have to be updated prior to each saccade by using efference copy to compensate for saccadic eye displacement (*eye displacement model*).[8] To test these two models, we started the double-step task from different initial orbital positions (0°, 10° left, 10° right). The spatiotopic model predicts that the second saccade is dysmetric whenever it starts from contralateral craniotopic hemispace. In contrast, the eye displacement model predicts that the second saccade is dysmetric after each first saccade in contralateral direction (FIG. 1).

METHODS

We investigated 10 patients with chronic postischemic lesions of the right posterior parietal cortex around the middle and posterior portion of the intraparietal sulcus where previous lesion and functional magnetic resonance imaging (fMRI) studies had identified a cortical location that is critical for the double-step task[3,9] (age of lesions: 1–24 months). We also evaluated 10 age-related healthy adults for control. Five patients had mild visual hemineglect.

Horizontal eye movements were recorded using infrared reflection oculography with the head fixed on a table-mounted system (AMTech, Weinheim). For visual stimulation, we used a red laser point, projected onto a screen (distance of 114 cm) and moved by a mirror galvanometer. The two peripheral targets of each double-step trial were presented successively at 6° right and 6° left of current eye fixation (or vice versa, or at 5° and 9°) for 140 and 100 ms, respectively. Then subjects had to fixate the remembered target positions in darkness. Initial orbital positions were 0°, 10° right, or 10° left on the horizontal meridian. Each combination of trials was presented 10 times in pseudorandom order.

RESULTS

Leftward saccades (FIG. 2A) were generally more dysmetric in the patients ($P < 0.01$), even the first saccades, although they could be performed according to retinal coordinates of the target. This reflects the well-known retinotopic deficit of contralateral visually guided saccades in posterior parietal lesions[3,10] and correlated

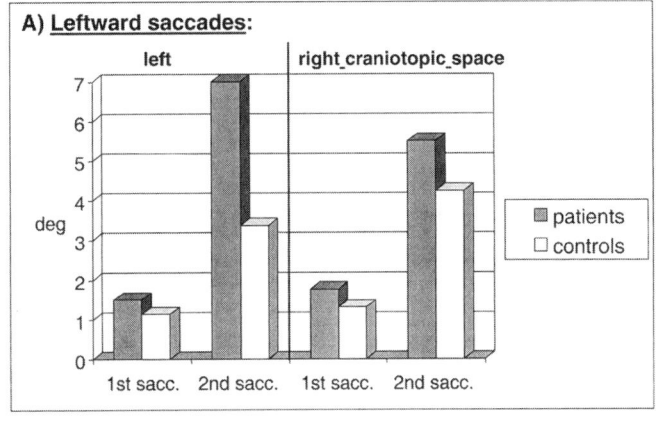

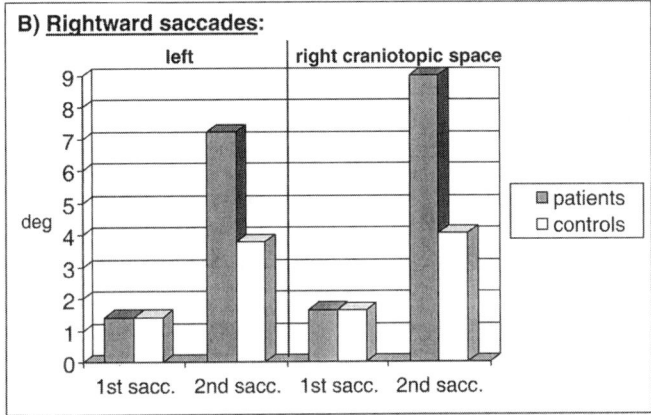

FIGURE 2. Mean error of post-saccadic eye position (in degrees of visual angle) with regard to target position, plotted separately for leftward (**A**) and rightward (**B**) first and second saccades, performed either in the left or in the right craniotopic hemispace.

with the severity of neglect. The deficit was more pronounced in left hemispace. A comparable finding was reported after temporal inactivation of the parietal eye field in monkeys.[11]

Rightward saccades (FIG. 2B) showed neither a retinotopic nor a craniotopic deficit. First saccades were normal. However, rightward second saccades (following a leftward first saccade) were grossly dysmetric, as compared to the control group ($P < 0.001$), even if the whole trial was performed in right craniotopic hemispace, as predicted by the eye displacement model.

CONCLUSIONS

Dysmetria of the second saccade in the double-step task is neither a retinotopic nor a craniotopic nor an absolute spatiotopic deficit, but a deficit of updating the spatial representation of the second target by using extraretinal information (efference copy) about first saccades in contralateral direction. It is thus a deficit of maintaining spatial constancy across leftward saccades. Our data confirm the predictions of the "eye displacement" model, thus arguing against an invariant spatiotopic coding of saccade goals in posterior parietal cortex.

REFERENCES

1. VON HOLST, E. & H. MITTELSTAEDT. 1950. Das Reafferenzprinzip. Naturwissenschaften **37:** 464–476.
2. BRIDGEMAN, B., A.H.C. VAN DER HEIJDEN & B.M. VELICHKOVSKY. 1994. A theory of visual stability across saccadic eye movements. Behav. Brain Sci. **17:** 247–292.
3. HEIDE, W., M. BLANKENBURG, E. ZIMMERMANN & D. KÖMPF. 1995. Cortical control of double-step saccades: implications for spatial orientation. Ann. Neurol. **38:** 739–748.
4. ANDERSEN, R.A. 1995. Encoding of intention and spatial location in the posterior parietal cortex. Cereb. Cortex **5:** 457–469.
5. GALLETTI, C., P.P. BATTAGLINI & P. FATTORI. 1993. Parietal neurons encoding spatial locations in craniotopic coordinates. Exp. Brain Res. **96:** 221–229.
6. DUHAMEL, J.-R., C.L. COLBY & M.E. GOLDBERG. 1992. The updating of the representation of visual space in parietal cortex by intended eye movements. Science **255:** 90–92.
7. COLBY, C.L. & M.E. GOLDBERG. 1999. Space and attention in parietal cortex. Annu. Rev. Neurosci. **22:** 319–349.
8. SCHLAG, J., M. SCHLAG-REY & P. DASSONVILLE. 1994. For and against spatial coding of saccades. *In* Visual and Oculomotor Functions. G. d'Ydewalle & J. van Rensbergen, Eds.: 3–17. Elsevier. Amsterdam.
9. HEIDE, W., F. BINKOFSKI, R.J. SEITZ, *et al.* 2001. Activation of fronto-parietal cortices during memorized triple-step sequences of saccadic eye movements: an fMRI study. Eur. J. Neurosci. **13:** 1177–1189.
10. PIERROT-DESEILLIGNY, C., S. RIVAUD, B. GAYMARD, *et al.* 1995. Cortical control of saccades. Ann. Neurol. **37:** 557–567.
11. LI, C.-S.R. & R.A. ANDERSEN. 2001. Inactivation of macaque lateral intraparietal area delays initiation of the second saccade predominantly from contralesional eye positions in the double-step task. Exp. Brain Res. **137:** 45–57.

Vestibular and Somatosensory Cortex Deactivation during Imagined Locomotion

A Functional Magnetic Resonance Imaging Study

KLAUS JAHN, ANGELA DEUTSCHLÄNDER, THOMAS STEPHAN, HARTMUT BRÜCKMANN, MICHAEL STRUPP, AND THOMAS BRANDT

Ludwig-Maximilians University, Klinikum Grosshadern, Department of Neurology, Marchioninistrasse 15, 81377 Munich, Germany

KEYWORDS: locomotion; motor imagery; functional imaging; vestibular system

INTRODUCTION

Locomotion is a complex motor performance based on spinal generators under the control of several distinct and separate supraspinal centers that initiate locomotion or modify locomotion speed. Sensory systems, such as the visual and the vestibular systems, contribute to the maintenance of direction and balance, particularly during locomotion at slow speed.[1] Studies on the differential effects of vestibular and visual perturbations during walking and running showed that running was significantly less dependent on sensory cues.[2,3] We hypothesized that vestibular sensorimotor control might be inhibited during highly automated locomotion such as running. This may prevent potentially adverse sensorimotor effects on an optimized spinal motor locomotion program. The aim of the present functional magnetic resonance imaging (fMRI) study was to determine whether the inhibition of the vestibular system during locomotion can be visualized as deactivation (blood oxygen level–dependent [BOLD] signal decrease) of the vestibular cortex. The imagining of standing, walking, and running was chosen because actual locomotion is methodologically incompatible with our imaging setup.

METHODS

Thirteen healthy subjects (mean age: 27.3 years) were trained to perform (eyes open) and imagine (eyes closed) four different conditions: lying (rest condition), standing, walking, and running. Functional imaging was done immediately after the training using a Siemens Magnetom Vision 1.5-T scanner and echo-planar imaging (EPI) sequences. A total of 34 slices covered the whole brain. Subjects were instruct-

Address for correspondence: Klaus Jahn, M.D., Department of Neurology, Klinikum Grosshadern, Marchioninistrasse 15, 81377 Munich, Germany. Voice: +49-89/7095-2588; fax: +49-89/7095-5584.
klaus.jahn@lrz.uni-muenchen.de

ed to imagine the four different conditions on acoustic demand for 22.5 s. Each condition was tested 14 times. Data preprocessing (realignment, normalization) and statistical analysis was done using statistical parametric mapping software (SPM99; http://www.fil.ion.ucl.ac.uk/spm). BOLD signal increases and decreases were tested for statistical significance for each subject and for the group ($P < 0.001$).

RESULTS

BOLD signal decreases were found during the imagining of walking and running, but not during the imagining of upright stance in cortical areas attributed to the vestibular and acoustic systems (posterior insula, superior temporal gyrus, supramarginal gyrus; BA 40,42; FIG. 1). These deactivations were most pronounced during the imagination of running (166 voxels for running vs. 117 voxels for walking), and they had a right-hemispheric preponderance (134 voxels right vs. 32 voxels left). Further deactivations were found during the imagining of walking and running in the primary and secondary somatosensory cortical areas (postcentral gyrus, superior parietal lobule, precuneus; BA 3,5,7). The localizations of these deactivations are given in the form of Brodmann areas (BAs) and Montreal Neurological Institute MNI) coordinates in TABLE 1.

TABLE 1. Deactivations during imagined standing, walking, and running in fMRI

Area	BA	Voxel	T	x	y	z
Standing						
No deactivation						
Walking						
R postcentral gyrus and superior parietal lobule	5/7	68	6.38	22	−48	64
R supramarginal gyrus	40	117	6.03	54	−28	26
Running						
R medial frontal gyrus	9	27	6.43	20	36	20
R inferior frontal gyrus (triangular)	9	9	4.89	40	20	28
R posterior insula/Heschl	42	20	8.16	32	−30	18
R superior temporal gyrus/Heschl	42	114	4.77	68	−22	10
L posterior insula/Heschl	42	32	5.27	−34	−24	18
L precuneus	7	60	5.65	−12	−42	50
R postcentral gyrus	5	18	4.59	28	−44	72
R postcentral gyrus	3	7	4.36	20	−34	54

NOTE: BOLD signal decreases (deactivations) during the imagining of standing, walking, and running (compared to imagining of lying); group analysis, $n = 13$, $P < 0.001$). BA: Brodmann areas; V: number of voxels; T: T value; R: right hemisphere; L: left hemisphere. The MNI coordinates (x, y, z) are listed for all areas larger than five voxels.

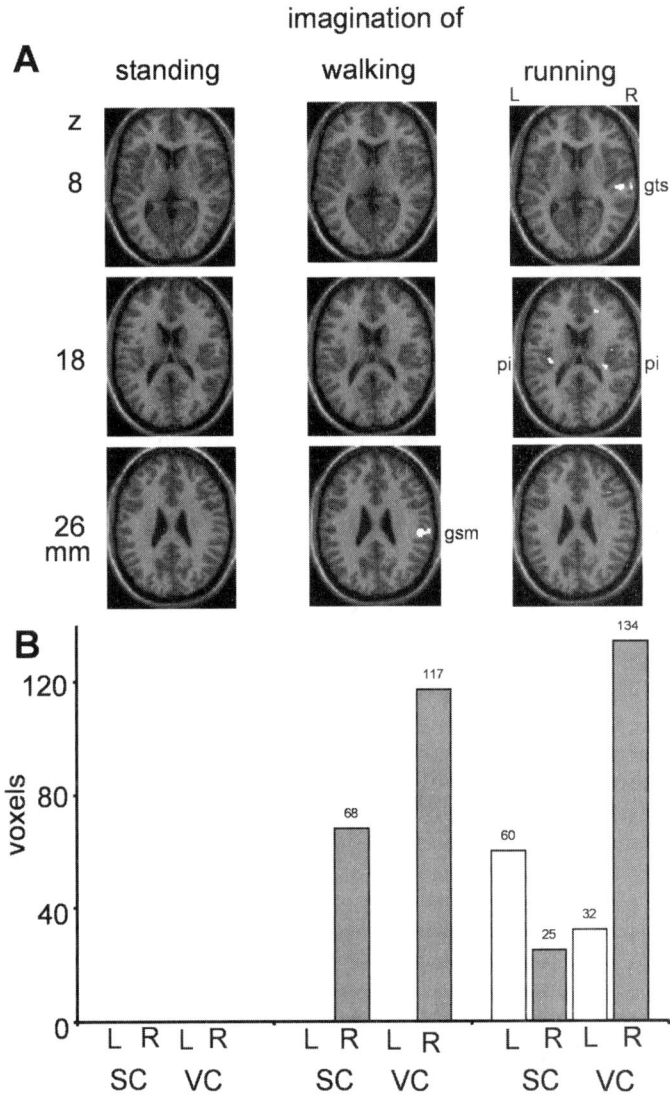

FIGURE 1. Deactivation in vestibular cortical (VC) and somatosensory cortical (SC) areas during imagined standing, slow walking, and running as compared to lying. (**A**) BOLD signal decreases (white) superimposed on the Montreal Neurological Institute (MNI) standard brain template (group analysis, 13 healthy subjects, $P < 0.001$). During imagining of standing (*left column*), no deactivations were found. During imagining of walking (*middle column*), BOLD signal decreases were located in the right supramarginal gyrus (gsm; BA 40) and right postcentral gyrus/superior parietal lobule (BA 5,7). During imagining of running (*right column*), deactivations were found bilaterally in the posterior insula (pi), right superior temporal gyrus (gts; BA 42), right postcentral gyrus (BA 3,5), and left precuneus (BA 7). MNI z-coordinates are provided on the left side. (**B**) Quantitative approach for de-

DISCUSSION

With fMRI, it was possible to visualize deactivations of the vestibular and somatosensory cortex during imagined locomotion. These deactivations were not found during imagined standing. Cluster sizes for deactivations of vestibular and somatosensory cortex areas were larger during imagined running than during imagined walking. This fits earlier findings about the inhibitory interaction between locomotion and vestibular function.[1,2] The findings of the current brain activation study also agree with the previous demonstration that actual and imagined locomotion suppress spontaneous nystagmus in patients with vestibular neuritis.[4] The major deactivations found in the posterior insula and retroinsular areas correspond best to the parieto-insular vestibular cortex (PIVC), as delineated electrophysiologically by Grüsser and colleagues[5] in monkeys. In humans, brain activation studies showed that cortical areas corresponding to the PIVC are activated by caloric and galvanic vestibular stimulation.[6] In summary, the current study shows that the inhibition of sensory signals during locomotion does not seem to be limited to peripheral and spinal mechanisms, but includes cortical representations of the somatosensory and the vestibular system. The right-hemispheric preponderance found in the current study confirms the right-hemispheric dominance of the vestibular system.[7]

ACKNOWLEDGMENTS

We are grateful to Judy Benson for copyediting the manuscript. This work was supported by the Deutsche Forschungsgemeinschaft.

REFERENCES

1. BRANDT, T., M. STRUPP & J. BENSON. 1999. You are better off running than walking with acute vestibulopathy. Lancet **355:** 233.
2. JAHN, K., M. STRUPP, E. SCHNEIDER, et al. 2000. Differential effects of vestibular stimulation on walking and running. NeuroReport 11: 1745–1748.
3. JAHN, K., M. STRUPP, E. SCHNEIDER, et al. 2001. Visually induced gait deviations during different locomotion speeds. Exp. Brain Res. **141:** 370–374.
4. JAHN, K., M. STRUPP & T. BRANDT. 2002. Both actual and imagined locomotion suppress spontaneous vestibular nystagmus. NeuroReport **13:** 2125–2128.
5. GRÜSSER, O.J., M. PAUSE & U. SCHREITER. 1990. Localisation and responses of neurons in the parieto-insular vestibular cortex of awake monkeys *(Macaca fascicularis)*. J. Physiol. **430:** 537–557.
6. BRANDT, T. & M. DIETERICH. 1999. The vestibular cortex: its locations, functions, and disorders. Ann. N.Y. Acad. Sci. **871:** 293–312.
7. BENSE, S., T. STEPHAN, T.A. YOUSRY, et al. 2001. Multisensory cortical signal increases and decreases during vestibular galvanic stimulation (fMRI). J. Neurophysiol. **85:** 886–899.

---

activations in sensory areas expressed by the number of deactivated voxels. BOLD signal decreases in BA 40 and 42 were attributed to the vestibular system (VC); in BA 3,5, and 7, to the somatosensory (SC) system. Numbers of voxels are given above columns (L for left-sided deactivations and R for right-sided deactivations). Deactivations showed a right-hemispheric preponderance in vestibular cortical areas and were most pronounced during the imagining of running.

Head Impulses in Three Orthogonal Planes of Space

Influence of Age

R. BRZEZNY,[a] S. GLASAUER,[b] O. BAYER,[b] C. SIEBOLD,[b] AND U. BÜTTNER[b]

[a]*Department of Neurology, Second School of Medicine, Charles University, Prague, Czech Republic*

[b]*Department of Neurology, Klinikum Grosshadern, Ludwig-Maximilians University, Munich, Germany*

KEYWORDS: vestibulo-ocular reflex (VOR); head-impulse testing; age; human; three-dimensional kinematics

INTRODUCTION

Increase in age leads to observable histological changes in nearly all anatomic structures involved in the vestibulo-ocular reflex (VOR).[1–6] Should reflex function depend directly on intact peripheral vestibular structures, then we might expect a decline in the VOR in response to anatomical loss. Alternatively, if the central compensatory mechanisms remain intact, the function of the VOR may remain relatively stable in spite of peripheral anatomical deterioration. Most studies indicate decreased gain with increasing age.[7–9] It has been recently shown that commonly used low-frequency stimuli are often insufficient to reveal vestibular impairment.[10] Vestibular loss, especially in chronic lesions, can be best demonstrated by the head-impulse test, which uses high accelerations.[11–13] Our aim is to test how aging affects function of rotational VOR response characteristics to transient rotational testing at high-acceleration head impulses, performed in all three orthogonal planes of stimulation.

METHODS

Subjects

We studied two age-segregated groups of randomly selected human subjects. The young group included nine subjects aged from 25 to 35 years; the elderly group, eight subjects aged from 61 to 81 years. All subjects were examined for any prior

Address for correspondence: R. Brzezny, Department of Neurology, Second School of Medicine, Charles University, Prague, Czech Republic. Voice: +420-22443-6801; fax: +420-22443-6820.
brzezny@fnmotol.cz

history of any condition or injury suggestive of vestibular disorder. Those with such histories were excluded from participation.

Procedure

We used unpredictable manually delivered head rotations with angular acceleration between 1000° and 13,000°/s^2 (head impulses) done in three orthogonal planes of space—yaw-horizontal, pitch-vertical, and roll-torsional—to test the three-dimensional input-output kinematics of the VOR. The subjects were seated in the center of a field coil system consisting of a cubic aluminum frame (side length: 140 cm) that produced three orthogonal magnetic fields (Remmel Systems, USA). Ocular rotation of the left eye around the horizontal (z-axis), vertical (y-axis), and the torsional (x-axis) was recorded with a dual search coil (Skalar, Delft, Netherlands). Three-dimensional search coil data were sampled at a rate of 1 kHz. One search coil was placed in the subject's left eye after adequate anesthesia of the conjunctiva with oxybuprocain-HCl. A second coil was thoroughly attached with an adhesive tape to the center of subject's forehead. Calibration has been described previously.[14] Subjects fixated a red laser dot (size: 0.1°) at the center of a screen placed 140 cm in front of the subject. Tests were performed in the dark with the laser dot being the only discernible point. Eye movements during the first 100 ms after each impulse onset (head velocity exceeded 20°/s) were analyzed. As measure for the gain of the VOR, we used the so-called gamma gain,[15] that is, the functionally relevant instantaneous gain for gaze stabilization. To compute the γ-gain, instantaneous eye velocity is first projected onto the head velocity vector. The γ-gain is the ratio of projected eye velocity to head velocity. For statistical analysis (repeated measures ANOVA), we used only the γ-gain at 40 ms after head-impulse onset. Examples of raw data are shown in FIGURE 1.

RESULTS

The repeated measures ANOVA revealed statistically significant age-related changes in VOR γ-gains [$F(1,15 = 9.9; P = 0.0066$] with elderly subjects showing lower VOR gains (young: 0.78 ± 0.02 SE; elderly: 0.67 ± 0.02 SE). Additionally, as expected, a highly significant effect of plane of stimulation [$F(2,30) = 45.0; P < 0.0001$] on VOR gain was found; that is, independent of age, vertical and horizontal gains were higher than torsional gain. No other effects or interactions reached significance. All results are presented in FIGURE 2.

CONCLUSION

Head-impulse testing disclosed age-related deterioration in γ-gains of the VOR in our group of subjects. The VOR age-dependent functional decline is seen in all planes of stimulation. However, the largest difference was found in the roll plane (torsional VOR); the smallest, in yaw (horizontal VOR). Lower gain values for torsional compared to horizontal and vertical VOR even in youth are possibly due to the torsional VOR being relatively unimportant in common daily activities.[15] If de-

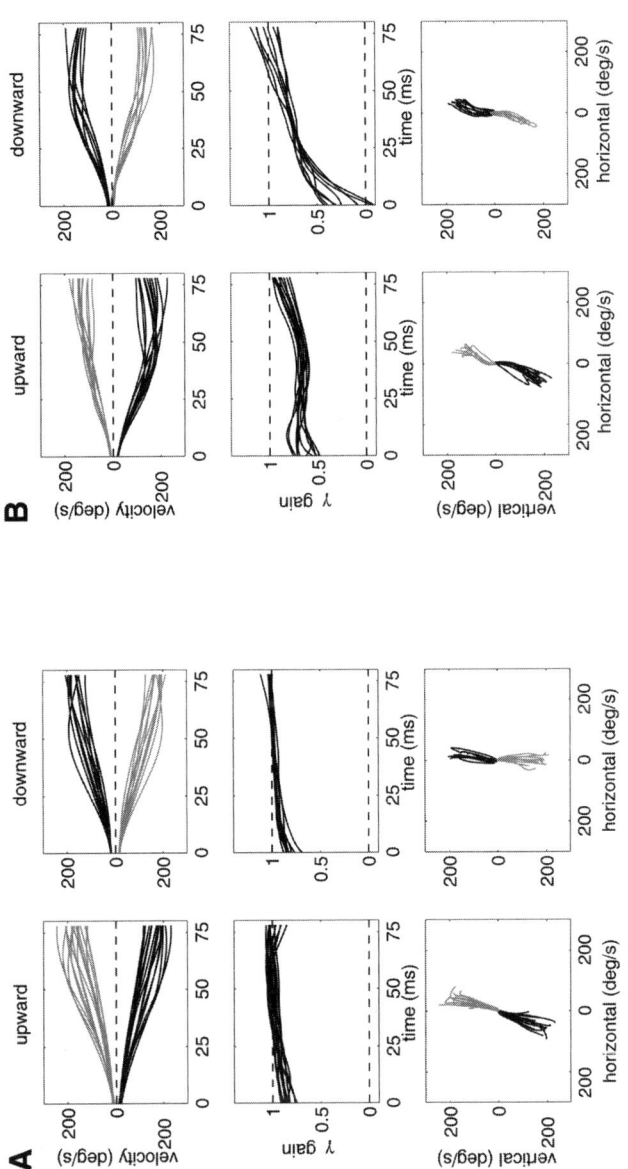

FIGURE 1. Examples of raw data (*black*: head velocity; *gray*: eye velocity) from one young subject (**A**, 35 years) and one old subject (**B**, 63 years). *Upper row*: all traces of vertical eye and head velocity over time. *Middle row*: γ-gains for vertical head impulses over time. *Lower row*: vertical versus horizontal eye and head velocity. The younger subject showed γ-gains (averaged over the median values of each time point) of 0.95 ± 0.07 for downward and 0.96 ± 0.07 for upward head impulses. The older subject showed γ-gains of 0.73 ± 0.29 for downward and 0.74 ± 0.10 for upward head impulses.

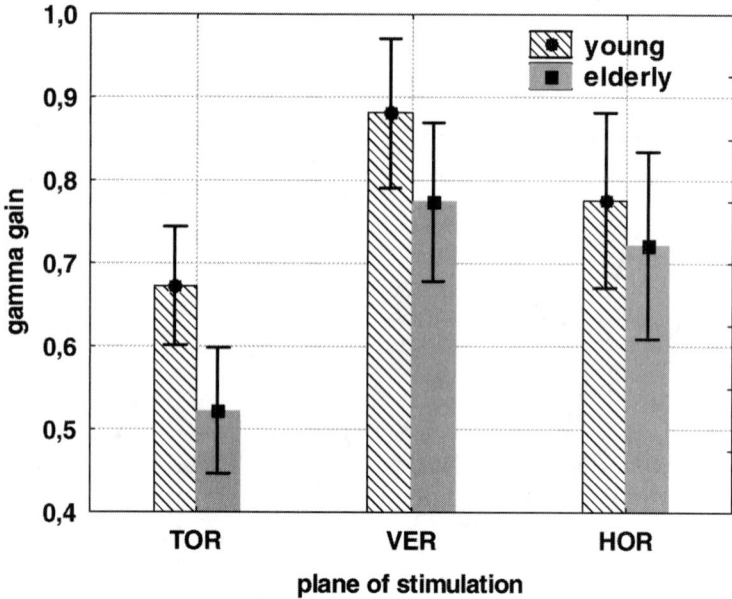

FIGURE 2. Results for VOR gain at $t = 40$ ms after head-impulse onset for all subjects in all three planes of stimulation. Young subjects (*circles*) showed significantly higher gains than elderly subjects (*squares*). *Symbols* and *bars* denote least-square means together with 95% confidence intervals.

cay of peripheral anatomical structures[1-5] involved in VOR would be the only factor for age-related gain decrease, a similar change in torsional and vertical gain would be expected, because torsional and vertical VOR share the same peripheral sensors and pathways. However, FIGURE 2 shows that the vertical gain decrease is smaller than the torsional gain decrease. These preliminary results suggest that vertical and horizontal, but not torsional, VOR response may, in the elderly, still be adaptively augmented by input from central vestibular structures, for example, from the cerebellum. Preserved function of those central structures in subjects above the age of 60 may thus be the chief factor responsible for our preliminary finding that differences in gain decrease depend on the plane of stimulation.

ACKNOWLEDGMENTS

This study was supported by the Mobility Fund of Charles University, Prague, Czech Republic; the Neuro-Euro Foundation, Czech Republic; and the Deutsche Forschungsgemeinschaft. We thank M. Hoshi, H. Lindeiner, and M. Kiss for help with data acquisition.

REFERENCES

1. ROSENHALL, U. 1973. Degenerative patterns in the aging human vestibular neuro-epithelia. Acta Otolaryngol. **76:** 208–220.
2. BERGSTROM, B. 1973. Morphology of the vestibular nerve. II. The number of myelinated vestibular nerve fibers in man at various ages. Acta Otolaryngol. **76:** 173–179.
3. RICHTER, E. 1980. Quantitative study of human Scarpa's ganglion and vestibular sensory epithelia. Acta Otolaryngol. **90:** 199–208.
4. PARK, J.J. et al. 2001. Age-Related change in the number of neurons in the human vestibular ganglion. J. Comp. Neurol. **431:** 437–443.
5. TANG, Y. et al. 2001. Age-Related Change of the Neuronal Number in the Human Medial Vestibular Nucleus: a Stereological Investigation. J. Vestib. Res. **11:** 357–363.
6. HALL, T.C. et al. 1975. Variations in the human Purkinje cell population according to age and sex. Neuropathol. Appl. Neurobiol. **1:** 267–292.
7. WALL, C., III et al. 1984. Effects of age, sex and stimulus parameters upon vestibulo-ocular responses to sinusoidal rotation. Acta Otolaryngol. **98:** 270–278.
8. PETERKA, R.J. et al. 1990. Age-related changes in human vestibulo-ocular reflexes: sinusoidal rotation and caloric tests. J. Vestib. Res. **1:** 49–59.
9. PAIGE, G.D. 1992. Senescence of human visual-vestibular interactions. I. Vestibulo-ocular reflex and adaptive plasticity with aging. J. Vestib. Res. **2:** 133–151.
10. WIEST, G. et al. 2001. Vestibular function in severe bilateral vestibulopathy. J. Neurol. Neurosurg. Psychiatry **71:** 53–57.
11. AW, S.T. et al. 1996. Three-dimensional vector analysis of the human vestibuloocular reflex in response to high-acceleration head rotations. II. Responses in subjects with unilateral vestibular loss and selective semicircular canal occlusion. J. Neurophysiol. **76:** 4021–4030.
12. SCHMID-PRISCOVEANU, A. et al. 2001. Caloric and search-coil head-impulse testing in patients after vestibular neuritis. J. Assoc. Res. Otolaryngol. **2:** 72–78.
13. HALMAGYI, G.M. et al. 1994. New tests of vestibular function. Baillieres Clin. Neurol. **3:** 485–500.
14. GLASAUER, S. et al. 2003. Three-dimensional eye position and slow phase velocity in humans with downbeat nystagmus. J. Neurophysiol. **89:** 338–354.
15. AW, S.T. et al. 1996. Three-dimensional vector analysis of the human vestibuloocular reflex in response to high-acceleration head rotations. I. Responses in normal subjects. J. Neurophysiol. **76:** 4009–4020.

Binocular Vertical-Torsional Spontaneous Nystagmus in a Midbrain Lesion Involving the Interstitial Nucleus of Cajal Indicates a Vestibular Imbalance of Vertical Semicircular Canals

CHRISTOPH HELMCHEN,[a] HOLGER RAMBOLD,[a] AND ULRICH BÜTTNER[b]

[a]*Department of Neurology, University of Luebeck, Luebeck, Germany*
[b]*Department of Neurology, University of Munich, Munich, Germany*

KEYWORDS: interstitial nucleus of Cajal; midbrain; vestibular imbalance; semicircular canals

INTRODUCTION

The interstitial nucleus of Cajal (iC) in the rostral midbrain is part of the vertical and torsional velocity-to-position integrator.[1] However, lesions of iC not only elicit vertical and torsional gaze-holding failure but also signs of vestibular imbalance consisting of static[2] and dynamic aspects, for example, nystagmus at "gaze straight ahead."[3–5] Contrary to expectations, given a common neural integrator deficit, rotation axes of the spontaneous nystagmus in both eyes at gaze straight ahead were disconjugate after iC lesions in macaque monkeys; that is, vertical and torsional components were not parallel in both eyes.[4] In the monkey, a comparison of the nystagmus with the eye muscle rotation axes revealed a coactivation of eye muscles similar to the effects of electrical stimulation of the anterior semicircular canal afferents.[4] We studied a patient with a midbrain infarction involving the iC who had clinically detectable asymmetric vertical-torsional nystagmus components on both eyes so that we could (1) compare the nystagmus rotation axes with the effects in the monkey lesion studies and (2) identify a vestibular imbalance of semicircular canal pathways.

PATIENT

The 64-year-old patient suffered from a sudden onset of vertigo, diplopia, oscillopsia, and gait unsteadiness. On clinical examination there was a vertical-torsional

Address for correspondence: Prof. Dr. C. Helmchen, Ratzeburger Allee 160, D-23538 Luebeck, Germany. Voice: +49-451-500-2927; fax: +49-451-500-2489.
helmchen_ch@neuro.mu-luebeck.de

Ann. N.Y. Acad. Sci. 1004: 478–481 (2003). © 2003 New York Academy of Sciences.
doi: 10.1196/annals.1303.056

spontaneous nystagmus with conjugate negative torsional (counterclockwise, intorsion of the right eye, and extorsion of the left eye) and downbeating components on both eyes. Vertical oculomotor range was reduced, and vertical saccades (upward more than downward) but not horizontal saccades were slowed. The vertical vestibulo-ocular reflex (VOR) elicited a normal range of vertical eye movements. The torsional VOR elicited quick phases in both direction. Vision was normal. Magnetic resonance imaging (MRI) showed a small unilateral midbrain lesion involving the left iC and the caudal part of the rostral interstitial nucleus of the medial longitudinal fascicle (riMLF). Fundus photography revealed pathological tonic ocular torsion of 14° on average.

After the patient had given her informed consent, binocular three-dimensional eye movements were recorded with the scleral search coil method (Remmel Labs, Ashland, MD) as described previously.[5] Scleral search coils (Combination annulus, Skalar, Delft, the Netherlands) were placed in each eye following topical anesthesia. The two eyes were calibrated using a combined offline *in vitro* and *in vivo* calibration that was used in previous studies.[5] The subject's head was comfortably stabilized in a natural upright position with a chin rest and a firm head support that kept the fore-

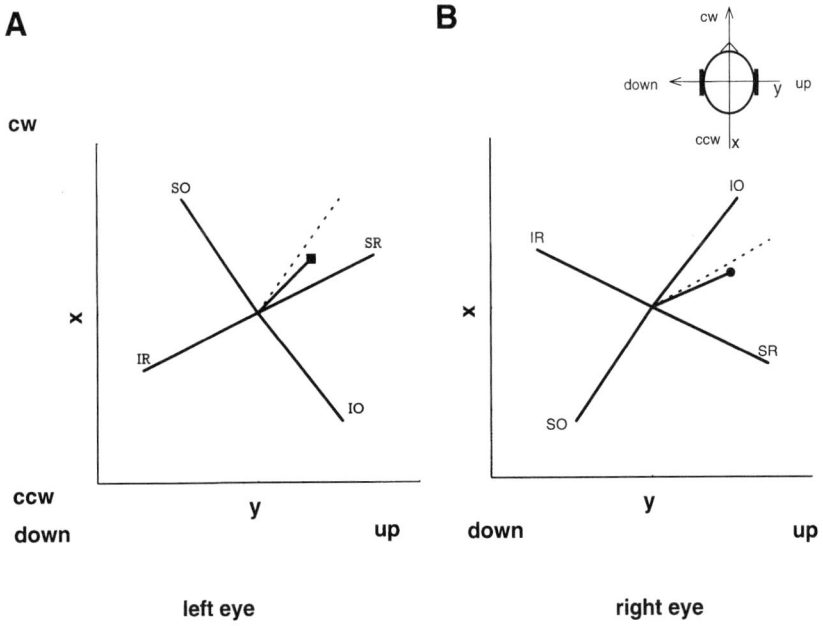

FIGURE 1. The mean rotation axes as normalized mean angular three-dimensional velocity of nystagmus slow phases (*short axes with symbols*) of the patient are shown in a torsional/vertical (*x/y*) projection. For better comparison, the eye muscle rotation axes are given by the *large axes*. The nystagmus rotation axes are closely aligned with the coactivation pattern (*dashed lines*) of IO/SR in the contralesional and SR/SO in the ipsilesional eye as it is elicited by stimulation of the semicircular canal afferents.[6] IO: inferior oblique; IR: inferior rectus; SO: superior oblique; SR: superior rectus muscle.

head stationary. For visual stimulation, a red laser spot (Lisa Laser Products, Kaltenberg, Germany) was front-projected by mirror galvanometers (GSI Lumonics) at target distances of 150 cm from the eyes. Spontaneous nystagmus on gaze straight ahead in darkness and spontaneous nystagmus on gaze straight ahead during fixation were recorded as well as visually guided saccades.

RESULTS

Search coil recordings revealed a conjugate negative torsional nystagmus with an exponential decrease of the slow phase with time constants ranging from 0.3 to 0.5 s for vertical and from 0.25 to 0.4 s for torsional components. Amplitudes of quick phases of nystagmus were on average 5° for torsional and 6° for vertical components. Vertical saccades were slowed to 160°/s on average for upward and downward gaze.

Slow phases of spontaneous nystagmus were analyzed if horizontal and vertical eye positions deviated less than 5° from gaze straight ahead. Rotation axes of slow phases of spontaneous nystagmus in gaze straight ahead position of the patient were calculated as mean angular velocity vectors (FIG. 1). The mean rotation axes around which the eye rotates are given by the normalized mean angular three-dimensional velocity of nystagmus slow phases in a torsional/vertical projection. The rotation axes were compared with the eye muscle rotation axes as derived from stimulation effects of semicircular canal afferents.[6] On the ipsilesional eye (FIG. 1A), there was a stronger torsional component with an axis which aligned best with a coactivation of the and superior rectus (SR) and superior oblique (SO) eye muscle. In contrast, the more vertical nystagmus component on the contralesional eye (FIG. 1B) aligned closely with the coactivation of the inferior oblique (IO) and superior rectus muscle.[6] Tonic ocular torsion did not significantly change the rotation axes. This pattern of binocular rotation axes resembles stimulation effects of the anterior semicircular canal afferents.

DISCUSSION

We provide further evidence that lesions of the iC not only elicit a neural integrator deficit but also a vestibular imbalance.[3,4] The coactivation pattern of eye muscles as derived from the rotation vector analysis of the nystagmus at gaze straight ahead in this patient resembles the stimulation effects of the anterior canal afferents in the animal experiment.[6] This pattern is compatible with the rotation axes after iC lesions in the monkey[4] and might be caused by a failure of the descending projections from iC to the vestibular nuclei.[7] This might functionally lead to an imbalance of the anterior semicircular canal signals between both vestibular nuclei, for example, by excitation of the ipsilesional anterior semicircular canal pathways. Thus, the hypothesis of a "descending mesencephalic integrator-OTR (ocular tilt reaction)"[2] with conjugate tonic ocular torsion requires an extension with respect to the semicircular canal imbalance as derived from the dysconjugacies of rotation axes of nystagmus at gaze straight ahead in iC lesions.

ACKNOWLEDGMENT

This work was supported by the Deutsche Forschungsgemeinschaft.

REFERENCES

1. CRAWFORD, J.D., W. CADERA & T. VILIS. 1991. Generation of torsional and vertical eye position signals by the interstitial nucleus of Cajal. Science **252:** 1551–1553.
2. BRANDT, T. & M. DIETERICH. 1998. Two types of ocular tilt reaction: the 'ascending' pontomedullary VOR-OTR and the 'descending' mesencephalic integrator-OTR. Neuro-ophthalmology **19:** 83–92.
3. HELMCHEN, C. et al. 1998. Deficits in vertical and torsional eye movements after uni- and bilateral muscimol inactivation of the interstitial nucleus of Cajal (IC) of the alert monkey. Exp. Brain Res. **119:** 436–452.
4. RAMBOLD, H., C. HELMCHEN & U. BÜTTNER. 2000. Vestibular influence on the binocular control of vertical-torsional nystagmus after unilateral lesions of the interstitial nucleus of Cajal (iC) in the alert monkey. Neuroreport **11:** 779–784.
5. HELMCHEN, C. et al. 2002. Localizing value of torsional nystagmus in small midbrain lesions. Neurology **59:** 1956–1964.
6. TOKUMASU, K., J.I. SUZUKI & K. GOTO. 1971. A study of the current spread on electric stimulation of the individual utricular and ampullary nerves. Acta Otolaryngol. **71:** 313–318.
7. CHIMOTO, S., Y. IWAMOTO & K. YOSHIDA. 1999. Projections and firing properties of down eye-movement neurons in the interstitial nucleus of Cajal in the cat. J. Neurophysiol. **81:** 1199–1211.

Vestibular Dysfunction in Acute Unilateral Hearing Loss

J. BOENKI,[a] H. RAMBOLD,[a] G. STRITZKE,[a] F. WISST,[b] B. NEPPERT,[c] AND C. HELMCHEN[a]

Department of [a]Neurology, [b]Otolaryngology, and [c]Ophthalmology, University of Luebeck, Luebeck, Germany

KEYWORDS: vestibular; hearing loss; head pulses

Acute unilateral hearing loss is a common syndrome affecting patients with a large age range.[1] It can be associated with vestibular loss, but it is unknown so far if acute unilateral hearing loss is always associated with vestibular impairment, and if incomplete vestibular dysfunction causes clinical symptoms. Discussion of the pathophysiology of the acute unilateral hearing loss is marked by controvers.[2-4] A neurolabyrinthitis of unknown origin and vascular disorders are the two pathomechanisms. Differential tests of the vestibular functions could help to establish a pathomechanism-based therapy because the vestibular deficits should be different with respect to the two pathomechanisms.

The study included 28 patients who presented with their first unilateral acute hearing loss over 30 dB (at more than one frequency) lasting over days. All patients were examined neurologically to exclude central vestibular disorders. In addition, they were examined by the otolaryngology department to exclude other vestibular diseases, such as Meniere's disease.

Auditory function was assessed by routine pure tone and speech audiometry. Eye movements at "gaze straight ahead" were recorded in the dark and in the light using the three-dimensional scleral search coil system (Remmel, Ashland, MD).[5] The semicircular canal function was characterized using the head-impulse test measured by three-dimensional scleral search coils.[6] The function of the utriculus was assessed by fundus photography and by the subjective visual vertical (SVV).[7] The sacculus function was examined 10 days after symptom onset by myogenic click-evoked potentials.[8] Stimulation was restricted to 100 dB normal hearing level (NHL) according to the guidelines of the Society of Otolaryngology in Germany.

Fifty percent of all patients showed—in addition to the acute hearing loss—a vestibular dysfunction that lasted for more than 10 days. Fifty-seven percent of patients with vestibular dysfunction complained of vertigo, 57% had a lateropulsion, and 50% had a spontaneous nystagmus to the contralesional side.

Address for correspondence: H. Rambold, Department of Neurology, University of Luebeck, Ratzeburger Allee 160, 23538 Luebeck, Germany. Voice: +451-500-3709; fax: +451 500 2489.
rambold_h@neuro.mu-luebeck.de

Fourteen percent of all patients showed a complete vestibular dysfunction, defined as impairment of all semicircular canals in addition to the otoliths. All those patients had a spontaneous nystagmus and complained of vertigo or lateropulsion.

Partial deficits of the vestibular labyrinth were found in 36% of all patients. Of these patients, 40% had a spontaneous nystagmus to the contralesional side, 30% complained of vertigo, 20% complained of dizziness, and 40% complained of lateropulsion. Altogether, 64% of the patients with partial vestibular dysfunction showed an impairment of the otoliths and 93% showed an impairment of the semicircular canals.

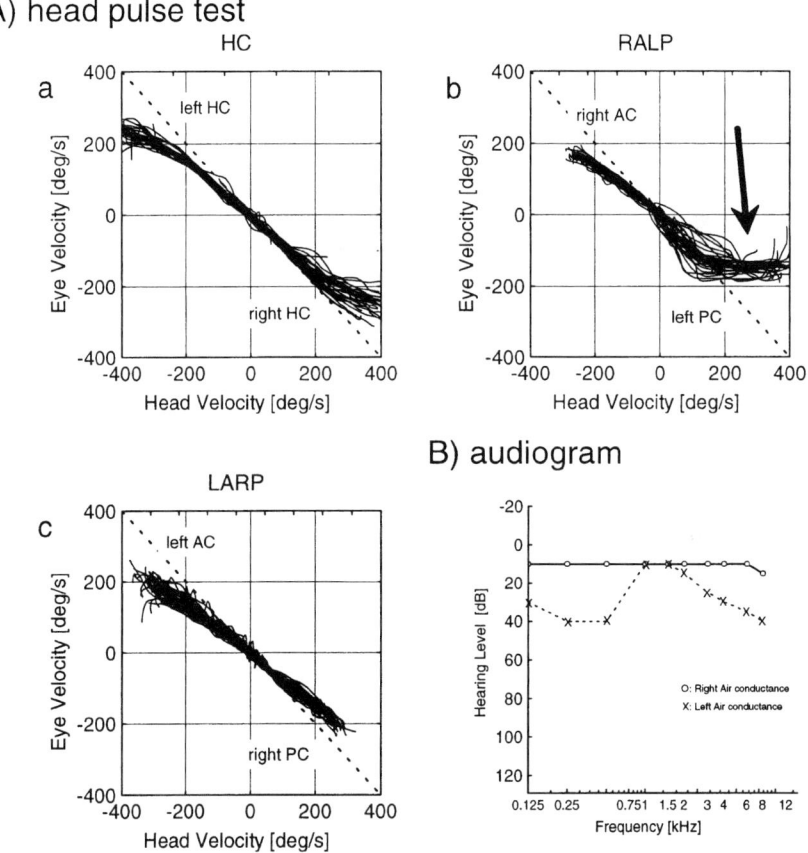

FIGURE 1. The head-impulse test of one patient with a partial vestibular impairment is shown in **A**, and the audiogram for air conductance is shown in **B**. In **a**, **b**, and **c**, eye-in-head velocity is plotted against head velocity. The tests of the six different semicircular canals show a left posterior canal paresis (*arrow*), whereas all other semicircular canals showed normal responses compared to the controls (not shown). In the audiogram (**B**), a hearing loss in the low-and high-frequency ranges of the left ear is found. HC: horizontal; AC: anterior; PC: posterior semicircular canal; RALP: right anterior and left posterior; LARP: left anterior and right posterior.

A distinct lesion pattern was prominent in this group: combined impairment of the cochlea and the posterior semicircular canal. Those patients were associated with higher age (mean age: 60 years) and vascular risk factors. The other patients with partial vestibular loss (mean age: 48 years) had a more scattered vestibular lesion pattern.

In acute unilateral hearing loss, a surprisingly high number of patients (50%) exhibited a vestibular dysfunction. Seventy-one percent of all patients with vestibular dysfunction were clinically symptomatic. In patients with incomplete vestibular dysfunction, 60% complained of signs of vestibular dysfunction.

The most common lesion pattern with a combined impairment of the posterior semicircular canal and the cochlea is consistent with the vascular supply of the labyrinth by the common cochlear artery. This might suggest that the lesion in those patients could be caused by a vascular pathomechanism.

REFERENCES

1. POSER, R. & H. HIRCHE. 1992. Randomisierte Doppelblindstudie zur Hörsturztherapie. HNO **40:** 396–399.
2. KIM, J.S., I. LOPEZ, P.L. DIPATRE, *et al.* 1999. Internal auditory artery infarction: clinicopathologic correlation. Neurology **52:** 40–44.
3. HOSTON, J.R. & R.W. BALOH. 1998. Acute vestibular syndrome. N. Engl. J. Med. **339:** 680–685.
4. LINSDAY, J.R. & W.G. HEMENWAY. 1956. Postural vertigo due to unilateral sudden partial loss of vestibular function. Ann. Otol. Rhinol. Laryngol. **65:** 692–706.
5. RAMBOLD, H., D. KÖMPF & C. HELMCHEN. 2001. Convergence retraction nystagmus: a disorder of vergence? Ann. Neurol. **50(5):** 677–681.
6. CREMER, P.D., G.M. HALMAGYI, S.T. AW, *et al.* 1998. Semicircular canal plane head impulses detect absent function of individual semicircular canals. Brain **121:** 699–716.
7. DIETERICH, M. & T. BRANDT. 1992. Cyclorotation of the eyes and the subjective visual vertical. *In* Clinical Neurology: Oculomotor Disorders of the Brainstem. Vol. 1(2): 301–316. 1st edit. U. Büttner & T. Brandt, Eds. Baillière Tindall. London.
8. WELGAMPOLA, M.S. & J.G. COLEBATCH. 2001. Vestibulocollic reflexes: normal values and the effect of age. Clin. Neurophysiol. **112:** 1971–1979.

Torsional Eye Movement Responses to Monaural and Binaural Galvanic Vestibular Stimulation

Side-to-Side Asymmetries

KLAUS JAHN,[a] ANDREA NAESSL,[a] MICHAEL STRUPP,[a] ERICH SCHNEIDER,[a] THOMAS BRANDT,[a] AND MARIANNE DIETERICH[b]

[a]*Department of Neurology, Klinikum Grosshadern, Ludwig-Maximilians University, Munich, Germany*

[b]*Johannes Gutenberg University, Mainz, Germany*

KEYWORDS: three-dimensional eye movements; video-oculography; galvanic vestibular stimulation

INTRODUCTION

Vestibular stimulation by head accelerations always involves multisensory activation of the vestibular, somatosensory, and visual systems. Over the past few years, galvanic vestibular stimulation (GVS) has become increasingly popular for testing vestibular function for clinical and research purposes.[1-3] Although GVS provides a nonphysiological stimulation, it is more selective than natural head accelerations and is thus an attractive tool for such tests.[4] Eye movement responses elicited by GVS mainly consist of torsional and horizontal components, as first described by Hitzig in 1871.[5] Animal experiments have shown that GVS increases the vestibular afferent spike frequency at the cathodal site and decreases it at the anodal site of stimulation.[6] As a continuation of a study on age-dependency of eye movement responses to GVS,[7] we analyzed side-to-side asymmetries in healthy subjects. It is necessary to know the normal range of asymmetry between left- and right-sided stimulation to interpret GVS responses in patients with vestibular diseases.

METHODS

Fifty-seven healthy subjects (age: 20–69 years; 33 females) gave their informed consent to participate in the study after being briefed about the experiments. Eye movements were measured by means of binocular video-oculography (VOG). The

Address for correspondence: Klaus Jahn, M.D., Department of Neurology, Klinikum Grosshadern, Ludwig-Maximilians University, Marchioninistrasse 15, 81377 Munich, Germany. Voice: +49-89/7095-2588; fax: +49-89/7095-5584.
klaus.jahn@lrz.uni-muenchen.de

eye position angles (including ocular torsion) were determined from a pair of artificial markers that were applied to the sclera just outside the left and the right edges of the iris.[8] Two infrared-sensitive cameras were used to capture and transfer digitized images of the eyes (sampling rate: 100 Hz) to a personal computer. A custom-made image processing software performed an online analysis of the captured images.[2] For galvanic stimulation, gold electrodes (diameter: 5 mm) were placed over both mastoid processes for binaural stimulation. For monaural stimulation, the second, indifferent electrode was placed at the posterior neck over the C7 spinous process. Rectangular, unipolar electrical direct current pulses of 10-s duration were delivered by a battery-powered current generator. After calibration (10° viewing angles), binaural (1 mA and 3 mA) and monaural (left and right, 3 mA) GVS was performed in each subject during fixation of a space-fixed target. Analysis was done off-line. After detecting torsional quick phases with an interactive software package, we determined mean values from the 10-s periods of stimulation for the following variables to characterize torsional nystagmus: slow-phase velocity (SPV), nystagmus frequency, quick-phase amplitude, and the tonic ocular torsion position (OTP) that would have been present without nystagmus. The last variable was determined by a nystagmus compensation algorithm.[2,9] A side-to-side ratio was calculated by dividing for each subject and each parameter the larger value from one side by the smaller value from the other side. For statistical analysis, means, standard deviations, and 95% confidence intervals were determined.

TABLE 1. Side-to-side ratio

	Mean	−95%	+95%
Ocular torsion position			
bi 1 mA	1.14	1.08	1.21
bi 3 mA	1.27	1.18	1.35
mo 3 mA cat	1.19	1.14	1.24
mo 3 mA an	1.18	1.12	1.24
Mean SPV			
bi 1 mA	1.31	1.16	1.47
bi 3 mA	1.44	1.32	1.57
mo 3 mA cat	1.41	1.25	1.57
mo 3 mA an	1.41	1.25	1.56
Amplitude			
bi 1 mA	1.28	1.10	1.47
bi 3 mA	1.48	1.36	1.61
mo 3 mA cat	1.42	1.22	1.62
mo 3 mA an	1.40	1.28	1.53
Frequency			
bi 1 mA	1.23	1.12	1.33
bi 3 mA	1.35	1.22	1.48
mo 3 mA cat	1.34	1.19	1.48
mo 3 mA an	1.34	1.14	1.55

ABBREVIATIONS: bi, binaural; mo, monaural; cat, cathodal; an, anodal.

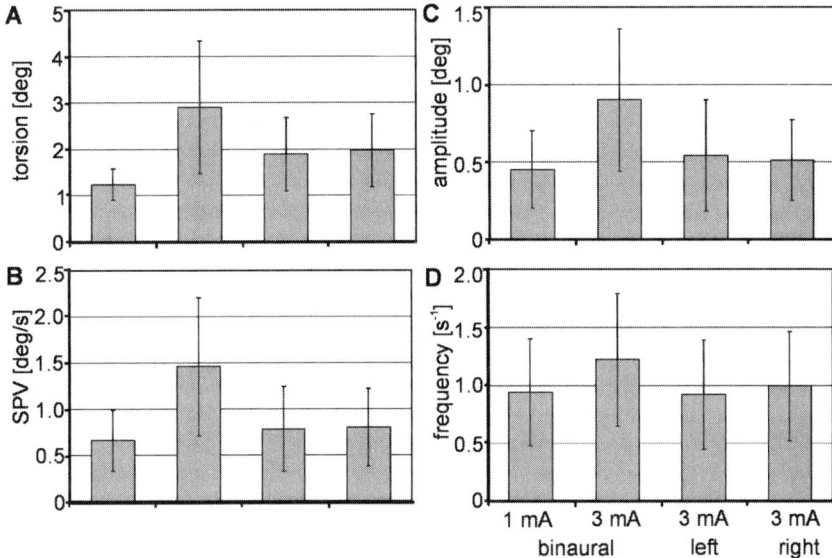

FIGURE 1. Eye movement responses to galvanic vestibular stimulation. Mean values for ocular torsion position (**A**), mean slow-phase velocity (**B**), amplitude (**C**), and frequency of torsional nystagmus (**D**). Four different stimulation conditions are shown: binaural 1 mA, binaural 3 mA, monaural cathode left 3 mA (*left*), and monaural cathode right 3 mA (*right*). Torsional eye movements were recorded during fixation of a stationary target. *Error bars* represent standard deviations.

RESULTS

Responses to GVS consisted of an ocular torsion to the side of the anode and superimposed torsional nystagmus with quick phases beating toward the cathode. FIGURE 1 shows mean values and standard deviations for binaural (1 mA and 3 mA) and monaural (3 mA left and right) stimulation. OTP and nystagmus were dependent on current strength. For 3 mA binaural stimulation (cathode left), mean values were 2.90 ± 1.43° for OTP, 1.46 ± 0.75°/s for nystagmus SPV, 0.90 ± 0.46° for nystagmus amplitude, and 1.22 ± 0.57 s^{-1} for nystagmus frequency. To quantify the asymmetry of responses in healthy subjects, a side-to-side ratio was calculated as described in the previous section. Mean values and 95% confidence intervals are given in TABLE 1. For monaural and binaural stimulation, mean differences between left- and right-sided stimulation were about 30%. There were no significant differences for asymmetry ratios between monaural and binaural stimulations or for the parameters analyzed (OTP, nystagmus). If cathodal and anodal stimulations were compared for the same ear, eye movements were about 10% larger with cathodal stimulation.

DISCUSSION

It is known that eye movement responses to GVS show large interindividual variability but good intraindividual reliability.[2,3,10,11] Explanations for increased interindividual variability have been proposed on the basis of the assumption of different thresholds for subpopulations of afferents,[10] a varying contribution of otolith input,[12] and interindividually different nystagmus frequencies and amplitudes.[2,9] In the present study, which included 57 healthy subjects, we showed that the normal range for side-to-side differences ranges from about 15% to about 45%. This has implications for the interpretation of GVS testing of vestibular nerve function in patients. With respect to age, an inverse U-shaped relation was found with increasing responses (OTP and nystagmus) from the third to the sixth decade and a decrease for older ages.[7] This was explained by the increased sensitivity of afferent nerve fibers, which compensates for hair cell loss beginning in childhood and continuing throughout life. Side-to-side ratios, however, increased only slightly and insignificantly with age (SPV and quick-phase amplitude).[7] The differential effect of cathodal and anodal stimulations reflects larger increases of resting discharge rates (cathode) compared with decreases (anode) according to Ewald's law.[13]

ACKNOWLEDGMENTS

We are grateful to Judy Benson for copyediting the manuscript. This work is part of A. Naessl's thesis at the University of Munich.

REFERENCES

1. WELGAMPOLA, M.S. & J.G. COLEBATCH. 2001. Vestibulocollic reflexes: normal values and the effect of age. Clin. Neurophysiol. **112:** 1971–1979.
2. SCHNEIDER, E., S. GLASAUER & M. DIETERICH. 2002. Comparison of human ocular torsion patterns during natural and galvanic vestibular stimulation. J. Neurophysiol. **87:** 2064–2073.
3. MACDOUGALL, H.G., A.E. BRIZUELA, A.M. BURGESS & I.S. CURTHOYS. 2002. Between-subject variability and within-subject reliability of the human eye-movement response to bilateral galvanic (DC) vestibular stimulation. Exp. Brain Res. **144:** 69–78.
4. DAY, B.L. 1999. Galvanic vestibular stimulation: new uses of an old tool. J. Physiol. **517:** 631.
5. HITZIG, E. 1871. Über galvanischen Schwindel. Reichertz und du Bois Reymond's Archiv 5.
6. GOLDBERG, J.M., C. FERNANDEZ & C.E. SMITH. 1982. Responses of vestibular-nerve afferents in the squirrel monkey to externally applied galvanic currents. Brain Res. **252:** 156–160.
7. JAHN, K., A. NAESSL, E. SCHNEIDER, *et al.* 2003. Inverse U-shaped curve for age dependency of torsional eye movement responses to galvanic vestibular stimulation. Brain **126:** 1579–1589.
8. CLARKE, A.H., A. ENGELHORN, C. HAMANN & U. SCHONFELD. 1999. Measuring the otolith-ocular response by means of unilateral radial acceleration. Ann. N.Y. Acad. Sci. **871:** 387–391.
9. SCHNEIDER, E., S. GLASAUER & M. DIETERICH. 2000. Central processing of human ocular torsion analyzed by galvanic vestibular stimulation. NeuroReport **11:** 1559–1563.

10. ZINK, R., S.F. BUCHER, A. WEISS, et al. 1998. Effects of galvanic vestibular stimulation on otolithic and semicircular canal eye movements and perceived vertical. Electroencephal. Clin. Neurophysiol. **107:** 200–205.
11. WATSON, S.R., A.E. BRIZUELA, I.S. CURTHOYS, et al. 1998. Maintained ocular torsion produced by bilateral and unilateral galvanic (DC) vestibular stimulation in humans. Exp. Brain Res. **122:** 453–458.
12. KLEINE, J.F., W.O. GULDIN & A.H. CLARKE. 1999. Variable otolith contribution to the galvanically induced vestibulo-ocular reflex. NeuroReport **10:** 1143–1148.
13. EWALD, R. 1892. Physiologische Untersuchungen über das Endorgan des Nervus octavus. Bergmann. Wiesbaden.

Barbecue Whole-Body Position Modulates Cerebellar Downbeat Nystagmus

SARAH MARTI, ANTONELLA PALLA, AND DOMINIK STRAUMANN

Department of Neurology, Zürich University Hospital, Zürich, Switzerland

KEYWORDS: downbeat nystagmus; ocular drift; gravity dependence; neuro-ophthalmology

Downbeat nystagmus is a frequent ocular motor sign in patients with lesions of the vestibulocerebellum.[1] Upward drift in cerebellar downbeat nystagmus is caused by two concurrent mechanisms[1,2]: (1) a gaze-evoked drift due to a leaky vertical neural integrator, and (2) an upward-directed velocity bias independent of vertical gaze eccentricity and already present with "gaze straight ahead." Recently, we have shown that the velocity bias, that is, the vertical drift in gaze straight ahead, consists of two components[3]: (1) a gravity-dependent component that sinusoidally modulates as a function of whole body position along the pitch plane, and (2) a gravity-independent component that is directed upward. The combination of these two components leads to an overall vertical drift that is minimal in supine and maximal in prone position. In the roll plane, however, no modulation of the vertical drift occurs; that is, the vertical velocity bias is approximately the same in upright and 90° ear-down body positions. Healthy subjects showed a similar sinusoidal modulation of the vertical drift velocity as a function of whole-body position, but in a scaled-down manner.

In upright and ear-down positions, the overall drift mainly consists of the gravity-independent component. In the supine position, the gravity-dependent component is directed downward and opposes the gravity-independent component, which is always directed upward. Thus, the overall vertical drift in both upright and ear-down positions is faster than in supine position. As a result, even though the gravity-dependent component modulates only along the pitch plane, changing whole-body position about the earth-horizontal yaw axis (barbecue rotation) should modulate downbeat nystagmus. Specifically, upward drift should be faster in the ear-down side positions than in the supine position.

FIGURE 1 confirms this hypothesis: vertical drift velocity during gaze straight ahead is plotted as a function of the angular whole-body position about the earth-horizontal yaw axis (barbecue position). In patients with cerebellar atrophy (left panel), the gravity-dependent component modulates sinusoidally and adds to a constant upward-directed, gravity-independent component. The overall drift is maximal in prone position and minimal in supine position, whereas in 90° side positions, the ve-

Address for correspondence: Sarah Marti, M.D., Department of Neurology, Zürich University Hospital, CH-8091 Zürich, Switzerland. Voice: +41-1-255-5564; fax: +41-1-255-4507.
sarah.marti@usz.ch

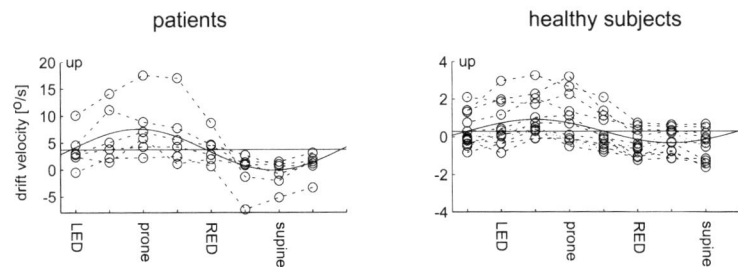

FIGURE 1. Vertical ocular drift velocity in gaze straight ahead as a function of whole-body angular position about the earth-horizontal yaw axis (barbecue position in 45° steps) and dual search coil recordings of right eyes. Median velocities of slow phases (*open circles* connected with dashed lines) are plotted for all subjects. First-harmonic sines (*solid lines*) were fitted through the pooled data. Offsets of sine fits are also indicated (*horizontal solid lines*). Note the different scaling of the ordinate in the two panels. *Left panel:* Patients with cerebellar downbeat nystagmus ($n = 6$). *Right panel:* Healthy subjects ($n = 12$).

locity of the overall drift is in between. In healthy subjects (right panel), there is no gravity-independent component, and thus the overall drift consists only of the gravity-dependent component. Therefore, the minimal overall drift is in the ear-down side positions.

At the bedside, it is not easy to observe downbeat nystagmus in prone position. In most cases, however, comparing the intensity of downbeat nystagmus between supine and ear-down side positions should be sufficient to demonstrate the influence of gravity on upward drift velocity. In patients with cerebellar atrophy, downbeat nystagmus increases when turning the head from supine position to the side.

ACKNOWLEDGMENTS

This work was supported by the Swiss National Science Foundation (No. 32-51938.97 SCORE A/No. 31-63465.00) and the Betty and David Koetser Foundation for Brain Research.

REFERENCES

1. ZEE, D.S., A. YAMAZAKI, P.H. BUTLER & G. GUCER. 1981. Effects of ablation of flocculus and paraflocculus of eye movements in primate. J. Neurophysiol. **46:** 878–899.
2. STRAUMANN, D., D.S. ZEE & D. SOLOMON. 2000. Three-dimensional kinematics of ocular drift in humans with cerebellar atrophy. J. Neurophysiol. **83:** 1125–1140.
3. MARTI, S., A. PALLA & D. STRAUMANN. 2002. Gravity dependence of ocular drift in patients with cerebellar downbeat nystagmus. Ann. Neurol. **52:** 712–721.

Two Opposite Effects of Nicotine on Downbeat Nystagmus: An Observation

CRISTIANA BORGES PEREIRA, MICHAEL STRUPP, VERA CARINA ZINGLER, AND THOMAS BRANDT

Department of Neurology, Klinikum Grosshadern, University of Munich, Germany

KEYWORDS: nicotine; downbeat nystagmus; etiology

INTRODUCTION

Downbeat nystagmus (DBN) is a central vestibular disorder that reflects a tone imbalance of the vestibuloocular reflex (VOR) in the pitch plane.[1] Several drugs have been proposed for the treatment of DBN, such as GABA agonists (baclofen and clonazepam), anticholinergic agents (scopolamine, benztropine, and thihexyphenidyl),[2,3] or the potassium channel blocker 3,4-diaminopyridine.[4] Other drugs such as carbamazepine, phenytoin, or lithium can themselves cause this disorder.[2] Interestingly, nicotine has been shown to induce upbeat nystagmus in healthy subjects after smoking a cigarette, but never DBN.[5,6] Therefore, the aim of this preliminary study was to test the effect of nicotine on patients with DBN.

PATIENTS AND METHODS

Six patients with DBN syndrome gave their written, informed consent to participate in the study. The experiments were done in accordance with the Helsinki II Declaration. None of the patients was taking medication. One patient was an occasional smoker (approximately five cigarettes per week); he did not smoke for 24 h before the measurement was made. Four patients had a progressive cerebellar disorder with additional cerebellar signs and symptoms (TABLE 1); cranial MRI showed significant cerebellar atrophy in three and ischemic lesions in one. The remaining two patients had a downbeat nystagmus syndrome with no associated neurological signs or symptoms and no brain pathology on MRI scans, that is, an "idiopathic DBN syndrome" (TABLE 1).

Eye movements were recorded in horizontal and vertical directions with an infrared camera at a resolution of 50 Hz (Mack Company, Pfaffenhofen, Germany) as described elsewhere.[5] A mask with the integrated camera was used to prevent any perception of ambient light. The data were recorded on a PC for further analysis.

Address for correspondence: Michael Strupp, M.D., Department of Neurology, Klinikum Grosshadern, Marchioninistrasse 15, D-81366 Munich, Germany. Voice: ++49-89-7095 2585; fax: 49-89-7095-5584 or -8883.

mstrupp@nefo.med.uni-muenchen.de

A) Cerebellar disorder

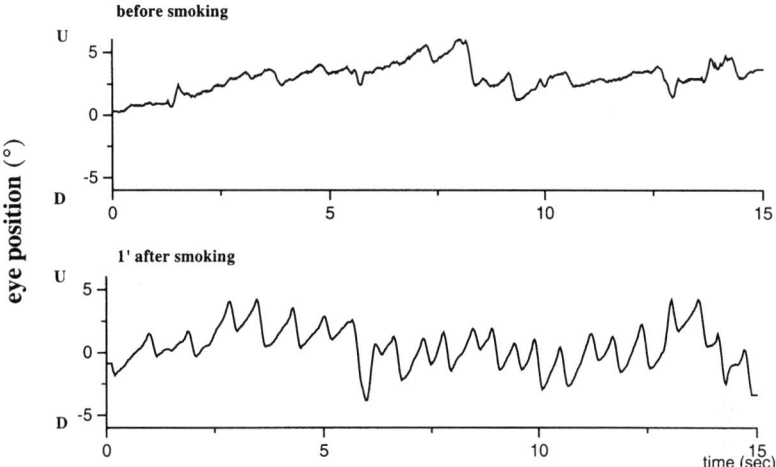

B) Idiopathic downbeat nystagmus syndrome

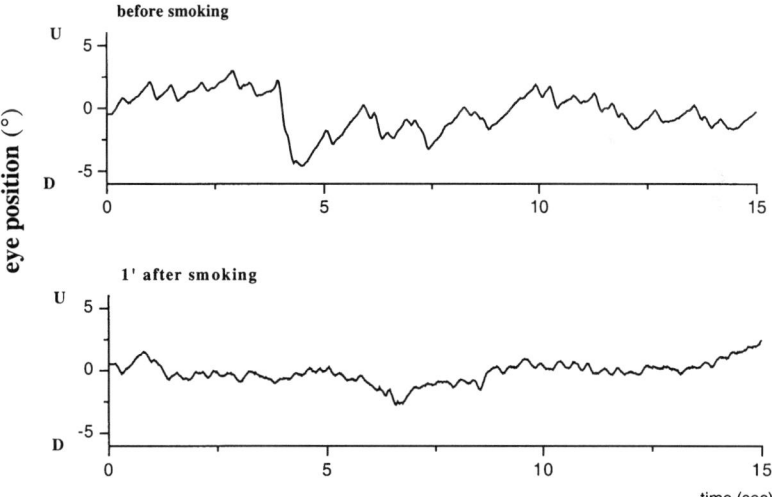

FIGURE 1. Original recording of vertical eye movement of a patient with DBN due to cerebellar disorder (**A**) or "idiopathic DBN" (**B**) before and 1 min after smoking a cigarette. SPV may be increased (**A**) or decreased (**B**). U, up; D, down; DBN, downbeat nystagmus; SPV, slow-phase velocity.

TABLE 1. Clinical details of patients with DBN and the effect of smoking on SPV of nystagmus

Group	Patient	Age	Age of symptom onset	Additional cerebellar signs/symptoms	MRI	SPV before smoking	SPV1' after smoking
Downbeat nystagmus with cerebellar atrophy/lesions	1	45	40	cerebellar ataxia, dysmetria	cerebellar atrophy	2°/s	7°/s
	2	59	57	cerebellar ataxia, dysartria	cerebellar atrophy	2°/s	2.5°/s
	3	67	67	cerebellar ataxia, dysartria	microangiopathy with cerebellar lesions	1°/s	1.5°/s
	4	63	54	cerebellar ataxia, dysartria	cerebellar atrophy	1°/s	2.5°/s
Idiopathic downbeat nystagmus syndrome	5	63	53	none	normal	11°/s	6.5°/s
	6	39	37	none	normal	5°/s	no nystagmus

Patients 1–4 had cerebellar disorders; patients 5–6 had idopathic DBN. All patients reported oscillopsia.

Measurements were made before and 1, 5, and 10 min after subjects smoked a filtered cigarette containing 0.9 mg nicotine and were repeated on the next day to monitor the reproducibility of the effects. The subjects remained seated with the head in the upright position and were instructed to look straight ahead without visual fixation.

RESULTS

Nicotine modulated downbeat nystagmus (reproducibly) in all subjects; however, it had diametrically opposite effects in different patients. The four patients with cerebellar atrophy or ischemic cerebellar lesions exhibited a transient *increase* in slow-phase velocity (SPV) by 50% to more than 100%; the absolute increase in SPV after smoking ranged from 0.5 to 5°/s. An example is shown in FIGURE 1A. In contrast, the two patients with "idiopathic DBN syndrome" showed a transient *decrease* in the SPV by approximately 50% (range of decrease of SPV after smoking: 4.5–5°/s; FIG. 1B and TABLE 1). The effect was maximal when first measured within 1 min after smoking but gradually decreased on subsequent recordings. Accordingly, patients with an increase of SPV reported a transient increase of oscillopsia, whereas patients with a decrease of SPV reported a transient attenuation of oscillopsia.

DISCUSSION

Downbeat nystagmus is assumed to result from an imbalance in the central VOR pathways. It is caused by either a bilateral lesion of the flocculus, which leads to an increase in tonic excitatory activity from the anterior semicircular canal to the superior recti eye muscles, or a lesion on the floor of the fourth ventricle between the vestibular nuclei, which interrupts the tonic excitatory activity from the posterior canal to the inferior recti eye muscles.[1]

The four patients with cerebellar atrophy or cerebellar ischemic lesions most likely suffered from a floccular disinhibition. The lesional dysfunction in the two remaining patients might be caused by a deficit of the excitatory activity to the inferior recti. DBN, when caused by a lesion between the vestibular nuclei, is usually a permanent syndrome, because it involves the commissural fibers necessary for central compensation of a vestibular tone imbalance. DBN with high SPV was present in these two patients for 2 years (5°/s) and 10 years (11°/s), respectively. How can such diametrically opposite effects of nicotine on the two types of clinical downbeat nystagmus be explained?

Nicotinic receptors have been detected in hair cells of the vestibular end-organs[7] and in all parts of the vestibular nuclei, particularly in the neurons in the medial and lateral nuclei that project to the cerebellum and spinal cord (for references, see Vidal et al.[8]). Nicotinergic action is always excitatory.[9] At sites of denervation neurons develop a denervation hypersensitivity by expressing more receptors.[10] One would expect therefore that nicotine effects are relatively stronger at such sites.

Based on anatomical and physiological findings, our data are compatible with the following (speculative) hypotheses. (1) Because of a partial denervation of the excitatory posterior canal input to the inferior recti, nicotine increases the deficient excitatory input in DBN, thereby diminishing the nystagmus. (2) In contrast, in DBN caused by a cerebellar disinhibition of the anterior canal input to the superior recti, nicotine further enhances the tone imbalance by increasing the excitatory activity, thereby increasing the nystagmus. Because our data are preliminary, further studies in patients with DBN syndrome due to defined structural cerebellar lesions are necessary to test these hypotheses.

CONCLUSION

The effect of nicotine on downbeat nystagmus after smoking a cigarette was measured in four patients with cerebellar disorder (cerebellar atrophy or ischemic cerebellar lesions in cranial MRI) and in two with "idiopathic" downbeat nystagmus (i.e., no other cerebellar signs or symptoms and normal cranial MRI). Nicotine had diametrically opposite effects on the two groups: it significantly increased SPV in the first group and decreased it in the second. Nicotinergic action is always excitatory. These contrary effects can be attributed to the different action that the compound has at different denervated sites of the vestibuloocular reflex in the pitch plane.

ACKNOWLEDGMENTS

We thank Ms. J. Benson for copyediting the manuscript. This study was supported by the Alfried Krupp von Bohlen und Halbach-Stiftung and the Alexander von Humboldt-Stiftung (C.B.P.).

REFERENCES

1. BALOH, R.W. & J.W. SPOONER. 1981. Downbeat nystagmus: A type of central vestibular nystagmus. Neurology **31:** 304–310.
2. LEIGH, R.J. & S. RAMAT. 1999. Neuropharmacologic aspects of the ocular motor system and the treatment of abnormal eye movements. Curr. Opin. Neurol. **12:** 21–27.
3. BÜTTNER, U. & L. FUHRY. 1999. Drug therapy of nystagmus and saccadic intrusions. Adv. Otorhinolaringol. **55:** 195–227.
4. STRUPP, M., O. SCHÜLER, S. KRAFCZYK, et al. 2003. Treatment of downbeat nystagmus with 3,4-diaminopyridine—a placebo-controlled, double-blind study. Neurology **61:** 165–170.
5. PEREIRA, C.B., M. STRUPP, TH. EGGERT, et al. 1999. Nicotine-induced nystagmus: 3-D analysis and dependence on head position. J. Neurol. **246:** 65.
6. SIBONY, P.A., C. EVINGER & K.A. MANNING. 1987. Tobacco-induced primary-position upbeat nystagmus. Ann. Neurol. **21:** 53–58.
7. ISHIYAMA, A., I. LOPEZ & P.A. WACKYM. 1995. Distribution of efferent cholinergic terminals and α-bungarotoxin binding to putative nicotinic acetylcholine receptors in the human vestibular end-organs. Laryncoscope **105:** 1167–1172.
8. VIDAL, P.P., N. VEBERT, M. SERAFIN, et al. 1999. Intrinsic physiological and pharmacological properties of central vestibular neurons. Adv. Otorhinolaringol. **55:** 26–81.
9. HILLE, B. 2001. Ionic Channels of Excitable Membranes. 3rd edit. Sunderland, MA.
10. FROEHNER, S.C. 1993. Regulation of ion channel distribution at synapses. Annu. Rev. Neurosci. **16:** 347–368.

Three-Dimensional Aspects of Spontaneous Nystagmus in Dorsolateral Medullary Infarction

HOLGER RAMBOLD AND CHRISTOPH HELMCHEN

Department of Neurology, University of Luebeck, 23538 Luebeck, Germany

KEYWORDS: nystagmus; dorsolateral medulla infarction; vestibular; semicircular canals

In the early phase of dorsolateral medullary infarction, nystagmus often can be observed at gaze straight ahead with a mixed torsional, horizontal, and vertical direction.[1,2] A feasible pathomechanism would be a vestibular imbalance[2,3] caused by a lesion of the vestibular nuclei or their commissural pathways in the dorsal medulla. However, it is still unclear whether the nystagmus is caused by an imbalance of the central pathways of the semicircular canals[1] or of the otoliths.

To elucidate these two hypotheses, we recorded binocular three-dimensional eye (scleral search coil)[4] movements of four patients with dorsolateral medullary infarction under head-restrained conditions and analyzed the rotation axes of the slow phases in the light and dark in their relationship to the eye muscle rotation axes.

A vestibular imbalance induces a nystagmus with a linear slow phase. Slow phases of our patients were linear or consisted of an initial exponential increase or decrease followed by a linear decline. The exponential and the linear part of the slow phase were separated using a fit (least square minimization) of the eye positions with $E(t) = E(0) + k1*e^{(1/tc*t)} + vel*t$ (E: eye position; t: time; E(0): eye position at start; k1: constant; vel: linear eye velocity; tc: time constant). The linear eye velocity (vel) was expressed as angular velocity and normalized. The smallest three-dimensional angle to each eye muscle was calculated. The slow-phase axes were corrected for tonic ocular torsion as previously reported.[5]

To test for a vestibular imbalance, we compared the eye muscle activation pattern of our patients with predicted patterns of the otoliths or of the semicircular canals.[6,7] The least three-dimensional angle deviation of the individual eye muscles from the vestibular axes were calculated.

The linear slow-phase axes showed a pattern of eye muscle activation that was different in each eye. The smallest deviation was found to the superior oblique muscle of the contralesional eye and the inferior oblique and inferior rectus muscle of

---

Address for correspondence: Holger Rambold, Department of Neurology, University of Luebeck, Ratzeburger Allee 160, 23538 Luebeck, Germany. Voice: +49 451-500-3709; fax: +49 451-500-2489.

rambold_h@neuro.mu-luebeck.de

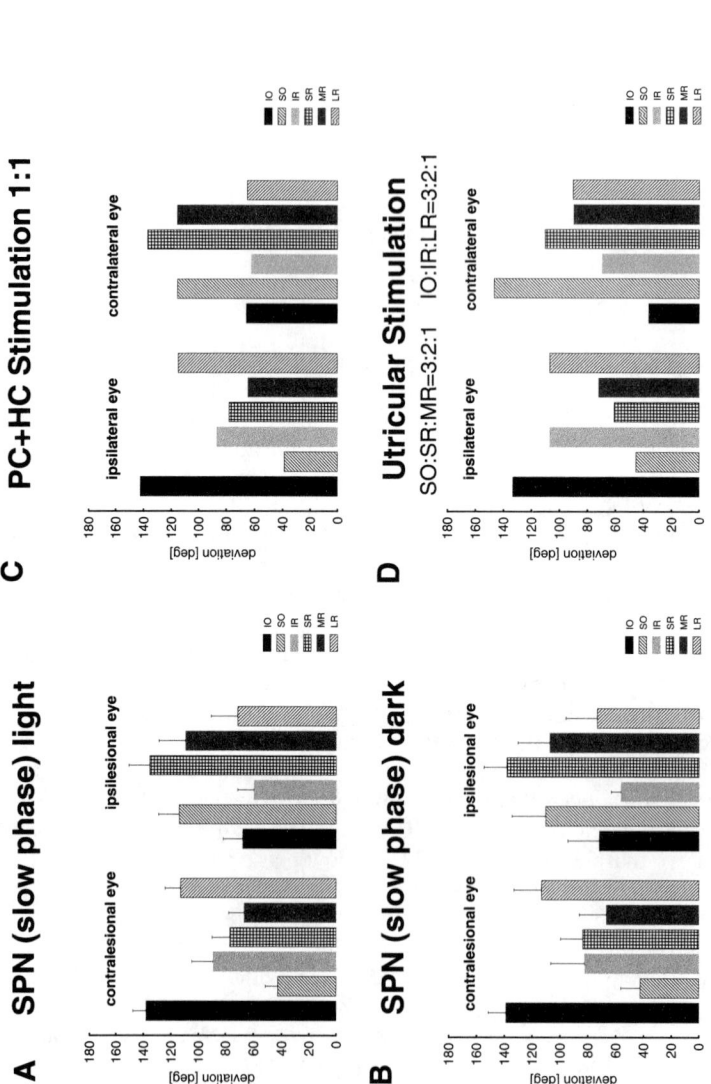

FIGURE 1. Deviation in degrees (mean: *boxes*; standard deviation: *whiskers*) of the linear, binocular nystagmus slow-phase axes (SPN) from the individual eye muscles at gaze straight ahead in the light (A) and in the dark (B). For comparison, the axis deviation of the combined stimulation of the contralesional horizontal and posterior semicircular canals from the eye muscle axes is shown in (C). In (D), the deviation of the hypothetical utricular contralateral stimulation axes from the eye muscle axes is plotted. The used ratios for muscle activation are given in the figures. The muscle axes activation pattern of the eye movements is best explained by a horizontal and posterior semicircular canal activation. HC, horizontal; PC, posterior semicircular canal; IO, inferior oblique; IR, inferior rectus; SO, superior oblique; SR, superior rectus; MR, medial rectus; LR, lateral rectus eye muscle.

the ipsilesional eye (FIG. 1). This muscle activation pattern could be explained by an approximately 1:1 horizontal and posterior semicircular canal activation of the contralesional side.[6] Combination of other semicircular canals or the axis of a hypothetical utricular stimulation did not properly explain the axis of the eye movements (FIG. 1D). There was no significant difference if the nystagmus was analyzed in the light or dark. Correcting for the tonic ocular torsion did not change the slow-phase axes deviation from the eye muscle axes to more than 5°.

The data support the hypothesis that spontaneous nystagmus in dorsolateral medullary syndrome is caused by a semicircular canal imbalance as suggested by Morrow and Sharpe[2] rather than an otolith imbalance. More specially, our analysis indicates a nystagmus pattern whose slow phases resemble a stimulation of the horizontal and posterior semicircular canal of the contralateral semicircular canals.

ACKNOWLEDGMENT

This work was supported by Deutsche Forschungsgemeinschaft (He 2489/2-7).

REFERENCES

1. GRESTY, M.A., A.M. BRONSTEIN, T. BRANDT & M. DIETERICH. 1992. Neurology of otolith function. Peripheral and central disorders. Brain **115:** 647–673.
2. MORROW, M.J. & J.A. SHARPE. 1988. Torsional nystagmus in the lateral medullary syndrome. Ann. Neurol. **24:** 390–398.
3. BALOH, R.W., R.D. YEE & V. HONRUBIA. 1981. Eye movements in patients with Wallenberg's syndrome. Ann. N.Y. Acad. Sci. **374:** 600–613.
4. RAMBOLD, H., D. KÖMPF, & C. HELMCHEN. 2001. Convergence retraction nystagmus: a disorder of vergence? Ann. Neurol. **50:** 677–681.
5. RAMBOLD, H., C. HELMCHEN & U. BÜTTNER. 2000. Vestibular influence on the binocular control of vertical-torsional nystagmus after lesions in the interstitial nucleus of Cajal. Neuroreport **11:** 779–784.
6. BLANKS, R.H., I.S. CURTHOYS & C.H. MARKHAM. 1975. Planar relationships of the semicircular canals in man. Acta Otolaryngol. **80:** 185–196.
7. TOKUMASU, K., J.I. SUZUKI & K. GOTO. 1971. A study of the current spread on electrical stimulation of the individual utricular and ampullary nerves. Acta Otolaryngol. **71:** 313–318.

Nonlinear Nystagmus Processing Causes Torsional VOR Nonlinearity

E. SCHNEIDER,[a] S. GLASAUER,[b] T. BRANDT,[a] AND M. DIETERICH[c]

Ludwig-Maximilians University, [a]Department of Neurology and
[b]Center for Sensorimotor Research, D-81377 Munich, Germany
[c]Johannes Gutenberg-University, D-55131 Mainz, Germany

KEYWORDS: vestibulo-ocular reflex; nystagmus; model; ocular torsion; beating field; nonlinearity; quick phase

INTRODUCTION

The eye movement component that rotates around the line of sight, i.e., the ocular torsion, is in many aspects different from horizontal and vertical eye movements. While ocular torsion is mediated only by reflexive pathways like the torsional vestibulo-ocular and optokinetic reflexes (TVOR and OKN, respectively), horizontal and vertical components are also subject to intentional control mechanisms that are mediated by the saccadic and the pursuit systems. Dynamic properties of torsional eye movements are also very distinct. While horizontal and vertical VOR components show a gain close to unity and a small neural integration leakage with a time constant around $\tau = 30$ s, the TVOR shows a smaller gain of 0.4 and also a greater leakage with $\tau = 2$ s.[1] During slow head rotations in roll, the TVOR is even less compensatory. At small stimulation levels the gain drops to a value of 0.2 and proves thus to be nonlinear, i.e., to depend on the stimulus magnitude.[2,3] In a recent study,[3] we hypothesized that this nonlinearity might be the result of a nonlinear processing of nystagmus quick phases rather than a nonlinearity in direct or integrator TVOR pathways. In the present study, we experimentally tested this hypothesis by measuring ocular torsion responses at different head rotation speeds. In addition to the conventional approach of analyzing slow-phase velocity (SPV) gains, we also analyzed properties of nystagmus quick phases. This method proved to be suitable for determining whether nonlinear processing of nystagmus frequency is responsible for the TVOR nonlinearity.

METHODS

TVOR responses to passive, whole-body rotations in roll around an earth-vertical axis were measured in seven subjects by means of video-oculography.[3] The subjects

---

Address for correspondence: E. Schneider, Department of Neurology, Ludwig-Maximilians University, Marchioninistr. 23, D-81377 Munich, Germany. Voice: +49-(0)89-7095-4830.
eschneider@nefo.med.uni-muenchen.de

were seated on a rotating chair, and a forehead rest restrained their heads to a nose-down position so that the naso-occipital axis was aligned in parallel with the axis of rotation. Thus, the effective stimulus acted mainly on the semicircular canals and not on the otoliths. A dim fluorescent dot located 0.5 m in front on the naso-occipital axis was used for fixation in an otherwise totally dark room. The stimuli consisted of step-ramp angular velocity profiles with a duration of 16 s. The initial velocity step was varied from 3° to 50°/s in five logarithmically spaced steps. On the basis of these step amplitudes, the superimposed acceleration ramps were adjusted to maintain the initial cupula deviation constant (FIG. 3, top). In this model-based approach of stimulus design, a cupular time constant of $\tau = 6$ s was assumed.[4] Each stimulation amplitude was administered four times in a block of sequentially alternating directions, and the blocks were applied in random order. For each subject and each velocity amplitude (v), mean values over the four stimulus repetitions were calculated for the frequency (f) and amplitude (a) of nystagmus quick phases as well as for the gains of SPV and nystagmus intensity ($i = f \cdot a$). Exponential functions of the form $f(v) = c \cdot (1 - e^{-v/v_c})$ were fitted in a least squares sense to these values (FIG. 1). Based on the results of these fits, a model was implemented in MATLAB Simulink

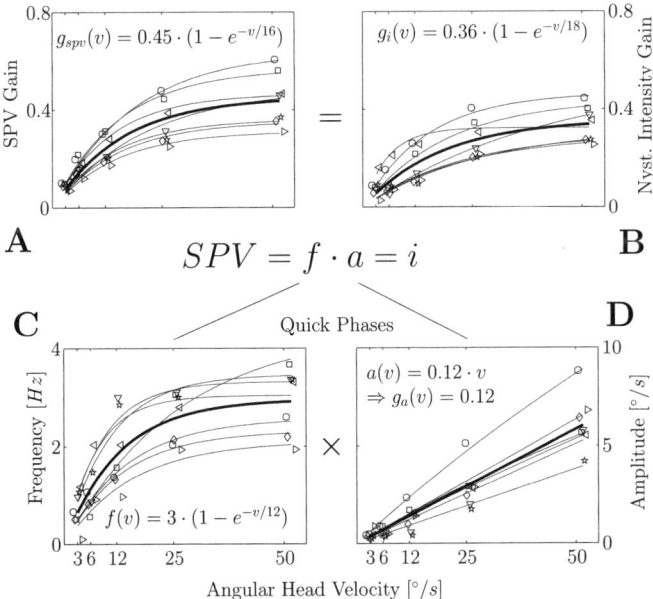

FIGURE 1. Nonlinear characteristics of the TVOR. Ocular torsion with subjects in a nose-down position was measured at roll angular head velocities (v), denoted with ticks on the x-axis. A nonlinear (exponential) gain dependency similar in shape was observed for the gains of both slow phase velocity (SPV, **A**) and nystagmus intensity (i, **B**). While quick phase amplitude (a, **D**) depended linearly on angular velocity, nystagmus frequency (f, **C**) showed the same nonlinear characteristic as the SPV gain. Thus, the reason for TVOR nonlinearity can be found in the frequency generation of torsional nystagmus. The functions displayed in each plot were fitted to subject data (*thin lines*) and to all recordings (*thick lines*).

to numerically simulate the observed torsional eye movements. The model consisted of the cupula mechanics, a leaky (τ = 2 s) torsional (neural) integrator,[1,5] and a nystagmus burst generator.

RESULTS AND DISCUSSION

We measured an SPV gain nonlinearity of the TVOR (FIG. 1), which was in agreement with an earlier report on the SPV gain of ocular counterroll in response to rotations around an earth-horizontal axis.[2] However, in the present study, the effective stimulation acted only on the semicircular canals and not on the otoliths. Therefore, we can conclude that the observed nonlinearity is mainly a property of canal-driven TVOR pathways alone. The dependency of SPV gain (g) on initial head velocity (v) was best described by the equation $g(v) = 0.45 \cdot (1 - e^{-v/v_c})$. From least square fits a velocity constant of v_c = 16°/s was determined, i.e., at v > 3 the SPV gain approaches the known TVOR gain of 0.45,[1,6] which means that only above 48°/s does the gain become constant and thus linear. Since in theory, average SPV and nystagmus intensity are identical (SPV = $a/\Delta t = a \cdot f = i$), we consequently observed a similar nonlinearity for the nystagmus intensity gain (FIG. 1B).

Which factor of the nystagmus intensity product $i = f \cdot a$ caused the TVOR nonlinearity? Since quick phase amplitudes a were linearly scaled with head velocity, only the nystagmus frequency f was left as the main suspect, and indeed, f showed a similar nonlinear dependency on stimulus magnitude as SPV (FIG. 1C). At $v > 3 \cdot v_c$, f approaches a value of $f_{max} \approx 3$ Hz, which is in agreement with other reports on typical values for nystagmus frequency.[7]

Based on a well-established model of the TVOR,[1,5] a new model was developed that additionally included a hypothetical nystagmus burst generator with a nonlinear characteristic (FIG. 2). A conventional analysis of the SPV gain alone would not have revealed the localization of the nonlinearity. A nonlinear scaling of the integrator input, for example, would have led to the same SPV gain characteristics. Only the detailed quick-phase analysis revealed the possible site of the nonlinearity: the frequency generator, whose input alone was scaled with the (nonlinear) function $f(v)$ = $1 - e^{-v/12}$. Furthermore, our data indicate that the frequency of the generated bursts as well as the amplitude of the quick phases for this type of stimulation are dependent solely on the vestibular information coming from the canal afferent input. Additional dependencies such as eye movement information processing[7] by feedback are not necessary to simulate adequate nystagmus properties. While the characteristics of the model were derived from our data, its predictions apply to other types of stimulation as well. Sinusoidal high-frequency TVOR stimulations, for example, would induce only little or no nystagmus. This indeed has been reported before.[8] Since head impulses fall in the same category of stimulation, they would not show the observed type of nonlinearity, because the nonlinearity would only become apparent in the presence of nystagmus. A number of attempts to model horizontal nystagmus on the basis of anatomical and neurophysiological findings can be found in the literature.[8,9] Our model, however, concentrates on the observed behavioral aspects of torsional nystagmus, which is believed to share brainstem circuitry with vertical but not with horizontal nystagmus.[10] Therefore, our model only partly resembles functionalities of known brainstem and midbrain structures like burster-

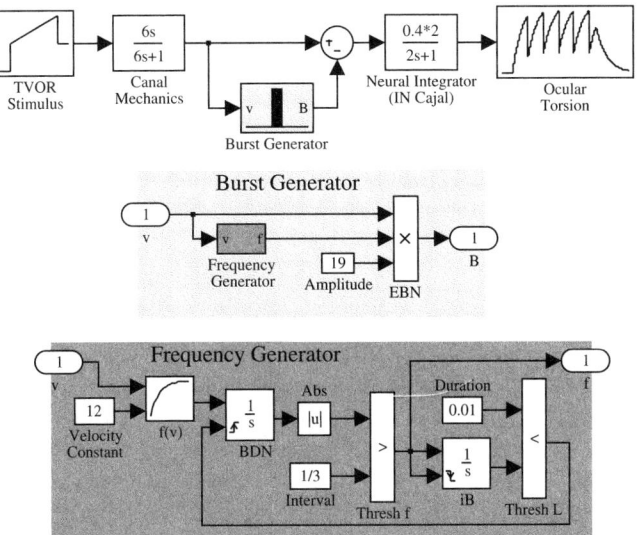

FIGURE 2. Hypothetical model of TVOR nystagmus generation. A known TVOR model[1,5] (*top*) was extended by a hypothetical nystagmus burst generator (*light gray boxes*) whose input is driven only by afferent information (v) from the canals. Burst amplitudes are linearly scaled with this input at the level of the excitatory burst neuron (EBN), while the input to the frequency generator (*dark gray boxes*) is scaled with the experimentally determined nonlinearity $f(v)$. The result of this operation is fed into a resettable integrator whose output resembles aspects of burster-driving neuron (BDN) functionality.[11,12] The integration continues until a threshold value is reached, which in turn triggers the start of the burst. The burst duration is determined by a second step of integration which resets the first integrator after another threshold value is reached. Bursts are then subtracted from the neural integrator input. The Simulink notation was used to formulate the model. For reasons of clarity the model was additionally subdivided into cascaded Simulink subsystems (*gray boxes*), and the noise generators used in the simulations of FIGURE 3 were not shown.

driving neurons (BDN)[11,12] or the interstitial nucleus of Cajal. BDN neurons are believed to constitute the first stage of vestibular processing in the network responsible for nystagmus generation.[13] For reasons of simplicity, the properties of these neurons were not modeled in every detail, but instead a minimal set of basic mathematical operations was used to simulate the observed effects on ocular torsion.

Model simulations (FIG. 3) could reproduce the main aspects of not only our present data. At small stimulation levels (FIG. 3, upper plots), an infrequent occurrence of quick phases together with a shift of the beating field toward the slow-phase direction can be observed. A similar observation was reported before for galvanic and natural vestibular stimulations of low intensities.[3] At the highest stimulation level (FIG. 3, bottom plot), the offset could even be reversed: in the given sample data, it was shifted in the direction of the quick phases. This was probably due to an overcompensating nystagmus intensity. Such shifts of the beating field were previously regarded as static ocular counterroll responses to otolith fiber activation by galvanic

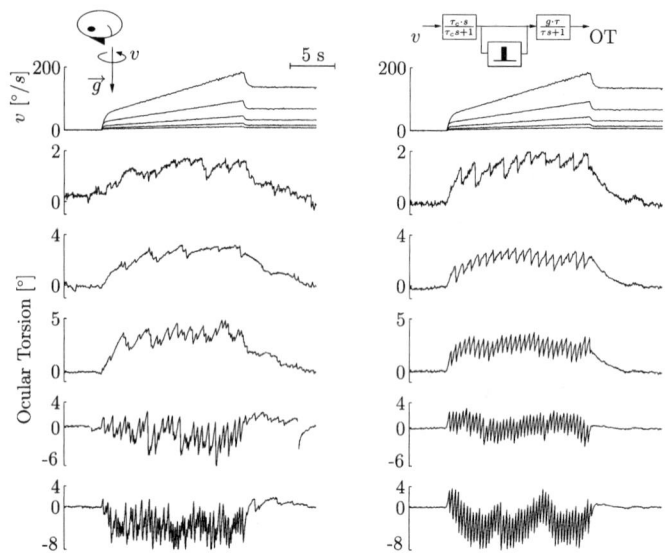

FIGURE 3. Original OT (*left*) and model simulation (*right*) in response to step-ramp stimuli (*top*). With increasing amplitude of step-ramp stimulus (*top*), increasing nystagmus frequencies and quick phase amplitudes can be observed (*left*). At small stimulus magnitudes a shift of the beating field in the direction of the slow phases is induced. This can be confused with a tonic OT. Model simulations are able to reproduce main aspects of the original OT recordings (*right*). For better comparison of experimental and simulation data, noise generators were added to the model. Beside measurement noise, the intervals between quick phases were randomized by adding Gaussian noise[7] to the BDN output.

vestibular stimulation.[14] Our data and simulations show that canal information alone is sufficient to induce torsional offset positions. A torsional offset induced by inadequate nystagmus-generating mechanisms might also have implications for the interpretation of the pathologic ocular torsions observed, for example, during vestibular imbalances. Indeed, monocular static torsion has been described in dorsolateral medullary infarctions, which involve vestibular nuclei (Wallenberg's syndrome). This was attributed to either posterior or anterior semicircular canal pathways being affected.[15] Further, in patients with vestibular nystagmus due to a peripheral tone, imbalance nystagmus disappears in the course of vestibular compensation.[16] The compensation of nystagmus together with a still present vestibular input (imbalance) might lead to an offset of ocular torsion.

CONCLUSION

Contrary to the common belief that static ocular torsion relies on otolith input, the present data and simulation support the view that a purely canal-induced TVOR can lead to torsional offset positions due to a lack of adequate quick-phase generation.

ACKNOWLEDGMENTS

This study was supported by Fritz-Thyssen-Stiftung and Deutsche Forschungsgemeinschaft (SFB 462, DI 379/4-1). We are grateful to Judy Benson for critically reading the manuscript.

REFERENCES

1. SEIDMAN, S.H., R.J. LEIGH, R.L. TOMSAK, et al. 1995. Dynamic properties of the human vestibulo-ocular reflex during head rotations in roll. Vision Res. **5:** 679–689.
2. PETERKA, R.J. 1992. Response characteristics of the human torsional vestibuloocular reflex. Ann. N.Y. Acad. Sci. **656:** 877–879.
3. SCHNEIDER, E., S. GLASAUER & M. DIETERICH. 2002. Comparison of human ocular torsion patterns during natural and galvanic vestibular stimulation. J. Neurophysiol. **87:** 2064–2073.
4. DAI, M., A. KLEIN, B. COHEN, et al. 1999. Model-based study of the human cupular time constant. J. Vestib. Res. **9:** 293–301.
5. ROBINSON, D.A. 1981. The use of control system analysis in the neurophysiology of eye movements. Annu. Rev. Neurosci. **4:** 463–503.
6. TWEED, D., D. SIEVERING, H. MISSLISCH, et al. 1994. Rotational kinematics of the human vestibuloocular reflex. I. Gain matrices. J. Neurophysiol. **72(5):** 2467–2479.
7. TRILLENBERG, P., D.S. ZEE & M. SHELHAMER. 2002. On the distribution of fast-phase intervals in optokinetic and vestibular nystagmus. Biol. Cybern. **87:** 68–78.
8. GALIANA, H.L. 1991. A nystagmus strategy to linearize the vestibulo-ocular reflex. IEEE Trans Biomed. Eng. **38(6):** 532–543.
9. CHUN, K.S. & D.A. ROBINSON. 1978. A model of quick phase generation in the vestibuloocular reflex. Biol. Cybern. **28:** 209–221.
10. VILIS, T., K. HEPP, U. SCHWARZ, et al. 1989. On the generation of vertical and torsional rapid eye movements in the monkey. Exp. Brain Res. **77:** 1–11.
11. OHKI, Y., H. SHIMAZU & I. SUZUKI. 1988. Excitatory input to burst neurons from the labyrinth and its mediating pathway in the cat: location and functional characteristics of burster-driving neurons. Exp. Brain Res. **72:** 457–472.
12. KITAMA, T., Y. OHKI, H. SHIMAZU, et al. 1995. Site of interaction between saccade signals and vestibular signals induced by head rotation in the alert cat: functional properties and afferent organization of burster-driving neurons. J. Neurophysiol. **74:** 273–287.
13. VAN BEUZEKOM, A.D. & J.A.M. VAN GISBERGEN. 2001. Interaction between visual and vestibular signals for the control of rapid eye movements. J. Neurophysiol. **88:** 306–322.
14. ZINK, R., S. STEDDIN, A. WEISS, et al. 1997. Galvanic vestibular stimulation in humans: Effects on otolith function in roll. Neurosci. Lett. **232(3):** 171–174.
15. DIETERICH, M. & T. BRANDT. 1992. Wallenberg's syndrome: lateropulsion, cyclorotation, and subjective visual vertical in thirty-six patients. Ann. Neurol. **31(3):** 399–408.
16. CURTHOYS, I.S. & G.M. HALMAGYI. 1995. Vestibular compensation: a review of the oculomotor, neural, and clinical consequences of unilateral vestibular loss. J. Vestib. Res. **5(2):** 67–107.

3,4-Diaminopyridine Improves Head-Shaking Nystagmus Caused by Neurovascular Cross-Compression

M. STRUPP, V. QUERNER, T. EGGERT, A. STRAUBE, AND T. BRANDT

Department of Neurology, University of Munich, Klinikum Grosshadern, Munich, Germany

KEYWORDS: head-shaking nystagmus; 3,4-diaminopyridine; cross-compression; eighth nerve

INTRODUCTION

There is good evidence that head-shaking nystagmus (HSN) may indicate (1) a peripheral tone imbalance of the vestibuloocular reflex[1] (e.g., due to a semicircular canal paresis), (2) a central vestibular tone imbalance leading to a direction-dependent asymmetric charge/discharge of the velocity storage mechanism due to nonlinearities,[1] or (3) a "latent" (compensated) vestibular tone imbalance, because HSN was also found in healthy control subjects.[2] We report on a patient who had severe HSN, most likely caused by a neurovascular cross-compression of the eighth nerve. Presumably, this led to a transient conduction block which significantly improved after treatment with the potassium channel blocker 3,4-diaminopyridine (3,4-DAP).[3]

CASE REPORT

A 55-year-old automobile mechanic had had severe episodes of HSN and oscillopsia for 1.5 years. During this time, he experienced "jumping images" after repeated head-shaking, but not when keeping his head still. He also developed an increasingly progressive hypacusis and intermittent tinnitus in the right ear. He reported no falls or episodes of rotatory or postural vertigo.

A pronounced rotatory nystagmus to the left after horizontal HS was the main finding of neurological testing. Up-and-down HS, HS in the planes of the other vertical semicircular canals, or keeping the head turned to the side or in a head-hanging position did not cause nystagmus. Auditory-evoked potentials showed that waves I and II were reduced and wave III prolonged in the right ear. An audiogram revealed a right-sided sensorineural hypacusis. MRI showed a cross-compression of an ante-

---

Address for correspondence: Michael Strupp, M.D., Department of Neurology, Klinikum Grosshadern, Marchioninistrasse 15, D-81366 Munich, Germany. Voice: ++49-89-7095-3678; fax: ++49-89-7095-6673.
mstrupp@nefo.med.uni-muenchen.de

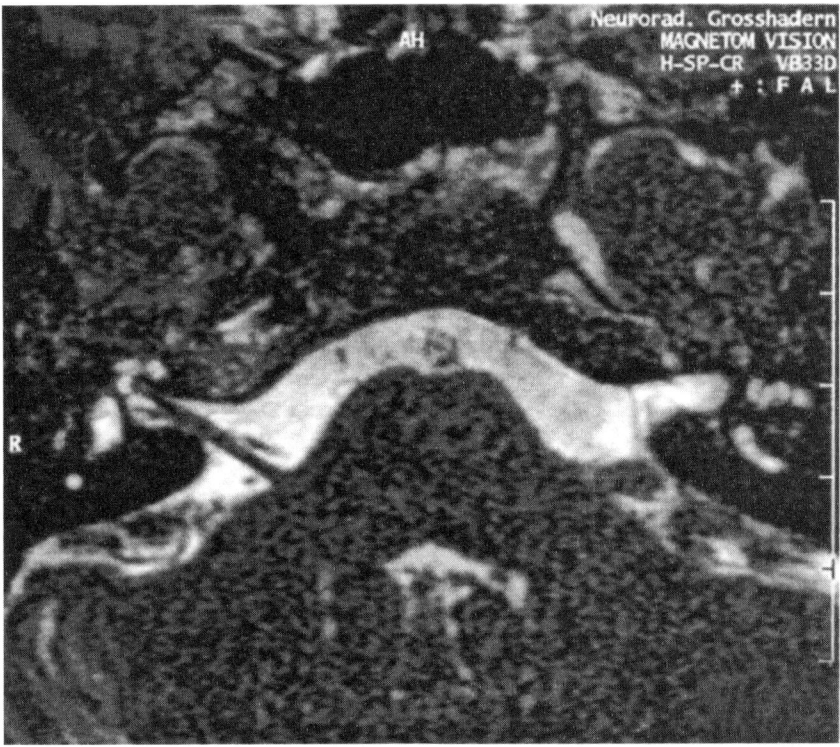

FIGURE 1. Cranial MRI (constructive interferences in steady state sequence) revealed a cross-compression of an anterior inferior cerebellar artery loop with the root entry zone of the eighth nerve on the right side.

rior inferior cerebellar artery (AICA) loop with the root entry zone of the right eighth nerve (FIG. 1).

Scleral search-coil recording (Remmel Labs) made after five horizontal HS maneuvers (FIG. 2A) revealed a rotatory nystagmus to the left which lasted 15 s (PI, peak slow-phase velocity 70°/s), followed by a rotatory nystagmus to the right after a latency of 4 s (PII, duration: 1–2 min). Posturography (Kistler Platform) after the patient performed 5 or 10 horizontal HS maneuvers while standing upright on foam rubber with eyes open showed a pronounced tendency to fall, which lasted about 10 s (FIG. 3A).

Administration of Tegretal (200 mg/day) had no effect on the nystagmus. Ingestion of the potassium channel blocker 3,4-DAP (15 mg), however, significantly reduced the oscillopsia and the peak slow-phase velocity of the HSN fell from 70°/s to 20°/s (FIG. 2B). Posturography showed less body sway after the ingestion of 3,4-DAP (FIG. 3B), and the patient was able to stand after horizontal HS without any aid.

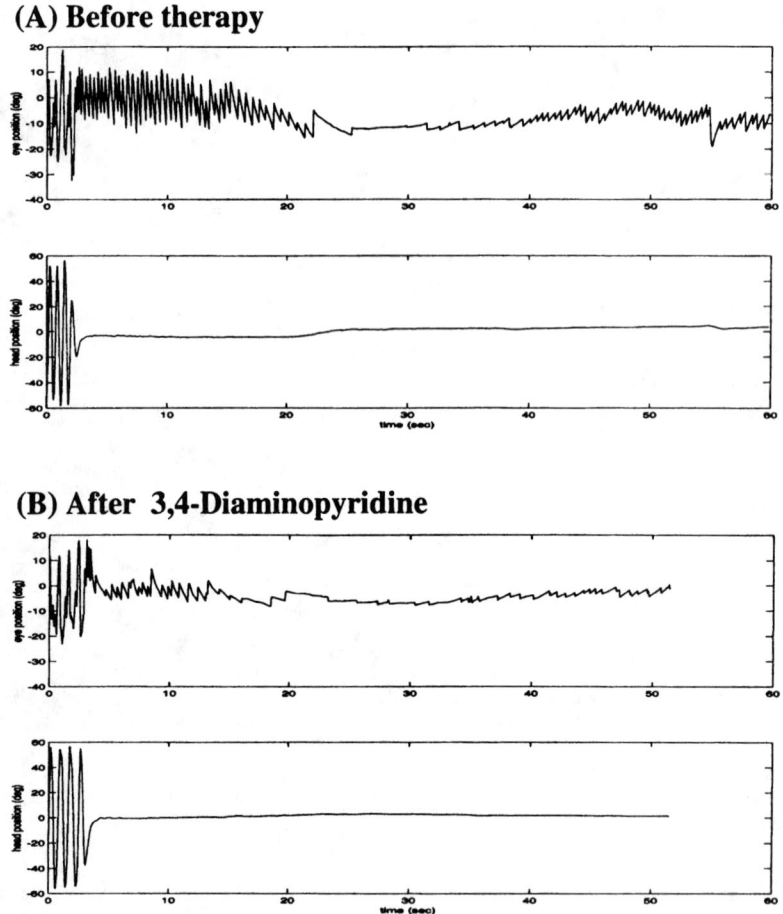

FIGURE 2. Scleral search-coil recording during and after five head-shaking maneuvers in the horizontal plane shows the horizontal trace of the eye movements (*top*) and the corresponding horizontal trace of the head movements (*bottom*): (**A**) before therapy and (**B**) 30 min after ingestion of 3,4-DAP.

DISCUSSION

The leftward direction of rotatory HSN agrees with the diagnosis of a transient conduction block of the right eighth nerve due to a mechanical irritation by the AICA loop, which caused the HSN. How can the effects of 3,4-DAP be explained? Since the early 1950s, it has been known that 3,4-DAP blocks potassium currents, mainly the so-called A-current, the delayed-rectifier, and other potassium channels.[3] By inhibiting these potassium currents, 3,4-DAP increases, for example, the duration of the action potential, thereby improving axonal conduction of action potentials and

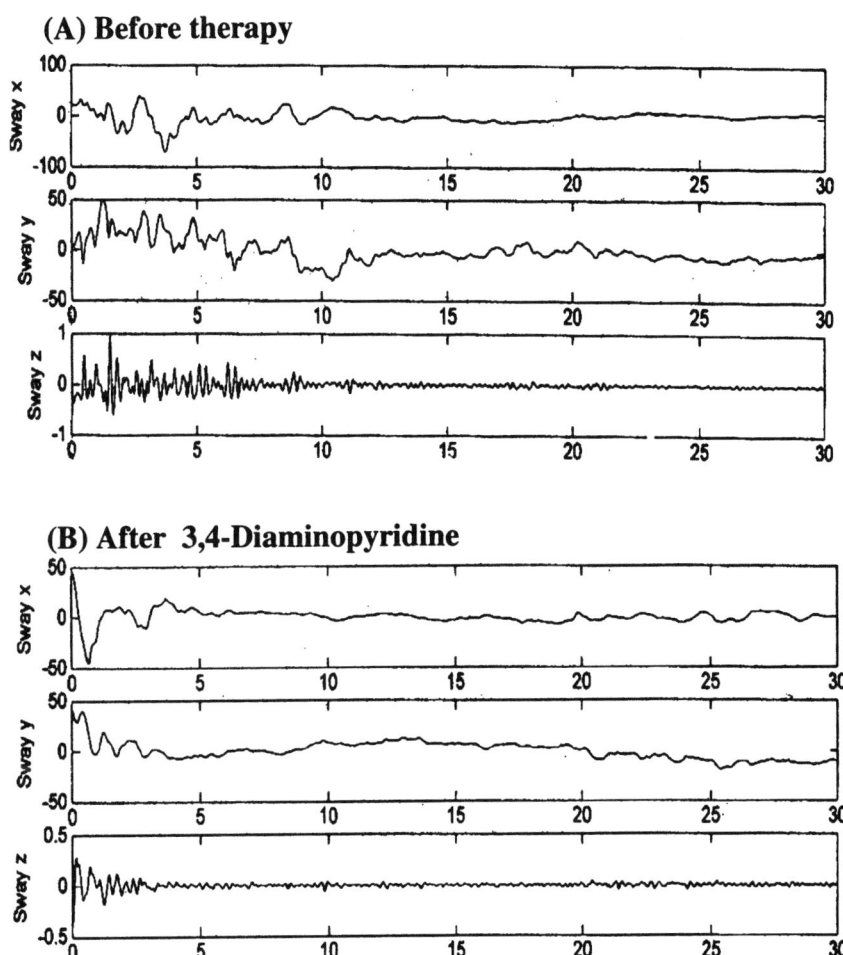

FIGURE 3. Posturographic recording of the patient standing on a foam-rubber padded force measuring platform with eyes open immediately after head-shaking. Original recordings of the body sway for the planes x, y, and z: (**A**) before therapy, (**B**) 45 min after ingestion of 3,4-DAP.

the release of neurotransmitters. Thus, 3,4-DAP has been used to improve action potential conduction in multiple sclerosis[4] as well as neurotransmission in Lambert-Eaton myasthenic syndrome.[5] The improvement of the symptoms and the reduction of HSN after 3,4-DAP can, therefore, most likely be attributed to increased axonal transmission to the eighth nerve, because 3,4-DAP prolongs the duration of the action potentials by blocking the axonal K^+ channels (A-current). Therefore, 3,4-DAP can be used to treat certain forms of neurovascular compression syndromes, if carbamazepine fails to improve symptoms. These findings also indicate that compression of the proximal eighth nerve can cause not only an excitation (as assumed to occur in most patients with vestibular paroxysmia[6]) but also a transient blockade of the interaxonal conduction.

REFERENCES

1. HAIN, T.C. & J. SPINDLER. 1993. Head-shaking nystagmus. *In* The Vestibulo-Ocular Reflex and Vertigo. J.A. Sharpe & H.O. Barber, Eds.: 217–228. Raven. New York.
2. ASAWAVICHIANGIANDA, S., M. FUJIMOTO, M. MAI, *et al.* 1999. Significance of head-shaking nystagmus in the evaluation of the dizzy patient. Acta Otolaryngol. (Stockh.) Suppl. **540:** 27–33.
3. HILLE, B. 2001. Ionic Channels of Excitable Membranes. 3rd edit. Sinauer Associates. Sunderland, MA.
4. BEVER, C-T.J., P.A. ANDERSON, J. LESLIE, *et al.* 1996. Treatment with oral 3,4 diaminopyridine improves leg strength in multiple sclerosis patients: results of a randomized, double-blind, placebo-controlled, crossover trial. Neurology **47:** 1457–1462.
5. SANDERS, D.B., J.M. MASSEY, L.L. SANDERS & L.J. EDWARDS. 2000. A randomized trial of 3,4-diaminopyridine in Lambert-Eaton myasthenic syndrome. Neurology **54:** 603–607.
6. BRANDT, T. & M. DIETERICH. 1994. Vestibular paroxysmia: vascular compression of the 8th nerve? Lancet **343:** 798–799.

Solving the Redundancy Problem for Unrestricted Reaching Movements: A Comparison of Patients with Cerebral Infarcts and Healthy Controls

THOMAS EGGERT,[a] TEKLA TIHANYI,[a,b] AND ANDREAS STRAUBE[a]

[a]*Department of Neurology, LMU-Munich, Munich, Germany*
[b]*Department of Biomechanics, Semmelweis University, Budapest, Hungary*

KEYWORDS: motor control; arm; Donders' law; joint coordination; pointing; human

INTRODUCTION

The many rotatory possibilities of the human arm allow it to reproduce one location of the hand by a large variety of arm positions. If some of these arm positions are more suitable for an intended hand position than others, the motor control system should avoid the unsuitable positions. Therefore, in a repetitive motor task, the redundancy problem of having many ways to point, should be resolved by reducing the degrees of freedom of the final arm position. The dimension of the redundancy problem can be defined as the maximum number of degrees of freedom that can be eliminated in a motor task. Several authors have addressed the one-dimensional redundancy problem that shoulder torsion is not directly restricted in many pointing tasks.[1,2] They found that for the shoulder joint Donders' law (reduction of the degrees of freedom from 3 to 2) was consistently valid only during pointing with a specific elbow extension. In general, however, across different angles of elbow extension and forearm torsion, the shoulder joint did not comply with Donders' law. In these studies, the restriction on elbow extension was directly imposed by the experimental condition. In contrast, during natural reaching, elbow extension and forearm torsion are limited indirectly by the restrictions imposed on hand position and orientation. This can lead to situations in which the dimension of the redundancy to be solved is much higher than one.

To investigate how the human motor control system solves redundancy problems of higher dimension, we examined human subjects during an unrestricted reaching task, in which they were instructed to control the position of the hand. Our aim was

Address for correspondence: Dr. T. Eggert, Department of Neurology, Klinikum Grosshadern, Marchioninistrasse 23, 81377 Munich, Germany. Voice: 49-89-7095-4834; fax: 49-89-7095-4801.
eggert@brain.nefo.med.uni-muenchen.de

Ann. N.Y. Acad. Sci. 1004: 511–515 (2003). © 2003 New York Academy of Sciences.
doi: 10.1196/annals.1303.064

to study the reduction of the degrees of freedom for all seven joint angles of arm and hand in healthy subjects and patients with a slight central paresis.

METHODS

Ten healthy controls and 10 patients with slight arm paresis due to lesions of the cerebral hemispheres were examined during a repetitive pointing task with the eyes open and closed. The three-dimensional position of six markers on shoulder, elbow, wrist, and hand were sampled by an ultrasonic device (Zebris, Isny, Germany) at 28 Hz and transformed to the following seven joint angles: shoulder torsional, horizontal, and vertical (ST, SH, SV), forearm torsion (FT), elbow extension (EE), hand vertical (HV), and hand horizontal (HH).

Subjects were instructed to extend the arm from a fixed starting position into a straight forward position (FIG. 1). The task was to repeatedly put the hand as precisely as possible in the same location in space. No external target or any other explicit instruction about the final hand position, orientation, or velocity was given. In a fully illuminated room, each subject performed 30 movements with the eyes open and 30 movements with the eyes closed.

The end of the movement was defined as the moment when the velocity of SV dropped below 10% of peak velocity. Final hand position (horizontal and vertical) was defined as the two-dimensional Cartesian position of the hand in the frontal-parallel plane at the end of the movement (HP_x, HP_y). Final arm position was defined as the vector of joint angles at the end of the movement. Variance of the final hand position was defined as the mean variance of horizontal and vertical final hand position [cm^2]. Variance of final arm position was defined as the mean of the variances of the components of final arm position [deg^2]. Statistical evaluation of the data were

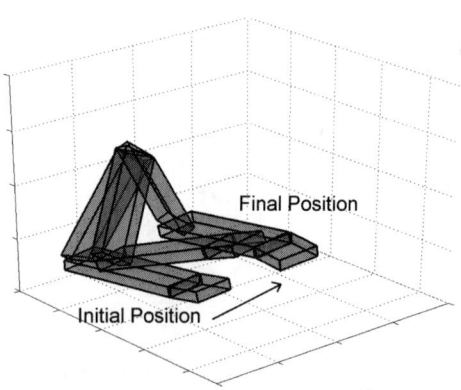

FIGURE 1. Reconstruction of the arm position on the basis of the three-dimensional positions of six markers attached to the arm. Shown are the initial, the final, and one intermediate arm position.

performed by means of an ANOVA with the within-subjects factor *condition* (eyes open, eyes closed) and the between subjects factor *group* (controls/patients).

RESULTS

Variability of Final Hand Position

The variability of the final hand position showed a main effect of the factor *condition* (F[1,18] = 13.57; $P < 0.002$) and an interaction between the two factors *condition* and *group* (F[1,18] = 6.49; $P < 0.02$). FIGURE 2A shows that patients repeated positioning of the hand less precisely with eyes closed than with eyes open (Scheffe: $P < 0.004$). With eyes open, there was no difference between groups.

Variability of Final Arm Position

The variance of final arm position was split into one part that could be explained on the basis of the final hand position by means of a multiple, quadratic regression and a second part, the residual variance. For the regression, two independent variables (HP_x and HP_y) and seven dependent variables (ST, SH, SV, FT, EE, HV, and HH at the end of the movement) were used. The residual variance shows how much the final arm position varied for a fixed final hand position. With eyes closed and eyes open, the total and the explained amount of the joint angle variability are very similar between patients and controls. The ANOVA was performed on the dependent variables total, explained and residual variance of final arm position. There was no significant effects or interactions of the factors *condition* and *group*. Approximately 50% of the total variance of final arm position was explained by the variance of final horizontal and vertical hand position (FIG. 2B).

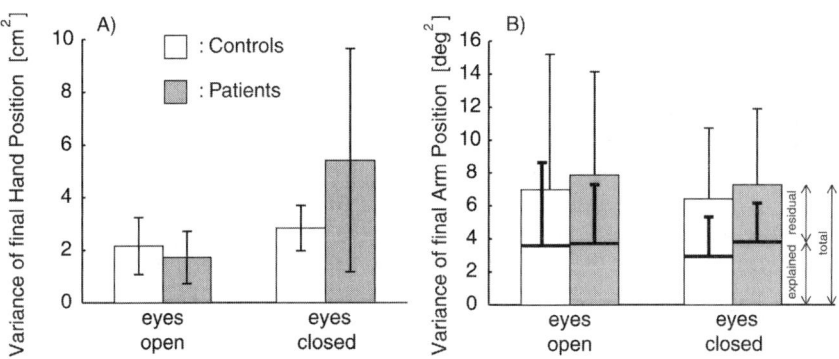

FIGURE 2. (**A**) Mean ± standard deviation between subjects of the variance of final hand position. (**B**) Bars and thin whiskers show the mean ± standard deviation between subjects of the variance of final arm position. Each *bar* is divided in the explained and the residual variance of final hand position (see text). Thick whiskers indicate the standard deviation of the explained variance.

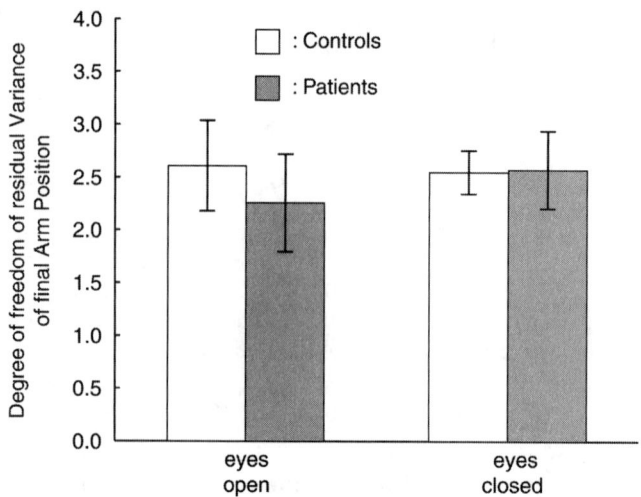

FIGURE 3. The degree of freedom of the residual variance of final arm position. With eyes open, patients tended to have fewer degrees of freedom.

Principle Component Analysis of Residual Variance

Thus, the seven degrees of freedom of final arm position (seven joint angles) were not reduced to the two degrees of freedom of the final hand position. Otherwise, 100% of the total variance could have been explained. The dimension of the residual variance was examined by means of a principle component analysis.

The (7×7) covariance matrix of the residual noise of the final arm position (the noise that does not depend on the final position of the hand) has five nonzero eigenvalues. These five variances were normalized on their sum and sorted by descending size. Their cumulative sum was interpolated by a cubic spline. The degree of freedom then was defined by the number of principle components, whose accumulated variance equaled 90% of the residual variance.

For 9 of 10 controls and for all patients, the residual variance was nonspherical (Mauchly: $P < 0.01$). The ANOVA of the degree of freedom showed only a marginally significant interaction between the two factors *condition* and *group* ($F[1,18] = 3.8$; $P < 0.07$). FIGURE 3 shows that patients, in contrast with controls, tended to have a smaller degree of freedom with eyes open than with eyes closed (Scheffe: $P < 0.18$; Fisher LSD: $P < 0.03$). With eyes closed, the degree of freedom of the final arm position was approximately 2.5 and did not differ between patients and controls. Thus, the maximum degree of freedom (5) was reduced by approximately 50%.

CONCLUSION

The ability to precisely reach was impaired in patients with slight paresis due to lesions of the cerebral hemispheres. However, the precision by which the final hand position determines the final arm position was the same for controls and patients.

Thus, despite their imprecise hand position, patients did not have any particular difficulty solving the redundancy problem. With eyes closed, the degree of freedom of the residual variance did not differ between controls and patients. In contrast, under visual control patients tended to have fewer degrees of freedom. This suggests that the patients can visually control the degrees of freedom of arm position. This might be a strategy for compensating for the increased variability of final hand position.

ACKNOWLEDGMENT

The study was supported by a grant of the EU (Marie-Curie training site).

REFERENCES

1. STRAUMANN, D., T. HASLWANTER, M.C. HEPP-REYMOND & K. HEPP. 1991. Listing's law for eye, head and arm movements and their synergistic control. Exp. Brain Res. **86:** 209–215.
2. MEDENDORP, W.P., J.D. CRAWFORD, D.Y. HENRIQUES, *et al.* 2000. Kinematic strategies for upper arm-forearm coordination in three dimensions. J. Neurophysiol. **84:** 2302–2316.

Common Reference System for Estimation of the Postural and Subjective Visual Vertical

K. JAGGI-SCHWARZ AND B.J.M. HESS

Department of Neurology, University of Zürich, 8091 Zürich, Switzerland

KEYWORDS: spatial orientation; neck afferents; semicircular canal–otolith interactions

INTRODUCTION

When tilted subjects are asked to set a luminous line to the perceived earth-vertical in a dark surrounding, they systematically underestimate the true direction of earth-vertical at large tilt angles, a phenomenon first described by Aubert (A-phenomenon).[1] At small tilt angles, subjects usually overestimate the direction of earth-vertical. Overestimation has been first reported by Müller, who termed the notion of E-phenomenon.[2] Since these first reports, this rather remarkable error behavior has been studied extensively.[3–7] The prevailing notion in most earlier studies was that the erroneous estimation of verticality results from otolith signals, which are thought to represent the major input for spatial orientation, and their interaction with somatosensory signals. To bring the subjects into tilted positions, most investigators used slow tilt velocities or waited for some time to prevent interaction with semicircular canal activity. Here, we tested the hypothesis that vestibular cues about self-orientation relative to gravity are most reliable when both the semicircular canals and the otolith organs are optimally activated. To compare the error behavior in estimations of the visual vertical and perceived body position, we used self-controlled passive tilts at constant velocity or acceleration.

METHODS

Ten to 18 subjects (6–12 men, 4–6 women) between 25 and 56 years participated in this study after having given written informed consent according to a protocol approved by the ethic committee of the Canton of Zurich. The medical case history showed that subjects had normal hearing and no otological or neurological disorders.

Address for correspondence: K. Jaggi-Schwarz, Department of Neurology, University of Zürich, 8091 Zürich, Switzerland. Voice: +41-1-255-5596; fax: +41-1-255-4507.
karin.jaggi@nos.usz.ch

EXPERIMENTAL SETUP AND PROTOCOL

Subjects sat comfortably on a chair mounted on a three-dimensional turntable with three servocontrolled motor driven axes (Acutronic, Switzerland). They were secured with safety belts and evacuation pillows. The head was positioned at the rotation center and restrained with an individually molded mask (Sinmed BV, the Netherlands). For estimating the subjective visual vertical, a luminous line consisting of an array of LEDs was mounted in front of the subject (visual angle: 21.2°, luminance 0.7 cd/m^2). A rotary knob allowed remote control of the line's angular orientation. After setting the luminous line, subjects pressed a button to indicate end of task and trigger digital reading of the line angle.

In a first series of experiments, the subjects had either to align a randomly set luminous line with the perceived earth-vertical direction ($n = 18$) or to estimate their orientation in degrees, for example, 90° left meant left ear-down ($n = 10$), after being tilted to the side in steps of 10° up to 60° and to 90° (acceleration: ±180°/s^2, peak velocity: 100°/s). Both tasks started 2 s after tilt onset. Afterward, subjects were returned to the initial upright position and the room light was switched on for approximately 10 s for reorientation. In a second series ($n = 10$), the subjects, while being tilted, had to estimate their position, which was previously verbally declared by the examiner. When satisfied, they pressed a button to stop chair rotation, to trigger digital reading of tilt position, and to initiate the luminous line-setting task. As in the first series, they had to align a randomly set luminous line with the perceived earth-vertical. The luminous line adjustments had to be executed as quickly and as accurately as possible, which happened within approximately 2.55 s (±1.1 s). Thereafter, subjects were returned to the initial upright position, and the room light was switched on for approximately 20 s for reorientation while the examiner announced the next tilt angle. The chair was either tilted at slow constant velocity tilts (acceleration: ±0.05°/s^2, peak velocity: 0.5°/s) or at constant acceleration (acceleration: ±3°/s^2, peak velocity: 100°/s). All paradigms were performed in total darkness. The angular orientation of the line (error <1°) and the subject's roll position (error <0.1°) were sampled at a rate of 833 Hz (Cambridge Electronics Device 1401 Plus) and stored on a PC hard disk for off-line analysis with MatLab (The Math Works, Inc.). Data were analyzed using the Friedman and Kruskal-Wallis nonparametric tests.

RESULTS

In the verbal estimation paradigm, we found that subjects underestimated (A-effect) body-tilt angles in the range of ±20° and ±60° (FIG. 1, gray line). Interestingly, the luminous line paradigm (FIG. 1, black line) showed in a similar tilt range overestimations (E-effect). This finding prompted us to combine estimation of body position with the luminous line paradigm in self-controlled tilt experiments with different tilt profiles. To our surprise, the luminous line paradigms showed an E-effect for both tilt profiles, which was larger in the constant velocity paradigm (FIG. 2A, thin black line) than in the constant acceleration roll tilt paradigm (FIG. 2B, thin black line). It is apparent that the mean error curves show a significantly larger A-effect (FIG. 2A, thick black line) for the position estimation in the velocity paradigm than in the acceleration paradigm (FIG. 2B, thick black line; Friedman-Test: $P < 0.05$

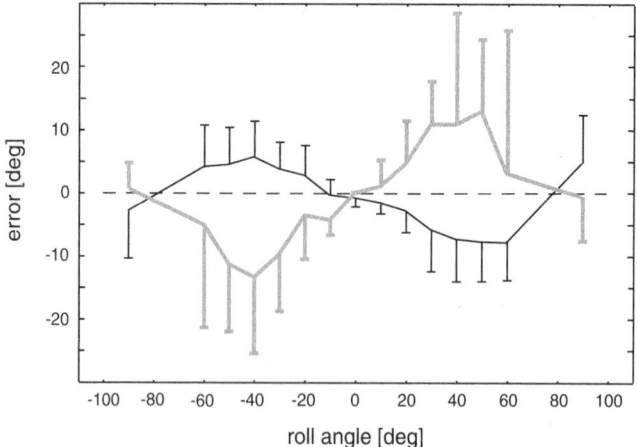

FIGURE 1. Comparison of mean error curves (±1 SD) for luminous line and verbal estimation paradigms. Average verbal estimations underestimate true body position (*solid gray line*) approximately in the same range where the luminous line paradigm shows overestimation (*solid black line*).

for all tilt angles; exceptions with $P > 0.05$ were at −40°, ±10°, 0°). Moreover, the resulting mean of position estimation and luminous line setting errors, plotted against the requested roll position, revealed that there is almost no difference between the velocity and acceleration paradigm (FIG. 2A and B, thick gray lines). This is also shown by a high correlation between the two paradigms ($R^2 = 0.73$, $P < 0.0001$). Finally, both error curves show minimal deviations from the zero in the range of ±45° roll tilt due to almost equal errors in luminous line settings and body-tilt estimations.

DISCUSSION

To challenge the capacity of vestibular self-orientation mechanisms, we used high-velocity and acceleration tilts that efficiently activate both the otolith organs and semicircular canals. With this procedure, we expected that estimation of self-orientation in space should be improved or even become veridical. We found an overall improvement, although there was still over- and underestimation. We attribute part of these persistent perceptual errors to activation of neck muscles by the vestibular system, appropriate for righting the head,[8–10] which might generate a bias towards earth-vertical in a head-fixed situation. However, vestibular-neck interactions cannot be the only factor, because otherwise the E-effect would increase with tilt angle up to a saturation level. We assume that somatosensory inputs (hidden in the A-effect) are another important factor, which predominates at larger tilt angles and over time. Surprisingly, the luminous line settings in the self-controlled tilt paradigm showed a much larger E-effect with constant velocity tilts than with constant acceleration tilts

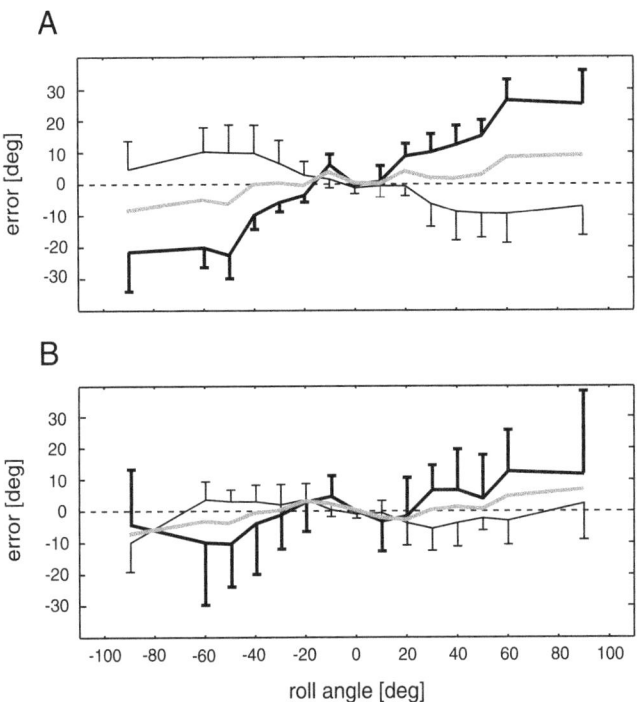

FIGURE 2. Estimations of body position and visual vertical and the resulting mean error. (**A**) Estimation errors plotted against the requested tilt angles during constant velocity roll tilts. Luminous line setting errors: *thin black line*; body position estimation errors: *thick black line*, resulting mean of position and luminous line setting errors: *thick gray line*. (**B**) Same format as in **A** but during constant acceleration roll tilts.

(FIG. 2A, B). At this point, we speculate that during slow tilts, with the head restrained, the E-effect becomes even larger because the long-lasting slow tilts lead to adaptation and/or misinterpretation of somatosensory, proprioceptive, and/or visceral signals, which have a larger impact under this condition even at smaller tilt angles. This impact is much smaller during accelerated rapid tilts, where the vestibular information is more precise. Thus, the reduction of the E-effect might be caused by the concomitant otolith-canal activation (FIG. 2B). During slow tilts, the range of actually reached positions was in the mean underestimated by approximately 25% of the desired positions. One explanation could be that tilt estimation failed because of disruption of sensory integration. The slow tilt velocity used in this study is a very unusual stimulus that is bound to lead to adaptation of somatosensory signals. Another remarkable result was the minimal difference between the acceleration and velocity paradigms when comparing the resulting mean of position estimation and luminous line setting errors as a function of the desired roll positions (FIG. 2A,B, thick gray lines). The high correlation between the two curves strongly suggests that estimations of visual vertical and body position use the same reference, which appears to be close to veridical in the range of approximately ±45°. It is the range at which the spatial reference might be determined predominantly by the otoliths, whereas for larger tilts a bias develops and increases up to 10°. This bias reflects probably a predominance of nonvestibular cues.

ACKNOWLEDGMENT

This study was supported by the Betty and David Koetser Foundation for Brain Research.

REFERENCES

1. AUBERT, H. 1861. Eine scheinbare bedeutende Drehung von Objekten bei Neigung des Kopfes nach rechts oder links. Arch. f. Pathol. Anat. **20:** 381–393.
2. MÜLLER, G.E. 1916. Über das Aubertsche Phänomen. Zeitschr. f. Sinnesphysiol. **49:** 109–246.
3. CURTHOYS, I.S. 1996. The role of ocular torsion in visual measures of vestibular function. Brain Res. Bull. **40:** 399–403.
4. MAST, F. & T. JARCHOW. 1996. Perceived body position and the visual horizontal. Brain Res. Bull. **40:** 393–397.
5. MITTELSTAEDT, H. 1983. A new solution to the problem of the subjective vertical. Naturwissenschaften **70:** 272–281.
6. STOCKWELL, C.W. & F.E. GUEDRY, JR. 1970. The effect of semicircular canal stimulation during tilting on the subsequent perception of the visual vertical. Acta Otolaryngol. **70:** 170–175.
7. VAN BEUZEKOM, A.D. & J.A. VAN GISBERGEN. 2000. Properties of the internal representation of gravity inferred from spatial-direction and body-tilt estimates. J. Neurophysiol. **84:** 11–27.
8. KANAYA, T. *et al.* 1995. Control of the head in response to tilt of the body in normal and labyrinthine-defective human subjects. J. Physiol. **489:** 895–910.
9. ROY, J.E. & K.E. CULLEN. 2001. Selective processing of vestibular reafference during self-generated head motion. J. Neurosci. **21:** 2131–2142.
10. WILSON, V.J. & J.G. MELVILL-JONES. 1979. Mammalian Vestibular Physiology. Plenum. New York.

Lateropulsion in Wallenberg's Syndrome Decreases with Increasing Locomotion Speed

KLAUS JAHN, MICHAEL STRUPP, AND THOMAS BRANDT

Ludwig-Maximilians University, Klinikum Grosshadern, Department of Neurology, Marchioninistrasse 15, 81377 Munich, Germany

KEYWORDS: locomotion; walking and running; vestibular control; Wallenberg's syndrome

INTRODUCTION

Patients with acute ischemic stroke of the dorsolateral medulla oblongata (Wallenberg's syndrome) present with a clinical syndrome that includes lateropulsion of the body, falls, and gait deviation to the side of the lesion.[1] These symptoms are associated with a tilt of perceived verticality and caused by a vestibular tone imbalance in the roll plane due to involvement of vestibular nuclei.[2] Prompted by an earlier finding that gait deviation in patients with acute unilateral peripheral vestibular failure (vestibular neuritis) was dependent on locomotion speed,[3] the differential effects of walking and running on lateropulsion were tested in patients with acute Wallenberg's syndrome.

METHODS

Twelve patients with acute dorsolateral infarction of the medulla oblongata (mean age, 50 years; range, 25–71 years, five women) participated in the study after being briefed about the experiments. The diagnosis of Wallenberg's syndrome was based on the clinical presentation and the demonstration of the typical ischemic medullary lesion on MRI. Patients were tested 3 to 10 days after the onset of symptoms. They were instructed to (1) walk straight ahead very slowly, (2) walk straight ahead as fast as they could, and (3) to run straight ahead with eyes open. The gait trajectories of five patients were recorded using two infrared sensitive cameras that detected a circular set of infrared light-emitting diodes attached to the trunk of the subject as described elsewhere.[4] The remaining seven patients were tested in the hospital ward with a digital video camera. To quantify mean gait deviation, we determined an angle between the straight-ahead axis and a line from the starting point

---

Address for correspondence: Klaus Jahn, M.D., Department of Neurology, Klinikum Grosshadern, Marchioninistrasse 15, 81377 Munich, Germany. Voice: +49-89/7095-2588; fax: +49-89/7095-5584.

klaus.jahn@lrz.uni-muenchen.de

to the patient's position after 5 s of locomotion. For statistical analysis a paired two-sided *t*-test was used.

RESULTS

All patients included in the study were able to walk with eyes open without support. They all showed reproducible gait deviation to the side of their lesion (seven left, five right). Five patients were too anxious to run and therefore were tested only during slow and fast walking. Mean angular deviation after 5 s of locomotion was 43.5 ± 19.1° ($n = 12$; range, 15–80 degrees) for slow walking, 22.8 ± 17.8° ($n = 12$; range, 0–60°) for fast walking, and 13.6 ± 13.7° ($n = 7$; range, 0–40°) for running. Mean and individual gait deviations are given in FIGURE 1. In the paired *t*-test, the difference in angular deviation was significant between slow and fast walking ($P < 0.001$), and between fast walking and running ($P = 0.034$). Further to these quantitative data, all patients reported that they felt more confident at higher locomotion speed. In fact, some were surprised how well they performed running, which they had not tried since the onset of their acute disorder.

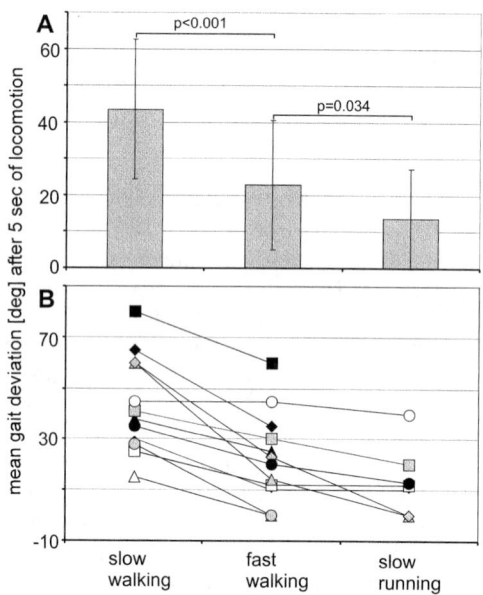

FIGURE 1. Gait deviation in Wallenberg's syndrome is dependent on locomotion speed and pattern. (**A**) Mean angular deviation toward the side of brainstem lesion after 5 s of locomotion with eyes open in 12 patients. *Error bars* represent standard deviations. Significance levels for the differences between slow walking and fast walking as well as between fast walking and running as indicated (paired *t*-test). The smallest deviation was observed with running, although the distance covered was longest after 5 s. (**B**) Individual gait deviations for the 12 patients. Each symbol represents one subject.

DISCUSSION

The data demonstrate that the dependency of gait deviation on locomotion speed (slow and fast walking) and locomotion pattern (walking and running) holds for both peripheral and central vestibular disorders. In earlier studies, we tested patients with vestibular neuritis and healthy subjects in whom an experimental transient vestibular tone imbalance (postrotatory or galvanic vestibular stimulation) was induced. Patients and subjects showed less deviation from the intended straight path when running than when walking. This was explained by the assumption that a highly automated spinal locomotion program for running operates largely independently of sensory control, whereas control of slow walking relies more on sensory input.[3,5] The latter view is supported by the neurophysiological finding that monosynaptic stretch reflexes from the legs are inhibited during locomotion.[6,7] Similarly, one can assume that with increasing speed of locomotion misleading input from the peripheral or central vestibular system is suppressed, thereby alleviating lateropulsion in patients with Wallenberg's syndrome. There is further experimental evidence for an inhibitory interaction between locomotor activity and the vestibular system. In patients with vestibular neuritis, spontaneous nystagmus is suppressed during locomotion,[8] and deactivation of the parietoinsular vestibular cortex was found during imagined locomotion.[9]

ACKNOWLEDGMENTS

We are grateful to Judy Benson for copyediting the manuscript. The work was supported by the Deutsche Forschungsgemeinschaft (Str384/4, SFB 462 A6).

REFERENCES

1. WALLENBERG, A. 1895. Acute Bulbäraffection (Embolie der Art. cerebelli post. inf. sinistr.). Arch. Psychiat. Nervenkr. **27:** 504–540.
2. DIETERICH, M. & T. BRANDT. 1993. Ocular torsion and tilt of subjective visual vertical are sensitive brainstem signs. Ann. Neurol. **33:** 392–399.
3. BRANDT, T., M. STRUPP & J. BENSON. 1999. You are better off running than walking with acute vestibulopathy. Lancet **355:** 233.
4. JAHN, K., M. STRUPP, E. SCHNEIDER, et al. 2001. Visually induced gait deviations during different locomotion speeds. Exp. Brain Res. **141:** 370–374.
5. JAHN, K., M. STRUPP, E. SCHNEIDER, et al. 2000. Differential effects of vestibular stimulation on walking and running. Neuroreport **11:** 1745–1748.
6. DIETZ, V. 1992. Human neuronal control of automatic functional movements: interaction between central programs and afferent input. Physiol. Rev. **72:** 33–69.
7. FAIST, M., V. DIETZ & E. PIERROT-DEEILLINGNY. 1996. Modulation, probably presynaptic in origin, of monosynaptic Ia excitation during human gait. Exp. Brain Res. **109:** 441–449.
8. JAHN, K., M. STRUPP & T. BRANDT. 2002. Both actual and imagined locomotion suppress spontaneous vestibular nystagmus. Neuroreport **13:** 2125–2128.
9. JAHN, K., A. DEUTSCHLÄNDER, T. STEPHAN, et al. 2003. An fMRI study of vestibular and somatosensory cortex deactivation during imagined locomotion. Ann. N.Y. Acad. Sci. **1004:** this volume.

Eye–Head Coordination

Challenging the System by Increasing Head Inertia

NADINE LEHNEN, STEFAN GLASAUER, AND ULRICH BÜTTNER

Department of Neurology with Centre of Sensorimotor Research, Klinikum Grosshadern, Ludwig-Maximilians University, Munich, Germany

KEYWORDS: eye–head coordination; head inertia

Under natural conditions, coordinated movements of eye and head are used to shift gaze toward new visual targets. In humans, combined eye–head saccades bring gaze to the target by a fast saccadic eye movement together with a slower head movement. After gaze reaches the target, it is stabilized at this position by the vestibuloocular reflex (VOR), which has been attenuated or shut off during the gaze displacement.[1,2] The interaction of eye and head during the gaze shift is far from clear. In particular, it remains questionable whether there is a single gaze error command as opposed to the eye and the head being driven by separate signals with distinct feedback loops. Moreover, the role of the various feedback systems is still debated. To further disclose interactions between eye and head, we investigated how gaze shifts are affected by changes in one of their components—the head.

The head moment of inertia of 11 normal human subjects with no known eye or head movement disorder was 2.5-fold increased using a helmet with a mass attached to it. Without and with head load, subjects performed horizontal gaze shifts toward shortly flashed targets in the complete dark. Required gaze shifts always crossed the midline (straight ahead). The subjects' left eye as well as their head rotation was measured in three axes with the search-coil-in-magnetic-field technique as previously described.[3] The primary gaze shift toward the target was analyzed.

In all subjects, the increased head moment of inertia significantly slowed down the head (FIG. 1A) and decreased the head contribution, that is, the head amplitude at the end of the primary gaze shift (FIG. 1B). In 9 of 11 subjects, these changes in head dynamics did not affect the retinal error at the end of the gaze shift (FIG. 1C) nor did they significantly change its duration.

Our results show that considerable changes in the head dynamics caused by an increase in head inertia do not affect the retinal error at the end of the gaze shift. Moreover, the head load does not significantly change the gaze shift duration. This last result conflicts with findings in cats where the gaze saccade duration increased

---

Address for correspondence: N. Lehnen, Department of Neurology, Klinikum Grosshadern, LMU München, 81377 München, Germany. Voice: 49-89-7095-4831; fax: 49-89-7095-4801.
nadine.lehnen@campus.lmu.de

Ann. N.Y. Acad. Sci. 1004: 524–526 (2003). © 2003 New York Academy of Sciences.
doi: 10.1196/annals.1303.067

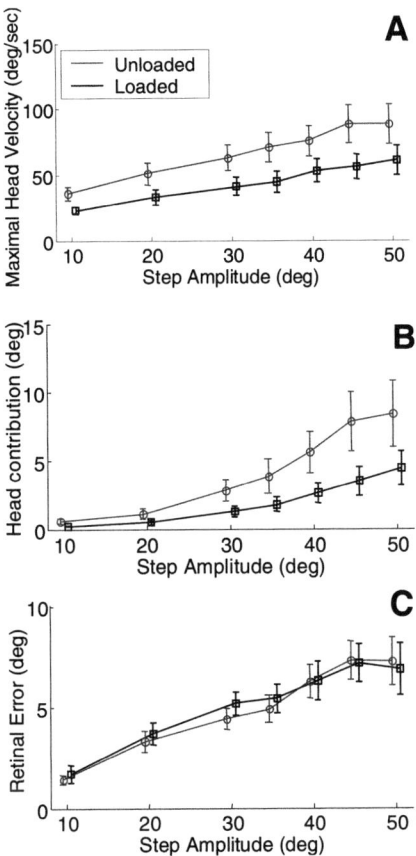

FIGURE 1. Comparison of loaded (*black squares*) and unloaded (*gray circles*) conditions. Mean ± SEM are given for each target step amplitude. (**A**) Maximal head velocity (mean, SEM) significantly decreased when the head inertia was increased (loaded condition). (**B**) Head contribution, the amplitude of the head at the end of the gaze shift, significantly decreased in the loaded condition. (**C**) However, even though changes in head contribution exceeded 5°, retinal error (9 of 11 subjects) with or without head load was not significantly different.

to account for the changes in head movement dynamics.[4] According to our results and consistent with previous studies,[5] in humans, increased head load does not affect gaze shift performance.

The present findings cannot be accounted for by learning due to visual feedback, because the latter was excluded by flashing the target. Thus, to bring gaze equally close to the target despite the lower head amplitude at the end of the gaze shift, other feedback mechanisms, vestibular or proprioceptive, must be at work.

REFERENCES

1. TABAK, S., J.B. SMEETS & H. COLLEWIJN. 1996. Modulation of the human vestibuloocular reflex during saccades: probing by high-frequency oscillation and torque pulses of head. J. Neurophysiol. **76:** 3249–3263.
2. GUITTON, D. & M. VOLLE. 1987. Gaze control in humans: eye-head coordination during orienting movements to targets within and beyond the oculomotor range. J. Neurophysiol. **58:** 427–459.
3. GLASAUER, S., M. HOSHI, U. KEMPERMANN, et al. 2003. Three-dimensional eye position and slow phase velocity in humans with downbeat nystagmus. J. Neurophysiol. **89:** 338–354.
4. COIMBRA, A.J., P. LEFEVRE, M. MISSAL & E. OLIVIER. 2000. Difference between visually and electrically evoked gaze saccades disclosed by altering the head moment of inertia. J. Neurophysiol. **83:** 1103–1107.
5. GAUTHIER, G.M., B.J. MARTIN & L.W. STARK. 1986. Adapted head- and eye-movement responses to added-head inertia. Aviat. Space Environ. Med. **57:** 336–342.

Perception and Pursuit

The Link between Object Motion Perception and the Motor Control of Ocular Pursuit

G. SCHWEIGART,[a] T. MERGNER,[a] AND G.R. BARNES[b]

[a]*Neurological University Clinic, 79106 Freiburg, Germany*

[b]*Department of Optometry and Neuroscience, University of Manchester Institute of Science and Technology, Manchester, United Kingdom*

KEYWORDS: motion perception; pursuit eye movements; sensorimotor control; model; human

INTRODUCTION

Motion of the image of a visual object across the stationary retina creates retinal slip, which is the basis of the target motion perception. However, when the object is tracked by the eyes, retinal slip may become very small, yet this perception persists, albeit diminished.[1] During pursuit, it is believed that target motion perception results from an internal signal representing eye movement.[2] This internal signal has been considered to contribute also to the control of pursuit.[3,4] Although there is considerable evidence of a link between perception and pursuit there are also conditions in which this link appears to break down. In humans, a moving background strongly affects target motion perception but hardly affects pursuit.[5,6] We have used a range of target and background motion conditions to measure target motion perception and compare it with the motor control of pursuit.

METHODS

Normal subjects ($n = 6$) were seated at the centre of a cylindrical screen (radius, 1 m). A red target (diameter, 0.5°; at eye level) and a background pattern (black-and-white patches) were projected onto the screen. They were independently rotated in the horizontal plane with a "raised cosine" velocity profile. Three stimulus frequencies ($f = 0.05$, 0.2, and 0.8 Hz) were used, each with four different peak angular displacements (A = 2°, 4°, 8°, or 16°). Corresponding peak velocities (V) ranged from 0.2°/s (0.05 Hz, 2°) to 25.6°/s (0.8 Hz, 16°). Five different stimulus combinations were used (see FIG. 1a–e): (a) "background double": background and target were ro-

Address for correspondence: G. Schweigart, Neurological University Clinic, Breisacher Strasse 64, 79106 Freiburg, Germany. Voice: 49-761-270-5230; fax: 49-761-270 5416.
schweiga@nz.ukl.uni-freiburg.de

tated in the same direction, but background with double the amplitude; (b) "background with": the background was rotated by the same amount and in the same direction as the target; (c) "background stationary": target rotated; (d) "background counter": the background rotated by the same amount as the target, but in the opposite direction; and (e) "background-only (Duncker's condition)": the target was stationary while the background was rotated. Subjects had to attentively fixate or track, respectively, the stationary (e) or moving target (a–d). After each stimulus, subjects delivered verbal estimates of perceived peak velocity of the target in space ("magnitude estimation"). Estimates were based on prior training sessions in which subjects learnt how to grade perceived velocity. Normalizing the estimates to a *standard stimulus* (f = 0.2 Hz/V = 3.2°/s/A = 8°) allowed measures of perceptual gain (*standard* estimates assumed veridical[7]).

RESULTS

Perceptual target velocity gain is plotted in FIGURE 1a–e (symbols). In the background stationary condition (FIG. 1c), gain was close to unity in the midvelocity

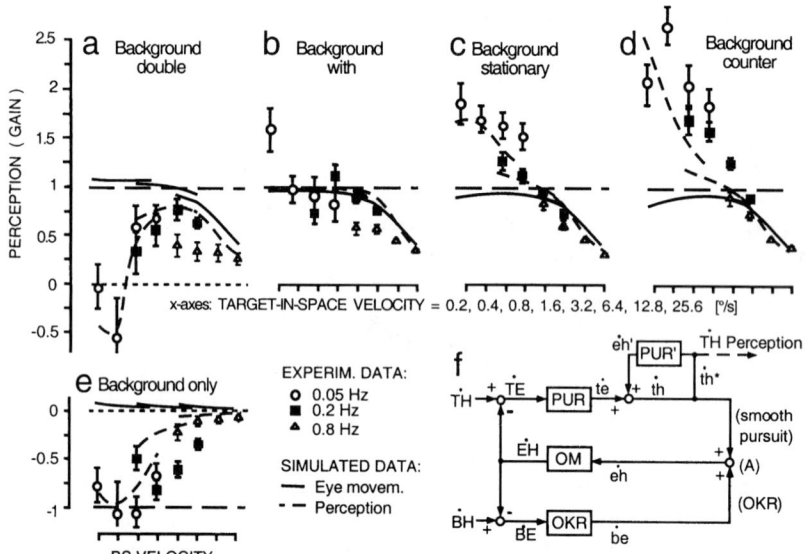

FIGURE 1. (**a–e**) Velocity estimates of target motion in space (TS) for different background motion conditions as a function of target velocity (abscissae, logarithmic scale, in °/s) for three stimulus frequencies (0.05, 0.2, 0.8 Hz; mean ± 1 SE). (**a–d**) Although TS was the same across all panels, background in space motion (BS) was modified from *left to right panels* as indicated above each panel. Veridical estimates would yield a gain of unity (*dashed horizontal lines*). (**e**) Target stationary, background moving (Duncker's condition); veridical, a gain of zero. (**f**) Model of pursuit-contingent target motion (velocity) perception. B'H, T'H, background-/target-to-head; OM, oculomotor plant.

range (approximately 3.2°/s), but was overestimated at low target velocity. In contrast, velocity was underestimated at high velocity (similar in a–d). In the background counter condition (FIG. 1d), the increase in gain with decreasing velocity was more pronounced than with background stationary. In the Background with condition (FIG. 1b), the 0.2- and 0.05-Hz estimation curves were level at approximately unity gain (exception, 0.2°/s). In the Background double condition (FIG. 1a), perceptual gain decreased with decreasing stimulus velocity. The direction of perceived target-in-space motion even reversed (negative gain values). Results from the background-only condition (Duncker; FIG. 1e) are plotted as a function of background-to-target velocity. Gain increased considerably with decreasing velocity, yielding the traditional Duncker's induced motion illusion.[5]

DISCUSSION

The data presented in FIGURE 1a–e show that the perception of target velocity (dashed curves, fits to simulation data) is not directly related to eye velocity (solid curves). However, the characteristics of perception bear a close resemblance to a premotor eye pursuit signal, as we show by reference to our pursuit model (for details, see Schweigart et al.[7,8]).

The upper part of the model (FIG. 1f) represents target pursuit control, which consists of a closed-loop negative feedback system with target-to-eye velocity (T˙E, retinal slip), representing the input and eye-in-head velocity (E˙H) the output. T˙E is processed by internal dynamics (PUR), giving t˙e, which is then modified by an internal positive feedback loop, which increases the gain associated with the target[9,10] and yields the internal target-related drive signal target-to-head (t˙h). The lower half of the model represents the optokinetic drive originating from background motion relative to the eye (B˙E, transformed by internal dynamics in box OKR to b˙e). Alone, it would produce optokinesis. These two sources (t˙h and b˙e) compete at summing junction A, producing the final ocular motor drive signal e˙h. Selectively boosting the gain of t˙e (through t˙h*) allows eye velocity control to be dominated by target velocity and not by background velocity.[6,8]

We posit that the t˙h signal not only controls pursuit, but also represents the source of target velocity perception. This is supported by simulations of the model in FIGURE 1a–e, where predicted perceptual gain is shown separately for the different background motion conditions (broken curves) together with predicted smooth pursuit gain (solid curves). The model effectively simulates the wide range of perceptual gain changes found experimentally, including Duncker's induced motion, whilst giving smooth eye pursuit gains that are hardly affected by the background. How does this difference arise? This can be illustrated by reference to the *background stationary* condition. As the eye pursues the target, it crosses the background and creates an opposing background-to-eye signal (b˙e). To maintain pursuit gain close to unity, this background drive must be opposed by a corresponding increase in the target-related drive signal t˙h, which comes in by t˙h*. A copy of t˙h*, we postulate, is the source of target motion perception. Perceptual gain increases as target velocity decreases because the background becomes stronger,[6,8] an effect that is clearly evident in the "Duncker" condition (FIG. 1e). Findings in the other stimulus conditions can be explained analogously.

Our findings shed new light on visual perception of target motion and its linkage to ocular pursuit. We suggest that perception is linked to action through the internal "attention and effort" loop (t˙h*) required to produce appropriate boosting of the target-related eye control. It includes a component to overcome the background, which is not present in the motor response itself.

ACKNOWLEDGMENTS

This work was supported by Deutscher Akademischer Austauschdienst 313/British German Academic Research Collaboration (ARC) Programme, ARC 1000 from the British Council, and Deutsche Forschungsgemeinschaft Me 715/5-1.

REFERENCES

1. AUBERT, H. 1886. Die Bewegungsempfindung. Pflügers Arch. **39:** 347–370.
2. BRIDGEMAN, B. 1995. A review of the role of efference copy in sensory and oculomotor control systems. Ann. Biomed. Eng. **23:** 409–422.
3. YOUNG, L.R. 1977. Pursuit eye movements—what is being pursued? *In* Control of Gaze by Brain Stem Neurons. R. Baker & E. Berthoz, Eds.: 29–36. Elsevier. North Holland. New York.
4. WYATT, H.J. & J. POLA. 1979. The role of perceived motion in smooth pursuit eye movements. Vision Res. **19:** 613–618.
5. DUNCKER, K. 1929. Über induzierte Bewegung. Psychol. Forsch. **12:** 180–259.
6. WORFOLK, R. & G.R. BARNES. 1992. Interaction of active and passive slow eye movement systems. Exp. Brain Res. **90:** 589–598.
7. SCHWEIGART, G., T. MERGNER & G.R. BARNES. 2003. Object motion perception is shaped by the motor control mechanism of ocular pursuit. Exp. Brain Res. **148:** 350–365.
8. SCHWEIGART, G., T. MERGNER & G. BARNES. 1999. Eye movements during combined pursuit, optokinetic and vestibular stimulation in macaque monkey. Exp. Brain Res. **127:** 54–66.
9. ROBINSON, D.A., J.L. GORDON & S.E. GORDON. 1986. A model of the smooth pursuit eye movement system. Biol. Cybern. **55:** 43–57.
10. BARNES, G.R. & T. HILL. 1984. The influence of display characteristics on active pursuit and passively induced eye movements. Exp. Brain Res. **56:** 438–447.

Haptic Subjective Vertical Shows Context Dependence

Task and Vision Play a Role during Dynamic Tilt Stimulation

WILLIAM GEOFFREY WRIGHT AND STEFAN GLASAUER

Department of Neurology with Center of Sensorimotor Research, Klinikum Grosshadern, Ludwig-Maximilians University, Munich, Germany

KEYWORDS: subjective vertical; context dependence; dynamic roll tilt

INTRODUCTION

Perceiving one's vertical is an integral part of efficiently functioning in an environment physically polarized along that dimension. How one determines the direction of gravity is not a task left only to inertial sensors, such as the vestibular organs, rather as numerous studies have shown, this task is influenced visually[1,2] and somatosensorily.[3–5] In addition, there is evidence that higher order cognitive effects such as expectancies[6] and context[7] are critical in perception of the vertical. One's ability to integrate these various inputs during normal activity is not generally questioned, one's doubts being satisfied by observing a waiter navigating a crowded restaurant with a tray balanced on one hand, neither tripping or dropping an entree. But how these various sources are integrated is still debated.

Most research focuses on subjective vertical perception used visual matching/alignment tasks,[2,3] verbal reports,[4] or saccadic eye movements[8] as a dependent measure. Although a motor task involving a joystick or indicator to be aligned with gravity without visual feedback is used much less frequently, there is good evidence that individuals easily orient limbs to an external gravity-aligned coordinate axis while being statically tilted.[9,10]

By exposure to a dynamic situation,[11] the central nervous system should be no more challenged by the task of determining the subjective vertical than during static conditions, because our spatial orientation systems were likely selected for just that. In addition, the sensitive calibration between visual and other sensory input also must have been key to its selection. This sensory interaction can be tested by changing the relation between the various sources. With the advent of virtual reality technology, a complex and "natural" visual stimulus is achievable and is easily

Address for correspondence: William Geofrey Wright, Department of Neurology with Center of Sensorimotor Research, Klinikum Grosshadern, Ludwig-Maximilians-University, Munich, Germany. Voice: 49-89-7095-4800; fax: 49-89-7095-4801.
gwright@alumni.brandeis.edu

manipulable. How one tests perception of verticality is also a pertinent question when researching spatial orientation systems. The system's performance may be better indicated by a task of higher relevance to its normal function. In other words, the dependent measure can be made more or less relevant to real-world tasks. With an experimental design that attempts to mimic natural conditions, the current study focuses on two main topics. First, how does manipulation of the visual inputs during passive roll-tilt affect one's sense of body orientation? And second, how does changing the task used to measure subjective vertical affect one's performance?

METHODS

Eight subjects were exposed to dynamic, sinusoidal, passive roll-tilt motion about the nasooccipital axis centered at ear level. Subjects were asked to indicate the perceived direction of gravity by continuously keeping a joystick (two tasks: cylindrical metal handle or glass full of water) vertical. The two tasks were tested in each of four visual conditions (darkness, in-phase, 180° out-of-phase, stationary) during ±20° tilt at 0.08 Hz in a counterbalanced fully nested repeated measures design. Exposure to the visual input was via a head-mounted display (Kaiser Electro Optics Proview-80 with an 80° diagonal field of view) with a visual input supplied from the perspective of a high-resolution minicamera mounted on the single-axis roll tilt machine at the center of rotation such that no linear visual motion occurred. Subjects sat with their head supported firmly in place. Three-dimensional motion of the joystick and the concurrent angle of tilt of the machine was measured using Intersense IS-600 Mark 2 Precision Motion Tracker. The different visual conditions were tested by mounting the camera in various positions on the tilt machine (in-phase: camera perspective same as subject's; 180° out-of-phase: camera facing backward relative to the subject; stationary: camera earth-fixed). Before the experiment, subjects were shown how to keep the joystick vertical, instructed to hold it tightly so that it could not be used as pendulum, and, in the case of the glass, were reminded that it would spill if it were not maintained vertical. During the experiment, unbeknownst to the subject, the glass was covered. Although the mass of glass and metal joystick differed by less than 23%, the difference in rotational inertia (which may be the more relevant property) was less than 15%, with the glass of water being greater in both cases. Subjects received no visual feedback of hand position during any conditions. Perfect indication of gravity (SV) would be seen if zero tilt was indicated. Subjects could either overcompensate or undercompensate for actual roll tilt. If the subject did not compensate for roll tilt at all and maintained the joystick aligned with their intrinsic longitudinal body axis, their compensation for tilt would have been zero and tilt excursion would 40° (see y axis in FIG. 1). The subject's indication of SV, the dependent measure, was calculated as the absolute peak-to-peak difference for each cycle of motion. Perfect indication of gravity would be equal to zero peak-to-peak difference.

RESULTS

The main findings are reported in FIGURE 1. A significant main effect of task was found ($F_{1,7} = 41.8$, $P < 0.0005$), and planned comparisons show the effect of task is

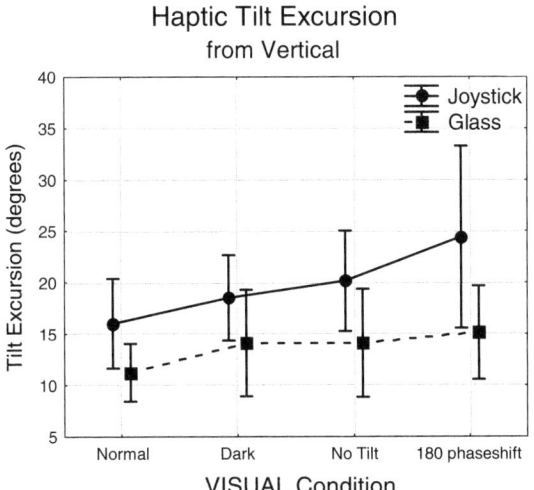

FIGURE 1. Tilt excursion of joystick (*circles*) and glass of water (*squares*) during four visual conditions (eight subjects; bars: 95% confidence intervals) during dynamic roll tilt stimulation. A tilt excursion of zero degrees indicates full compensation for the ±20° tilt. Using the glass, subjects significantly better indicated the subjective haptic vertical. In the normal visual condition (visual-vestibular concordance), subjects performed significantly better than in any other condition.

significant during all visual conditions ($P < 0.05$). Specifically, the ability to indicate the haptic subjective vertical is significantly more aligned with gravity when a full glass of water was used as a joystick rather than the solid, cylindrical, metal handle. A significant main effect of visual condition was also found ($F_{3,5} = 6.14$, $P < 0.05$). Planned comparisons show that in the visual condition with visual-vestibular concordance, subjects compensated for roll-tilt significantly better than all other visual conditions ($P < 0.05$). There was, however, no difference among visual conditions, darkness, phase-shifted discordant visual-vestibular, or the stationary visual scene. Across subjects, there was a greater tendency to undercompensate for tilt; however, there was no systematic pattern across visual condition or task, and some subjects displayed both behaviors within and between conditions.

DISCUSSION

The primary findings show that a subject's ability to indicate the haptic subjective vertical without visual feedback of the hand is significantly improved by the type of task used as a dependent measure. Although subjects showed surprisingly poor performance in indicating the direction of gravity with the metal joystick (<60% compensation for roll tilt), they performed significantly better when using a glass full of water as an indicator in all conditions. It is clear from this result that holding the glass of water improves one's ability to indicate the gravitational vertical, and we propose that a context-dependent motor skill is invoked.

The role of context dependence in motor skills recently has gained more attention.[12,13] In the current study, it is likely by increasing the relevance of the task to maintaining object verticality automatically induced a motor skill that most people master at an early age. Because task order was counterbalanced across four visual conditions, this provides further evidence that this motor proficiency is automatically induced, because subjects showed no ability to invoke this skill with the metal handle even directly after performing a water-glass trial.

The poor performance of indicating the vertical in the current study was unexpected because both semicircular canal and otolith responses at the chosen frequency (0.08 Hz) are close to veridical, and static tilt up to 20° is indicated without errors.[8] It was not surprising that subjects could maintain joystick alignment with the gravity better when visual input was concordant with the actual motion of the tilt machine. However, the expectation that viewing a complex, natural scene via head-mounted display would induce a compelling sense of vection regardless of its concordance with inertial stimulation was not found. There was no clear evidence of visual capture. We suggest that the level of stimulation of the vestibular and somatosensory input may be too high here to simply be "outweighed" by the discordant visual input.

ACKNOWLEDGMENT

This research was partially supported by a grant from the Deutscher Akademischer Austauschdienst.

REFERENCES

1. DICHGANS, J. *et al.* 1972. Moving visual scenes influence the apparent direction of gravity. Science **178:** 1217–1219.
2. MITTELSTAEDT, H. 1986. The subjective vertical as a function of visual and extraretinal cues. Acta Psychol. **63:** 63–85.
3. MITTELSTAEDT, H. & E. FRICKE. 1988. The relative effect of saccular and somatosensory information on spatial perception and control. Adv. Otorhinolaryngol. **42:** 24–30.
4. GUEDRY, F.E. 1974. Psychophysics of vestibular sensation. *In* Handbook of Sensory Physiology, Vol. 6. Part II. H.H. Kornhuber, Ed.: 1–154. Springer Verlag. New York.
5. LACKNER, J.R. & A. GRAYBIEL. 1979. Parabolic flight: loss of sense of orientation. Science **206:** 1105–1108.
6. WERTHEIM, A.H., B.S. MESLAND & W. BLES. 2001. Cognitive suppression of tilt sensations during linear horizontal self-motion in the dark. Perception **30:** 733–741.
7. LACKNER, J.R. & A. GRAYBIEL. 1983. Perceived orientation in free fall depends on visual, postural, and architectural factors. Aviat. Space Environ. Med. **54:** 47–51.
8. VAN BEUZEKOM, A.D. & J.A.M. VAN GISBERGEN. 2000. Properties of the internal representation of gravity inferred from spatial-direction and body-tilt estimates. J. Neurophysiol. **84:** 11–27.
9. DARLING, W.G. & R. BARTELT. 2003. Kinesthetic perception of visually specified axes. Exp. Brain Res. **149:** 40–47.
10. DARLING, W.G. & J.M. HONDZINSKI. 1999. Kinesthetic perceptions of earth- and body-fixed axes. Exp. Brain Res. **126:** 417–430.

11. GLASAUER, S. 1995. Linear acceleration perception: frequency dependence of the hilltop illusion. Acta Otolaryngol. Suppl. **520:** 37–40.
12. COHN, J.V., P. DIZIO & J.R. LACKNER. 2000. Reaching during virtual rotation: context specific compensations for expected coriolis forces. J. Neurophysiol. **83:** 3230–3240.
13. MILNER, A.D. & R.T. DYDE. 2003. Why do some perceptual illusions affect visually guided action, when others don't? Trends Cogn. Sci. **7:** 10–11.

Hoffmann, K.-P., 10–18
Horn, A.K.E., 19–28, 40–49, 414–417
Huonker, R., 457–464

Jaggi-Schwarz, K., 516–520
Jahn, K., 352–358, 469–472, 485–489, 521–523
Johanson, C., 183–195

Kalla, R., 316–324
Kaneko, C.R.S., 262–270, 451–456
Keller, E.L., 29–39
Kipiani, E., 241–251
Klam, F., 271–282
Kleine, J., 241–251, 252–261
Klier, E.M., 122–131
Koene, A., 389–393
Kömpf, D., 465–468
Krafczyk, S., 352–358
Kumar, A.N., 337–346, 394–398
Kurkin, S., 262–270

Landau, K., 347–351
Lehnen, N., 524–526
Leigh, R.J., 337–346, 394–398
Ling, L., 61–68, 158–168
Luan, H., 169–182
Lutz, S., 440–445

Magnusson, A.K., 422–423
Marti, S., 490–491
Marx, E., 283–288, 446–450
McCrea, R.A., 169–182
Mergner, T., 303–315, 527–530
Messoudi, A., 414–417
Missal, M., 29–39
Mohr, C., 229–240
Mustari, M.J., 196–205, 381–384, 399–403

Naessl, A., 485–489
Navarro-Lopez, J.D., 424–428
Neiss, W.F., 418–421
Neppert, B., 482–484

Ono, S., 196–205, 381–384, 399–403

Palla, A., 347–351, 490–491
Pawlowski, M., 457–464
Pélisson, D., 69–77, 377–380
Pereira, C.B., 492–496
Phillips, J.O., 158–168

Querner, V., 506–510
Quinet, J., 404–408

Rambold, H., 229–240, 478–481, 482–484, 497–499
Raphan, T., 78–93, 359–376
Rauch, E., 409–413
Rottach, K.G., 465–468

Sackerer, B., 465–468
Sato, F., 262–270
Schautzer, F., 316–324,
Schneider, E., 352–358, 485–489, 500–505
Schneider, W.X., 289–296
Schulz, P., 409–413
Schwaiger, M., 434–439, 440–445
Schweigart, G., 527–530
Sharpe, J.A., 111–121
Shelhamer, M., 94–110
Shupak, A., 297–302
Siebold, C., xiii–xiv, 158–168, 241–251, 473–477
Sparks, D.L., 220–228
Sprenger, A., 229–240, 465–468
Stephan, T., 283–288, 434–439, 440–445, 446–450, 469–472
Straka, H., 429–433
Straube, A., 506–510, 511–515
Straumann, D., 347–351, 490–491
Streppel, M., 418–421
Stritzke, G., 482–484
Strupp, M., 316–324, 352–358, 409–413, 469–472, 485–489, 492–496, 506–510, 521–523

Takeichi, N., 262–270, 451–456
Tal, D., 297–302
Tchelidze, T., 241–251
Tham, R., 422–423
Theil, D., 409–413
Thurtell, M.J., 325–336

INDEX OF CONTRIBUTORS

Tihanyi, T., 511–515
Trigo, J.A., 1–9
Tusa, R.J., 196–205, 381–384
Tweed, D., 111–121

Wahle, P., 19–28
Walker, M.F., 94–110
Weber, K.P., 347–351
Wilden, A., 241–251
Wisst, F., 482–484

Wong, A.M.F., 111–121
Wright, W.G., 531–535

Yajeya, J., 424–428
Yakushin, S.B., 78–93

Zee, D.S., 94–110
Zingler, V.C., 492–496